T0252106

Thieme

Textbook of Diabetic Neuropathy

F. Arnold Gries, M.D.

Professor emeritus
German Diabetes Research Institute
at the Heinrich Heine University
Clinical Department
Düsseldorf, Germany

Norman E. Cameron, Ph.D.

Professor
Diabetic Complications Lab
Department of Biomedical Sciences
Institute of Medical Sciences
Aberdeen University
Aberdeen, Scotland

Phillip A. Low, M.D., FRACP, FRCP

Professor
Department of Neurology
Mayo Clinic
Rochester, MN, USA

Dan Ziegler, M.D.

Professor
German Diabetes Research Institute
at the Heinrich Heine University
Clinical Department
Düsseldorf, Germany

With contributions by

H. Andersen
J.C. Arezzo
J.W. Baynes
G.J. Biessels
G.B. Bolli
P. Bottini
A.J.M. Boulton
V. Bril
N.E. Cameron
M.A. Cotter
P.J. Dyck
S.E.M. Eaton
J. Eckel
T. Erbas
C.G. Fanelli
C. Feinle
E.L. Feldman
W.H. Gispen
F.A. Gries
J. Hilsted
M. Horowitz
J. Jakobsen
K.L. Jones
W. Kennedy
J. Jervell
P.A. Low
D. Luft
R.A. Malik
C.J. Mathias
G. Menzinger
A.P. Mizisin
B. Neundörfer
D.O'Donovan
S. Pampanelli
T.S. Park
C.R. Pierson
G. Pittenger
F. Porcellati
H.C. Powell
W. Rathmann
P. Rösen
M. Samsom
R. Schmidt
L. Scionti
J.E. Shaw
A.A.F. Sima
M. Skeen
V. Spallone
K. Stansberry
M.J. Stevens
C. Stief
R. Straub
K.A. Sullivan
G. Sundkvist
M. Taskiran
S. Tesfaye
P.K. Thomas
A. Veves
A.I. Vinik
J.D. Ward
P. Watkins
G. Wendelschafer-Crabb
D. Ziegler
P. Zimmet

139 Illustrations
93 Tables

Thieme
Stuttgart · New York

Library of Congress Cataloging-in-Publications Data
is avaible from the publisher

© 2003 Georg Thieme Verlag,
Rüdigerstraße 14, D-70469 Stuttgart, Germany
http://www.thieme.de
Thieme New York, 333 Seventh Avenue,
New York, N. Y. 10001 U.S.A.
http://www.thieme.com

Cover design: Martina Berge, Erbach-Ernsbach
Typesetting by Satzpunkt Bayreuth, Bayreuth
Printed in Germany by Grammlich, Pliezhausen

ISBN 3-13-127581-2 (GTV)
ISBN 1-58890-005-3 (TNY)

1 2 3 4 5

Important Note: Medicine is an ever-changing science undergoing continual development. Research and clinical experience are continually expanding our knowledge, in particular our knowledge of proper treatment and drug therapy. Insofar as this book mentions any dosage or application, readers may rest assured that the authors, editors, and publishers have made every effort to ensure that such references are in accordance with **the state of knowledge at the time of production of the book.**

Nevertheless, this does not involve, imply, or express any guarantee or responsibility on the part of the publishers in respect to any dosage instructions and forms of applications stated in the book. **Every user is requested to examine carefully** the manufacturers' leaflets accompanying each drug and to check, if necessary in consultation with a physician or specialist, whether the dosage schedules mentioned therein or the contraindications stated by the manufacturers differ from the statements made in the present book. Such examination is particularly important with drugs that are either rarely used or have been newly released on the market. Every dosage schedule or every form of application used is entirely at the user's own risk and responsibility. The authors and publishers request every user to report to the publishers any discrepancies or inaccuracies noticed.

Some of the product names, patents, and registered designs referred to in this book are in fact registered trademarks or proprietary names even though specific reference to this fact is not always made in the text. Therefore, the appearance of a name without designation as proprietary is not to be construed as a representation by the publisher that it is in the public domain.

This book, including all parts thereof, is legally protected by copyright. Any use, exploitation, or commercialization outside the narrow limits set by copyright legislation, without the publisher's consent, is illegal and liable to prosecution. This applies in particular to photostat reproduction, copying, mimeographing or duplication of any kind, translating, preparation of microfilms, and electronic data processing and storage.

Preface

It has long been known that diabetics are prone to characteristic diseases of the kidneys (P. Kimmelstiel and C. Wilson 1936), eyes (E. Jaeger 1853), and nerves (J. Rollo 1798). However, it wasn't until insulin therapy became established and large numbers of patients with long-term diabetes were examined that the syndrome-like character of these complications became recognized in the mid-20th century. Because the incidence of complications rises with the duration of the diabetes, it was once common to speak in terms of a "late diabetic syndrome." Today the preferred term is "chronic diabetic complications." These complications basically determine the quality of life and life expectancy of persons with diabetes. Their prevention is an important focal point of modern diabetes management.

Chronic diabetic complications are firmly entrenched in the consciousness of patients and their therapeutic teams. In the past, diabetic neuropathy (DNP) was usually relegated to the role of a neglected stepsister. But this attitude in no way reflects its impact on quality of life, problems of diabetes management, sequelae such as oligosymptomatic myocardial ischemia and diabetic foot syndrome, disease costs, or the prognosis for survival. One reason for the tendency to underestimate DNP may be that the functional disturbances of the nervous system can run a subclinical course for some time. The patient has no obvious distress, and the physician finds evidence of the neuropathy only by conducting specific tests. The physician's efforts may lack focus due to the absence of a positive nosologic definition and generally accepted diagnostic criteria and standards, and because the clinical manifestations of DNP are so diverse. Finally, therapeutic options for DNP were, until recently, unsatisfactory.

For many years, then, DNP was not a matter of serious concern in any of the clinical or theoretical biomedical disciplines. This changed only during the last three decades. In 1978, the first international symposium was held dealing with autonomic DNP. The proceedings of that conference were published by Thieme Verlag (Gries et al. Aspects of Autonomic Neuropathy. Stuttgart–New York: Thieme; 1980). Within a decade, an international group formed and began to organize and publish symposia within the framework of the International Diabetes Federation Congresses, which are held every three years. A special expression of the growing interest in DNP was the founding of NEURODIAB, the Diabetic Neuropathy Study Group of the European Association for the Study of Diabetes (EASD) in 1989. Since that time, this group has staged annual meetings at a high scientific level, attended by scientists from all over the world. This study group may well be the most effective channel for the rapid, critically attended exchange of information on advances in DNP research.

Scientific conferences are held mainly for the purpose of discussing new research results. Accordingly, the publications stemming from these conferences are geared toward the research interests of the authors. Information on state-of-the-art knowledge and techniques is presented in a highly selective way.

Our goal is to present a systematic review that covers both the physiology of the nervous system and the pathology and pathophysiology of the various forms of DNP. Given the past inadequacies of pharmacotherapy, we explore the pathology and pathophysiology of DNP from various aspects, since they provide the basis for the development and evaluation of medical therapies. Against this background, special emphasis is placed upon the clinical presentation of DNP. Finally, we address the socioeconomic aspects of DNP and offer thoughts on a structured approach to treatment. This chapter includes guidelines for the diagnosis and outpatient management of diabetic peripheral neuropathy. They are consensus guidelines. After the manuscript was completed, evidence-based guidelines on sensorimotor and autonomic DNP were issued by the German Diabetes Association in cooperation with various professional societies. They include recommendations on the responsibilities of the various care levels (general practitioner, internist, diabetologist, neurologist, hospital). Unfortunately, these guidelines could not be incorporated into the present work.

All the chapters conclude with an extensive reference list for further reading, although we did not attempt to make the list complete. We beg the indulgence of readers who find no mention of their own important contributions. We also admit that our ideal concepts for the book have not been perfectly realized, and therefore we are grateful for any constructive comments or criticisms.

The preparation of this book demanded a great deal of effort from many distinguished experts in their fields. We gratefully acknowledge the team spirit of our authors and their outstanding contributions.

We express thanks to our publisher, especially Clifford Bergman, M.D. and Mr. Gert Krüger and their teams, for their support and dedication in the editing and publication of this book.

Fall 2002

F. Arnold Gries
Norman E. Cameron
Phillip A. Low
Dan Ziegler

Contributors

Henning Andersen, M.D., Ph.D.
Neurologisk Afdeling
Arhus Kommunehospital
Arhus, Denmark

Joseph C. Arezzo, Ph.D.
Department of Neuroscience
Albert Einstein College of Medicine
R.F. Kennedy Center
New York, USA

John W. Baynes, Ph.D.
Carolina Distinguished Professor
Department of Chemistry and Biochemistry
University of South Carolina
Graduate Science Research Center
Columbia, SC, USA

G.J. Biessels, M.D.
Department of Neurology
Universitair Medisch Centrum Utrecht
Utrecht, The Netherlands

Geremia B. Bolli, M.D.
Istituto di Medicina Interna
Scienze Endocrine e Metaboliche
Università di Perugia
Perugia, Italy

Paolo Bottini, M.D.
Department of Internal Medicine
Umbertide Hospital
Umbertide, Italy

Andrew J.M. Boulton, M.D.
Professor
Department of Medicine
Manchester Royal Infirmary
Manchester, UK

Vera Bril, B.Sc., M.D., FRCP(C)
Division of Neurology
Toronto General Hospital
Toronto, Canada

Norman E. Cameron, Ph.D.
Professor
Diabetic Complications Lab
Department of Biomedical Sciences
Institute of Medical Sciences
Aberdeen University
Aberdeen, Scotland

Mary A. Cotter, Ph.D.
Professor
Department of Biomedical Sciences
Institute of Medical Sciences
University of Aberdeen
Aberdeen, Scotland

Peter J. Dyck, M.D.
Professor
Department of Neurology
Mayo Clinic
Rochester, MN, USA

Simon E.M. Eaton, M.D.
Diabetes Research Unit
Royal Hallamshire Hospital
Sheffield, UK

Jürgen Eckel, M.D.
Deutsches Diabetes-Forschungsinstitut
Heinrich Heine Universität
Düsseldorf, Germany

Tomris Erbas, M.D.
Department of Endocrinology and Metabolism
Hacettepe Medical School
Hacettepe University
Sihhiye Ankara, Turkey

Carmine G. Fanelli, M.D.
University of Perugia
Perugia, Italy

Christine Feinle, Ph.D.
University of Adelaide Department of Medicine
Royal Adelaide Hospital
Adelaide, SA, Australia

Eva L. Feldman, M.D., Ph.D.
Department of Neurology
University of Michigan Medical Center
Ann Arbor, MI, USA

W.H. Gispen, M.D.
Professor
Rudolf Magnus Institute of Neuroscience
University of Utrecht
Utrecht, The Netherlands

F. Arnold Gries, M.D.
Professor emeritus
German Diabetes Research Institute
at the Heinrich Heine University
Düsseldorf, Germany

Jannik Hilsted, M.D.
Professor
Department of Endocrinology
Hvidovre Hospital
Hvidovre, Denmark

Michael Horowitz, M.D., Ph.D.
Department of Medicine
Royal Adelaide Hospital
Adelaide, SA, Australia

Johannes Jakobsen, M.D.
Arhus Kommunehospital
Universitetshospital Arhus Amt
Arhus, Denmark

Karen L. Jones, M.D.
Department of Medicine
Royal Adelaide Hospital, University of Adelaide
Adelaide, SA, Australia

William Kennedy, M.D.
Professor
University of Minnesota
Minneapolis, MN, USA

Jak Jervell, M.D.
Professor Emeritus
Oslo University
Oslo, Norway

Phillip A. Low, M.D., FRACP, FRCP
Professor
Department of Neurology
Mayo Clinic
Rochester, MN, USA

Dieter Luft, M.D.
Professor
Abt. Innere Med. IV
Med. Univ. Klinik
Tübingen, Germany

Rayaz A. Malik, M.D.
Department of Medicine
Manchester Royal Infirmary
Manchester, UK

Christopher J. Mathias, D.Phil., D.Sc., FRCP
Pickering Unit
St. Mary's Hospital
Imperial College School of Medicine
London, UK

Guido Menzinger, M.D.
Professor
Cattedra di Endocrinologia
Div. Malattie Dismetaboliche
Universita di Roma Tor Vergata
Roma, Italy

Andrew P. Mizisin, Ph.D.
Department of Pathology
School of Medicine
University of California, San Diego
La Jolla, CA, USA

Bernhard Neundörfer, M.D.
Professor
Neurolog. Klinik der Universität
Erlangen, Germany

Deirdre O'Donovan, M.D.
Department of Medicine
Royal Adelaide Hospital
Adelaide, SA, Australia

Simone Pampanelli, M.D.
University of Perugia
Perugia, Italy

Tae Sun Park, M.D.
Division of Endocrinology
Department of Internal Medicine
Chonbuk Nat, Univ. Med. School
Chonbuk, Korea

Christopher R. Pierson, M.D.
Department of Pathology
Wayne State University
Detroit, MI, USA

Gary Pittenger, Ph.D.
Associate Professor
Departments of Internal Medicine
and Pathology/Anatomy
The Strelitz Diabetes Institutes
Eastern Virginia Medical School
Norfolk, VA, USA

Francesca Porcellati, M.D.
Dipartimento di Medicina Interna e Scienze Endocrine
University of Perugia
Perugia, Italy
Henry C. Powell, M.D., D.Sc.
Department of Pathology
University of California San Diego
La Jolla, CA, USA

Wolfgang Rathmann, MSPH, M.D.
Department of Biometrics and Epidemiology
Deutsches Diabetesforschungsinstitut
Heinrich-Heine-Universität
Düsseldorf, Germany

Peter Rösen, M.D.
Professor
Deutsches Diabetesforschungsinstitut
Heinrich-Heine-Universität
Düsseldorf, Germany

Melvin Samsom, M.D.
Gastrointestinal Motility Unit
University Hospital Utrecht
Utrecht, The Netherlands

Robert Schmidt, M.D., Ph.D.
Department of Pathology
Washington University
School of Medicine
St. Louis, MO, USA

Luciano Scionti, M.D.
Department of Internal Medicine
University of Perugia
Perugia, Italy

Jonathan E. Shaw, M.D.
International Diabetes Institute
Caulfield, VIC, Australia

Anders A.F. Sima, M.D., Ph.D.
Department of Pathology
Wayne State University
Detroit, MI, USA

Mark Skeen, M.D.
Neurology Department
Naval Medical Regional Center
Portsmouth, VA, USA

Vincenza Spallone, Ph.D.
Department of Internal Medicine
Tor Vergata University
Rome, Italy

Kevin Stansberry, M.D.
Diabetes Research Institute
Norfolk, VA, USA

Martin J. Stevens, M.B.B.Ch.
Division of Endocrinology and Metabolism
Department of Internal Medicine
University of Michigan
Ann Arbor, MI, USA

Christian Stief, M.D.
Professor
Urologische Klinik
Mediz. Hochschule Hannover
Hanover, Germany

Rainer Straub, M.D.
Professor
Klinik u. Poliklinik f. Innere Medizin I
Klinikum d. Univ. Regensburg
Regensburg, Germany

Kelli A. Sullivan, Ph.D.
Department of Neurology
University of Michigan
Ann Arbor, MI, USA

Göran Sundkvist, M.D., Ph.D.
Professor
Department of Endocrinology
Malmö University Hospital
University of Lund
Malmö, Sweden

Mustafa Taskiran, M.D.
Deptartment of Endocrinology
Hvidovre University Hospital
Hvidovre, Denmark

Solomon Tesfaye, M.D.
Diabetes Research Institute
Royal Hallamshire Hospital
Sheffield, UK

P.K. Thomas, M.D.
Professor emeritus
University Department of Clinical Neurology
London, UK

Aristidis Veves, M.D.
Beth Israel Deaconess Medical Center
Boston, MA, USA

Aaron I. Vinik, M.D., Ph.D.
Director, Diabetes Research Institute
The Diabetes Institute
Norfolk, VA, USA

John D. Ward, M.D., FRCP, B.Sc.
Professor emeritus
Diabetes Research Unit
Royal Hallamshire Hospital
Sheffield, UK

Peter Watkins, M.D., FRCP
Department of Diabetes
King's College Hospital
London, UK

Gwen Wendelschafer-Crabb, M.D.
University of Minnesota
Minneapolis, MN, USA

Dan Ziegler, M.D.
Professor
German Diabetes Research Institute
at the Heinrich Heine University
Düsseldorf, Germany

Paul Zimmet, M.D., Ph.D.
Professor/Director
International Diabetes Institute
Caulfield, VIC, Australia

Contents

1 Diabetes Mellitus: An Introduction

F.A. Gries, J. Eckel, P. Rösen, and D. Ziegler

The aim of this introduction is to provide a general understanding of diabetes mellitus and its impact on the diabetic individual. It will focus on aspects of epidemiology, pathobiochemistry, prevention, and therapy. Given the scope covered, selectivity and bias of topics and citations have been accepted as unavoidable.

Definition

The term "diabetes mellitus" comprises a number of chronic diseases characterized by hyperglycemia due to absolute or relative insulin deficiency. Hyperglycemia is only the most obvious biochemical marker of complex metabolic disorders that affect carbohydrate, lipid, protein, and electrolyte metabolism and may impair numerous organs and functions of the organism.

Diagnosis

The diagnosis of diabetes mellitus is based on classical symptoms (weight loss, polyuria, thirst, muscular weakness and fatigue) and persistent hyperglycemia. Glucosuria and elevated glycosylated hemoglobin (HbA_{1c}) levels should not be used for diagnosis. The criteria for diagnosis of hyperglycemia and the classification of diabetes mellitus are not uniformly accepted. Some physicians use the criteria of the United States National Diabetes Data Group of 1979 [1], which was endorsed by the World Health Organization Study Group on Diabetes Mellitus in 1985 [2], while others prefer the criteria of the Expert Committee on the Diagnosis and Classification of Diabetes Mellitus of the American Diabetes Association 1998 [3] (Table 1.**1**).

The criteria published in 1998 tend to diagnose diabetes in younger and more obese subjects than the WHO 1985 criteria, while subjects with postprandial hyperglycemia, microalbuminuria, and those with other predictors of cardiovascular disease are less likely to receive this diagnosis despite the fact that they are at similar risk of premature death [4–8].

Classification

The diabetes mellitus classification of 1979 [1] was based "in large part on the pharmacological treatment used in its management." This was reflected in the terms "insulin-dependent diabetes mellitus" (IDDM) and "non-insulin-dependent diabetes mellitus" (NIDDM) and the further subdivision of patients with the

Table 1.**1** Criteria for the diagnosis of diabetes according to the World Health Organization [2] and the American Diabetes Association [3]

World Health Organization	American Diabetes Association
Clinical:	
Increased thirst and urine volume, unexplained weight loss, established by casual blood glucose	Polyuria, polydipsia and unexplained weight loss plus casual plasma or capillary blood glucose ≥ 200 mg/dl (11.1 mmol/l)
or	or
Biochemical:	
Casual venous plasma glucose[a] > 200 mg/dl (11.1 mmol/l), fasting venous or capillary plasma glucose[b] ≥ 140 mg/dl (7.8 mmol/l) *and* 2 h venous or capillary plasma or capillary whole blood glucose[c] ≥ 200 mg/dl (11.1 mmol/l) after glucose load[d]	Fasting plasma glucose ≥ 126 mg/dl (7.0 mmol/l) or capillary blood glucose ≥ 110 mg/dl or 2 h plasma or capillary blood glucose ≥ 200 mg/dl (11.1 mmol/l) during an oral glucose tolerance test

a Values for capillary plasma >220 mg/dl, for venous whole blood >180 mg/dl, for capillary whole blood >200 mg/dl
b Value for venous and capillary whole blood ≥ 120 mg/dl
c Value for venous whole blood ≥180 mg/dl
d Performed as described by WHO 1985 [2] using a glucose load containing the equivalent of 75 g anhydrous glucose dissolved in water

latter into obese and nonobese. The typing of 1998 is based on etiology and pathogenetic mechanisms (Table 1.**2**). About 50 different types of diabetes mellitus have been identified, the majority of cases being type 1, type 2, or gestational diabetes mellitus.

There is a great similarity between type 1 diabetes and IDDM and between type 2 diabetes and NIDDM. However, these pairs of terms should not be used indiscriminately as being respectively synonymous. Type 1 diabetes mellitus may for a limited time after manifestation remain non-insulin-dependent, particularly when it begins in an adult (latent autoimmune diabetes in adults, LADA; see page 10). On the other hand, NIDDM, like any type of diabetes mellitus, may become insulin-dependent at an advanced or critical stage.

Table 1.**2** Shortened version of the classification of diabetes according to the Expert Committee on the Diagnosis and Classification of Diabetes mellitus [3]

I.	Type 1 diabetes (β-cell destruction, usually leading to absolute insulin deficiency)
	A. Immune-mediated
	B. Idiopathic
II.	Type 2 diabetes (may range from predominantly insulin resistance with relative insulin deficiency to a predominantly secretory defect with insulin resistance)
III.	Other specific types
	A. Genetic defects of β-cell function
	B. Genetic defects in insulin action
	C. Disease of the exogenic pancreas
	D. Endocrinopathies
	E. Drug- or chemical-induced
	F. Infections
	G. Uncommon forms of immune-mediated diabetes
	H. Other genetic syndromes sometimes associated with diabetes
IV.	Gestational diabetes (GDM)

Epidemiology

Epidemiological research on diabetes mellitus is hampered by methodological problems. The criteria and methods for both the diagnosis and the classification of diabetes mellitus have changed over time. Population-based studies are rare, studies based on subgroups are usually biased, and even random samples are not always representative. The epidemiology of diabetes mellitus shows considerable regional variation, so that when data from different regions are compared, the ethnicity, gender, and age structure of the groups that had been studied need to be considered – but frequently these have not been communicated. These problems are more relevant to studies on type 2 respectively NIDDM than type 1 respectively IDDM.

Type 1 Diabetes/IDDM

The *incidence* of IDDM varies considerably with geography and ethnicity. In Japan, China, and in African Americans the incidence (number of new cases per 100 000 person-years) in the age group of 0–14 years is below 5. In most European regions it is about 10–20 per 100 000 person-years, and in Finland and Sardinia it is above 30 [2,9,10,11].

The highest incidence of IDDM is found in children below the age of 15, but IDDM or type 1 diabetes may become manifest at any age. The estimated incidence in adults is about half that observed in children of the respective population. However, the figure may be much higher if cases of LADA are included, which may comprise about 10 % of all patients initially diagnosed as having type 2 diabetes mellitus [12]. Worldwide a trend to increasing incidence in children and adolescents has been observed [13–15]. According to a Finnish study the incidence is increasing more in younger than older age groups [16]. Firstborn children are at highest risk. The risk increases with the age of the mother [17].

Reliable data about the *prevalence* of IDDM/type 1 diabetes mellitus are not available. Type 1 diabetes is associated with genetic as well as environmental factors. The rising incidence can hardly be explained by a change in the gene pool, so environmental factors must be playing a major role. However, it is impossible at present to decide what these environmental factors are.

The *life expectancy* of IDDM subjects is reduced. The number of lost years of life depends on the age at diagnosis (it is highest in early-onset IDDM) and on the quality of care as well as on chronic complications [18–20]. In the USA, mortality "among males was 5.4 times higher and in females it was 11.5 times higher than in the total US population." "Among people with age at diagnosis < 30 years, IDDM reduces life expectancy by at least 15 years." In 70–90 % the cause of death is related to diabetes [21]. In long-term type 1 diabetes vascular complications are the most important predictors and causes of death[22–24] (Table 1.**3**). In the USA, ketosis has been the cause of death in about 10% of people with IDDM who died at 0–44 years of age. Hypoglycemia may be the undiagnosed cause of sudden death. It was noted as an underlying cause of death in about 1 of 300 deaths due to diabetes [25]. Others have estimated that 2–4 % of all deaths in IDDM subjects are due to hypoglycemia [26].

Type 2 Diabetes/NIDDM

Type 2 diabetes mellitus is by far the most common type of diabetes. By extrapolation from the incidence of diabetic retinopathy in recently diagnosed subjects it may be concluded that the disease will manifest a couple of years before it is diagnosed. Most cases are diagnosed in individuals under the age of 60 years. The highest prevalence is found in the age group of 65–75 years.

Since type 2 diabetes develops insidiously, it is difficult to determine its incidence. Most reliable are *prevalence* data of clinical NIDDM/type 2 diabetes and of impaired glucose tolerance (IGT), which is assumed to precede clinical NIDDM/type 2 diabetes. Considerable regional differences exist in the prevalence of NIDDM/type 2 diabetes depending on relative body weight, life style, ethnic origin, nutritional habits, social status, education, and the age structure of the population [27, 28]. Type 2 diabetes/NIDDM used to be the disease of affluent societies in highly developed industrialized regions. This is no longer true. The highest prevalence is now found in Fiji, Micronesia, and among the Pima Indians. There is a worldwide trend towards both increasing prevalence and incidence and a lowering of the age at manifestation. It has been predicted that the number of diabetic subjects worldwide will double during the next two decades. This will be due not only to a rising incidence but also to increasing life expectancies in the growing world population.

Type 2 diabetes is associated with an increased mortality. In western countries the loss of life years is about 30% of normal life expectancy (Table 1.**4**). Because the NIDDM/type 2 diabetes population is older as a whole, the average absolute number of lost years is smaller than in type 1 diabetes and becomes insignificant in the very old. The main cause of death is cardiovascular disease [22, 29] (Table 1.**3**).The association between blood glucose control and the risk of dying is rather weak [30].

Table 1.**3** Causes of death by type of diabetes

Cause of death	Type 1 [24] (%)	Type 2 [24] (%)	Type 2 [21] (%)
Ischemic heart disease	27	34	40
Stroke	10	9	10
Other cardiovascular disease	5	7	15
Renal disease	18	11	–
Diabetes	4	3	13
Cancer	10	14	13
Gastrointestinal disease	4	7	–
Infectious disease	3	2	4 (combined)
Respiratory disease	3	2	
Other	14	11	5
Total	100	100	100

After [21,24]

Other types of diabetes mellitus, such as gestational diabetes mellitus (GDM), maturity-onset diabetes in the young (MODY), malnutrition-related diabetes mellitus (MRDM), and endocrine syndromes associated with diabetes mellitus will not be discussed in this chapter.

Table 1.**4** Age-related loss of years of life in diabetes mellitus (predominantly type 2)

Age (years)	Marks 1971	Goodkin 1975	Panzram 1981	Wolter 1986	Schneider 1991
40–49	8	10	7–8	6–12	16[a]
50–59	6	6	5–6	4–9	10
60–69	4	5	4	2–6	4
≥70			3		1.5–3

From [432], rounded value

Etiology and Pathogenesis of Diabetes

Type 1 Diabetes

More than 20 different regions of the human genome show some linkage with type 1 diabetes mellitus [31]. Many of these *genes* carry a risk, others protect.

The strongest linkage is seen for the major histocompatibility complex, which is located on chromosome 6 (IDDM1 locus). The importance of some HLA class II genes (e.g., DR 7, DR 9, DQA1 0301, DQB1 0201) differs among ethnic groups [9], as may be true for HLA class I genes. The physiological role of HLA molecules is to present foreign and self antigens to T lymphocytes and to other cells involved in the initiation of insulitis. The region of the insulin genes on chromosome 11p15 (IDDM2 locus) may also be involved. The importance of other type 1 diabetes mellitus-associated gene loci remains open.

Even in monozygotic twins the concordance for diabetes is not more than 50%, which indicates the importance of nongenetic factors. Environmental factors have been mainly studied in laboratory animals. The spontaneous diabetic NOD mouse is the star model, where numerous modulations of the environment or immunomodulatory protocols have been reported to lower the incidence of diabetes mellitus [32]. The ease of this success in preventing diabetes in a mouse model means that the observations cannot be simply transferred to the human situation.

In humans some seasonal variations of *incidence* with peaks in winter and early spring have been reported [11,33], but they seem to be absent in HLA-DR 3-positive and very young children [15]. The introduction of cow-milk-based diets before 3 months of age has been accused as a diabetogenic factor, but the epidemiological data remain controversial [34]. A homology of bovine serum albumin and human islet proteins and of immunogenic epitopes on β casein A1 which resemble β-cell epitopes (immunogenic mimicry) have been suggested to be responsible for the induction of insulitis. Prospective or controlled intervention studies comparing feeding with cow-milk proteins and breastfeeding will be needed to answer this question [34]. Nitrosamines, various toxins, and infection with rubella, German measles, mumps, coxsackievirus B_1, Epstein–Barr virus, and cytomegalovirus have also been discussed as possible causes. With the exception of congenital rubella virus infection [35], definite evidence of a causal role remains to be established.

Type 1 diabetes mellitus is an insulin deficiency syndrome caused by β-cell destruction. This is the result of an immune-mediated disease which leads to chronic inflammation of the islets of Langerhans, called *insulitis*. Various types of mononuclear cells are involved. On the basis of animal experiments, two types of insulitis may be distinguished [36–38]:

- *Benign Th-2* (T-helper-2 cell) *type insulitis* is characterized by secretion of interleukin (IL)-4, IL-10, and IL-13 and absence of aggressive immune cells. Cellular infiltration is located in the periphery of the islets and little β-cell destruction is seen.
- *Destructive Th-1* (T-helper-1 cell) *type insulitis* is characterized by secretion of interferon (IFN)-γ, tumor necrosis factor (TNF)-α, and IL-2 and the presence of cytotoxic T cells and activated macrophages, which migrate into the islets and cause β-cell damage by induction of apoptosis or necrosis.

As a rule, insulitis is a chronic process which may begin in early childhood [39]. Its earliest sign seems to be the appearance of islet autoantibodies in blood, which may be detected many years before clinical diabetes can be diagnosed. Whether insulitis will proceed to clinical diabetes, and how rapidly this may occur, seems to depend on a variety of hitherto hypothetical immune modulatory factors. Th-2 cytokines

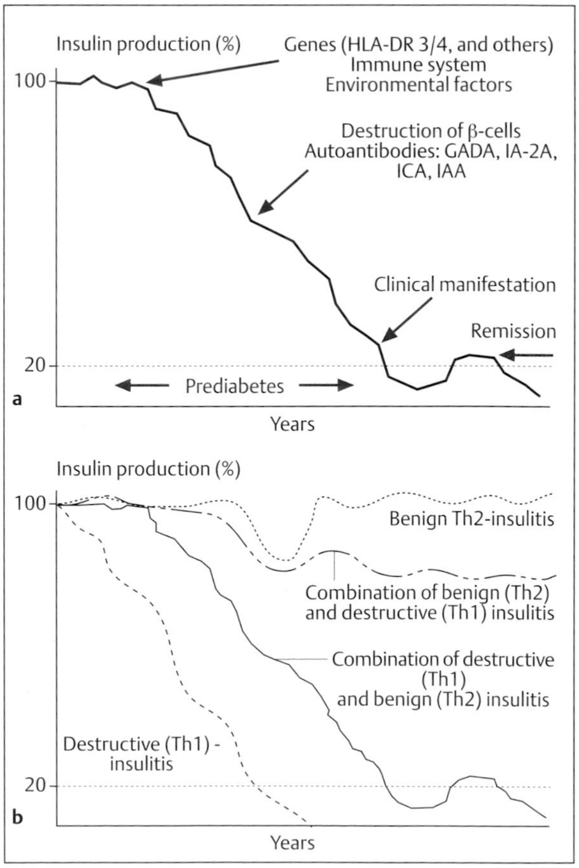

Fig. 1.1a, b Development of type 1 diabetes mellitus. **a** Insulin secretion in relation to clinical signs. **b** Insulin secretion in relation to type of insulitis. (Adapted by permission from Martin and Kolb [43])

suppress Th-1 cells and vice versa [40,41]. If the Th-2/Th-1 balance is shifted towards a Th-1 dominance, β-cell destruction will proceed until insulin release has dropped so low that blood glucose can no longer be regulated within the normal range, and clinical diabetes will become manifest [42] (Fig. 4.**1**).

In recent-onset diabetes, histological analysis of the pancreas shows infiltration by mononuclear cells, mostly T lymphocytes and monocytes/macrophages. Insulin-producing β cells are preferentially attacked. Other lobules of the pancreas may contain either completely insulin-deficient small islets which consist of A, D, and PP cells (A cells secrete glucagon, D cells somatostatin, and PP cells pancreatic polypeptide) or apparently normal islets. Such normal islets may persist for several years after diagnosis and could explain the remission or "honeymoon" phase and different grades of severity of the disease.

B lymphocytes and islet cell autoantibodies are not essential for β-cell destruction [433]. In the early stages of insulitis, glucose metabolism and stimulated insulin secretion are normal. When stimulated, early insulin secretion drops in autoantibody-positive subjects to the 1st percentile of normal, this indicates a loss of more than 80% of the β cells and the manifestation of diabetes mellitus in the very near future [44] .

Type 2 Diabetes

Genes and Determination Factors

Type 2 diabetes mellitus is a heterogeneous group of disorders that result from the combination of insulin resistance and impaired insulin secretion. Their etiology "may range from predominantly insulin resistance with relative insulin deficiency to a predominantly secretory defect with insulin resistance" [3]. A widely accepted pathogenetic model assumes that diabetes develops in carriers of *susceptibility genes* if they are exposed to determination factors. The idea of a genetic basis is supported by both twin studies and differences in prevalence between ethnic groups [45]. The genetic influence is stronger than in type 1 diabetes (Table 1.**5**). Multiple candidate genes have been nominated, including "thrifty genes" related to the metabolic syndrome [47,48], but the type 2 diabetes genes are not yet established. The mutations that have been found in MODY [49] play no role in ordinary type 2 diabetes.

Most *determination* factors are related to insulin resistance (Table 1.**6**). Some of these factors, such as age, are beyond our control, but most can be influenced. Of outstanding importance is the metabolic syndrome, which was first described in 1967 [50] (Table 1.**7**). Its multifactorial etiology is not yet fully understood [52]. The metabolic syndrome precedes and accompanies overt diabetes. Its components also constitute risk factors for vascular complications. This explains why many subjects already show angiopathies at the time of diagnosis of diabetes mellitus. For this reason, it is reasonable to expand the concept of type 2 diabetes to the early disorders of the preclinical phase, which traditionally have been neglected.

Obesity is closely related to physical inactivity. Both physical inactivity and obesity are associated with type 2 diabetes [53–56]. The relationship is most pronounced in the visceral (android, truncal, abdominal central) type of obesity [57–59]. This type of obesity is in its turn related to aging [60] and to physical inactivity [61]. Increasing abdominal adipose tissue

Table 1.**5** Risk of diabetes in various populations

Population	IDDM	NIDDM	IGT
General population	1/500	1/40	1/20
HLA DR3 or DR4	1/150		
HLA DR3 / DR4	1/40		
Siblings of a diabetic person			
All	1/14	1/8	1/4
HLA haplotype nonidentical	1/100		
HLA haplotype identical	1/6		
Children of diabetic parent(s)			
Both parents diabetic	1/25	1/8	
Mother diabetic	1/40-50		
Father diabetic	1/20		
Twin of a diabetic person			
Dizygote	1/20	1/8	
Homozygote	1/3	9/10 –10/10	

From [46]

IDDM, insulin-dependent diabetes mellitus; NIDDM, non-insulin-dependent diabetes mellitus; IGT, impaired glucose tolerance

Table 1.6 Determination factors of type 2 diabetes mellitus

Family history of diabetes mellitus
Age
Metabolic syndrome
Physical inactivity
Western life style
Diabetogenic drugs
Endocrinopathies and pregnancy

mass and weight gain are predictors of impaired glucose tolerance, dyslipoproteinemia, hypertension, and hyperuricemia [55]. Weight reduction predicts improvement of these risk factors [62] and of life expectancy [63]. This direct relationship indicates that obesity and physical activity are causal determininants rather than being accidentally associated with these disorders.

The importance of life style has been shown in longitudinal studies on, for example, Indians who emigrated to South Africa [64], and Japanese people who emigrated to North America [65], where they developed not only obesity but also diabetes. Thus, a genetic predisposition to diabetes may be revealed only under the influence of a diabetogenic life style. This concept has been confirmed in other populations [66,67] and by intervention studies (see p. 19). It has also been suggested that fetal malnutrition may predispose to the metabolic syndrome [68–71], but this hypothesis has been challenged [72,73].

Insulin Sensitivity

In the majority of type 2 diabetic individuals *insulin resistance* seems to be a very early or indeed the primary metabolic disorder [74–76]. In the general population insulin sensitivity varies over a wide range. The variation between members of a family is smaller than that between families [91], indicating a genetic determination.

The mechanisms of insulin resistance most likely involve polygenic defects [76] (Table 1.**8**), which cannot be discussed in this chapter. However, insulin resistance may also be acquired [77]. Some factors that enhance insulin resistance are identical with determination factors of type 2 diabetes (Table 1.**6**).

The biochemistry of insulin resistance has been extensively studied. Insulin acts through binding to a specific receptor which is composed of two extracellular insulin-binding α-subunits (135 kDa) and two cytoplasmic β-subunits (95 kDa) that carry a tyrosine kinase domain. Insulin binding initiates a conformational change which results in the activation of a tyrosine kinase. Important substrates of this kinase are the receptor itself and the insulin receptor substrates IRS-1 to IRS-4. Processes which are not completely understood connect the hormone to different signaling cascades which trigger either metabolic or mitogenic stimulation (Fig. 1.**2**).

The effects of insulin are cell-specific (Table 1.**9**). Insulin stimulates glucose uptake and glycogen synthesis in muscle. Insulin resistance of the muscle may precede impaired glucose tolerance. It usually begins with

Table 1.7 The metabolic syndrome originally [50] and today

1969	2000
Obesity	[a]Obesity, abdominal type
	[a]Insulin resistance
Hyperinsulinemia	Hyperinsulinemia
Impaired glucose tolerance	[a]Impaired glucose tolerance, type 2 diabetes
	Dyslipoproteinemia
Hypertriglyceridemia	[a]Hypertriglyceridemia [a]Low-HDL cholesterol Small, dense LDL
Hyperlipidacidemia	Hyperlipidacidemia
Abnormal adipose tissue metabolism	Hypertension Activated hemostasis Platelet activation Low PAI-1 Low thromboplastin Hyperfibrinogenemia Hyperuricemia Hyperandrogenemia in women [a]Albuminuria

[a] WHO criteria [51]

HDL, High-density lipoprotein; LDL, low-density lipoprotein; PAI-1, plasminogen activator inhibitor-1

Table 1.8 Causes and candidate genes of primary insulin resistance

Insulin receptor
Insulin binding site (α-subunit)
Tyrosine kinase activity (β-subunit)
Insulin receptor substrate
IRS-1 (polymorphism) [79,80]
Glucose utilization
GLUT-4 (decreased expression and/or translocation) [81]
Glycogen synthase?
Hexokinase II?
Others
Rad [82]
Glucagon receptor [83]
Fatty acid binding protein (FABP) [84]
β_3-Adrenergic receptor [85]
Tumor necrosis factor α (TNF-α) [86–88]
Calpain-10 [89]

Adapted from [78]

an impairment of nonoxidative glucose metabolism; later, oxidative glucose metabolism is also involved [91–93]. These defects may contribute to postprandial hyperglycemia.

It has been suggested that genetically determined insulin resistance of the muscle is the primary defect in the majority of type 2 diabetic individuals [74,94]. However, in cell culture, muscle cells from lean, non-diabetic, insulin-resistant subjects do not preserve their insulin resistance, suggesting that environmental factors may be of pivotal importance in the insulin sensitivity of muscle [95].

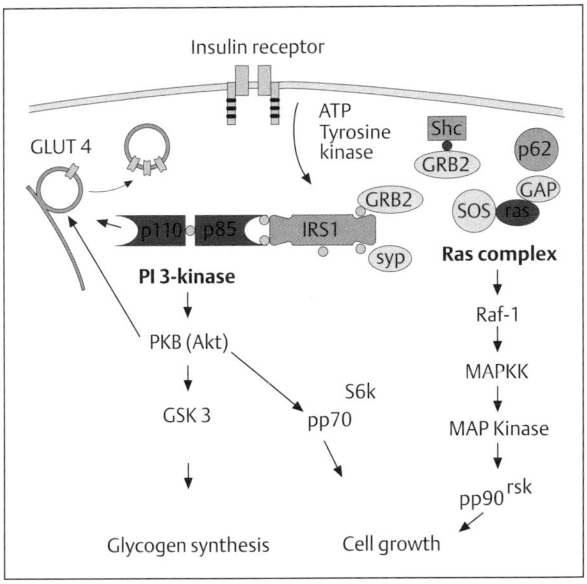

Fig. 1.2 Hypothetical insulin signaling pathways. Insulin signaling is initiated at the level of the insulin receptor. The insulin receptor tyrosine kinase activity leads to tyrosine phosphorylation of insulin receptor substrates (IRS1, IRS2, Shc). The phosphotyrosine residues of these proteins transfer the signal via SH2 domains and adapter molecules (Grb2, SOS, Syp) onto signal mediators like PI-3 kinase and the RAS complex. The PI-3 kinase pathway leads to translocation of glucose transporter 4 GLUT-4) and stimulation of glycogen synthesis; the RAS complex is a mediator for the activation of the MAP kinase, which is important for insulin-dependent cell growth and protein synthesis. (Adapted by permission from Holman and Kasuga [90] and from J. Eckel, personal communication)

PI 3-kinase, phosphatidylinositol 3-kinase; IRS, insulin receptor substrate; Shc, adaptor protein Shc; SH2, Src homology 2; PKB, protein kinase B; SOS, son-of-sevenless; Ras, small GTP-binding protein; Raf proteins, serine-threonine kinases with homology to PKC; MAP kinase, mitogen activated protein kinase; GSK3, glycogen synthase kinase 3; GRB2, growth factor receptor binding protein 2; Syp, SH2 domain-containing protein-tyrosine-phosphatase

Table 1.9 Effects of insulin on different tissues

Effect	Tissue
Stimulation of membrane transport	
Glucose	Muscle, adipose tissue
Amino acids	Muscle, adipose tissue
Ions	Muscle, adipose tissue, liver
Stimulation of synthesis	
Glycogen	Muscle, adipose tissue
Protein	Muscle, adipose tissue, lactating mammary gland
Fatty acids	Liver, adipose tissue, lactating mammary gland
Triglycerides	Liver, adipose tissue, lactating mammary gland
Inhibition of	
Lipolysis	Adipose tissue
Proteolysis	Muscle, liver
Gluconeogenesis and glucose production	Liver
Cell proliferation and differentiation	Stem cells, preadipocytes, fibroblasts Differentiated cells?

In the *liver* insulin suppresses gluconeogenesis and hepatic glucose release. Insulin resistance may unleash hepatic glucose output, which plays a role in fasting hyperglycemia.

In *adipocytes* insulin inhibits lipolysis and stimulates glucose uptake, lipid synthesis, and esterification of fatty acids. Therefore, insulin resistance results in elevated plasma free fatty acids (FFA), which in their turn contribute to insulin resistance, increased gluconeogenesis, hepatic glucose output, and very-low-density lipoprotein (VLDL) production.

The mechanism of the relationship between *obesity* and insulin resistance is still a matter of debate. FFA could play a major role [100]. High plasma FFA concentrations induce insulin resistance in muscle and liver [96]. The augmentation of adipose mass results in increased FFA release. Since visceral fat cells are metabolically more active and more sensitive to lipolytic stimuli, the increase of FFA is most pronounced in persons with visceral obesity. This is in line with the high diabetes rate in this type of obesity.

At the molecular level, the Randle mechanism, the inhibition of the glycogen synthase [96], the inhibition of the insulin signal cascade [97], or genomic effects which could be mediated through peroxisome proliferator-activated receptor (PPAR)-α have been discussed as possibly implicated in insulin resistance [98].

The Randle mechanism, also called the glucose–fatty acid cycle, postulates an inhibition of muscular glucose utilization by FFA [99]. Its relevance in humans is debated [92,100]. FFA are also important stimulators of hepatic gluconeogenesis and hepatic glucose output [101], which is unleashed in early impaired glucose tolerance [102]. This effect allows the enhanced hepatic glucose output to be explained without postulating genuine hepatic insulin resistance.

Another link between obesity and insulin resistance could be related to the hormonal activity of *adipose tissue*. Fat cells produce a variety of molecules with endocrine and paracrine activity. Some of them, including leptin, estrogens, IGF-1, FFA, and complement factors are released into the circulation. The cytokines TNF-α, interleukin-6, and angiotensinogen or angiotensin may act locally. Since metabolically active fat cells are located not only in adipose tissue but also inside the muscle, in close vicinity to myocytes, signals from these fat cells may have effects on adipocytes or muscle cells without being detectable in the circulation.

There is some evidence that signals released from fat cells are involved in insulin resistance. In laboratory animals the expression of TNF-α in adipocytes is linked to insulin resistance [86]. This cytokine stimulates phosphorylation of the serine residues of IRS-1, leading to reduced activity of the insulin receptor tyrosine kinase [88,103]. An inhibition of insulin signaling at the phosphatidylinositol 3-kinase (PI-3 kinase) level has been shown in human fat cells [88]. It could explain why TNF-α inhibits insulin-stimulated glucose transporter 4 (GLUT-4) expression and translocation [88,104,105] and may thereby impair glucose utilization. In obesity and type 2 diabetes, the expression of TNF-α and its receptors is increased in adipose and muscle tissue [86,104].

Physical activity has major effects on glucose and lipid metabolism. The sequence of metabolic changes during exercise can be summarized as follows: white muscle fiber metabolism dominates during the first few minutes of exercise. During endurance exercise red fibers dominate. Their aerobic glycolysis is increased and all endogenous and exogenous substrates are oxidized. Muscle and liver glycogen is mobilized and used up. Glucose uptake may increase up to 20-fold. Serum insulin decreases, indicating enhanced insulin sensitivity. After about 10 minutes' exercise, oxidation of FFA becomes more important and may increase to up to 50-fold of the basal level. Finally, energy metabolism is fueled mainly by FFA and β-hydroxybutyrate/acetoacetate. After strenuous exercise (e. g., marathon), plasma FFA may stay elevated and glucose uptake may remain reduced for several hours ("post-exercise insulin resistance"). A paradoxical increase in blood glucose is seen after short-term exhaustive exercise, which is the result of stress hormone release [106,107].

Increased insulin sensitivity during exercise is due to increased muscular blood flow with greater insulin delivery to muscle, opening of closed capillaries, which enhances the surface area for glucose uptake, and translocation of glucose transporters, mainly GLUT-4 [108]. Physical training stimulates GLUT-4 synthesis [109]. Enhanced insulin sensitivity vanishes in periods of physical inactivity. This occurs as early as after a few days of strict bed rest.

Clinical experience shows that in poorly controlled diabetic individuals insulin sensitivity is decreased. It improves when metabolic control is restored towards normal. This *metabolic insulin resistance* has been described by the term "glucose toxicity." The mechanism of glucose toxicity is not fully understood. One explanation is increased synthesis of glucosamine, which could cause insulin resistance by inhibition of the translocation of GLUT-4 in muscle [110–112]. Glucosamine seems also to inhibit glucose-induced insulin secretion [110]. Thus, this metabolite would mimic both the major pathogenetic mechanisms in type 2 diabetes. However, since poor metabolic control is characterized by high plasma FFA levels, the aforementioned effects of plasma FFA on liver and muscle metabolism could also explain some signs of metabolic insulin resistance.

Insulin Secretion

Instead of postulating insulin resistance and peripheral underutilization of glucose as the primary defect, some investigators have proposed that impaired insulin secretion and impaired suppression of hepatic glucose production are the important determinants of glucose intolerance [102,113]. Gerich [114] based his view on the evaluation of insulin secretion after an oral glucose load. In subjects with impaired glucose tolerance, and even more in those with clinical NIDDM, early insulin secretion is reduced and late insulin secretion increased [115]. Defective early insulin release is responsible for impaired glucose tolerance, which on its part triggers late hyperinsulinemia. The suppression of hepatic glucose production is impaired [102,116], resulting in increased hepatic glucose output. Under steady-state conditions this is equal to increased glucose disposal. Indeed, forearm muscle glucose uptake is not impaired in person with impaired glucose tolerance [116]. From these observations, Gerich concluded that peripheral insulin resistance cannot be an important pathogenetic factor [114].

Hepatic glucose output is directly related to fasting plasma glucose, supporting the view that the liver plays a major role in fasting hyperglycemia. However, increased hepatic glucose output may not be a primary defect. As mentioned before, increased hepatic glucose output can be explained as a response to enhanced lipolysis, with the primary defect being ascribed to insulin resistance of the adipocyte.

Recently, in order to elucidate the sequence of events, body weight and body composition, insulin secretion, insulin action, and endogenous glucose output were continuously monitored in a longitudinal study over several years in Pima Indians in whom normal glucose tolerance progressed to diabetes [117]. Progression to impaired glucose tolerance was associated with an increase in body weight and fat mass and a decline in both early insulin response to a glucose stimulus and insulin-stimulated glucose disposal. Progression to diabetes was accompanied by progression of these two disorders and, in addition, by an increase in basal endogenous glucose output. Subjects who retained a normal glucose tolerance in spite of weight gain (nonprogressors) were insulin-resistant but improved their early insulin secretion. According to this study, the ability to improve early insulin secretion decides progression to diabetes. Increased endogenous glucose output is a later event in the development of type 2 diabetes [117].

Genes responsible for defects of early insulin secretion and insulin secretory capacity have not yet been identified. However, the familial nature of type 2 diabetes leaves little doubt that they play a role. On the other hand, secretory defects may also be acquired due to glucose toxicity or hyperlipacidemia [118]. Thus, there is evidence for primary genetic and secondary environmental influences on insulin secretion and insulin sensitivity, respectively.

Clinical Picture of Diabetes Mellitus

Acute Symptoms

Mild hyperglycemia usually does not cause symptoms and may not be noticed by the patient, but severe hyperglycemia will always cause clinical symptoms.

People with untreated diabetes develop progressive hyperglycemia. When the renal threshold for plasma glucose of about 7 mmol/l is surpassed, glucose is excreted with the urine. Glucosuria goes along with osmotic diuresis and results in large urine volume, thirst, exsiccosis, and electrolyte disorders. Together with these effects of insulin deficiency, electrolyte imbalance is accentuated by cellular loss and renal excretion of potassium. Protein synthesis is lowered and accelerated proteolysis results in protein loss from muscle and other tissues. Increased amino acid levels in blood may be utilized for energy metabolism and gluconeogenesis. Lipid storage is blocked, while lipolysis is increased. This results in the massive appearance of FFA in blood. They are in part incorporated into lipoproteins, thus inducing hyper- and dyslipidemia. FFA also swamp into the energy metabolism. This process is enhanced by elevated levels of plasma glucagon, which activates the enzyme carnitine-palmitoyl-transferase (CPT-1) and the transport of long-chain fatty acids into the mitochondria. Here they compete with glucose for the oxidative chain, thus decreasing glucose oxidation. The supply of FFA is greater than the energy need. The FFA surplus is only degraded to the level of β-hydroxybutyrate and α-ketoglutarate, which may accumulate and cause ketoacidosis.

FFA also stimulate gluconeogenesis and hepatic glucose output, they modulate signal chains (e. g., PI-3 and IRS phosphorylation depressed, PKC activated), and contribute to metabolic insulin resistance (pages 6–8).

These disorders result in the classical symptoms of insulin deficiency: polyuria, thirst, polydipsia, exsiccosis, muscle wasting, loss of lipid stores, weight loss, polyphagia, fatigue, and nausea. At diagnosis, about 1% of the subjects have developed ketoacidosis with hyperventilation and eventual coma.

Type 1 Diabetes

Five phases of type 1 diabetes mellitus may be distinguished.

Prediabetes is characterized by the presence of islet cell autoantibodies in blood serum without metabolic disorders. Clinically important types are antibodies against islet cell cytoplasm (ICA), glutamic acid decarboxylase(LGAD), and tyrosinphosphatase (IA-2) (Table 1.**10**). Islet cell autoantibodies can often be detected many years before clinical manifestation. Transient presence of antibodies may have no relevance, but persisting antibodies indicate that type 1 diabetes will follow with a probability that increases if more than one autoantibody is detected and if they are present at high titers. In antibody-positive persons they should be monitored once or twice per year. Tests for insulin secretory capacity may have additional predictive value [44].

At *manifestation* symptoms are more frequent in younger than in older individuals. In young subjects it may be only hours or a few days from the first signs until a serious clinical syndrome develops. In later adulthood, the progression from insulin deficiency to overt clinical diabetes is often retarded [120–122]. The clinical picture of these people may resemble that of type 2 diabetes, but they are islet cell antibody-positive and will usually need insulin during the first year after diagnosis. It can be expected that about 10% of newly diagnosed diabetic subjects originally classified as having type 2 in fact have this form of type 1 diabetes [12]. The term "latent autoimmune diabetes inadults" (LADA) has been used to describe this subgroup.

Table 1.**10** Islet cell specific autoantibodies in type 1 diabetes. Prevalence at manifestation

Antibodies to	Prevalence (%)
Islet cell cytoplasm (ICA, IgICA, ICCA)	60–90
Glutamic acid decarboxylase (GAD)	70–90
IA-2	70–90
IA-2β	> 50%
Insulin (IAA)	20–100
Proinsulin (PAA)	10–20
BSA	60–100
ICA 69	60
38-kDa insulin granules	> 30
Glucose transporter	80–100
Carboxy peptidase H	30–50
Polar antigen	30–50
52-kDa protein	> 30
150-kDa protein	80–100
Islet cell surface (ICSA)	60–80

Adapted from [120]

Frequently the manifestation of type 1 diabetes seems to be precipitated by coincident diseases that increase the insulin requirement, such as infections, pregnancy, hyperthyroidism, glucocorticoid treatment, or severe somatic stress (myocardial infarction, major surgery, etc.).

In about two-thirds of subjects a *remission* will follow the initiation of therapy. The required insulin dose decreases and metabolism stabilizes due to some recovery of insulin and C-peptide secretion together with improved insulin sensitivity. The remission period can be prolonged by experimental immunomodulatory therapy [123]. However, sooner or later the individual will become C-peptide-negative. After some weeks or months, remission is usually followed by a *relapse* and the development of *irreversible clinical diabetes*, which under unfavorable conditions may proceed to *end-stage diabetes* with chronic complications.

If diabetes mellitus is suspected, the diagnosis should immediately be checked by laboratory tests. If the diagnosis is confirmed, it is advisable to start therapy and normalize the metabolism promptly, because this seems to improve the chances of inducing a remission [124].

Treated type 1 diabetes mellitus is not associated with hypertension, lipid disorders, or obesity. However, this does not rule out their existence at diagnosis or that they may develop later. The further course of the disease is determined by the lability of the metabolism, problems of insulin substitution, glucose monitoring, hypoglycemia, and hyperglycemia. The quality of metabolic control is the main determinant of the prognosis.

Type 2 Diabetes

In the majority of cases the disease begins as a metabolic syndrome. In this early stage most symptoms are reversible. Progression to clinical diabetes is not inevitable. The progress of the blood glucose disorder from impaired fasting glucose or impaired glucose tolerance to overt diabetes may take years. Even when diagnostic criteria are reached, hyperglycemia may not cause the classical symptoms, and glucosuria may be minimal or lacking due to an elevated renal threshold. Other symptoms will often be misinterpreted as a normal attribute of aging. Thus, it may take a couple of years until diabetes is diagnosed.

In contrast to type 1 diabetes mellitus, glucose metabolism in type 2 diabetes mellitus is usually fairly stable. However, treatment is usually more difficult than in type 1 diabetes because it requires life-style changes. The disorder tends to increasing severity, and over the years it becomes more and more difficult to achieve near-normal metabolic control [125]. As in the case of type 1 diabetes, the prognosis of type 2 diabetes depends on the quality of metabolic control. However, in addition to glucose metabolism, the other components of the metabolic syndrome such as obesity, hypertension, and dyslipoproteinemia, and life style are equally important.

Chronic Complications

The chronic complications of diabetes – mainly microangiopathy, neuropathy, and macroangiopathy – are major problems, because they determine the prognosis and quality of life of the patients. Although the details of their pathogenesis are not fully understood, there is no doubt that the diabetic condition is the major cause. Epidemiological studies have shown that their incidence increases with poor metabolic control [126–132] and can be reduced by lowering HbA_{1c} [127,130,131,133]; however, the beneficial effect of strict metabolic control on macroangiopathy is rarely significant [127,130,133–135]. Many proposals have been put forward to explain "diabetes the risk factor," which forms a network of potentially pathogenetic mechanisms. Recent articles have covered specific topics and the reader is referred to these publications [136–145]. It is not the aim of this short introduction to add another review.

In addition to insulin deficiency/hyperglycemia, other pathogenic factors such as adverse life style, hypertension, lipid disorders, proteinuria, unfavorable hemorrheology, and activated hemostasis are also involved. These will be mentioned in the context of the various clinical manifestations.

The following section outlines the role of hyperglycemia in the pathogenetic network leading to microangiopathy [146–149].

Introduction to the Pathogenesis of Microangiopathy

Hyperglycemia has three important effects that are to some extent interdependent: nonenzymatic *glycation*, activation of the *polyol pathway*, and generation of *reactive oxygen species* (ROS).

The formation of early glycation endproducts (Schiff base and Amadori products) is reversible, but glycated long-lived molecules like DNA and matrix/basement membrane proteins may undergo irreversible cross-linking and other not yet fully understood complex reactions to form *advanced glycation endproducts* (AGE).

This process leads to considerable changes in their three-dimensional structure and function. Glycated LDL (low-density lipoproteins) are more atherogenic than nonglycated LDL. The charge of matrix proteins may be altered, leading to increased permeability, and basement membrane proteins may become resistant to degradation and increase in thickness and stiffness. AGE may impair the relaxation of vessels by quenching nitric oxide [150]. Moreover, they favor coagulation and thrombosis and initiate atherosclerosis by stimulating macrophages to express AGE receptors (RAGE) and to release cytokines such as TNF-α, IL-1, and IGF.

The activation of the *polyol pathway* leads to the accumulation of sorbitol, which is followed by myoinositol depletion and inactivation of Na^+-K^+-ATPase channels. In addition, the production of fructose and sorbitol, which contribute to the formation of AGE, is increased.

There is much evidence that both advanced glycation endproducts (AGE) and high glucose are able to induce the generation of *ROS* in various types of vascular cells and that this process plays an important role in the initiation of vascular complications in diabetes. In addition to the autoxidation of glucose, three different mechanisms of ROS production are presently under debate:

1. Activation of a membrane-bound, macrophage-like NADH-oxidase. Activation of NADH-oxidase in endothelial cells and smooth muscle cells has been reported in subjects with hypertension and hypercholesterolemia. AGE and angiotensin II are strong activators of this enzyme in vascular cells.
2. Alternatively, it has been suggested that the electron flux in endothelial nitric oxide synthase (NOS III) becomes uncoupled in diabetes and hyperglycemia. In this uncoupled state the electrons flowing from the reductase domain to the oxygenase domain of the NOS complex are diverted to molecular oxygen rather than to L-arginine. In line with this assumption, production of ROS was prevented in human and rat endothelial cells in the presence of inhibitors of NOS.
3. Recently, Nishigawa et al. [146] demonstrated in cultured bovine aortic endothelial cells that in hyperglycemic conditions the mitochondrial electron flux becomes uncoupled from ATP synthesis, resulting in increased ROS production. ROS production was prevented by various uncouplers of the mitochondrial electron chain and overexpression of the uncoupling protein (UCP-2). The activation of protein kinase C, the polyol pathway, the transcription factor NFκB, and the increased formation of AGE and glucosamine were clearly dependent on the formation of ROS, suggesting that at least in these cultured endothelial cells the formation of ROS is the central, initiating step for the transformation of endothelial cells into an active, prothrombotic state. According to these observations, an accelerated substrate flow from either glucose or fatty acids seems to be the final cause for the generation of ROS and oxidative stress.

Against this background, the great importance of accelerated conversion of glucose to fructose by the so-called sorbitol pathway and the changes in the cellular redox state by these processes is obvious. The conversion of glucose consumes NADPH and leads to increased flow of NADH to mitochondria. Since an important cofactor of glutathione peroxidase is diminished, the regeneration of glutathione is impaired, which may limit the antioxidative capacity of the cells and contribute to the occurrence of oxidative stress in diabetes.

The generation of ROS seems to be the initiating factor for a number of processes known to be relevant to the development of vascular complication:

1. Activation of protein kinase C (PKC). The activation of PKC in cells and tissues that take up glucose independently of insulin is mediated not only by a hyperglycemia-dependent increase in diacylglycerol (DAG), but also by the enhanced formation of ROS. Activation of PKC seems to be a common downstream mechanism to which multiple cellular and functional abnormalities in the diabetic vascular tissue can be attributed, including changes in vascular blood flow, vascular permeability, extracellular matrix components, and cell growth.
2. Activation of redox-sensitive transcription factors by AGE and hyperglycemia. AGE formation has so far mostly been in discussion as a process of protein modification. From recent studies it follows, however, that interactions of AGE-modified proteins with specific AGE receptors serve not only to eliminate AGE proteins, but also to induce signal transaction pathways which lead to the generation of ROS, depletion of cellular antioxidant defense mechanisms (e. g., glutathione, ascorbate) and the activation of redox-sensitive transcription factors such as NFκB [144,151]. The activation of NFκB and presumably also other redox-sensitive transcription factors promotes the expression of a variety of kinins, such as the procoagulant tissue factor, endothelin-1, and the adhesion molecules VCAM-1 (vascular cellular adhesion molecule 1), ICAM-1 (intercellular adhesion molecule 1), and MCP-1 (monocyte chemoattracting protein 1), all of which have been found to be increased in the diabetic state. The concept of AGE-induced oxidative stress which activates transcription factors could explain the concomitant occurrence of oxidative stress and changes in the dynamic endothelial balance from an anticoagulant to a procoagulant state, from vasodilatation to vasoconstriction and impaired microcirculation.
3. Activation of the hexosamine pathway and activation of the transcription factor SP-1. ROS have been shown to inhibit glyceraldehyde 3-*P*-dehydrogenase. In consequence, more glucose will be metabolized to glutamine 6-phosphate. This molecule has been shown to play a role in the induction of insulin resistance. It also enhances glycosylation and activation of the transcription factor SP-1, which accelerates synthesis of plasminogen activator inhibitor 1 (PAI-1) and transforming growth factor β_1 (TGF-β1), both of which contribute to the pathogenesis of vascular complications by changes in the hemostatic balance and remodeling processes of the vessel wall.
4. Quenching of nitric oxide. Oxidative stress seems thereby to initiate a vicious cycle reinforcing the imbalance in the redox state of cells and the generation of ROS. These therefore counterbalance the cytoprotective effects of nitric oxide on microcirculation, on the permeability and adhesiveness of the vessel wall, and growth inhibition of smooth muscle cells.
5. Taken together, ROS activate interrelated processes and mechanisms which play a major role in the development of vascular complications in diabetes. However, it must be borne in mind that the outcome of the processes may vary depending the site affected (large vessels, resistance vessels, capillaries).

Following the metabolic concept of pathogenesis, one would expect that the extracellular changes are ubiquitous systemic disorders and that all insulin-independent cells (for only these are exposed to intracellular hyperglycemia) are affected. However, microangiopathy is clinically evident only in the kidney and the eye, and is thought to play a role in neuropathy. Microangiopathy usually begins with reversible functional disorders and may end with irreversible loss of organ function. For this reason, early detection (screening) and monitoring are of paramount importance.

Retinopathy

Epidemiology

The prevalence of diabetic retinopathy is highest in early-onset insulin-treated diabetic subjects and lowest in late-onset non-insulin-treated diabetic subjects. The prevalence increases with the duration of diabetes. In early-onset insulin-treated subjects proliferative diabetic retinopathy is rarely seen within the first five years of diabetes, but after 15 years it is found in 25% of patients and after 20 years in more than 50%. Beyond 20 years, almost 100% of people with diabetes mellitus will develop diabetic retinopathy [152]. In late-onset diabetes retinopathy may be observed at the time the diabetes is diagnosed, but proliferative diabetic retinopathy is rare. The 10-year incidence and progression rates reflect these trends (Table 1.**11**). Macular edema is more common in late-onset diabetes [153]. Senile cataracts, which will not be further discussed, appear earlier in life and progress faster than in nondiabetic subjects.

Pathology

Diabetic retinopathy is a disease of the retinal vasculature. In the early stages capillary blood flow is increased. The capillary basement membrane is thickened, its composition and charge are altered, its permeability to blood-borne particles and molecules is

Table 1.11 Ten years cumulative incidence of diabetic retinopathy or progression to proliferative diabetic retinopathy (PDR)

Diabetic group	10-Year incidence (%)	10-Year progression to PDR (%)
Younger-onset taking insulin:		
Male	93	29
Female	85	31
Total	89	30
Older-onset taking insulin:		
Male	77	25
Female	80	23
Total	79	24
Older-onset not taking insulin:		
Male	69	7
Female	65	12
Total	67	10

Data from the Wisconsin Epidemiologic Study of Diabetic Retinopathy [434]

increased, and pericytes are lost. This process is related to hyperglycemia [127, 130–132] and modified by hypertension [158, 159], smoking [160,161], and pregnancy [162–164].

An early morphological sign is the presence of microaneurysms. These have been interpreted as abortive attempts to vascularize ischemic areas. Other early signs are intraretinal (flame-shaped or dotted) hemorrhages and lipoprotein deposits (hard exudates). They are indicative of increased capillary permeability, which could be due to modified LDL, free radical damage of endothelial cells, or AGE formation in the endothelial matrix proteins, which attract platelets and macrophages and stimulate the expression of vascular permeability factor (VPF) and other cytokines. Disruption and fenestrations of the endothelial layer and vascular proliferation may occur. Another important clinical sign of vascular permeability is focal or diffuse macular edema.

A later morphological sign is capillary closure. This may be caused by the activated hemostasis with expression of adhesion molecules in platelets and leukocytes as well as by procoagulatory changes of the endothelium and matrix areas exposed to the blood flow because of endothelial disrupture.

Capillary closure is followed by ischemia, which is a potent trigger of new vessel formation. This process is normally suppressed by collagen IV, but it is stimulated by collagen fragments, fibronectin, and local growth factors such as vascular endothelial growth factor (VEGF; secreted in response to hypoxia), fibroblast growth factor (FGF), and TGF-β. Formation of new vessels may not be restricted to the retina. They may grow into the preretinal space and vitreous and eventually cause retinal detachment. New vessel formation may also occur in the iris, where it causes rubeosis iridis and possibly neovascular glaucoma.

Classification

For the purposes of therapy and prognosis, diabetic retinopathy may be classified according to the Early Treatment Diabetic Retinopathy Study Research Group [165] as follows:

1. Background retinopathy, characterized by microaneurysms, hard exudates, generalized venous dilatation, intraretinal hemorrhages, and occasional cotton wool spots (retinal infarcts). Background diabetic retinopathy does not necessarily progress to more advanced stages.
2. Preproliferative retinopathy, characterized by localized irregularities of venous caliber (beading), which are strong predictors of neovascularization; venous looping and reduplication; multiple (≥ 5) cotton wool spots; and intraretinal microvascular abnormalities (IRMAs—abnormally branched vessels within the retina).
3. Proliferative retinopathy, characterized by abnormal new vessels growing into the preretinal space, vitreous, or, occasionally, on the iris. Bleeding from these vessels, retinal detachment due to contraction of fibrotic structures that develop in the hemorrhages, and neovascular glaucoma may cause impairment of vision.

Another cause of impaired vision is maculopathy due to capillary leakage (edematous, wet maculopathy) or to ischemia (dry maculopathy).

Management

The different classes of diabetic retinopathy require different action depending on the risk of loss of vision. In general, the best primary prevention is near-normal metabolic control, normal blood pressure, and giving up smoking [127,130,158,159,166,167]. In secondary prevention, abrupt normalization of poor metabolic control of long duration should be avoided because of the so-called normoglycemic re-entry phenomenon [168,169]. Dyslipoproteinemia increases the risk of hard exudates, maculopathy [170], and vascular proliferations [171] and should be effectively treated. Guidelines for ophthalmological intervention have been developed (for references see [172–174]). The most important technical methods of treating diabetic retinopathy are photocoagulation and vitreous surgery, which may save useful vision in up to 70% of cases of severe proliferative diabetic retinopathy. A difficult problem is dry (ischemic) maculopathy. Treatments based on improving the microcirculation are still experimental [175].

Any diabetic person requires an ophthalmological checkup at diagnosis and annually thereafter.

Background retinopathy should be monitored every 6 months. Referral to the ophthalmologist is indicated soon in the case of preproliferative diabetic retinopathy or maculopathy. Referral is urgent if new vessels develop, particularly if they originate from the optic disk. Immediate referral is indicated if retinal detachment, vitreous hemorrhage, or neovascular glaucoma is suspected.

Nephropathy

Diabetic nephropathy is a microvascular disease of the glomerulus (diabetic glomerulosclerosis). It begins with hyperfiltration followed by proteinuria, hypertension, and progressive renal failure. The pathogenesis and clinical course of diabetic nephropathy are better known in type 1 than in type 2 diabetes. They appear to be similar but not identical.

Epidemiology

The prevalence of microalbuminuria or any more advanced stage of nephropathy in IDDM increases during the first 20 years after diagnosis (or, in children, after puberty) to > 50% and levels off thereafter. During this time only about half of the microalbuminuric subjects will develop macroproteinuria and only a minority will develop endstage renal disease [176]. The cumulative incidence of persistent macroproteinuria is about 35% in both IDDM and NIDDM. However, endstage renal disease after 30 years of diabetes is more often present in IDDM (> 20%) than in NIDDM (10%) [177–179]. About 30–50% of all patients on chronic dialysis have diabetes (which does not imply that the reason is always the diabetes). Since type 2 diabetes is much more frequent than type 1 diabetes, it contributes the majority of these subjects.

The incidence and progression of diabetic nephropathy are related to metabolic control [127,130–133] and blood pressure [158,159]. A threshold phenomenon was postulated [180], but was rejected [181,182]. Mortality is high in subjects with diabetic nephropathy. Microalbuminuria has been identified as a strong predictor of cardiovascular disease.

In proteinuric subjects coronary artery disease is about 15 times more frequent than in diabetic subjects without proteinuria [154], and cardiovascular mortality is increased nine-fold [183,184]. Ten-year survival of subjects with persistent proteinuria used to be only 20–50% [179,185]. Antihypertensive treatment and renal replacement therapy have effectively improved the prognosis. In recent studies, eight-year survival after the onset of persistent proteinuria rose to 70–87% [176,186,187].

Before renal replacement therapy was available, the main cause of death in subjects with proteinuria was uremia. About 25% died from myocardial infarction or stroke. Renal replacement therapy reduced deaths from uremia but increased deaths from cardiovascular causes [188].

Pathology

As in diabetic retinopathy, there is no doubt about the influence of hyperglycemia on the development of diabetic nephropathy. However, the causal relationship is less clear. There is no linear relation between the cumulative incidence of any sign of diabetic nephropathy and the duration of diabetes, and more than half of diabetic subjects never develop such nephropathy [176,189]. Normal kidneys transplanted into diabetic recipients may develop typical lesions, but the rate of development varies and is independent of metabolic control [155]. These observations suggest that hyperglycemia is necessary but not sufficient for the development of diabetic nephropathy. Other important pathogenetic factors are hypertension, protein intake, renal hemodynamics, smoking, and genetics.

The hyperglycemia-related pathogenetic effects discussed on pages 11 and 12 are also found in diabetic nephropathy. In addition, synthesis of the glucosaminoglycan heparan sulfate and glycoproteins is impaired [136]. These molecules contribute to the negative charge of the glomerular capillary membranes and are involved in the selectivity of glomerular filtration, which consequently may be reduced. Hemodynamics are another important pathogenetic factor. The impact of hypertension on diabetic nephropathy has been shown in epidemiological and antihypertensive treatment studies [156–159,190,191]. A significant example of direct jeopardizing of the kidney by hypertension is seen in people with unilateral renal artery stenosis, where only the kidney with the patent artery develops glomerulosclerosis [155].

Evidence for a genetic influence comes from family studies. Siblings of probands with nephropathy develop signs of nephropathy several times more often than do siblings of probands without nephropathy [192,193]. Recently epidemiological studies showed an increased incidence of diabetic nephropathy at level of a protein intake exceeding 20% of total energy [194], suggesting a pathogenetic role of nutritional protein.

The clinical picture of diabetic nephropathy is dominated by functional disorders, which may be classified according to Mogensen [195] (Table 1.**12**). The functional disorders correspond to morphological changes. The early increase in glomerular filtration rate has been explained by the ubiquitously increased blood flow and peripheral vasodilation. It correlates to increased kidney size, glomerular volume, and capillary filtration surface area.

Microalbuminuria develops without apparent morphological changes. It seems to be caused by increased glomerular capillary pressure and a loss of negative

Table 1.**12** Diabetic nephropathy: stages and clinical characteristics

Stage		Glomerular filtration rate	Urinary albumin excretion rate	Blood pressure	Time since diagnosis of diabetes (years)
1	Hyperfunction	High	Normal	Normal	Initially
2	Latency	Normal/high	Normal	Normal	0–?
3	Microalbuminuria	Normal	20–200 μg/min 30–300 mg/day	Normal Increasing	5–15
4	Persistent proteinuria	Normal/ decreasing	<300 mg/day	Elevated	10–15
5	Renal failure	Decreased	>300 mg/day	Elevated	15–30

Adapted from [195]

charge of the glomerular basement membrane. When the pores of this membrane enlarge, filtration selectivity is lost, and (macro-)proteinuria develops. With mesangial expansion due to continuous deposition of indigestible matrix proteins (formation of AGE on collagen, laminin, fibronectin) and thickening of the endothelial layer, vascular obstruction will occur, which results in a decrease of the filtering area. Histological studies show diffuse or nodular glomerulosclerosis [196–198]. In this situation blood pressure increases, glomerular filtration rate decreases, and progressive renal failure with end stage renal disease will develop.

Management

It is essential to detect diabetic nephropathy at a reversible stage. At Mogensen's stages 1–3 (Table 1.**12**) the disorders are reversible and renal function may be kept normal if effectively treated. In stages 4 and 5 it may only be possible to delay or possibly halt progression.

The most relevant diagnostic sign is microproteinuria. Microalbuminuria screening should be started not later than five years after diagnosis of type 1 diabetes, and at the time of diagnosis of type 2 diabetes. For correct diagnosis and follow-up monitoring, quantitative determination of albumin in urine collected over precisely measured time periods is essential. An albumin excretion rate (AER) below 30 mg per 24 hours (20 μg/min) is considered normal, whereas an AER above 300 mg per 24 hours (200 μg/min) is considered to define macroalbuminuria or proteinuria. In between these two extremes is the range of microalbuminuria. Alternatively, the urinary albumin/creatine ratio may be determined [189].

Prevention and treatment of diabetic nephropathy is based on achieving near-normal metabolic control [127,129–131,199–202], lowering elevated blood pressure to values below 130/80 mmHg [157,158, 191], a normal protein intake of 0.8–1.2 g/kg body weight [203,204], cessation of smoking (if applicable), and diagnosis and treatment of nondiabetic renal or urinary tract disease.

In normotensive diabetic subjects ACE inhibitors do not reliably prevent the development of microalbuminuria [205]. In normotensive patients with microalbuminuria, captopril and calcium channel blockers [206–212] retard the progression of nephropathy. In hypertensive subjects both the ACE inhibitor captopril and the β-adrenergic blocker atenolol retard the development of microalbuminuria [158,206]. In hypertensive diabetic subjects with micro- or macroalbuminuria, lowering blood pressure with ACE inhibitors, β-adrenergic blockers, or calcium channel blockers retards the progression of albumin excretion [213–221]. While the UK Prospective Diabetes Study (UKPDS) suggested that blood pressure reduction itself may be more important for nephroprotection than the type of drug used for treatment, recent secondary prevention studies in type 2 diabetic subjects suggest that inhibition of the renin–angiotensin system may be more advantageous than other antihyperintensive therapy. In studies with ACE inhibitors [222] and with angiotensin receptor blockers [223–225] the nephroprotective effect was beyond that attributable to blood pressure control.

Cardiovascular risk is increased at any stage of diabetic nephropathy, and the majority of patients with such nephropathy will die not of uremia but of macrovascular complications [183,184,188,226]. Prevention of these complications is mandatory, and risk factors for macroangiopathy other than hypertension should also be treated.

Diabetic nephropathy is accompanied by lipid disorders which are believed to contribute essentially to the high cardiovascular risk [227]. Treatment of dyslipoproteinemia is mandatory, as are "stop smoking" programs for smokers.

Platelet aggregation inhibition with aspirin is recommended in diabetic patients with albuminuria [228]. Radiopaque media should only be used after careful hydration of the patient [229].

Patients with endstage renal disease will need renal replacement therapy. Chronic hemodialysis, peritoneal dialysis (intraperitoneal, continual ambulatory), and renal transplantation in combination with pancreas transplantation [230] are presently the methods of choice. The prognosis of patients who have undergone transplantation has recently been improved but still is not as good as in nondiabetic subjects [176,187,230].

Almost 100% of patients with endstage renal disease also have diabetic retinopathy and/or diabetic neuropathy. Monitoring and treatment of these complications is equally important.

Macroangiopathy

The term "macroangiopathy" was introduced by Lundbaek [231] to draw attention to the fact that large-vessel disease in diabetes is not just a matter of atherosclerosis occurring in a diabetic subject, but is a facet of diabetic angiopathy as important as microangiopathy. The major clinical complications of macroangiopathy are coronary artery disease, stroke, and amputation. Only coronary artery disease will be discussed in more detail in this chapter.

Epidemiology

Due to the insidious course of macroangiopathy and the difficulties of early diagnosis, reliable population-based data on its incidence and prevalence are lacking. Some epidemiological data on the clinical manifestations are available [232]. The figures for their incidence and prevalence in diabetes depend on their occurrence in the general population to which they belong and differ considerably between countries [233]. However, clinical, epidemiological [154,234–236], and autopsy studies [237,238] and cause-of-death statistics [29,239] agree that the figures are higher in people with type 1 diabetes/IDDM and type 2 diabetes/NIDDM than in the general population. After 30 years of IDDM, cardiovascular disease accounts for two-thirds of all deaths [21]. Macroangiopathy develops earlier in life and occurs almost independently of gender [154,240]. The increase in risk is higher in women than in men [236,241,242]. Thrombotic complications of macroangiopathy are the leading cause of death in diabetes [29,243–245].

Coronary artery disease is 3.3 times more frequent in diabetic than in nondiabetic people [246]. Myocardial infarction is 3.7 times more frequent in diabetic men and 5.9 times more frequent in diabetic women [242]. In another study [247] the increase was 6.7 times in type 2 and 12.2 times in type 1 diabetic women. The higher risk of women goes along with more atherogenic lipid profiles (see below). The standardized mortality rate (corrected for age and gender) for any heart disease is 9.1 times higher if diabetes mellitus is diagnosed before the age of 30 and 2.3 times higher if it is diagnosed later [248]. As a rough estimate, in western societies about half of diabetic people die of premature cardiac death. Stroke is about twice as frequent as in the general population, and two out of three amputations are performed in diabetic people.

Pathology

The histology of lesions in the arterial wall of diabetic subjects is similar to what is seen in the general population. However, lesions tend to be located in more distal regions of the vasculature. In diabetic subjects, the established sequence of early events in atherogenesis seems to be the same as in nondiabetic subjects: -adhesion of monocytes to endothelial cells, mediated by VCAM-1-penetration of monocytes into the vessel wall, mediated by MCP-1-activation of monocytes to form macrophages/foam cells/fatty streaks, mediated by MCSF (macrophage colony stimulating factor). The classical risk factors of atherosclerosis are also effective in diabetes mellitus [135,154,249–251], and diabetes enhances the impact of these risk factors. Hyperglycemia contributes to the pathogenesis of macroangiopathy. However, the correlation with the duration of diabetes and HbA_{1c} is weak. There must be additional specific risk factors in diabetic people, which are absent or only weakly expressed in nondiabetic people (Table 1.**13**).

Activated hemostasis seems to play an important role. It results from increased plasma coagulation and decreased fibrinolysis together with a loss of physio-

Table 1.**13** Risk factors of atherosclerosis and diabetic macroangiopathy

Classical risk factors of atherosclerosis	Additional specific risk factors of diabetic macroangiopathy
Hypertension, systolic and diastolic	Hyperglycemia
Dyslipidemia	Abnormal lipoproteins
Obesity	Platelet activation
Smoking	Endothelial dysfunction
Stress	Hypercoagulation (increased fibrinogen and PAI-1)
Physical inactivity	Albuminuria
Family history of atherosclerosis	Hyperhomocystinemia
Age	Insulin?
Previous myocardial infarction	Duration of diabetes?

logical endothelial platelet resistance, increased thrombogenicity of the subendothelial matrix, and platelet activation [138,140,252–255]. The plasma factors involved in hypercoagulation have been summarized by Ceriello [256,257]: increase of plasma fibrinogen, factor VII and VIII, α_2-macroglobulin, and PAI-1, decrease of protein C, protein S, and prostacycline, and increase in the activity of factor X, antithrombin III, heparin cofactor II, and von Willebrand factor. Only some of the mechanisms underlying these disorders are known, e. g., the regulation of PAI-1 by TNF-α, insulin, VLDL, AGE, and endothelial injury [258].

Platelet activation, which is well documented [259–261], is in part constitutional and results from the priming of megakaryocytes [262,263]. However, it may also be induced reactively by LDL [264] and by endothelial injury through thromboxane A_2, which is increased in diabetes [265]. Platelet activation goes along with increased expression of adhesion molecules. It favors thrombogenesis and the formation of circulating aggregates of platelets and platelets with leukocytes that are large enough to occlude small vessels [266]. This process is promoted by dyslipoproteinemia [267]. The expression of adhesion molecules contributes to the unfavorable rheological properties of the blood.

After interaction of activated platelets with injured endothelial cells, various growth factors are released which are known to be involved in atherogenesis, such as platelet-derived growth factor (PDGF), TGF-β, endothelium-derived relaxing factor (EDRF), endothelin-1, and others [268]. Thus, platelet activation may favor thrombogenesis, atherogenesis, capillary occlusion, and microvascular proliferation.

Endothelial dysfunction is another key factor in the pathogenesis of diabetic angiopathies [140,269]. The balanced interaction between blood and vessel wall, which regulates blood flow, hemostasis and vessel wall metabolism, is disturbed in diabetes. Loss of normal endothelial function and activation of abnormal reactions [270] may initially be caused by endothelial injury, and this may finally result in loss of cellular integrity and in cell death.

Endothelial dysfunction is a ubiquitous defect which is not limited to the regions of clinical angiopathy. Its early clinical marker seems to be microalbuminuria.

Blood flow is mainly regulated by vasodilatory EDRF (EDRF = nitric oxide) and the prostaglandin derivative prostacyclin, while endothelin-1, angiotensin II and the platelet factors thromboxane and serotonin are vasoconstrictive. In diabetes the balance of this system is disturbed. The main cause seems to be nitric oxide quenching by AGE [150] and other oxidative stress [271,272].

Lipids and lipoproteins are predictors of coronary artery disease [273]. Discussions of their role in the pathogenesis of atherosclerosis usually emphasize high triglycerides and cholesterol and low HDL-cholesterol levels. These abnormalities are frequently observed in diabetes, and their impact on risk of coronary artery disease is at least as high as in the nondiabetic population [274–278]. The significance of postprandial hypertriglyceridemia in diabetes may have been underestimated in the past [279–281]. Insulin substitution favors an antiatherogenic lipoprotein pattern [282]. In well-controlled type 1 diabetes, lipids tend to be fairly normal. By contrast, dyslipidemia is usually observed as a part of the metabolic syndrome in obese subjects with impaired glucose tolerance and type 2 diabetes [276]. It also develops in poorly controlled type 1 diabetes and in subjects with nephropathy [283,284] (Table 1.**14**). Lipid abnormalities seem to be more pronounced in women than in men [285,286].

In the presence of insulin and under the influence of high serum glucose, free fatty acids, and amino acids, VLDL synthesis is increased in the liver. Peripheral triglyceride uptake is delayed because of low lipoprotein lipase activity, resulting in hypertriglyceridemia. Hypertriglyceridemia correlates with PAI-1 activity and is associated with low HDL-cholesterol and alterations in the metabolism of other lipoproteins.

In addition to these quantitative alterations, the generation of abnormal lipoproteins seems to be very important [287,288]. The dyslipoproteinemia of diabetes is characterized by the formation of triglyceride-rich particles (VLDL1) and abnormal LDL [274,289, 290]. Small, dense LDL (LDL III) are susceptible to lipid oxidation and strongly related to cardiovascular risk [291–295]. Another effect is the lowering of cardioprotective HDL2, usually measured as low HDL-cholesterol [290,296–298].

Lipoproteins are also subject to glycation of their apoproteins and phospholipids [227]. Glycation promotes lipid oxidation and markedly changes the functional properties of lipoproteins. They become

Table 1.**14** Lipid and lipoprotein patterns in diabetes mellitus

Condition	Serum lipoproteins				
	Total cholesterol	TG	VLDL	LDL	HDL
Type 1 diabetes					
Well controlled	↔	↔	↔	↔	↔
Poorly controlled	↑	↑	↑	↑	↔↓
Type 2 diabetes					
Well controlled	↔↑	↑	↑	↔↑	↓
Poorly controlled	↑	↑	↑	↑	↓
Diabetic nephropathy	↑	↑	↑	↑	↓

TG, total triglycerides; VLDL, very-low-density lipoprotein; LDL, low-density lipoprotein; HDL, high density lipoprotein immunogenic and bind to specific scavenger receptors. This excludes them from the regulated lipid metabolism [299] and drains them into foam cell formation. They also act as stimulators of kinin release from endothelial cells and monocytes/macrophages. Thus, diabetic dyslipoproteinemia is related to a variety of factors that may enhance the risk of macroangiopathy [290,295,298].

The correlation of insulin and its precursors with macroangiopathy has received much attention [300]. It has been shown that insulin stimulates the migration, proliferation, LDL binding, and cholesterol synthesis of vascular smooth muscle cells. It may also raise blood pressure by enhancing sodium reabsorption and the sympathetic tone of vessel walls. Insulin is a prerequisite of increased VLDL synthesis, which is an important early step in the development of dyslipoproteinemia. Insulin, proinsulin, and hypertriglyceridemia stimulate PAI-1 synthesis in endothelial cells and liver and inhibit fibrinolysis [301]. However, the possible role of insulin in the pathogenesis of macroangiopathy remains a matter of debate. It may make a difference whether insulin is being used to restore insulin deficiency or whether it occurs as hyperinsulinemia in insulin-resistant states.

Clinical Picture and Management of Coronary Heart Disease

Considering the high mortality associated with myocardial infarction and the high risk of reinfarction, primary and secondary prevention of coronary heart disease (CHD) is of utmost importance.

In both types of diabetes mellitus, myocardial infarction and macroangiopathy are related to metabolic control, but a significant lowering of risk by lowering HbA_{1c} alone could not be shown [127,130]. Treatment of obese type 2 diabetic subjects with metformin significantly lowered the incidence of myocardial infarction [133], indicating that this drug has not only antidiabetic effects, but also others. In type 2 diabetes myocardial infarction is also associated with hypertension [159]. However, as shown in the UKPDS [158], which used calcium channel and β-receptor blockers, lowering of blood pressure by itself was not able to reduce significantly the risk of myocardial infarction. In contrast, studies with ACE inhibitor ramipril significantly lowered the risk of myocardial infarction, stroke, and cardiovascular death [222,302], indicating that other than blood pressure lowering effects must be important.

Primary and secondary prevention with aspirin has been recommended [138,303,304], and dyslipidemia should also be treated. In secondary prevention, clinical data showed that β-blockers [305] and ACE inhibitors [306,307] were beneficial.

From the list of known risk factors (Table 1.**13**) it is evident that primary prevention of macroangiopathy should pay attention to more than just the risk factors considered in the Diabetes Control and Complications Study (DCCT) and UKPDS. The need for a holistic view [308] is underlined by intervention studies in diabetic populations [309,310].

In myocardial infarction in diabetic subjects, most frequently the left coronary artery is occluded, and often two or three arteries are involved. The lesions tend to be localized distally; unstable plaques are frequent.

The most frequent complications of myocardial infarction in diabetes mellitus are left ventricular dysfunction, congestive heart failure, cardiogenic shock, arrhythmias, and sudden death [311–313]. Silent infarction is frequent and seems to be more closely related to the severity of the coronary artery disease than to cardiac autonomic neuropathy [314–316].

The prognosis depends on age, acute metabolic control, and duration of diabetes [317–319]. Early and late mortality is increased 1.5- to 2.5-fold in men and fourfold in women [29,320]. Recently one-year mortality was reduced by infusion of glucose with insulin and potassium [321]. The benefit of thrombolytic therapy is debated [322,323]. A considerable reduction of late mortality has been achieved by surgical therapy [324]. The indication for interventional therapy of myocardial infarction in diabetes is the same as in the general population. In most studies the early mortality associated with percutaneous transluminal coronary angioplasty, stent implantation, and coronary bypass surgery was no higher than in nondiabetic subjects, but long-term survival is still lower [325–330].

In addition to coronary artery disease, diabetic subjects may have cardiac problems even when the coronary arteries are intact. They have been attributed to diabetic cardiomyopathy and microvascular dysfunction characterized by reduced coronary flow reserve [331,332].

■ Management of Diabetes Mellitus

Prevention

Since diabetes mellitus has taken on epidemic dimensions, with an incidence that continues to rise, prevention is indispensable if we are to gain control of this disease. In the etiology of both types of diabetes, genes and environmental factors complement one another. Genes will most likely not become the target of preventive measures in the foreseeable future. However, environmental factors could offer the chance for successful intervention.

At present we do not know the environmental factors involved in the pathogenesis of type 1 diabetes mellitus. Ongoing prevention studies are aiming at the elimination of potential triggers of the autoimmune process and intervention studies at the level of the insulitis, or the basic mechanisms of autoimmunity [43,333,334]. The results remain to be seen.

In type 2 diabetes mellitus the determination factors are known (Table 1.**6**). Only early detection and treatment of the metabolic syndrome will reverse the epidemic trend of type 2 diabetes and its major complications. Among the factors that can be influenced, adverse life style, obesity, and physical inactivity are highly significant [53–56,335–338]. Their correction is the best prevention and causal treatment of type 2 diabetes mellitus.

Societies with increasing prevalence of type 2 diabetes seem to be characterized by a Western life style that includes little physical activity and in which overeating is common. Therefore, prevention of type 2 diabetes should start with population-wide awareness campaigns and counseling about a healthy life style. The management of "civilization-dependent" diseases is not just a medical problem but also a cultural one. The particular situations in different geographic regions must be taken into account. Voluntarily changing a life style which people have found comfortable and pleasant is a life-long task. It is not enough to face people with rational arguments. They need to be offered emotional rewards as well. The ideal would be to make healthy life style fashionable [339].

Various strategies have been proposed in the past [340]. Holistic approaches have been the most promising [337,338]. They have proved to be effective under study conditions, but the epidemic trend has not yet been reversed. One reason for the failure may be that intervention is usually targeted at adults, whereas a life style is often shaped in childhood and prevention should be started at that age.

Treatment

Treatment Aims

The primary goals of treatment are identical for all types of diabetes mellitus (Table 1.**15**).

The impact of diabetes both on the affected subjects and their families and on the health services is important. *Mortality* is increased. Although recent studies have shown that the prognosis can be improved, it appears to be difficult to replicate the study experiences in the diabetic population in general. For economic reasons this will be impossible in developing regions of the world.

Quality of life is decreased. Reduced life expectancy and the risk of disabling complications frighten many diabetic people, even though their fear may remain unconscious. It is a strain for many diabetic people tointegrate regular self-management into their daily lives. It is burdensome to have to abstain from certain social activities and pleasures, to accept the limitation of fitness and working capacity, and to realize that society tends to consider people with diabetes less reliable and fit for use. Being diabetic may also impair one's chances of employment, and the cost of health insurance may be higher than normal. Psychological problems, both obvious and hidden, and social discrimination are important causes of reduced quality of life.

Table 1.**15** Primary goals of diabetes management

Relief of symptoms
Improvement of quality of life
Prevention of acute and chronic complications
Reduction of mortality
Treatment of accompanying disorders
Prevention of discrimination
Prevention of psychological, social and economic problems

Chronic complications of diabetes are a major burden. This is evident in respect of loss of vision, renal failure, or diabetic neuropathies with pain, the diabetic foot syndrome, and autonomic failure such as erectile dysfunction. *Concomitant diseases* such as the metabolic syndrome also constitute a burden.

The best way to avoid complications of diabetes and early death seems to be near-normal metabolic control, with effective treatment of hypertension, dyslipoproteinemia, and adverse life style (Table 1.**16**). Both fasting and postprandial hyperglycemia are predictors of chronic complications [3,7,341,342]. For prevention of chronic complications, the Kumamoto study elaborated the following glycemic thresholds: HbA_{1c} < 6.5 %, fasting blood glucose <110 mg/dl (<11.1 mmol/l), 2-hour postprandial glucose > 180 mg/dl (< 10 mmol/l).

Basically, the goals shown in Table 1.**16** are valid for all types of diabetes mellitus except for gestational diabetes. They may be modified under certain conditions, for example, if strict metabolic control would mean an increased risk of hypoglycemia, if life expectancy is short for other reasons than diabetes, or in geriatric patients with multiple morbidity in whom diabetes is a second-order problem. Sometimes these goals may also be incompatible with well-being, because changing a comfortable life style will often be necessary to achieve the goals. In these cases a compromise should be agreed upon between the diabetic patient and his/her care team.

Near-normal metabolic control plays a pivotal role not only in chronic, but also in acute hyperglycemia of people who have not had diabetes mellitus. Such conditions occur frequently after major surgery or other major somatic stress such as multiple trauma or severe burns. In the past, these critically ill people were usually treated only in the presence of hyperglycemia exceeding 200 mg/dl (11 mmol/l) with the aim of keeping blood glucose below this level. This standard of treatment is insufficient, since a recent study has shown that lowering morning blood glucose from an average of 153 mg/dl (8.5 mmol/l) to 103 mg/dl (5.7 mmol/l) reduces mortality by almost 50 % [343]

Table 1.**16** Medical goals of diabetes management according to Deutsche Diabetes Gesellschaft [344]

Capillary blood glucose		
Postprandial	130–160 mg/dl	7.2–8.9 mmol/l
Fasting	90–120 mg/dl	5.0–6.7 mmol/l
Bed time	110–140 mg/dl	6.1–7.8 mmol/l
HbA_{1c} (%)	6.5	
Triglycerides (mg/dl)	≤150 mg/dl	≤1.71 mmol/l
LDL cholesterol (mg/dl)	≤130 mg/dl	≤3.45 mmol/l
HDL cholesterol (mg/dl)	≥40 mg/dl	≥1.04 mmol/l
BMI (female/male)	25/26	
Blood pressure (mmHg)	≤140/85	
	120/80[a]	
Healthy life style		
Well-being		

[a] In subjects with microangiopathy

Nonpharmacological Treatment

The goals of treatment can seldom be attained by conventional *methods of patient care*, where the doctor makes out a prescription and the patient has to follow it. In order to keep metabolism in a near-normal range, it is necessary to check actual glycemic control frequently, often several times a day. Values that are too high or too low must be corrected, and to plan treatment according to the events of the day. These daily therapeutic measures are unpredictable and cannot be carried out by doctors and their team, only by the diabetic subjects (or those around them) themselves. Consequently, people with diabetes should no longer be seen as "patients" "suffering from" their disease, but must become active partners of their doctors (Table 1.**17**). To be qualified for this role, they must be knowledgeable and motivated to take on the responsibility for managing their own diabetes. Teaching, training, and empowerment of people with diabetes mellitus is thus believed to be essential, even though this has not always been proven [345–348].

The role of the doctors and their team will be to teach people with diabetes, design therapeutic options for the individual diabetic person, and arrange regular checkups (Table 1.**17**). Their role is also to encourage and support the patients, give ongoing advice, and help in acute and chronic problems. However, the doctors cannot take responsibility for the correctness of daily management and for therapeutic failures due to noncompliance on the part of the patients.

Teaching should enable the diabetic subjects (and if possible people in their social environment) to understand the disease and its treatment and to detect and

Table 1.**17** Nonpharmacological management of diabetes mellitus

A. The role of the patients:
Learn about diabetes
Develop health consciousness and self-management behavior
Set goals for your therapy
Express and discuss your wishes and expectations with your health care team
Control and correct yourself regularly
Adopt a healthy life style
Profit from the expertise of your health care team
Don't "suffer" from your diabetes
Decide to want what you have realized as being good for you
B. The role of the doctor and the diabetes team:
Teaching and training, ongoing advice, back-up, empowerment, and motivation of the persons with diabetes
Discussion and consensus on goals of individual therapy
Design of individual therapy
Nutrition counseling and self-management plan

Table 1.18 Topics for teaching and training of people with diabetes

What does diabetes mellitus mean? (causes, symptoms, natural course, prevention, rights and roles)
Sensible eating (what to eat, nutrients and energy content, metabolic effect, shopping, cooking)
Physical activity (pros and cons of different activities, metabolic and cardiovascular effects, joint loading, monitoring)
Self-monitoring (blood glucose, body weight, skin, blood pressure, how and when to do, how to document)
Hypoglycemia (causes, symptoms, prevention, treatment)
a Oral antidiabetic drugs (action, when to take, side effects)
a Isulin (action, how to inject, pens and other devices, schedule, dosage)
Care of skin and feet (how to examine, instruments for care)
a Not smoking (importance, how to give up smoking)
Blood pressure (importance, measurement, how, when, actions at high blood pressure)
Chronic complications (symptoms, regular check-ups, risk, prevention, treatment)
When to contact the doctor or diabetes care team
Special situations (traveling, being ill)
Social problems (driver's license, insurance, diabetes risk of descendants)

a If reasonable

manage complications early on (Table 1.**18**). Transferring knowledge and abilities is important. More important, however, is empowerment. The diabetic persons should not simply take on the doctors recommendations, but should develop their own health beliefs. Instead of obeying prescriptions, they should want to attain good control and wish to practice self-monitoring, treatment adaptation, and a healthy life style. In other words, they should be able to develop appropriate self-care behavior.

An important aim of patient teaching and training is regular *self-monitoring* of blood glucose, body weight, skin, particularly of the feet, and blood pressure (Table 1.**19**). Urinary glucose determination is inadequate as the only method. Aglucosuria does not constitute proof of good metabolic control, because the renal threshold for glucose may be far above the treatment goal. Furthermore, only blood glucose self-monitoring can show the risk of hypoglycemia, which is the greatest obstacle to strict metabolic control.

Nutrition of diabetic people should contain no more than 30% of energy as fat and only 10% as saturated fatty acids. This is much less than is usually consumed in Western diets. Protein intake should not exceed 20% of energy. The majority of energy intake should be in the form of carbohydrates, preferentially complex carbohydrates. However, trained people with good metabolic control may also take some sugar (about 50 g per day) in several portions combined with food rich in fibers. Alcohol should be limited to 15 g per day for women and 30 g per day for men. Salt should be used in moderation [203,349]. About 80% of diabetic people are obese. For these people, restriction of energy intake combined with physical activity is essential in order to achieve slow but continuous weight loss. Nutritional advice must aim to keep eating enjoyable and to help diabetic subjects to satisfy their nutritional preferences within the limits of sensible eating.

Nonpharmacological treatment is the basis for management of all types of diabetes mellitus. Whether it will be successful depends not only on the commitment of the doctor and his team, but also on the cultural background and the all-round educational level of the diabetic person. Only educated, well-trained, independent-minded patients will claim their right

Table 1.19 Rules for self-monitoring of metabolic parameters

- Blood glucose testing is preferable for metabolic control. It is mandatory for patients on insulin or oral antidiabetic drugs that stimulate insulin secretion. It is a vital safeguard against hypoglycemia. Perform urine ketone tests during illness or when blood glucose increases above 20 mmol/l. Document all results.

- In well-controlled, stable patients:
  Fasting, before main meals, at bedtime, 1–2 times per week.
- In poorly controlled, unstable patients or during illness:
  Fasting, postprandially, before meals, at bedtime, daily until stabilized.
- During intensified insulin treatment:
  Before each insulin dose, if necessary postprandially.
- If hypoglycemia is suspected.

Other self-monitoring:
- Check body weight, inspect feet at least weekly.
- Check blood pressure, if normal monthly, if elevated more often, possibly several times per day until targets of control are achieved.
- Record special events.

to choose among different therapeutic options, will know what kind of service they are entitled to demand from the health care system, and will realize what they themselves have to contribute to the management of their diabetes. Only these patients will have a realistic chance of effective diabetes management and a good long-term prognosis.

The benefit of nonpharmacological treatment has been shown. Weight reduction reduces mortality considerably [63]. Teaching improves metabolic control and may reduce the need for pharmacotherapy [347,350]. Well-established tools of pharmacological treatment of diabetes cannot be used without teaching, training, and empowerment of the patient.

Pharmacological Treatment of Type 1 Diabetes

General Aspects

The person with type 1 diabetes mellitus needs insulin from the very start of the disease. It is useless and may be dangerous to try a treatment without insulin. Different types of insulin treatment are presently practiced, which may be described as: (1) conventional insulin therapy, (2) intensified or functional insulin therapy, either by means of multiple subcutaneous injections, or by continuous subcutaneous insulin infusion. Other therapies, such as intraperitoneal or intraportal insulin infusion, are still experimental.

Conventional insulin therapy is characterized by a prescribed insulin formulation, dosage, and time of application. The quality of metabolic control is monitored by the diabetes care team. The patient performs blood glucose self-monitoring to prevent hypoglycemia but not as a basis for adapting treatment. Nutrition is inflexible, as the amount of carbohydrates and the time of eating are fixed in order to compensate for the blood glucose-lowering effect of insulin and physical work, and are mainly dictated by the pharmacokinetics of the injected insulin. Metabolic control in type 1 diabetes is poorer with conventional therapy than it is with intensified therapy [127]. For this reason, conventional therapy should be avoided in type 1 diabetes. For type 2 diabetes, it may be satisfactory.

By contrast, *intensified (functional) insulin therapy* is flexible. This aims to imitate physiological insulin secretion (but without combining insulin with C-peptide and amylin and without releasing insulin into the portal vein). The nutrition-independent (basal) insulin requirement is covered by an injection of long-acting insulin or several injections of intermediate-acting insulin or by continuous subcutaneous infusion at a basal insulin rate. In addition, bolus insulin is given to correct hyperglycemia or to cover nutrition-dependent insulin requirements. This method allows nutrition and physical activity to remain variable and also allows immediately correction of blood glucose deviations. However, it requires frequent self-monitoring of blood glucose and the diabetic subject must be able to adjust the insulin properly. The risk of weight gain is increased.

Practical Aspects

When type 1 diabetes mellitus is diagnosed, the patients need much attention, because they need to realize that they have acquired a life-long disease that will change their life. Usually the diagnosis is made because of deranged metabolism. These patients should initially be treated as inpatients. The ketoacidotic patient must be treated as an emergency case. The initial inpatient period should be used for intensive teaching and training which will be continued on an outpatient basis. To make insulin therapy easier, the use of insulin pens should be favored.

If insulin therapy is not initiated on a ward, it may for the purpose of training be started as conventional insulin therapy.

Conventional insulin therapy (CT) is usually performed with intermediate-acting human NPH insulin (NPH = neutral protamine Hagedorn) or mixtures of human NPH insulin and short-acting regular insulin (Table 1.**20**). Since the duration of action of NPH insulin is less than 24 hours it must be given twice a day or more often. Because there is a delay before NPH insulin begins to act, it is usually given 30–45 minutes before breakfast and dinner. In view of the nutrition-dependent insulin need over the course of the day, about two-thirds of the daily dose is given in the morning and one-third in the evening. If the postprandial blood glucose increment is unacceptably high, mixed insulins are given in the morning or also in the evening. The proportion of regular insulin in mixtures may be chosen anywhere in the range between 10% and 50%.

To compensate for the action of insulin, carbohydrate intake must be properly distributed over the day. The dietary regimen also depends on physical activity and must be developed by trial and error. As a proposal to start with, total daily carbohydrate intake may be divided in eight parts with two-eighths given at breakfast, one-eighth about 3–4 hours later, one-eighth at lunch, one-eighth in the afternoon, two-eighths at dinner, and one-eighth at bedtime. Unless there is an emergency, it is advisable to start insulin therapy with a low dose. The effect of this very first dose should be monitored by repeated blood glucose measurements. Thereafter, the insulin dose may be swiftly adjusted.

Given the appropriate social and educational background in the patient, type 1 diabetes should be treated with *intensified insulin therapy (ICT)* from the very beginning. At first, the diabetes care team will be responsible for the enterprise, while the patient is learning. After the teaching and training phase, the diabetic subject will take over responsibility step by step. According to the basis/bolus concept, basal insulin needs

Table 1.**20** Pharmakokinetic data of insulin formulations

	Action profile (hours)[a]		
	Onset	Peak	Duration
Short-acting human insulin analogues			
Lispro	0.3–0.5	0.5–1.5	3–4
Aspart	0.3–0.5	0.5–1.5	3–4
Human insulins			
Regular	0.3–0.8	1–5	5–8
NPH	0.5–1.0	2–6	11–16
Long-acting insulin analogue			
Glargine	1–2	–	18–24
Mixed insulins[b]			
10–50 % regular 50–90 % NPH	0.3–0.80	1–6	10–18
Pump insulin	0.2–0.5	–	–[c]

NPH, neutral protamine Hagedorn.
[a] Depending on dosage;
[b] depending on mixture;
[c] depending on infusion time

will be covered by two to three injections of NPH. The aim is to guarantee a permanent, fairly constant supply with insulin without causing hypoglycemia and to take into account the circadian variation of the insulin demand. Since the insulin demand usually begins to increase in the early morning at 3–4 A.M., the last dose of NPH is often given at bed time. The basal insulin dose is usually about 50% of the total daily insulin dose, or 0.7–1.0 U per hour. If it is difficult to find the right dosage, this can be tested over a 24-hour fasting period with close blood glucose monitoring. However, this procedure is rarely necessary.

The bolus injection should be used for correction of hyperglycemia. It should also be related to carbohydrate intake and should take account of the fact that in a circadian pattern the need for a carbohydrate unit is highest at breakfast time, being then about 1.3 times as high as in the afternoon and evening. The bolus is given subcutaneously either in the form of regular human insulin 15–30 minutes before the meal or in the form of the insulin analogues insulin lispro or insulin aspart at the beginning of the meal. If food intake is unpredictable, the injection of the fast-acting insulin analogues may be given immediately after the meal according to how much was actually eaten.

On average, 1.3–1.5 U insulin are needed to compensate for 10–12 g carbohydrates or for a hyperglycemia of 40–50 mg/dl. Vice versa, about 10–12 g carbohydrates are needed to elevate blood glucose by 40–50 mg/dl. Insulin therapy should always be accompanied by blood glucose monitoring, preferably self-monitoring by the diabetic subject (see Table 1.**19**).

In *continuous subcutaneous insulin infusion* (CSII), pump insulin is infused by means of a programmable precision insulin pump and infusion system. The action kinetics of pump insulin are similar to those of subcutaneously injected insulin. The amounts of basal and bolus insulin and the timing of the infusion are similar to those in ICT. CSII has the advantage that the action kinetics remain constant as long as the infusion site is not changed and that basal insulin infusion can exactly be adjusted to the circadian needs. The risk of hypoglycemia is usually lower than with ICT, but unnoticed pump errors with loss of insulin supply may result in rapidly developing ketoacidosis. Other technical problems can usually be easily solved without any danger to the patient.

For emergency treatment of ketoacidosis and other unusual situations, treatment handbooks should be consulted.

Various insulins and insulin analogues are available to meet the different pharmacokinetic requirements (Table 1.**20**). Insulin should be given strictly subcutaneously. Intracutaneous injection or injection into tendons and muscle sheaths will delay insulin action, while injection into the muscle will accelerate the action. The kinetics of insulin action also depend on the region into which insulin is injected-relatively fast in the abdominal region and slower in the arm or thigh. Even in the same region, the peak time of insulin action may vary considerably from day to day. The action of regular insulin starts much slower than physiological insulin secretion. For this reason, regular insulin should be given 15–30 minutes before meals. The duration of action is longer than the average duration of food digestion and absorption and usually requires a snack 3–4 hours after the injection in order to avoid hypoglycemia.

New insulins have been developed with the aim of improving the concept of physiological insulin substitution. Insulin glargine is a 30^{B}-Arg-Arg insulin analogue with almost constant insulin kinetics over 24 hours [351]. The risk of hypoglycemia can be kept low. Insulin glargine seems to be useful as basal insulin in ICT and may be used for the evening dose in type 2 diabetes.

For meal-time insulin demand the bioavailability of regular subcutaneously injected human insulin is too sluggish. Two insulin analogues avoid this problem: insulin lispro (28^B-lysine–29^B-proline human insulin) and insulin aspart (28^B-aspartic acid human insulin). The action kinetics of these insulin analogues are fast enough to allow treatment without an interval between injection and meal and without a snack between main meals [352,353]. No benefit with regard to the risk of hypoglycemia could be established [354]. These analogues have also been used in CSII treatment [355].

Recently inhaled insulin was developed as a noninvasive alternative to subcutaneous insulin administration. From a proof-of-concept study in type 1 diabetic individuals [356] and an observation study in patients with type 2 diabetes [357] it was concluded that inhaled insulin may offer a practical, noninvasive alternative to insulin injections, because it maintains glycemic control without major side effects and may provide greater patient satisfaction than subcutaneously injected insulin. These first clinical studies will stimulate the development of this new form of insulin therapy [358,359].

The insulin analogues glargine, lispro, and aspart have only recently been introduced into clinical practice. Data on their long-term safety and benefit are not yet available and must be awaited before their advantages and disadvantages can be finally assessed. This may not be a theoretical argument, since the binding properties of the analogues to the insulin and IGF-1 receptors are not always identical with those of human insulin [360–362]. However, postmarketing surveys of more than a million treatment-years have provided no evidence for any increase in mitogenic risk with lispro (T. Krause, personal communication, 2001).

While the DCCT [127] has clearly shown that intensified insulin therapy is superior to conventional insulin therapy, no long-term studies in type 1 diabetic subjects using combinations of insulin and oral drugs such as metformin or α-amylase inhibitors are available.

Pharmacological Treatment of Type 2 Diabetes

Glucose Metabolism

About 25 % of newly diagnosed type 2 diabetic individuals can initially have their condition controlled by nonpharmacological treatment [125]. The others need additional pharmacological therapy. Metabolic control deteriorates continuously from the very start of the disease. For this reason, the number of subjects who need drugs will increase, and those who were initially

Table 1.**21** Dosage of oral antidiabetic drugs

Drug	Single dose (mg)	Max. daily dose (mg)	Doses/day
α-Amylase inhibitors			
Acarbose	50–300	900	1–3
Miglitol	50–300	900	1–3
Biguanide			
Metformin	500–850	2550	1–3
Sulfonylurea, β-cell stimulators			
Glibenclamide[a]	1.75–7	20	1–2
Glimepiride	1–6	8	1
Glibornuride	12.5–25	75	1–3
Gliclazide	40–160	240	1–2
Glyburide	3–6	12	1–2
Glisoxepide	2–8	16	1–2
Glinides, β-cell stimulators			
Repaglinide	0.5–4	16	2–4
Nateglinide	120	360	3
Glitazones, insulin sensitizers			
Rosiglitazone	2–8	8	1–2
Pioglitazone	15–30	45	1

[a] Micronized

on monotherapy will eventually need combination drug therapy [125].

Five classes of oral antidiabetic drugs (Table 1.**21**) and insulin (Table 1.**20**) are available for pharmacological treatment of type 2 diabetes.

The competitive α-amylase inhibitors (acarbose, miglitol) delay digestion of complex carbohydrates. By this mechanism they reduce the postprandial rise of glucose, serum insulin, and gastric inhibitory polypeptide (GIP) and stimulate release of glucagon-like peptide 1 (GLP-1) [363]. The antidiabetic effect is seen promptly after the first dose. Their efficacy is well documented [364–368].

Major adverse drug effects are flatulence, abdominal discomfort, and bloating, which usually occur during the first 2–3 weeks of treatment, particularly if the dosage is increased too rapidly. These effects are promptly reversible after discontinuation of treatment but may cause noncompliance problems. It is therefore strongly recommended to start with a very low dose (e. g., 50 mg acarbose at breakfast) and titrate the dose very slowly upwards according to how it is tolerated. Other adverse events are very rare. Monotherapy with α-amylase inhibitors does not cause hypoglycemia nor weight gain [365–368]. There is no risk of tachyphylaxia. These drugs may be combined with sulfonylurea, metformin, or insulin. Their effect is additive. If hypoglycemia occurs during combination therapy, monosaccharides must be given as antidote.

The main metabolic effect of *metformin* is inhibition of hepatic glucose production, with little effect on peripheral insulin sensitivity [369,370]. The molecular mechanisms of this effect are not known. Fasting and daytime blood glucose are reduced by metformin. It may take a couple of days or even weeks until the full therapeutic effect has developed.

The antidiabetic effect of metformin alone [133,371,372] and in combination [373,374] is well documented.

Metformin monotherapy does not cause hypoglycemia or weight gain. There is no risk of tachyphylaxia. The drug may be combined with insulin, glitazones, glinides, sulfonylurea, and α-amylase inhibitors. In combination with sulfonylurea or insulin it is able to reduce weight gain [133].

However, in the UKPDS, the addition of metformin treatment to poorly controlled patients receiving sulfonylurea significantly increased the risk of diabetes-related and all-cause mortality [133]. A recent retrospective analysis has cast further doubt on the benefit of this combination [375]. This finding of the UKPDS has been criticized on methodological grounds [376] and the relevance of this observation has been questioned. The American Diabetes Association decided not to change the guidelines on the pharmacological treatment of hyperglycemia in NIDDM [377], because the study had not provided assurance about the risk or benefit of the combination of sulfonylurea and metformin.

A rare but possibly fatal adverse event is lactic acidosis. The risk of this complication increases with overdose or reduced elimination of metformin (serum creatinine > 1.2 mg/dl) and in all conditions in which lactate production is increased or lactate utilization decreased, such as shock, sepsis, hypoxia, alcohol abuse, or narcosis. Ketosis may be aggravated by metformin. Frequent but harmless adverse events include reversible gastrointestinal discomfort and diarrhea. The contraindications for metformin must be carefully taken into account.

Sulfonylurea stimulates endogenous insulin secretion, leading to a decrease in postprandial and fasting blood glucose. The effect is mediated by the closing of ATP-dependent potassium channels in the plasma membrane of pancreatic β cells. This mechanism explains why the efficacy of sulfonylurea depends on the existence of an endogenous insulin reserve. Although administration of sulfonylurea makes the β cells more sensitive to glucose stimulation, the impaired first-phase insulin secretion, which is the most important defect in type 2 diabetes, is not restored [378,379].

The efficacy of sulfonylurea tends to vanish during long-term therapy (late or secondary failure). This may be due to progressive exhaustion of the endogenous insulin reserve. To manage this problem sulfonylurea may be combined with insulin, glitazones, and α-amylase inhibitors. The antidiabetic effect of sulfonylurea treatment alone or in combination is well documented [380,381].

The most frequent adverse event is hypoglycemia, which may begin insidiously and last longer than a day. Sulfonylurea-treated patients usually experience weight gain. Other adverse events are rare. Drug interactions which modulate the efficacy of sulfonylurea are frequent [382].

New oral drugs have recently been developed in order to better mimic physiological insulin secretion and to improve insulin sensitivity.

The *glinides* (repaglinide and nateglinide) are benzoic acid derivatives which belong to a new class of insulin secretagogues referred to as "prandial glucose regulators." Compared with glibenclamide these drugs are rapidly absorbed and excreted (t_{max} of plasma concentration: glibenclamide 300 minutes [383], repaglinide 45 minutes [384], nateglinide 45–60 minutes [385]; $t_{1/2}$ of plasma elimination: glibenclamide nine hours [383], repaglinide one hour [384], nateglinide one hour [385]. These drugs bind to specific receptors on the pancreatic β cell, heart, and peripheral muscle cells. In comparison with glibenclamide and gliburide, the binding of nataglinide is much more specific for β cells [386].

The mechanism of action, action profile, and pharmacokinetics of repaglinide and nateglinide are similar but not identical [387]. The binding of repaglinide or nateglinide is rapidly followed by closing of ATP-dependent K^+ channels, discontinuous depolarization of the cell membrane, and Ca^{++} influx, resulting in a rapid insulin release of short duration. In vitro, the insulin-stimulatory effect of repaglinide is enhanced by the presence of physiological concentrations of glucose. Under these conditions repaglinide is several times more potent than glibenclamide [386]. After stimulation with glinides the kinetics of postprandial insulin secretion are more similar to physiological insulin secretion than they are after stimulation with sulfonylurea [388,389].

These drugs cut off postprandial glucose peaks, lower HbA_{1c}, and can be effectively combined with metformin [390–392].

In poorly controlled type 2 diabetic patients formerly treated with metformin, repaglinide monotherapy was as effective as metformin. The combination of repaglinide or nateglinide with metformin seems to be superior to monotherapy [391–393].

Adverse effects of glinides are hypoglycemia, gastrointestinal symptoms, blurred vision, and, rarely, elevated liver enzymes and hypersensitive reactions of the skin. Interactions with drugs metabolized by the cytochrome P450 system may occur. Efficacy is modulated by drug interaction in a similar way as with sulfonylurea.

The *thiazolidinediones (glitazones)* rosiglitazone and pioglitazone are called "insulin sensitizers." They lower blood glucose by improving the insulin sensitivity of liver, adipose tissue, and muscle [394,395]. Glitazones develop their metabolic effect through binding to the peroxisome proliferator-activated nuclear receptor-γ (PPAR-γ). This glitazone-activated receptor may become effective as a transcription factor for proteins involved in the regulation of glucose and lipid metabolism. Glitazones improve insulin signaling by increasing the phosphorylation of the insulin receptor, the insulin receptor substrate 1 (IRS-1), and phosphatidylinositol-3 (PI-3) kinase [395]. They also stimulate the expression of glucose transporters GLUT-1 and GLUT-4 [397,398], enhance glucose utilization [399], and suppress hepatic glucose output [400]. Rosiglitazone inhibits the expression of the leptin gene in rat adipocytes [401,402] and stimulates the expression of uncoupling proteins 1 and 3 (UCP1 and UCP3) in preadipocytes [403]. Pioglitazone reduces the expression of TNF-α in muscle and adipose tissue [404]. This effect may be responsible for the favorable influence on the insulin receptor tyrosine kinase and the serine phosphorylation of the insulin receptor [405]. However, a reduced availability of free fatty acids in blood and tissues may also improve insulin sensitivity [406]. The significance of the glitazone effects on proliferation and differentiation of various cell types is unknown. A possible beneficial effect may be inhibition of LDL-induced growth of vascular smooth muscle cells [407].

Adverse effects of glitazones include fluid retention, edema, cardiac failure, anemia, and slight increase in LDL cholesterol and body weight.

Troglitazone, which has been withdrawn from the market, showed severe (fatal) liver toxicity. Rosiglitazone and pioglitazone have been claimed not to be liver toxic, but cases of new liver disease during therapy with rosiglitazone have been reported [408–411], and minor functional disorders may occur. There is at present no proof of a causal relationship, but careful monitoring of liver function is indicated.

Interactions with drugs metabolized by the cytochrome P450 system are possible. Since glitazones have a broad spectrum of effects (there are more than those mentioned in this chapter) and since not all the genes regulated by PPAR-γ seem to be completely known, their safety profile cannot be definitively assessed.

Significant lowering of blood glucose has been reported with glitazones used alone [412]. However, the effect is smaller than with metformin or sulfonylurea [413]. Better effects are seen in combination with metformin [414], sulfonylurea [415], and possibly insulin [416]. At present most clinical information is available only in the form of abstracts. The official regulations for the use of glitazones differ between countries.

The efficacy of the new drugs has only been tested using surrogate markers such as blood glucose and HbA_{1c}. Cardiac benefits have been claimed [417], but so far none of these drugs has been tested in large-scale, long-term prospective studies on safety and efficacy such as the UKPDS using ultimate clinical endpoints or other patient-oriented outcomes.

For most clinicians *insulin* monotherapy is a second choice in type 2 diabetes mellitus, usually in the form of conventional insulin therapy. Since type 2 diabetes is associated with insulin resistance, high doses are usually necessary [418,419].

The insulin dose may be reduced by the addition of oral antidiabetic drugs [381,420,421]. Recently, intensified insulin treatment has been recommended [422]. However, the metabolic control achieved using different insulin regimens was comparable [423,424]. The most important adverse effects of insulin in the treatment of type 2 diabetes are hypoglycemia and weight gain. Weight gain may be reduced by combining insulin with metformin [133,425].

Clinical Aspects

Pharmacological therapy should be evidence-based, achieve the goals of therapy, be safe and causal rather than symptomatic, easy and comfortable for the patient, and inexpensive. Only two landmark studies on pharmacological therapy of type 2 diabetes mellitus have used mortality and diabetes-related morbidity as ultimate endpoints. The Kumamoto study [131,426] evaluated the effects of intensive insulin therapy on prevention and progression of retinopathy, nephropathy, and neuropathy, and studied the cost–benefit relationship. The UKPDS [130,133,368] compared standard and intensive treatment with human insulin, chlorpropamide, glibenclamide and other sulfonylurea drugs, metformin, and acarbose. Three aggregate endpoints were used: (1) any diabetes-related endpoint, which includes various cardiac diseases, renal failure, amputations, and eye problems; (2) diabetes-related death; and (3) all-cause mortality. The UKPDS also analyzed the cost–benefit relationship and treatment of hypertension.

The main points that can be drawn from these studies are:

1. Intensive blood glucose lowering therapy with glibenclamide, metformin, or insulin (NB not with chlorpropamide [130]) delays the onset and progression of microvascular complications in type 2 diabetes.
2. The HbA_{1c} lowering potency of these drugs was comparable.
3. Intensive treatment of obese type 2 diabetic subjects with metformin can also reduce the risk of macrovascular complications.

In none of the studies was diabetes management ideal. The goals of blood glucose control were rarely met, the rates of chronic complications of diabetes remained high, and adverse events were frequent during sulfonylurea and insulin treatment. The need for combination therapy was realized [125], but the addition of metformin to sulfonylurea had adverse effects. Other combinations were not systematically studied. New drugs could not be investigated. These shortcomings make it difficult to select the best therapy for each individual patient solely on the basis of these important studies. For this reason, the therapeutic options will now also be considered from the practical and pathophysiological points of view.

Intensive treatment with sulfonylurea or insulin has adverse effects. It increases the risk of hypoglycemia. In the past this used to be a minor problem, but it becomes a question of safety and quality of life if the goal of therapy is near-normoglycemia. The other adverse effect is weight gain. Most type 2 diabetic subjects are overweight and are advised to lose weight. The patients experience both hypoglycemia and weight gain as causing distress and impairing their quality of life [130]. Weight gain is a precipitating factor for diabetes and a macrovascular risk factor. Therefore, it is legitimate to ask whether the benefit of lowering HbA_{1c} by insulin or glibenclamide is not jeopardized by the risk of this side effect. Therapy with either drug alone may not be a first choice.

Another concern is the fact that neither human insulin nor sulfonylurea corresponds with the pathogenetic defects of type 2 diabetes. They do not restore early insulin secretion because they are too sluggish; that is, the meal-related early phase of insulin action comes too late and the postprandial insulin action lasts too long.

Both types of drugs may overcome insulin resistance but they do not restore insulin sensitivity. If insulin sensitivity improves, this is not a direct drug effect but a nonspecific effect of lowering blood glucose and decreasing glucose toxicity. In the future, rather than insulin and sulfonylurea, rapid- and short-acting insulin analogues and glinides should be considered to initiate a more physiological insulin substitution, and metformin and glitazones to improve insulin sensitivity. However, the new drugs urgently need to be evaluated in controlled prospective studies using hard endpoints.

Intensive treatment with oral drugs or insulin over three years will lower HbA_{1c} below 7 % in only half of the patients. In the majority, combination therapy is indicated. Combinations of oral antidiabetic drugs

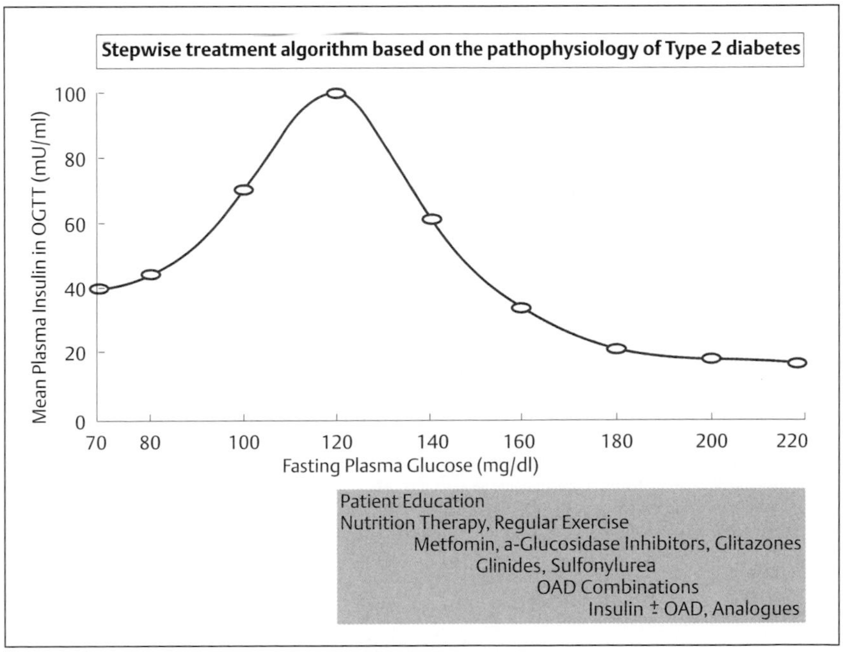

Fig. 1.3 Proposed stepwise treatment algorithm based on the pathophysiology of type 2 diabetes. For the rationale of this proposal, see text. The warnings with respect to possible unknown long-term side effects must be taken into account. (Modified after Matthaei et al. [395])

have already been discussed. The *combination of insulin with oral antidiabetic drugs* may be even more important. The combination of insulin with sulfonylurea has been extensively studied [381,420,421,427,428]. It is convenient and may save some insulin. If postprandial hyperglycemia after breakfast is the main problem, the morning sulfonylurea dose may be replaced by regular or mixed insulin or short-acting insulin analogues. If fasting hyperglycemia is the main problem, the evening oral antidiabetic drug dose may be replaced by NPH insulin at bedtime. Metabolic control can be improved by various combinations without increasing the risk of hypoglycemia [423,424,427,428]. The combination of insulin with metformin is also possible. This combination offers the advantage of avoiding weight gain [133,425].

A proposed rationale for the selection of drugs in the treatment of type 2 diabetes mellitus is given in Figure 1.**3**.

Metabolic Syndrome

The outstanding significance of treating the metabolic syndrome to prevent type 2 diabetes mellitus has already been discussed. The metabolic syndrome usually persists in clinical type 2 diabetes, and therefore its treatment remains important.

The impact of overweight/obesity and the importance of weight reduction have been repeatedly confirmed. Weight reduction is not easy. Even more difficult is maintaining reduced body weight over long periods of time. The ideal aim is normal body weight, which will very seldom be achieved. However, much lesser weight reduction is also beneficial [53, 54, 62, 336]. In support of nonpharmacological treatment with nutrition and physical activity, two drugs have recently been introduced: the intestinal lipase inhibitor orlistat, which reduces nutritional fat absorption, and the serotonin/norepinephrine reuptake inhibitor sibutramine, which is an appetite suppressant. Both drugs have been shown to enhance weight loss during conventional weight reduction programs. Orlistat may inhibit absorption not only of fat but also of lipid-soluble drugs and essential nutrients. Sibutramine may evoke psycho-neurological symptoms and increase arterial blood pressure. The drug also has the drawback of a variety of contraindications and drug interactions.

The beneficial effect of lowering elevated blood pressure and specific drug effects on nephropathy and coronary artery disease have already been discussed. The UKPDS [158] has shown that lowering blood pressure from 154/87 to 144/82 mmHg significantly reduced diabetes-related endpoints by 24%, microvascular endpoints by 37%, and stroke by 44%. The epidemiological analysis of this study offers the conclusion that the lowest risk will be "in those with systolic blood pressure less than 120 mm Hg" [159].

Dyslipoproteinemia that does not respond to weight reduction should be corrected by pharmacological therapy. Statins are the first-choice drug if serum cholesterol is elevated. They have favorable effects on small, dense LDL and lower the risk of macroangiopathy complications [429,430]. Fibrates (and analogues) should be favored if triglycerides are increased. These drugs also lower plasma fibrinogen and are beneficial for hypercoagulation and impaired microcirculation. However, the combination of statins and fibrates (and analogues) should definitely be avoided, because it increases the risk of myositis and other severe adverse drug effects.

Prophylactic treatment of hypercoagulation with aspirin or other drugs that reduce platelet aggregation has been recommended [228,304].

Treatment of the metabolic syndrome requires lifestyle changes. Physical activity should be integrated into everyday life, and every smoker should be offered a course in giving up smoking.

This kind of broad approach has been proven to be effective both in preventing [337, 338] and in managing [431] type 2 diabetes mellitus. The task for the future will be to integrate this experience into public health.

References

[1] National Diabetes Data Group. Classification and diagnosis of diabetes mellitus and other categories of glucose intolerance. Diabetes 1979; 28: 1039–57.

[2] World Health Organization. Diabetes mellitus: Report of a WHO Study Group. Geneva: World Health Organization; 1985.

[3] American Diabetes Association. Report of the Expert Committee on Diagnosis and Classification of Diabetes Mellitus. Diabetes Care 1998; 21 (suppl 1): S5–19.

[4] The DECODE Study Group on behalf of the European Diabetes Epidemiology Group. Consequences of the new criteria for diabetes in older men and women – the DECODE study (Diabetes epidemiology: Collaborative analysis of diagnostic criteria in Europe). Diabetes Care 1999; 22: 1667–71.

[5] The DECODE Study Group on behalf of the European Diabetes Epidemiology Group. Glucose tolerance and cardiovascular mortality: comparison of fasting and 2-hour diagnostic criteria. Arch Intern Med 2001; 161: 397–404.

[6] Rathmann W, Giani G, Mielck A. Cardiovascular risk factors in newly diagnosed abnormal glucose tolerance: comparison of 1997 ADA and 1985 WHO criteria. Diabetologia 1999; 42: 1268–9.

[7] Tominaga M, Eguchi H, Manaka H, Igarashi K, Kato T, Sekikawa A. Impaired glucose tolerance is a risk factor for cardiovascular disease, but not impaired fasting glucose. Diabetes Care 1999; 22: 920–4.

[8] Balkau B. The Decode study: Diabetes epidemiology: collaborative analysis of diagnostic criteria in Europe. Diabetes Metab (Paris) 2000; 26: 282–6.

[9] Ekoe JM. Epidemiology and etiopathogenesis of IDDM in other ethnic groups. In: Alberti KGMM, DeFronzo RA, Keen H, Zimmet P, editors. International textbook of diabetes mellitus. Chichester: John Wiley and Sons Ltd; 1992: 129–45.

[10] Green A, Gale EAM, Patterson CC, for the EURODIAB ACE Study Group. Incidence of childhood-onset insulin-dependent diabetes mellitus: The EURODIAB ACE Study. Lancet 1992; 339: 905–9.

[11] Karvonen M, Tuomilehto J, Libman I, La Porte R, for the World Health Organization DIAMOND Project Group. A review of the recent epidemiological data on the worldwide incidence of type 1 (insulin-dependent) diabetes mellitus. Diabetologia 1993; 36: 883–92.

[12] Schiel R, Mueller UA. GAD autoantibodies in a selection-free population of insulin treated diabetic patients: indicator of a high prevalence of LADA? Diab Res Clin Pract 2000; 49: 33–40.

[13] Neu A, Kehrer M, Hub R, Ranke MB. Incidence of diabetes in German children aged 0–14 years. Diabetes Care 1997; 20: 530–3.

[14] Onkamo P, Väänänen S, Karvonen M, Tuomilehto J. Worldwide increase in incidence of type I diabetes—the analysis of the data on published incidence trends. Diabetologia 1999; 42: 1395–403.

[15] Rosenbauer J, Herzig P, Kries R von, Neu A, Giani G. Temporal, seasonal and geographical incidence patterns of type 1 diabetes mellitus in children under 5 years of age in Germany. Diabetologia 1999; 42: 1055–9.

[16] Karvonen M, Pitkäniemi J, Tuomilehto J, the Finnish Childhood Diabetes Registry Group. The onset age of type 1 diabetes in Finnish children has become younger. Diab Care 1999; 22: 1066–70.

[17] Bingley PJ, Douek JF, Rogers CA, Gale EAM, on behalf of the BOX (Bart's-Oxford) Study Group. Influence of maternal age at delivery and birth order on the risk of type 1 diabetes in childhood: prospective population based family study. BMJ 2000; 321: 420–4.

[18] Deckert T, Poulsen JE, Larsen M. Prognosis of diabetics with diabetes onset before the age of thirty one, I: Survival, causes of death, and complications. Diabetologia 1978; 14: 363–70.

[19] Rossing P, Hougaard P, Borch-Johnsen K, Parving HH. Predictors of mortality in insulin dependent diabetes: 10 year observational follow-up study. BMJ 1996; 313: 779–84.

[20] Borch-Johnsen K, Kreiner S, Deckert T. Mortality of type 1 (insulin-dependent) diabetes mellitus in Denmark: a study of relative mortality in 2930 Danish type 1 diabetic patients diagnosed from 1933–1972. Diabetologia 1986; 29: 767–72.

[21] American Diabetes Association. Diabetes 1996 vital statistics. Alexandria, Va: American Diabetes Association, 1996.

[22] Diabetes Epidemiology Research International (DERI) Mortality Study Group: International evaluation of cause-specific mortality and IDDM. Diabetes Care 1990; 14: 55–60.

[23] Portuese E, Orchard T. Mortality in insulin-dependent diabetes mellitus. In: Harris MI, Cowie CC, Stern MP, Boyko EJ, Reiber GE, Bennett PH, editors. Diabetes in America. 2nd ed. Bethesda, Md: National Institutes of Diabetes and Digestive and Kidney Diseases; 1995: 221–32. NIH publication no. 95-1468.

[24] Stephenson JM, Kenny S, Stevens LK, Fuller JH. Lee E, and the WHO Multinational Study Group. Proteinuria and mortality in diabetes: the WHO multinational study of vascular disease in diabetes. Diabet Med 1995; 12: 149–55.

[25] Centers for Disease Control. Diabetes surveillance 1993. Atlanta, Ga: US Department of Health and Human Services, Public Health Service, Centers for Disease Control; 1993.

[26] Tattersall RB, Gale EAM. Mortality. In: Frier BM, Fisher BM, editors. Hypoglycaemia and diabetes: clinical and physiological aspects. London: Edward Arnold, 1993.

[27] Zimmet P, Dowse G, Finch C, Serjeantson S, King H. The epidemiology and natural history of NIDDM: lessons from the South Pacific. Diabet Metab Rev 1990; 6: 91–124.

[28] Bennet PH, Bogardus C, Tuomilehto J, Zimmet P. Epidemiology and natural history of NIDDM: non-obese and obese. In: Alberti KGMM, DeFronzo RA, Keen H, Zimmet P, editors. International textbook of diabetes mellitus. Chichester: John Wiley and Sons Ltd; 1992: 147–76.

[29] Panzram G. Mortality and survival in type 2 (non-insulin-dependent) diabetes mellitus. Diabetologia 1987; 30: 123–31.

[30] Groeneveld Y, Petri H, Hermanst J, Springer MD. Relationship between blood glucose level and mortality in type 2 diabetes mellitus: a systematic review. Diabet Med 1999; 16: 2–13.

[31] Bain SC, Mijovic CH, Barnett AH. Genetic factors in the pathogenesis of insulin-dependent diabetes mellitus. In: Pickup J, Williams G, editors. Textbook of diabetes. Oxford: Blackwell Science; 1997: 13.1–13.13.

[32] Atkinson MA, Leiter EH. The NOD mouse model of type 1 diabetes: as good as it gets? Nat Med 1999; 5: 601–4.

[33] Levy-Marchal C, Patterson C, Green A, on behalf of the EURODIAB ACE Study Group. Variation by age group and seasonality at diagnosis of childhood type 1 diabetes in Europe. Diabetologia 1995; 38: 823–30.

[34] Wasmuth HE, Kolb H. Cow's milk and immune-mediated diabetes. Proc Nutr Soc 2000; 59: 573–9.

[35] Ginsberg-Fellner F, Fedun B, Cooper Z, et al. Interrelationships of congenital rubella and type 1 insulin-dependent diabetes mellitus. In: Jaworski MA, Molnar GD, Rajotte RV, Singh B, editors. The immunology of diabetes mellitus. Amsterdam: Elsevier; 1986: 279–86.

[36] Rabinovitch A. Immune regulatory and cytokine imbalance in the pathogenesis of IDDM. Diabetes 1994; 43: 613–21.

[37] Liblau RS, Singer SM, McDevitt HO. Th1 and Th2 CD4+ T cells in the pathogenesis of organ-specific autoimmune disease. Immunol Today 1995; 16: 34–8.

[38] Kolb H. Benign versus destructive insulitis. Diabetes Metab Rev 1997; 13: 139–46.

[39] Ziegler AG, Hummel M, Schenker M, Bonifacio E. Autoantibody appearance and risk for development of childhood diabetes in offspring of patients with type 1 diabetes: the 2 year analysis of the German BABYDIAB Study. Diabetes 1999; 48: 460–8.

[40] Katz JD, Benoist C, Mathis D. T helper cell subjects in insulin-dependent diabetes. Science 1995; 268: 1185–8.

[41] Healey D, Ozegbe P, Arden S, Chandler P, Hutton J, Cooke A. In vitro activity and in vitro specificity of CD4+ Th1 and Th2 cells derived from the spleens of diabetic NOD mice. J Clin Invest 1995; 95: 2979–85.

[42] Kallmann B, Hüther M, Tuber M, Feldkamp J, Bertrams J, Gries FA, Lampeter EF, Kolb H. Systemic bias of cytokine production toward cell-mediated immune regulation in IDDM and toward humoral immunity in Graves disease. Diabetes 1997; 46: 237–43.

[43] Martin S, Kolb H. Type 1 Diabetes: Immunopathogenese, Immunintervention und Immunprävention. In: Schatz H, editors. Diabetologie kompact. Berlin: Blackwell, 2001: 45–52.

[44] Verge CF, Gianani R, Kawasaki E, Yu L, Pietropaolo M, Jackson F, Chase HP, Eisenbarth GS. Prediction of type 1 diabetes in first-degree relatives using a combination of insulin, GAD, and ICA 512 bdc/IA-2 antibodies. Diabetes 1996; 45: 926–33.

[45] McKeigue PM. Ethnic variation in insulin resistance and risk of type 2 diabetes. In: Reaven G, Laws S, editors. Contemporary endocrinology: insulin resistance. Totowa, NJ: Humana Press Inc; 1999: 19–33.

[46] Vadheim CM, Rotter JI. Genetics of diabetes mellitus. In: Alberti KGMM, DeFronzo R, Keen H, Zimmet P, editors. International textbook of diabetes mellitus. Chichester: John Wiley & Sons; 1992: 31–98.

[47] Neel JV. Diabetes mellitus: a thrifty genotype rendered detrimental by "progress". Am J Hum Genet 1962; 14: 353–62.

[48] Dowse G, Zimmet P. The thrifty genotype in non-insulin-dependent diabetes. BMJ 1993; 306: 532–3.

[49] Pfeiffer AFH. Die verschiedenen Formen der Zuckerkrankheit und deren Genetik. In: Schatz H, editor. Diabetologie kompakt. Berlin: Blackwell, 2001: 5–13.

[50] Jahnke K, Daweke H, Liebermeister H, Schilling WH, Thamer G, Preiss H, Gries FA. Hormonal and metabolic aspects of obesity in humans. In: Östmann J, editor. Diabetes. Proceedings of the sixth congress of the International Diabetes Federation. Amsterdam: Exerpta Medica Foundation; 1969: 533–9.

[51] Alberti KGMM, Zimmet PZ, for the WHO Consultation. Definition, diagnosis and classification of diabetes mellitus and its complications. I: Diagnosis and classification of diabetes mellitus, provisional report of a WHO consultation. Diabet Med 1998; 15: 539–53.

[52] Poulsen P, Vaag A, Kyvik K, Beck-Nielsen H. Genetic versus environmental aetiology of the metabolic syndrome among male and female twins. Diabetologia 2001; 44: 537–43.
[53] Manson JE, Rimm EB, Stampfer MJ, Colditz JA, Willett WC, Krolewski AS, Rossner B, Hennekens CH, Speizer FE. Physical activity and incidence of non-insulin-dependent diabetes mellitus in women. Lancet 1991; 338: 774–8.
[54] Manson JE, Nathan DM, Krolewski AS, Stampfer MJ, Colditz GA, Willett WC, Hennekens CH. A prospective study of exercise and incidence of diabetes among US male physicians. JAMA 1992; 268: 63–7.
[55] Chan JM, Rimm EB, Colditz GA, Stampfer MJ, Willet WC. Obesity, fat distribution, and weight gain as risk factors for clinical diabetes in men. Diabetes Care 1994; 17: 961–9.
[56] Colditz GA, Willett WC, Rotnitzky A, Manson JE. Weight gain as a risk factor for clinical diabetes mellitus in women. Ann Intern Med 1995; 122: 481–6.
[57] Vague J. The degree of masculine differentiation of obesities: a factor determining predisposition to diabetes, atherosclerosis, gout, and uric calculous disease. Am J Clin Nutr 1956; 4: 20–7.
[58] Björntorp P. Abdominal obesity and the development of non-insulin-dependent diabetes mellitus. Diabetes Metab Rev 1988; 4: 615–22.
[59] Kissebah AH, Krakower GR. Regional adiposity and morbidity. Physiol Rev 1994; 74: 761–811.
[60] Kohrt WM, Kirvan JP, Staten MA, Bourey RE, King DS, Holloszy JO. Insulin resistance in aging is related to abdominal obesity. Diabetes 1993; 42: 273–81.
[61] Matsuzawa Y, Shimomura J, Nakamura T, Keno Y, Tokunaga K. Pathophysiology and pathogenesis of visceral fat obesity. In: Sakamoto N, Alberti KGMM, Hotta N, editors. Pathogenesis and treatment of NIDDM and its related problems. Amsterdam, Exerpta Medica, Int Congr Series 1057; 1994: 171.
[62] Lean MEJ, Powrie JK, Anderson AS, Garthwaite PH. Obesity, weight loss and prognosis in type 2 diabetes. Diabet Med 1990; 7: 228–33.
[63] Williamson DF, Thompson TJ, Thun M, Flanders D, Pamuk E, Byers T. Intentional weight loss and mortality among overweight individuals with diabetes. Diabetes Care 2000; 23: 1499–504.
[64] Omar MAK, Hammond MD, Seedat MA, Dyer RB, Rajput MC, Motala HA, Joubert SM. The prevalence of diabetes mellitus in a large group of South African Indians. S Afr Med J 1985; 67: 924–6.
[65] Fujimoto WY, Leonetti DL, Kinpour JL, Nevell-Morris L, Shuman WP, Stolov WC, Wahl PW. Prevalence of diabetes mellitus and impaired glucose tolerance among second generation Japanese-American men. Diabetes 1987; 36: 721–9.
[66] Cohen AM. Prevalence of diabetes among different ethnic Jewish groups in Israel. Metabolism 1961; 10: 50–8.
[67] O'Dea K. Diabetes in Australian aborigines: impact of the western diet and lifestyle. J Intern Med 1991; 232: 103–17.
[68] Barker DJP, Hales CN, Fall DHD, Osmond C, Phillips K, Clark PMS. Type 2 (non-insulin-dependent) diabetes mellitus, hypertension and hyperlipidaemia (syndrome X): relation to reduced fetal growth. Diabetologia 1993; 36: 62–7.
[69] Philipps DJW, Barker DJP, Barker CN, Hirst S, Ormond C. Thinness at birth and insulin resistance in adult life. Diabetologia 1994; 37: 150–4.
[70] Lithell HO, McKeigue PM, Berglund L, Mohsen R, Lithell UB, Lean DA. Relation of size at birth to non-insulin-dependent diabetes and insulin concentrations in men aged 50–60 years. BMJ 1996; 312: 406–10.
[71] Bo S, Cavallo-Perin P, Ciccone G, Scaglione L, Pagano G. The metabolic syndrome in twins: a consequence of low birth weight or of being a twin? Exp Clin Endocrinol Diabetes 2001; 109: 135–40.
[72] Matthews F, Yudkin P, Neil A. Influence of maternal nutrition on outcome of pregnancy: prospective cohort study. BMJ 1999; 319: 339–43.
[73] Matthews F, Yudkin P, Neil A. Author's reply. BMJ 2000; 320: 942.
[74] Groop LC. NIDDM an inherited disease of skeletal muscle energy metabolism? Exp Clin Endocrinol 1993; 101 (suppl 2): 294.
[75] Kahn CR. Insulin action, diabetogenes, and the cause of type II diabetes. Diabetes 1994; 43: 1066–84.
[76] Kahn CR, Vincent D, Doria A. Genetics of non-insulin-dependent (type II) diabetes mellitus. Annu Rev Med 1996; 47: 509–31.
[77] Karam JH. Reversible insulin resistance in non-insulin-dependent diabetes mellitus. Horm Metab Res 1996; 28: 440–4.
[78] Dugi K, Kassessinoff T, Nawroth PP. Type 2 Diabetes und genetische Defekte der β-Zellfunktion. In: Nawroth PP, editor. Kompendium Diabetologie. Berlin: Springer; 1999: 170–268.
[79] Zhang Y, Wat N, Stratton IM, Warren-Perry MG, Orho M, Groop L, Turner RC. UKPDS 19: Heterogeneity in NIDDM: separate contributions of IRS-1 and β3-adrenergic receptor mutations to insulin resistance and obesity respectively with no evidence for glycogen synthase gene mutations. Diabetologia 1996; 39: 1503–11.
[80] Grant PJ, Strickland MH, Mansfield MW. Insulin receptor substrate-1 gene and cardiovascular risk factors in NIDDM [letter]. Lancet 1995; 346: 841–2.
[81] Garvey WT, Huecksteadt TP, Mathaei S, Olefsky M. Role of glucose transporters in the cellular insulin resistance of type II non-insulin-dependent diabetes mellitus. J Clin Invest 1988; 81: 1528–36.
[82] Reynet C, Kahn CR. Rad: a member of the ras family overexpressed in muscle of type II diabetic humans. Science 1993; 262: 1441–4.
[83] Hager J, Hansen L, Vaisse C, Vionnet N, Philippi A, Poller W, Velho G, Carcassi C, Contu L, Julier C, et al. A missense mutation in the glucagon receptor gene is associated with non-insulin-dependent diabetes mellitus. Nat Genet 1995; 9: 299–304.
[84] Baier LJ, Sacchettini JC, Knowler WC, Eads J, Paolisso G, Tataranni PA, Mochizuki H, Bennett PH, Bogardus C, Prochazka M. An amino acid substitution in the human intestinal fatty acid binding protein is associated with increased fatty acid binding, increased fat oxidation, and insulin resistance. J Clin Invest 1995; 95: 1281–7.
[85] Walston J, Silver K, Bogardus C, Knowler WC, Celli FS, Austin S, Manning B, Strosberg AD, Stern M, Raben N, Sorkin JD, Roth J, Shuldiner AR. Time of onset of non-insulin-dependent diabetes mellitus and genetic variation in the β3-adrenergic receptor gene. N Engl J Med 1995; 333: 343–7.
[86] Hotamisligil GS, Spiegelman BM. Tumor necrosis factor alpha: a key component of the obesity-diabetes link. Diabetes 1994; 43: 1271–8.
[87] Shagizadeh M, Ong JM, Garvey WT, Henry RR, Kern PA. The expression of TNF-α by human muscle. J Clin Invest 1996; 97: 1111–6.
[88] Liu SL, Spelleken M, Röhrig K, Hauner H, Eckel J. Tumor necrosis factor-α acutely inhibits insulin signalling in human adipocytes. Diabetes 1998; 47: 515–22.
[89] Horikawa Y, Oda N, Cox NJ. Lix, Orho-Melander M, Hara M, Hinokio Y, Lindner TH, Mashima H, Schwarz PE, del Bosque-Plata L, Horikawa Y, Oda Y, Yoshinchi I, Colilla S, Polonsky KS, Wei S, Concannon P, Iwasaki N, Schulze J, Baier LJ, Bogardus C, Groop L, Boerwinkle E, Hanis CL, Bell GI. Genetic variation in the gene encoding calpain-10 is associated with type 2 diabetes mellitus. Nat Genet 2000; 26: 163–75.
[90] Holman GD, Kasuga M. From receptor to transporter: insulin signalling to glucose transport. Diabetologia 1997; 40: 991–1003.
[91] Lillioja S, Mott DM, Zawadzki JK, Young AA, Abbott WGH, Knowler WC, Bennett PH, Moll P, Bogardus C. In vivo insulin action is familial characteristic in non diabetic Pima Indians. Diabetes 1987; 36: 1329–35.
[92] Eriksson J, Franssila-Kallunki A, Ekstrand A, Saloranta C, Widen E, Schalin C, Groop L. Early metabolic defects in persons at increased risk for non-insulin-dependent diabetes mellitus. N Engl J Med 1989; 321: 337–43.
[93] DeFronzo R. The triumvirate β-cell, muscle, and liver: a collusion responsible for NIDDM. Diabetes 1988; 37: 667–87.
[94] Groop LC, Kankutr RTM, Schalin-Jäntti C, Eckstrand A, Nikula-Iljäs P, Widen E, Kuismanen E, Eriksson J, Franssila-Kallunki A, Saloranta C, Koskimies S. Association between polymorphism of the glycogen synthase gene and non-

insulin-dependent diabetes mellitus. N Engl J Med 1993; 328: 10–4.
[95] Krutzfeldt J, Kausch C, Volk A, Klein HH, Rett K, Häring HU, Stumvoll M. Insulin signaling and action in cultured skeletal muscle cells from lean healthy humans with high and low insulin sensitivity. Diabetes 2000; 49: 992–8.
[96] Colberg SR, Simeneau J, Icland Thaete F, Kelley DE. Skeletal muscle utilization of free fatty acids in women with visceral obesity. J Clin Invest 1995; 95: 1846–53.
[97] Dresner A, Laurent D, Marcucci M, Griffin ME, Dufour S, Cline GW, Slezak LA, Andersen DK, Hundal RS, Rothman DI, Petersen KF, Shulman GI. Effects of free fatty acids on glucose transport and IRS-1 associated phosphatidylinositol 3-kinase activity. J Clin Invest 1999; 103: 253–9.
[98] Kersten S, Seydoux J, Peters J, Gonzalez FJ, Desvergne B, Wahli W. Peroxisome proliferator-activated receptor-α mediates the adaptive response to fasting. J Clin Invest 1999; 103: 1489–98.
[99] Randle PJ, Garland PB, Hales CN, Newsholme EA. The glucose-fatty acid cycle. Its role in insulin sensitivity and the metabolic disturbances of diabetes mellitus. Lancet 1963; i: 785–9.
[100] Boden G Free fatty acids, insulin resistance, and type 2 diabetes mellitus. Proc Ass Amer Phys 1999, 111:241–8.
[101] Rebrin K, Steil GM, Getty L, Bergmann RN. Free fatty acid as a link in the regulation of hepatic glucose output by peripheral insulin. Diabetes 1995; 44: 1038–45.
[102] Bavenholm PN, Pigon J, Östenson CG, Efendic S. Insulin sensitivity of suppression of endogenous glucose production is the single most important determinant of glucose tolerance. Diabetes 2001; 50: 1449–54.
[103] Hotomisligil GS, Peraldi P, Budavari A, Ellis R, White MF, Spiegelman BM. IRS-1 mediated inhibition of insulin receptor tyrosine kinase activity in TNF-α and obesity induced insulin resistance. Science 1996; 271: 665–8.
[104] Hauner H, Petruschke T, Russ M, Eckel J. Effects of tumor necrosis factor alpha (TNF-α) on glucose transport and lipid metabolism of newly differentiated human fat cells in cell culture. Diabetologia 1995; 38: 764–71.
[105] Stephens JM, Pekala PH. Transcriptional repression of the GLUT-4 and C/EBP genes in 3T3-L1 adipocytes by tumor necrosis factor-α. J Biol Chem 1991; 266: 21839–45.
[106] Mitchell TH, Abraham G, Schiffrin A, Leiter LA, Marliss E. Hyperglycaemia after intensive exercise in IDDM subjects during continuous subcutaneous insulin infusion. Diabetes Care 1988; 11: 311–7.
[107] Gries FA. Nutrition and physical activity in diabetes. In: Fabris F, Pernigotti L, Ferrario E, editors. Sedentary life and nutrition. New York: Raven Press; 1990: 157–62.
[108] Wallberg-Henriksson H. Repeated exercise regulates glucose transport capacity in skeletal muscle. Acta Physiol Scand 1986; 127: 39–43.
[109] Dela F, Ploug T, Handberg A, Petersen LN, Larsen JJ, Mikines KJ, Galbo H. Physical training increases muscle GLUT-4 protein and mRNA in patients with NIDDM. Diabetes 1994; 43: 862–5.
[110] Giaccari A, Morviducci L, Zoretta D, Sbraccia P, Caiola S, Buongiorno A, Bonadonna RC, Tamburrano G. In vivo effects of glucosamine on insulin secretion and insulin sensitivity in the rat: possible relevance to the maladaptive response to chronic hyperglycaemia. Diabetologia 1995; 38: 518–24.
[111] Baron AD, Zhu JS, Zhu JH, Weldon H, Maianu L, Garvey WT. Glucosamine induces insulin resistance in vivo by affecting GLUT 4 translocation in skeletal muscle. Implications for glucose toxicity. J Clin Invest 1995; 96: 2792–801.
[112] Hawkins M, Hu M, Yu J, Eder H, Vuguin P, She L, Barcilai N, Leiser M, Backer JM, Rossetti L. Discordant effects of glucosamine on insulin-stimulated glucose metabolism and phosphatidylinositol-3-kinase activity. J Biol Chem 1999; 274: 31312–19.
[113] Pimenta W, Korytkowski M, Mitrakou A, Jenssen T, Yki-Järvinen H, Evron W, Dailey G, Gerich J. Pancreatic beta-cell dysfunction as the primary genetic lesion in NIDDM. JAMA 1995; 273: 1855–61.
[114] Gerich JE. Pathogenesis and treatment of type 2 (non-insulin-dependent) diabetes mellitus (NIDDM). Horm Metab Res 1996; 28: 404–412.
[115] Davies MJ, Rayman G, Grenfell A, Gray IP, Day JL, Hales CN. Loss of the first phase insulin response to intravenous glucose in subjects with persistent impaired glucose tolerance. Diabet Med 1994; 11: 434–6.
[116] Mitrakou A, Kelley D, Venemann T, Pangburn J, Reilly J, Gerich H. Role of reduced suppression of hepatic glucose output and diminished early insulin release in impaired glucose tolerance. N Engl J Med 1992; 326: 22–9.
[117] Weyer C, Bogardus C, Mott DM, Pratley RE. The natural history of insulin secretory dysfunction and insulin resistance in the pathogenesis of type 2 diabetes mellitus. J Clin Invest 1999; 104: 787–94.
[118] Paolisso G, Tagliamonte MR, Rizzo MR, Gualdiero P, Saccomanno F, Gambordella A, Guigliano D, Onofrio FD, Howard BV. Lowering fatty acids potentiates acute insulin response in first-degree relatives of people with type 2 diabetes. Diabetologia 1998; 41: 1127–32.
[119] Kolb H. Äthiopathogenese und Genetik. In: Berger M, editor. Diabetes mellitus. München: Urban & Schwarzenberg, 1995: 209–14.
[120] Groop LC, Bottazzo GF, Doniach D. Islet cell antibodies identify latent type 1 diabetes in patients 35–75 years at diagnosis. Diabetes 1986; 35: 237–41.
[121] Hother-Nielsen O, Faber O, Schwartz-Sörensen N, Beck-Nielsen H. Classification of newly diagnosed diabetic patients as insulin-requiring or non-insulin-requiring based on clinical and biochemical variables. Diabetes Care 1988; 1: 531–7.
[122] Niskanan L, Karjalainen J, Sarlund H, Siitonen O, Uusitopa M. Five-year follow-up of islet cell antibodies in type 2 (non-insulin-dependent) diabetes mellitus. Diabetologia 1991; 34: 402–8.
[123] Canadian–European Diabetes Study Group. Cyclosporin induced remission of IDDM after early intervention: association of 1 year of cyclosporin treatment with enhanced insulin secretion. Diabetes 1988; 37: 1574–82.
[124] Shah SC, Malone JI, Simpson NE. A randomized trial of intensive insulin therapy in newly diagnosed insulin-dependent diabetes mellitus. N Engl J Med 1989; 320: 550–4.
[125] Turner RC, Cull CA, Frighi V, Hohman RR, for the UK Prospective Diabetes Study (UKPDS) Group. Glycemic control with diet, sulfonylurea, metformin, or insulin in patients with type 2 diabetes mellitus. Progressive requirement for multiple therapies (UKPDS 49). JAMA 1999; 281: 2005–12.
[126] Brinchmann-Hansen O, Dahl-Jörgensen K, Sandvik L, Hanssen KF. Blood glucose concentrations and progression of diabetic retinopathy: the seven year results of the Oslo Study. BMJ 1992; 304: 19–22.
[127] The Diabetes Control and Complications Trial Research Group. The effect of intensive treatment of diabetes on the development and progression of long-term complications in insulin-dependent diabetes mellitus. N Engl J Med 1993; 329: 977–86.
[128] Amthor KF, Dahl-Jörgensen K, Berg TJ, Heier MS, Sandvik L, Aagenaes O, Hanssen KF. The effect of 8 years of strict glycaemic control on peripheral nerve function in IDDM patients: the Oslo Study. Diabetologia 1994; 37: 579–84.
[129] Reichard P, Pihl M, Rosenqvist U, Sule J. Complications in IDDM are caused by elevated blood glucose level: the Stockholm Diabetes Intervention Study (SDIS) at 10-year follow-up. Diabetologia 1996; 39: 1483–8.
[130] UK Prospective Diabetes Study (UKPDS) Group. Intensive blood glucose control with sulfonylureas or insulin compared with conventional treatment and risk of complications in patients with type 2 diabetes (UKPDS 33). Lancet 1998; 352: 837–53.
[131] Ohkubo Y, Kishikawa H, Araki E, Miyata T, Isami S, Motoyoshi S, Kojima Y, Furuyoshi N, Shichiri M. Intensive insulin therapy prevents the progression of diabetic microvascular complications in Japanese patients with non-insulin-dependent diabetes mellitus: a randomized prospective 6-year study. Diabetes Res Clin Pract 1995; 28: 103–17.
[132] Stratton IM, Adler AI, Neil AW, Matthews DR, Manley SE, Cull CA, Hadden D, Turner RC, Holman RR, on behalf of the UK Prospective Diabetes Study Group. Association of

glycaemia with macrovascular and microvascular complications of type 2 diabetes (UKPDS 35): prospective observational study. BMJ 2000; 321: 405–12.
[133] UK Prospective Diabetes Study (UKPDS) Group. Effect of intensive blood glucose control with metformin on complications in overweight patients with type 2 diabetes (UKPDS 34). Lancet 1998; 352: 854–65.
[134] Abraira C, Colwell J, Nuttwall F, Sawin CT, Hendersen W, Comstock JP, Emanuele NV, Levin SR, Pacold I, Lee HS, and the Veterans Affairs Cooperative Study on Glycemic Control and Complications in type 2 Diabetes (VA CSDM) Group. Cardiovascular events and correlates in the Veterans Affairs Feasability Trial. Arch Intern Med 1997; 157: 181–8.
[135] Ito H, Harano Y, Suzuki M, Hattori Y, Tacheuchi M, Inada H, Inoue J, Kawamori R, Murase T, Ouchi Y, Umeda F, Nawata H, Oim H, and the Multiclinical Study for Diabetic Macroangiopathy Group. Risk factor analysis for macrovascular complication in non obese NIDDM patients. Multiclinical Study for Diabetic Macroangiopathy (MSDM). Diabetes 1996; 45 (suppl 3): S19–23.
[136] Schleicher E, Nerlich A. The role of hyperglycaemia in the development of diabetic complications. Horm Metab Res 1996; 28: 367–73.
[137] Giardino J, Brownlee M. The biochemical basis of microvascular disease. In: Pickup J, William G, editors. Textbook of diabetes. Oxford: Blackwell Science; 1997: 42. 1-16.
[138] Gries FA, Petersen-Braun M, Tschöpe D, Loo J van de. Haemostasis and diabetic angiopathy: pathophysiology and therapeutic concepts. Stuttgart: Georg Thieme Verlag, 1993.
[139] Vlassara H, Bucala R. Advanced glycation and diabetes complications: an update. Diabetes Annu 1995; 9: 227–44.
[140] Tschöpe D, Rösen P. Gerinnungsstörungen bei metabolischem Syndrom und Typ 2 Diabetes. In: Mehnert H, editor. Herz, Gefäße und Diabetes. München: Medikon; 1997: 117–32.
[141] Baron AD, Quon MJ. Insulin action and endothelial function. In: Reaven GM, Laws A, editors. Insulin resistance. Totowa, NJ: Humana Press, 1999: 247–63.
[142] Laws A. Insulin resistance and dyslipidemia: implications for coronary heart disease risk. In: Reaven GM, Laws A, editors. Insulin resistance. Totowa, NJ: Humana Press, 1999: 267–80.
[143] Packer L, Rösen P, Tritschler HJ, King GL, Azzi A. Antioxidants in diabetes management. New York: Marcel Dekker; 2000.
[144] Nawroth PP, Borcea V, Bierhaus A, Joswig M, Schiekofer S, Tritschler HJ. Oxidative stress, NF-kB activation, and late diabetic complications. In: Packer L, Rösen P, Tritschler HJ, King GL, Azzi A, editors. Antioxidants in diabetes management. New York: Marcel Dekker; 2000: 185–204.
[145] Idris J, Gray S, Donelley R. Protein kinase C activation: isozyme-specific effects on metabolism and cardiovascular complications in diabetes. Diabetologia 2000; 44: 659–73.
[146] Nishigawa T, Edelstein D, Du XL, Yamagishi SI, Matsumura T, Kaneda Y, Yorek MA, Beebe D, Oates PJ, Hammes HP, Giardino I, Brownlee M. Normalizing mitochondrial superoxide production blocks three pathways of hyperglycaemic damage. Nature 2000; 404: 787–90.
[147] Du XL, Edelstein D, Rossetti L, Fantus IG, Goldberg H, Ziyadeh F, Wu J, Brownlee M. Hyperglycemia-induced mitochondrial superoxide overproduction activates the hexosamine pathway and induces plasminogen activator inhibitor-1 expression by increasing SP 1 glycosylation. Proc Natl Acad Sci USA 2000; 97: 12222–6.
[148] Koya D, King GL. Protein kinase C activation and the development of diabetic complications. Diabetes 1998; 47: 859–66.
[149] Rösen P, Nawroth PP, King G, Möller W, Tritschler HJ, Packer L. The role of oxidative stress in the onset and progression of diabetes and its complications: a summary of a congress series sponsored by UNESCO-MCBM, the American Diabetes Association and the German Diabetes Society. Diabetes Metab Res Rev 2001; 17: 189–212.
[150] Bucala R, Tracey A, Cerami A. Advanced glycosylation products quench nitric oxide and mediate defective endothelium-dependent vasodilation in experimental diabetes. J Clin Invest 1991; 87: 432–8.
[151] Bierhaus A, Schiekofer S, Schwaninger M, et al. Diabetes-associated sustained activation of the transcription factor nuclear factor-kappaB. Diabetes 2001; 50: 2792–808.
[152] Klein R, Klein BEK, Moss SE, Davis MD, DeMets DL. The Wisconsin epidemiologic study of diabetic retinopathy II. Prevalence and risk of diabetic retinopathy when age at diagnosis is less than 30 years. Arch Ophthalmol 1994; 102: 520–6.
[153] Klein R, Klein BEK, Moss SE, Cruickshank KJ. The Wisconsin Epidemiologic Study of Diabetic Retinopathy XV. The longterm incidence of macular edema. Ophthalmology 1995; 102: 7–16.
[154] Krolewski AS, Kosinski EJ, Warram JH, Leland OS, Busick EJ, Asmal AC, Rand LI, Christlieb AR, Bradley RF, Kahn CR. Magnitude and determinants of coronary artery disease in juvenile-onset, insulin-dependent diabetes mellitus. Am J Cardiol 1987; 59: 750–5.
[155] Mauer SM, Goetz FC, McHugh LE, Sutherland DER, Barbosa J, Najarian JS, Steffes MW. Longterm study of normal kidneys transplanted into patients with type 1 diabetes. Diabetes 1989; 38: 516–23.
[156] Parving HH, Hommel E, Smidt UM. Protection of kidney function and decrease of in albuminuria by captopril in insulin dependent diabetes with nephropathy. BMJ 1987; 297: 1086–91.
[157] Parving HH, Andersen M, Smidt UH, Hommel E, Mathiesen ER, Svendsen PA. Effect of antihypertensive treatment on kidney function in diabetic nephropathy. BMJ 1987; 294: 1443–7.
[158] UK Prospective Diabetes Study Group. Tight blood pressure control and risk of macrovascular and microvascular complications in type 2 diabetes: UKPDS 38. BMJ 1998; 317: 703–13.
[159] Adler AI, Stratton IM, Neil HAW, Yudkin JS, Mathews DR, Cull CA, Wright AD, Turner RC, Holman RR, on behalf of the UK Prospective Diabetes Study Group. Association of systolic blood pressure with macrovascular and microvascular complications of type 2 diabetes (UKPDS 36): prospective observational study. BMJ 2000; 321: 412–9.
[160] Sjolie AK. Ocular complications in insulin treated diabetes mellitus: an epidemiological study. Acta Ophthalmol 1985; 172 (suppl): 1–77.
[161] Mühlhauser I, Sawicki P, Berger M. Cigarette smoking as a risk factor for macroproteinuria and proliferative retinopathy in type 1 (insulin-dependent) diabetes. Diabetologia 1986; 29: 500–3.
[162] Klein BEK, Moss SE, Klein R. Effect of pregnancy on progression of diabetic retinopathy. Diabetes Care 1990; 13: 34–40.
[163] Rosenn B, Miodovnik M, Kranias G, Khoury J, Combs CA, Mimouni F, Siddiqi TA, Lipman MJ. Progression of diabetic retinopathy in pregnancy: association with hypertension in pregnancy. Am J Obstet Gynecol 1992; 166: 1214–8.
[164] Chew EY, Mills JL, Metzger BE, Remaley NA, Jovanovic-Petersen L, Knopp RH, Conley M, Rand L, Simpson JL, Holmes LB, Aorans JH. Metabolic control and progression of retinopathy. National Institute of Child Health and Human Development Diabetes in Early Pregnancy Study. Diabetes Care 1995; 18: 631–7.
[165] Early Treatment Diabetic Retinopathy Study Research Group. Grading diabetic retinopathy from stereoscopic color fundus photographs. An extension of the modified Airlie house classification. Early Treatment Diabetic Retinopathy Study Report number 10. Ophthalmology 1991; 98: 786–806.
[166] Chaturvedi N, Stephenson JM, Fuller JH. The relationship between smoking and microvascular complications in the EURODIAB IDDM Complications Study. Diabetes Care 1995; 18: 785–92.
[167] Mühlhauser I, Bender R, Bott U, Jörgens V, Grüsser M, Wagener W, Overmann H, Berger M. Cigarette smoking and progression of retinopathy and nephropathy in type 1 diabetes. Diabet Med 1996; 13: 536–43.
[168] Ballegooie E Van, Hooymans JMM, Timmerman Z, Reitsma WD, Sluiter WJ, Schweitzer NMJ, Doorenbos H. Rapid deterioratiion of diabetic retinopathy during treatment with continuous subcutaneous insulin infusion. Diabetes Care 1984; 7: 236–42.
[169] DCCT Research Group. Early worsening of diabetic retinopathy in the Diabetes Control and Complications Trial. Arch Ophthalmol 1998; 116: 874–86.

[170] Chew EY, Klein ML, Ferris FL, Remaley NA, Murphy RP, Chantry K, Hoggwerf BJ, Miller D, for the ETDRS Research Group. Association of elevated serum lipid levels with retinal hard exsudate in diabetic retinopathy. Early Treatment Diabetic Retinopathy Study (ETDRS). Report 22. Arch Ophthalmol 1996; 114: 1079–84.
[171] Davis MD, Fisher MR, Gangnon RE, Barton F, Aiello LM, Chew EY, Ferris FL, Knatterud GL, for the Early Treatment Diabetic Retinopathy Study Research Group. Risk factors for high-risk proliferative diabetic retinopathy and severe visual loss: Early Treatment Diabetic Retinopathy Study report #18. Invest Ophthalmol Vis Sci 39: 233–52.
[172] The Diabetic Retinopathy Study Research Group. Indications for photocoagulation treatment of diabetic retinopathy: Diabetic Retinopathy Study report no. 14. Int Ophthalmol Clin 1987; 27 (suppl4): 239–53.
[173] The Diabetic Retinopathy Vitrectomy Study Research Group. Early vitrectomy for severe vitreous hemorrhage in diabetic retinopathy. Four-year results of a randomized trial: Diabetic Retinopathy Vitrectomy Study Report no 5. Arch Ophthalmol 1990; 108: 958–64.
[174] Early Treatment Diabetic Retinopathy Study Research Group. Early photocoagulation for diabetic retinopathy. Early Treatment Diabetic Retinopathy Study Research Group (EDTRS) report number 9. Ophthalmology 1991; 98: 766–85.
[175] Widder RA, Brunner R, Walter P, Lüke C, Bartz-Schmidt KU, Heimann K, Borberg H. Improvement of visual acuity in patients suffering from diabetic retinopathy after membrane differential filtration: a pilot study. Transfus Sci 1999; 21: 201–6.
[176] Krolewski M, Eggers P, Warram JH. Magnitude of end-stage renal disease in IDDM: a 35-year follow-up study. Kidney Int 1996; 50: 2041–6.
[177] Krolewski AS, Warram JH, Christlieb AR, Busick EJ, Kahn CR. The changing natural history of nephropathy in type 1 diabetes. Am J Med 1985; 78: 785–94.
[178] Ballard DJ, Humphrey LL, Melton LJ, Frohnert PP, Chu C-P, O'Fallon WM, Palumbo PJ. Epidemiology of persistent proteinuria in type II diabetes mellitus. Population-based study in Rochester, Minn. Diabetes 1988; 37: 405–12.
[179] Humphrey LL, Ballard DJ, Frohnert PP, Chu CP, O'Fallon M, Palumbo PJ. Chronic renal failure in non-insulin dependent diabetes mellitus. A population based study in Rochester, Minn. Ann Intern Med 1989; 111: 788–96.
[180] Krolewski AS, Laffel LMB, Krolewski M, Quinn M, Warram JH. Glycosylated hemoglobin and risk of microalbuminuria in patients with insulin-dependent diabetes mellitus. N Engl J Med 1995; 332: 1251–5.
[181] Diabetes Control and Complications Trial Research Group. The absence of a glycemic threshold for the development of long-term complications: the perspective of the Diabetes Control and Complications Trial. Diabetes 1996; 45: 1289–98.
[182] Haffner SM. Is there a glycemic threshold? Arch Intern Med 1997; 157: 1791.
[183] Borch-Johnsen K, Kreiner S. Proteinuria: value as a predictor of cardiovascular mortality in insulin dependent diabetes mellitus. BMJ 1987; 294: 1651–4.
[184] Jensen T, Borch-Johnsen K, Kofoed-Enevoldsen A, Deckert T. Coronary heart disease in young type 1 (insulin-dependent) diabetic patients with and without diabetic nephropathy: incidence and risk factors. Diabetologia 1987; 30: 144–8.
[185] Moloney A, Turnbridge WMG, Ireland JT, Watkins PJ. Mortality from diabetic nephropathy in the United Kingdom. Diabetologia 1983; 25: 26–30.
[186] Parving HH, Hommel E. Prognosis in diabetic nephropathy. BMJ 1989; 29: 230–3.
[187] Matthiesen ER, Borch-Johnsen K, Jensen DV, Deckert T. Improved survival in patients with diabetic nephropathy. Diabetologia 1989; 32: 884–6.
[188] Brunner FP, Selwood NH. Profile of patient on RRT in Europe and death rate due to major causes of death groups. The EDTA Registration Committee. Kidney Int 1992; 38 (suppl): S4–15.
[189] Warram JH, Gearin G, Laffel L, Krolewski AS. Effect of duration of type I diabetes on the prevalence of stages of diabetic nephropathy defined by urinary albumin/creatinine ratio. J Am Soc Nephrol 1996; 7: 930–7.
[190] Ravid M, Savin H, Jutin I, Bental T, Lang R, Lishner M. Long-term effect of ACE inhibition on development of nephropathy in diabetes mellitus type II. Kidney Int 1994; 45 (suppl): S161–164.
[191] Mogensen CE, Keane WF, Bennett PH, Jerums G, Parving HH, Passa P, Steffes MW, Striker GE, Viberti GC. Prevention of diabetic renal disease with special reference to microalbuminuria. Lancet 1995; 346: 1080–4.
[192] Seaquist ER, Goetz FC, Rich S, Barbosa J. Familial clustering of diabetic kidney disease. Evidence for genetic susceptibility to diabetic nephropathy. N Engl J Med 1989; 320: 1161–5.
[193] Borch-Johnsen K, Norgaard K, Hommel E, Mathiesen ER, Jensen JS, Deckert T, Parving HH. Is diabetic nephropathy an inherited complication ? Kidney Int 1992; 41: 719–22.
[194] Toeller M, Buyken A, Heitkamp G, Brämswig S, Man J, Milne R, Gries FA, Keen H, and the EURODIAB IDDM Complications Study Group. Protein intake and urinary albumin excretion rates in the EURODIAB IDDM Complications Study. Diabetologia 1997; 40: 1219–26.
[195] Mogensen CE. Natural history of renal functional abnormalities in human diabetes mellitus: from normoalbuminuria to incipient and overt nephropathy. In: Brenner BM, Stein JH, editors. The kidney in diabetes mellitus. New York: Churchill Livingstone; 1989: 19–49.
[196] Steffes MW, Osterby R, Chavers B, Mauer SM. Mesangial expansion as a central mechanism for loss of kidney function in diabetic patients. Diabetes 1989; 38: 1077–81.
[197] Osterby R. Glomerular structural changes in type 1 (insulin-dependent) diabetes mellitus: causes, consequences and prevention. Diabetologia 1992; 35: 803–12.
[198] Osterby R, Gall MA, Schmitz A, Nielsen FS, Nyberg G, Parving HH. Glomerular structure and function in proteinuric type 2 (non-insulin-dependent) diabetic patients. Diabetologia 1993; 36: 1064–70.
[199] Wang PH, Lau J, Chalmers TC. Meta-analysis of effects of intensive blood-glucose control on late complications of type 1 diabetes. Lancet 1993; 341: 1306–9.
[200] Hasslacher C, Bostedt-Kiesel A, Kempe HP, Wahl P. Effect of metabolic factors and blood pressure on kidney function in proteinuria type 2 (non-insulin-dependent) diabetic patients. Diabetologia 1993; 36: 1051–6.
[201] Bangstad HJ, Osterby R, Dahl-Jorgensen K, Berg KJ, Hartman A, Hanssen KF. Improvement of blood glucose control in IDDM patients retards the progression of morphological changes in early diabetic nephropathy. Diabetologia 1994; 37: 483–90.
[202] Sawicki PT. Stabilization of glomerular filtration rate over 2 years in patients with diabetic nephropathy under intensified therapy regimens. Diabetes Treatment and Teaching Programmes Working Group. Nephrol Dial Transplant 1997; 12: 1890–9.
[203] European Diabetes Policy Group. A desktop guide to type 2 diabetes mellitus. Diabetic Med 1999; 16: 716–30.
[204] American Diabetes Association. Diabetic nephropathy. Diabetes Care 2000; 23 (suppl 1): S67–72.
[205] EUCLID Study Group. Randomized placebo-controlled trial of lisinopril in normotensive patients with insulin-dependent diabetes and normoalbuminuria or micro-albuminuria. Lancet 1997; 349: 1787–92.
[206] UKPDS Group. Efficacy of atenolol and captopril in reducing risk of macrovascular and microvascular complications in type 2 diabetes, UKPDS 39. BMJ 1998; 317: 713–20.
[207] Marre MJ, Chatellier G, Leblanc H, Guyene TT, Menard J, Passa P. Prevention of diabetic nephropathy with enalapril in normotensive diabetics with microalbuminuria. BMJ 1988; 297: 1092–5.
[208] Microalbuminuria Captopril Study Group. Captopril reduced the risk of nephropathy in IDDM patients with microalbuminuria. Diabetologia 1996; 39: 587–93.
[209] Sano T, Hotta N, Kawamura T, Matsumae H, Chaya S, Sasaki H, Nakayama M, Hara T, Matsuo S, Sakamoto N. Effects of long-term enalapril treatment on persistent microalbuminuria in normotensive type 2 diabetic patients: results of a 4-year, prospective, randomized study. Diabet Med 1996; 13: 120–4.

[210] Ahmad J, Siddiqui MA, Ahmad H. Effective postponement of diabetic nephropathy with enalapril in normotensive type 2 diabetic patients with microalbuminuria. Diabetes Care 1997; 20: 1576–81.
[211] Jungmann E, Haak T, Malanyn M, Mortasawi N, Unterstöger E, Scherberich J, Usadel KH: Vergleichsstudie zur Wirkung von Nitrendipin und Enalapril auf Mikroalbuminuria und Alpha-1-Mikroglobulin-Ausscheidung bei Patienten mit Typ 1 Diabetes mellitus. Diabetes Stoffw 1993; 2: 372–7.
[212] Crepaldi G, Casta Q, Deferrari G, Mangili R, Navalesi R, Santeusanio F, Spalluto A, Vanasia A, Villa MG, Nosadini R. The Italian Microalbuminuria Study Group in IDDM: Effect of lisinopril and nifedepine on the progression to overt albuminuria in IDDM patients with incipient nephropathy and normal blood pressure. The Italian Microalbuminuria Study Group in IDDM. Diabetes Care 1998; 21: 104–10.
[213] Bjorck S, Mulec H, Johnson SA, Norden G, Aurell M. Renal protective effect of enalapril in diabetic nephropathy. BMJ 1992; 304: 339–43.
[214] Lewis EJ, Hunsicker LG, Bani RP, Rhode RD. The effect of angiotensin-converting-enzyme inhibition on diabetic nephropathy. Collab Study Group. N Engl J Med 1993; 329: 1456–62.
[215] Ravid M, Savin H, Jutrin I, Bental T, Katz B, Lishner M. Long-term stabilizing effect of angiotensin-converting enzyme inhibition on plasma creatinine and on proteinuria in normotensive type II diabetic patients. Ann Intern Med 1993; 118: 577–81.
[216] Laffel LM, McGill JB, Gans DJ. The beneficial effect of angiotension-converting-enzyme inhibition on diabetic nephropathy. The Collaberative Study Group. Am J Med 1995; 99: 497–504.
[217] Slataper R, Vicknair N, Sadler R, Bakris G. Comparative effects of different antihypertensive treatments on progression of diabetic renal disease. Arch Intern Med 1993; 153: 973–80.
[218] Elving LD, Wetzels JFM, Lier HJJ van, Nobel E de, Berden JHM. Captopril and atenolol are equally effective in retarding progression of diabetic nephropathy. Results of a 2 year prospective, randomized study. Diabetologia 1994; 37: 604–9.
[219] Bakris GL, Copley JB, Vicknair N, Sadler R, Leurgans S. Calcium channel blockers versus other antihypertensive therapies on progression of NIDDM associated nephropathy. Kidney Int 1996; 50: 1641–50.
[220] Velussi M, Brocco E, Frigato F, Zolli M, Muollo B, Maioli M, Carraro A, Tonolo G, Tresu P, Cernigoi AM, Fioretto P, Nosadini R. Effects of cilazapril and amlodipine on kidney function in hypertensive NIDDM patients. Diabetes 1996; 45: 216–22.
[221] Böhlen L, DeCourten M, Weidmann P. Comparative study of the effect of ACE inhibitors and other antihypertensive agents on proteinuria in diabetic patients. Am J Hypertens 1994; 7: 84S–92S.
[222] Heart Outcomes Prevention Evaluation (HOPE) Study Investigators. Effects of ramipril on cardiovascular and microvascular outcomes in people with diabetes mellitus: results of the HOPE study and MICRO-HOPE substudy. Lancet 2000; 355: 253–9.
[223] Parving HH, Lehnert H, Bröckner-Mortensen J, Gonis R, Andersen S, Arner P, for the Irbesartan in patients with type 2 diabetes and microalbuminura study group. The effect of irbesartan on the development of diabetic nephropathy in patients with type 2 diabetes. N Engl J Med 2001; 345: 870–8
[224] Lewis EJ, Hunsicker LG, Clarke WR, Berl T, Pohl MA, Lewis JB, Ritz E, Atkins RC, Rohde R, Raz J, for the Collaborative Study Group. Renoprotective effect of the angiotensin-receptor antagonist irbesartan in patients with nephropathy due to type 2 diabetes. N Engl J Med 2001; 345: 851–60.
[225] Brenner BM, Cooper ME, DeZeeuw D, Keane WF, Mitch WE, Parving HH, Remuzzi G, Snapinn SM, Zhang Z, Shahinfar S, for the RENAAL Study Investigators. Effect of losartan on renal and cardiovascular outcomes in patients with type 2 diabetes and nephropathy. N Engl J Med 2001; 345: 861–9.
[226] Mattock MB, Keen H, Viberti GC, El-Gohari MR, Murrels TJ, Scott GS, Wing JR, Jackson PJ. Coronary heart disease and urinary albumin excretion rate in type 2 (non-insulin-dependent) diabetic patients. Diabetologia 1988; 31: 82–7.
[227] Bucala R, Makita Z, Vega G, Grundy S, Koschinsky T, Cerami A, Vlassara H. Modification of low density lipoprotein by advanced glycation endproducts contributes to the dyslipidaemia of diabetes and renal insufficiency. Proc Natl Acad Sci USA 1994; 91: 9441–5.
[228] American Diabetes Association. Aspirin therapy in Diabetes. Diabetes Care 2000; 23 (suppl 1): S61–62.
[229] Solomon R, Werner C, Mann DJ, DeSilva P. Effects of saline, mannitol, and fluid to prevent acute decreases in renal function induced by radiocontrast agents. N Engl J Med 1994; 331: 1416–20.
[230] Smets YFC, Westendorp RGJ, Pijl JW van der, deCharro FT, Ringers J, de Fijter JW, Lemkes HHPJ. Effect of simultaneous pancreas kidney transplantation on mortality of patients with type-1 diabetes mellitus and end-stage renal failure. Lancet 1999; 353: 1915–9.
[231] Lundbaek K. Introduction: Blood vessel disease in diabetes. In: Lundbaek K, Keen H, editors. Blood vessel disease in diabetes mellitus (V. Capri conference). Acta Diab Lat 1971; 8 (suppl 1): 3–4.
[232] Jarrett RJ. Epidemiology of macrovascular disease and hypertension in diabetes mellitus. In: Alberti KGMM, DeFronzo RA, Keen H, Zimmet P. International textbook of diabetes mellitus. Chichester: John Wiley & Sons; 1992:1459–70.
[233] The World Health Organisation Multinational Study of Vascular Disease in Diabetics. Prevalence of small vessel and large vessel disease in diabetic patients from 14 centers. Diabetologia 1985; 28 (suppl): 615–40.
[234] Klein R. Hyperglycemia and microvascular and macro-vascular disaease in diabetes. Diabetes Care 1995; 18: 258–68.
[235] Selby JV, Zhang D. Risk factors for lower extremity amputation in persons with diabetes. Diabetes Care 1995; 18: 509–16.
[236] Kannel WB. Prevalence, incidence, and mortality of coronary heart disease. In: Fuster V, Voss R, Topol EJ, editors. Atherosclerosis and coronary artery disease, vol 1. Philadelphia, Pa: Lippincott-Raven; 1996: 13–21.
[237] Bell ET. A post mortem study of vascular disease in diabetes. Arch Pathol 1952; 53: 444–62.
[238] Waller BF, Palumbo PJ, Lie T, Roberts WC. Status of the coronary arteries at necropsy in diabetes mellitus with onset after age 30 years. Am J Med 1980; 69: 498–506.
[239] Green A, Hougaard P. Epidemiological studies of diabetes mellitus in Denmark, V. Mortality and causes of death among insulin-treated diabetic patients. Diabetologia 1984; 26: 190–4.
[240] Donahue RP, Orchard TJ. Diabetes mellitus and macrovascular complications. An epidemiological perspective. Diabetes Care 1992; 15: 1141–55.
[241] Chan P, Pan WH. Coagulation activation in type 2 diabetes mellitus: the higher coronary risk of female diabetic patients. Diabetic Med 1995; 12: 504–7.
[242] Löwell H, Stieber J, Koenig W, Thorad B, Hörmann A, Gostomzyk J. Das diabetes-bedingte Herzinfarktrisiko in einer süddeutschen Bevölkerung: Ergebnisse der MONICA-Augsburg-Studien 1985–1994. Diabetes Stoffw 1999; 8: 11–21.
[243] Brand FN, Abbott RD, Kannel WB. Diabetes, intermittent claudication, and risk of cardiovascular events. Framingham Study. Diabetes 1989; 38: 504–9.
[244] Diabetes Epidemiology Research International Mortality Study Group. Major cross-country differences in risk of dying for people with IDDM. Diabetes Care 1991; 14: 40–54.
[245] Songer TJ, DeBerry K, LaPorte RE, Tuomilehto J. International comparisons of IDDM mortality. Diabetes Care 1992; 15 (suppl 1): 15–21.
[246] Rendel M, Kimmell DB, Bamisedun O, Fulmer J. The health care status of the diabetic population as reflected by physician claims to a major insurer. Arch Intern Med 1993; 153: 1360–6.
[247] Manson JH, Colditz GA, Stampfer MJ, Willet WC, Krolewski AS, Rosner B, Arky RA, Speizer FE, Hennekens CH. A prospective study of maturity onset diabetes mellitus and risk of coronary heart disease and stroke in women. Arch Intern Med 1991; 151: 1141–7.

[248] Moss SE, Klein R, Klein BE. Cause specific mortality in a population-based study of diabetes. Am J Publ Health 1991; 81: 1158–62.
[249] Hanefeld M, Fischer S, Julius U, Schulze J, Schwanebeck U, Schmechel H, Ziegelasch HJ, Lindner J, the DIS Group: Risk factors for myocardial infarction and death in newly detected NIDDM: the diabetes intervention study, 11-year follow-up. Diabetologia 1996; 39: 1577–83.
[250] Standl E, Balletshofer B, Dahl B, Weichenhain B, Stiegler H, Hörmann A, Holle R. Predictors of 10 year macrovascular and overall mortality in patients with NIDDM: the Munich General Practitioner Project. Diabetologia 1996; 39: 1540–5.
[251] Turner RC, Millns J, Neil HAW, Stratton IM, Mauley SF, Matthews DR, Holman RR, for the United Kingdom Prospective Diabetes Study Group. Risk factors for coronary artery disease in non-insulin-dependent diabetes mellitus: United Kingdom Prospective Diabetes Study (UKPDS 23). BMJ 1998; 316: 823–8.
[252] Kwaan HC. Changes in blood coagulation, platelet function, and plasminogen-plasmin system in diabetes. Diabetes 1992; 41 (suppl 2): 32–5.
[253] Vague P, Raccah D, Yuhan Vague I. Hemobiology, vascular disease, and diabetes with special reference to impaired fibrinolysis. Metabolism 1992; 41: 2–6.
[254] Colwell JA. Vascular thrombosis in type II diabetes mellitus. Diabetes 1993; 42: 8–11.
[255] Carter AM, Grant PJ. Vascular homeostasis, adhesion molecules, and macrovascular disease in non-insulin-dependent diabetes mellitus. Diabet Med 1997; 14: 423–32.
[256] Ceriello A, Giuliano D, Quatraro A, Marchi F, Barbanti M, Lefebvre P. Evidence for a hyperglycaemia-dependent decrease of antithrombin III-thrombin complex formation in humans. Diabetologia 1990; 33: 163–7.
[257] Ceriello A. Coagulation activation in diabetes mellitus: the role of hyperglycaemia and therapeutic prospects. Diabetologia 1993; 36: 1119–25.
[258] Panahloo A, Mohamed-Ali V, Lane A, Green F, Humphries SE, Yudkin JS. Determinants of plasminogen activator inhibitor-1 in treated type II diabetes and its relation to a polymorphism in the plasminogen activator inhibitor-1 gene. Diabetes 1995; 44: 37–42.
[259] Tschöpe D, Rösen P, Esser J, Schwippert B, Nieuvenhuis HK, Kehrel B, Gries FA. Large platelets circulation in an activated state in diabetes mellitus. Semin Thrombos Hemost 1991; 17: 433–8.
[260] Tschöpe D, Rösen D, Schwippert B, Gries FA. Platelets in diabetes: the role in the hemostatic regulation in atherosclerosis. Sem Thromb Hemostas 1993; 19: 122–8.
[261] Lupu C, Calb M, Ionescu M, Lupu F. Enhanced prothrombin and intrinsic factor X activation on blood platelets from diabetic patients. Thrombos Haemost 1993; 70: 579–83.
[262] Tschöpe D, Rösen P, Gries FA. The role of the megakaryocyte-platelet system for diabetic angiopathy: is metabolic control preventive therapy enough? Thromb Haemorrh Disorders 1992; 6: 1–8.
[263] Tschöpe D, Lampeter E, Schwippert B. Megakaryocytes and platelets in diabetes mellitus. Hämostaseologie 1996; 16: 144–50.
[264] Watanabe J, Wohltmann HJ, Klein RL, Colwell JA, Lopes-Virella MF. Enhancement of platelet aggregation by low density lipoprotein in patients with diabetes mellitus. Diabetes 1988; 37: 1652–7.
[265] Davi G, Catalano J, Averna M, Notarbartolo A, Strano A, Ciabattoni G, Patrono C. Thromboxane biosynthesis and platelet function in type II diabetes mellitus. N Engl J Med 1990; 322: 1769–74.
[266] Rauch U, Tschöpe D, Piolot R, Schwippert B, Benthake H, Ziegler D, Gries FA. Circulating inflammatory leukocyte-platelet co-aggregates associated with diabetic cardiovascular autonomic neuropathy [abstract]. Circulation 1995; 92 (suppl): 638.
[267] Tschöpe D, Hesse S, Rauch U, Schwippert B. Monocyte-platelet co-aggregation is associated with low HDL/high triglyceride dyslipoproteinaemia in NIDDM patients [abstract]. Diabetes 1996; 45 (suppl 2): 270A.
[268] Fuster V, Badimon L, Badimon JJ, Chesebro JH. The pathogenesis of coronary artery disease and the acute coronary syndromes. N Engl J Med 1992; 326: 242–50.
[269] Feener ED, King GL. Vascular dysfunction in diabetes mellitus. Lancet 1997; 350 (suppl I): SI9–13.
[270] Clarkson P, Celermajor DS, Donald AE, Sampson M, Sorenson KE, Adams M, Yue DK, Betteridge DJ, Deanfield JE. Impaired vascular reactivity in insulin-dependent diabetes mellitus is related to disease duration and low density lipoprotein cholesterol levels. Am J Coll Cardiol 1996; 28: 573–9.
[271] Cohen RA. Dysfunction of vascular endothelium in diabetes mellitus. Circulation 1993; 87 (suppl 5): 67–76.
[272] Lorenzi M. Glucose toxicity in the vascular complications of diabetes: the cellular perspective. Diab Metab Rev 1992; 8: 85–103.
[273] Laasko M, Lehto S, Penttila J, Pyörälä K. Lipids and lipoproteins predicting coronary heart disease mortality and morbidity in patients with non-insulin-dependent diabetes.Circulation 1993; 88: 1421–30.
[274] Stern MP, Haffner SM. Dyslipidemia in type 2 diabetes: implications for therapeutic intervention. Diabetes Care 1991; 14: 1144–59.
[275] International Task Force for Prevention of Coronary Heart Disease. Recommendations of the European Atherosclerosis Society: Prevention of coronary heart disease: scientific background and new clinical guidelines. Nutr Metab Cardiovasc Dis 1992; 2: 113–56.
[276] Laakso M. Epidemiology of diabetic dyslipidaemia. Diabetes Rev 1995; 3: 408–22.
[277] Manninen V, Tenkanen H, Koskinen P, Huttunen JK, Mäntari M, Heimonen OP, Frick MH. Joint effects of triglycerides and LDL cholesterol and HDL cholesterol concentrations on coronary heart disease risk in the Helsinki Heart Study. Implications for treatment. Circulation 1992; 85: 37–45.
[278] Hokanson JE, Austin MA. Triglyceride is a risk factor for coronary disease in men and women: a meta analysis of population based prospective studies [abstract]. Circulation 1993; 88: 510.
[279] Zilversmit DB. Atherogenesis: a postprandial phenomenon. Circulation 1979; 60: 473–85.
[280] Patsch JR, Miesenbeck G, Hopferwieser T, Hijhtberger V, Knapp E, Dunn KJ, Gotto AM, Patsch W. Relationship of triglyceride metabolism and coronary artery disease: studies in the postprandial state. Arterioscler Thromb 1992; 12: 1336–45.
[281] Tan KCB, Cooper MB, Ling KL, Griffin BA, Freeman DJ, Packard CJ, Shepherd J, Hales CN, Betteridge DJ. Fasting and postprandial determinants for the occurrence of small dense LDL species in non insulin dependent diabetic patients with and without hypertriglyceridaemia: the involvement of insulin, insulin precursor species and insulin resistance. Atherosclerosis 1995; 113: 273–87.
[282] Taskinen MR, Kuusi T, Helve E, Nikkila K, Yki-Järvinen H. Insulin therapy induces antiatherogenic changes of serum lipoproteins in non-insulin-dependent diabetes. Arteriosclerosis 1988; 8: 168–77.
[283] Winocour PH, Durrington PN, Irhola M, Hillier VF, Anderson DC. The prevalence of hyperlipidaemia and related clinical features in insulin-dependent diabetes mellitus. Q J Med 1989; 70: 265–76.
[284] Haaber AB, Kofoed-Enevoldsen A, Jensen T. The prevalence of hypercholesterolaemia and its relationship with albuminuria in insulin-dependent diabetic patients: an epidemiological study. Diabet Med 1992; 9: 557–61.
[285] Walden CE, Knopp RH, Wahl PW, Beach KW, Strandness E. Sex differences in the effect of diabetes mellitus on lipoprotein, triglyceride, and cholesterol concentrations. N Engl J Med 1984; 311: 953–9.
[286] Haffner SM, Mykkanen L, Stern MP, Paidi M, Howard BV. Greater effect of diabetes on LDL size in women than in men. Diabetes Care 1994; 17: 1164–71.
[287] Lopes-Virella MF, Virella G. Cytokines, modified lipoproteins, and arteriosclerosis in diabetes. Diabetes 1996; 45 (suppl 3): S40–4.
[288] Witztum JL. Role of modified lipoproteins in diabetic macroangiopathy. Diabetes 1997; 46 (suppl 2): S112–14.
[289] Lahdenperä S, Syränne M, Kahri J, Taskinen MR. Regulation of low-density lipoprotein particle size distribution in NIDDM and coronary disease: importance of serum triglycerides. Diabetologia 1996; 39: 453–61.

[290] Taskinen MR, Smith U. Lipid disorders in NIDDM: implications for treatment. J Intern Med 1998; 244: 361–70.
[291] Austin MA, Breslow JL, Hennekens CH, Buring JE, Willet WC, Krause RM. Low density lipoprotein subclass patterns and risk of myocardial infarction. JAMA 1988; 260: 1917–21.
[292] Graaf J De, Hak-Lemmers HLM, Hectors MPC, Demacker PNM, Hendricks JCM, Stalenhoef AFH. Enhanced susceptibility to in vitro oxidation of the dense low density lipoprotein subfraction in healthy subjects. Arterioscler Thromb 1991; 11: 298–306.
[293] Stewart MW, Laker MF, Dyer RG, et al. Lipoprotein compositional abnormalities and insulin resistance in type 2 diabetic patients with mild hyperlipidaemia. Arterioscler Thromb 1993; 13: 1046–52.
[294] Selby JV, Austin MA, Newman B, Zhang D, Quesenberry CP, Mayer EJ, Krauss RM. LDL subclass phenotypes and the insulin resistance syndrome in women. Circulation 1993; 88: 381–7.
[295] Grundy AM. Small LDL, atherogenic dyslipidaemia, and the metabolic syndrome. Circulation 1997; 95: 1–4.
[296] Gordon DJ, Probstfield JL, Garrison RJ, Neaton JD, Castelli WP, Knoke JD, Jacobs DR, Bangdiwala S, Tyroler A. High density lipoproteincholesterol and cardiovascular disease: four prospective American studies. Circulation 1989; 79: 8–15.
[297] Rönnemaa T, Laakso M, Kallio V, Pyörälä K, Marniemi J, Puukka P. Serum lipids, lipoproteins and apolipoproteins and the excessive occurrence of coronary heart disease in non-insulin-dependent diabetic patients. Am J Epidemiol 1989; 130: 632–45.
[298] Howard BV. Lipoprotein metabolism in diabetes. Curr Opin Lipidol 1994; 5: 216–20.
[299] Steinberg D, Parthasarathy S, Carew TE, Khou JC, Witztum JL. Beyond cholesterol: modifications of low density lipoprotein that increase its atherogenicity. N Engl J Med 1989; 320: 913–24.
[300] Nagi DK, Hendra TJ, Ryle AJ, Cooper TM, Temple RC, Clark PMS, Schneider AE, Hales CN, Yudkin JS. The relationships of concentrations of insulin, intact proinsulin and 32-33 split proinsulin with cardiovascular risk factors in type 2 (non-insulin-dependent) diabetic subjects. Diabetologia 1990; 33: 532–7.
[301] Panahloo A, Mohamed-Ali V, Lane A, Green F, Humphries SE, Yudkin JS. Determinants of plasminogen activator inhibitor-1 in treated type II diabetes and its relation to a polymorphism in the plasminogen activator inhibitor-1 gene. Diabetes 1995; 44: 37–42.
[302] Mann JFE, Gerstein HC, Pogue J, Bosch J, Yusuf S, for the HOPE Investigators. Renal insufficiency as a predictor of cardiovascular outcomes and the impact of ramipril: the HOPE randomized trial. Ann Intern Med 2001; 134: 629–36.
[303] Antiplatelet Trialists' Collaboration. Collaborative overview of randomized trials of antiplatelet therapy, I: Prevention of death, myocardial infarction, and stroke by prolonged antiplatelet therapy in various categories of patients. BMJ 1994; 308: 81–106.
[304] Colwell JA. Aspirin therapy in diabetes. Diabetes Care 1997; 20: 1767–71.
[305] Malmberg K, Herlitz J, Hjalmarson A, Ryden L. Effect of metoprolol on mortality and late infarction in diabetics with suspected acute myocardial infarction: retrospective data from two large studies. Eur Heart J 1989; 10: 423–8.
[306] Pfeffer MA, Braunwald E, Moye LA, Basta L, Brown EJ, Cuddy TE, Davis BR, Geltman EM, Goldman S, Flaker GC, Klein M, Lamas GA, Packer M, Rouleau J, Rouleau JL, Rutherford J, Wertheimer JH, Hawkins C, on behalf of the SAVE Investigators. Effect of captopril on mortality and morbidity in patients with left ventricular dysfunction after myocardial infarction: results of the survival and left ventricular enlargement trial. N Engl J Med 1992; 327: 669–77.
[307] Ball SG, on behalf of the AIRE Study Group. Effect of ramipril on mortality and morbidity of survivors of acute myocardial infarction with clinical evidence of heart failure: the acute infarction ramipril efficacy (AIRE) study. Lancet 1993; 342: 821–8.
[308] Yudkin JS. How can we best prolong life? Benefits of coronary risk factor reduction in non-diabetic and diabetic subjects. BMJ 1993; 306: 1313–8.
[309] Smith DA. Comparative approaches to risk reduction of coronary heart disease in Tecumseh non-insulin-dependent diabetic population. Diabetes Care 1986; 9: 601–8.
[310] Stamler J, Vaccaro O, Neaton JD, Wentworth D, for the Multiple Risk Factor Intervention Trial Research Group. Diabetes, other risk factors and 12-year cardiovascular mortality for men screened in the Multiple Risk Factor Intervention Trial. Diabetes Care 1993; 16: 434–44.
[311] Smith JW, Marcus FE, Serokman R. Prognosis of patients with diabetes mellitus after myocardial infarction. Am J Cardiol 1984; 54: 718–21.
[312] Karlson BW, Herlitz J, Hjalmarson A. Prognosis of acute myocardial infarction in diabetic and non-diabetic patients. Diabet Med 1993; 10: 449–54.
[313] Löwel H, Dinkel R, Hörmann A, Stieber J, Görtler E. Herzinfarkt und Diabetes: Ergebnisse der Augsburger Herzinfarkt-Follow-up Studie 1985–1993. Diabetes Stoffw 1996; 5 (suppl 1): 19–23.
[314] Scheidt-Nave C, Barrett-Connor E, Wingard DL. Resting electrocardiographic abnormalities suggestive of asymptomatic ischaemic heart disease associated with non insulin dependent diabetes mellitus in a defined population. Circulation 1990; 81: 899–906.
[315] Weiner DA, Ryan TJ, Parsons L, Fisher LD, Chaitman BR, Sheffield LT, Tristani FE. Significance of silent myocardial ischaemia during exercise testing in patients with diabetes mellitus: a report from the Coronary Artery Surgery Study (CASS) Registry. Am J Cardiol 1991; 68: 729–34.
[316] Airaksinen KEJ. Silent coronary artery disease in diabetes—a feature of autonomic neuropathy or accelerated atherosclerosis? Diabetologia 2001; 44: 259–66.
[317] Oswald GA, Corcoran S, Yudkin JS. Prevalence and risk of hyperglycaemia and undiagnosed diabetes in patients with acute myocardial infarction. Lancet 1984; i: 1264–7.
[318] Fava S, Aquilina O, Azzopardi J, Muscat HA, Fenech FF. The prognostic value of blood glucose in diabetic patients with acute myocardial infarction. Diabet Med 1996; 13: 80–3.
[319] Lawson EB, Zinman B. The effect of intensive insulin therapy on macrovascular disease in type 1 diabetes: a systematic review and metaanalysis. Diabetes Care 1998; 21: 82–7.
[320] Singer DE, Nathan DM, Andersson KM, Wilson PWF, Evans JC. Association of HbA1c with prevalent cardiovascular disease in the original cohort of the Framingham Heart Study. Diabetes 1992; 41: 202–8.
[321] Malmberg K, Norhammar A, Wedel H, Ryden L. Glycometabolic state at admission: important risk marker of mortality in conventionally treated patients with diabetes mellitus and myocardial infarction: long-term results from the diabetes and insulin-glucose infusion in acute myocardial infarction (DIGAMI) study. Circulation 1999; 99: 2626–32.
[322] Gray RP, Yudkin JS, Patterson DLH. Enzymatic evidence of impaired reperfusion in diabetic subjects after thrombolytic therapy for acute myocardial infarction—a role for plasminogen activator inhibitor ? Br Heart J 1993; 70: 530–6.
[323] Fibrinolytic Therapy Trialists (FTT) Collaborative Group. Indications for fibrinolytic therapy in suspected acute myocardial infarction: collaborative overview of early mortality and major morbidity results from all randomized trials of more than 1000 patients. Lancet 1994; 343: 311–22.
[324] Barzilay JI, Kronmal RA, Bittner V, Eaker E, Evans C, Forster ED. Coronary artery disease and coronary artery bypass grafting in diabetic patients aged ≥65 years: report from the Coronary Artery Surgery Study (CASS) Registry. Am J Cardiol 1994; 74: 334–9.
[325] Rahimtoola SH, Bennet AJ, Grunkemeier GL, Block P, Starr A. Survival at 15–18 years after coronary bypass grafting for angina in women. Circulation 1993; 88: 71–8.
[326] Carrozza JP, Kuntz RE, Fishman RF, Banin DS. Restenosis after arterial injury caused by coronary stenting in patients with diabetes mellitus. Ann Intern Med 1993; 118: 344–9.
[327] Risum O, Abdelnoor M, Svennevig JL, Levorstad K, Gullestad L, Bjornerheim R, Simonson S, Nitter-Hange S. Diabetes mellitus and morbidity and mortality risks after coronary artery bypass surgery. Scand J Thor Cardiovasc Surg 1996; 30: 71–5.

[328] BARI Investigators. Influence of diabetes on 5-year mortality and morbidity in a randomized trial comparing CABG and PTCA in patients with multivessel disease. Circulation 1997; 96: 1761–9.
[329] Abizaid A, Kornowski R, Mintz GS, Hong MK, Abizaid AS, Mehran R, Pichard AD, Kent KM, Satler LF, Wu H, Popma JJ, Leon MB. The influence of diabetes mellitus on acute and late clinical outcomes following coronary stent implantation. J Am Coll Cardiol 1998; 32: 584–9.
[330] Thourami WH, Weintraub WS, Stein B, Gebhart SSP, Craver JM, Jones EL, Guyton RA. Influence of diabetes mellitus on early and late outcome after coronary artery bypass grafting. Ann Thorac Surg 1999; 67: 1045–52.
[331] Nitenberg A, Valensi P, Sachs R, Dali M, Aptecar E, Attali J-R. Impairment of coronary reserve and Ach-induced coronary vasodilation in diabetic patients with angiopathically normal coronary arteries and normal left ventricular systolic function. Diabetes 1993; 42: 1017–25.
[332] Strauer BE, Motz W, Vogt M, Schwarztkopff B. Impaired coronary flow reserve in NIDDM. A possible role for diabetic cardiopathy in humans. Diabetes 1997; 46 (suppl 2): S119–24.
[333] Schernthaner G. Progress in the immunointervention of type 1 diabetes mellitus. Horm Metab Res 1995; 27: 547–54.
[334] Becker DJ, LaPorte RE, Libman I, Pietropaolo M, Dosch HM. Prevention of type 1 diabetes: is now the time ? J Clin Endocrin Metab 2000; 85: 498–506.
[335] Helmrich SP, Ragland DR, Leung RW, Paffenbarger RS. Physical activity and reduced occurrence of non-insulin-dependent diabetes mellitus. N Engl J Med 1991; 325: 147–52.
[336] Eriksson KF, Lindgräde F. Prevention of type II (non-insulin-dependent) diabetes mellitus by diet and physical exercise. Diabetologia 1991; 34: 891–8.
[337] Tuomilethto J, Lindström J, Eriksson JG, Valle TT, Hämäläinen H, Ilanne-Parikka P, Keinänen-Kinkaanniemi S, Uusitupa M, for the Finnish Diabetes Prevention Study Group. Prevention of type 2 diabetes mellitus by changes in lifestyle among subjects with impaired glucose tolerance. N Engl J Med 2001; 344: 1343–50.
[338] Hu FB, Manson JE, Stampfer MJ, Colditz G, Liu S, Solomon CG, Willett WC. Diet, lifestyle, and the risk of type 2 diabetes mellitus in women. N Engl J Med 2001; 345: 790–7.
[339] King H, Dowd JE. Primary prevention of type 2 (non-insulin-dependent) diabetes mellitus. Diabetologia 1990; 33: 3–8.
[340] Chiasson JL. Konzepte für primäre Prävention des nicht insulinabhängigen Diabetes mellitus (NIDDM). In: Hanefeld M, Leonhardt W, editors. Das metabolische Syndrom. Stuttgart: Gustav Fischer Verlag; 1996:89–95.
[341] Hanefeld M, Temelkowa-Kurktschiev T. The postprandial state and the risk of atherosclerosis. Diabet Med 1997; 14: S6–11.
[342] Shaw JE, Hodge AM, deCourten M, Chatson P, Zimmett PZ. Isolated post-challenge hyperglycaemia confirmed as a risk factor for mortality. Diabetologia 1999; 42: 1050–4.
[343] Berghe G van den, Wouters P, Weekers F, Verwaest C, Bruyninckx F, Schetz M, Vlasselaers D, Ferdinande P, Lauwers P, Bouillon R. Intensive insulin therapy in critically ill patients. N Engl J Med 2001; 345: 1359–67.
[344] Deutsche Diabetes Gesellschaft. Evidenzbasierte Diabetes-Leitlinie DDG—Diskussionsentwurf: Therapieziele und Behandlungsstrategien beim Diabetes mellitus. Diabetes Stoffw 1999; 8 (suppl 3): 25–36.
[345] Gries FA. Das Arzt-Patienten-Verhältnis bestimmt das Krankheitserlebnis und Management des Diabetes mellitus. In: Herpertz S, Paust R, editors. Psychosoziale Aspekete in Diagnostik und Therapie des Diabetes mellitus. Lengerich, Berlin: Pabst Science Publ; 1999: 125–36.
[346] Skinner TC, Cradock S. Empowerment: what about the evidence ? Pract Diab Int 2000; 17: 91–5.
[347] Assal JP, Mühlhauser I, Pernet A, Gfeller R, Jörgens V, Berger M. Patient education as the basis for diabetes care in clinical practice and research. Diabetologia 1985; 28: 602–13.
[348] Berger M, Jörgens V, Mühlhauser J, Zimmermann H. Die Bedeutung der Diabetikschulung in der Therapie des Typ 1 Diabetes. Dtsch Med Wochenschr 1983; 109: 424–30.
[349] The Diabetes and Nutrition Study Group (DNSG) of the European Association for the Study of Diabetes (EASD). Recommendations for the nutritional management of patients with diabetes mellitus. Eur J Clin Nutrit 2000; 54: 353–5.
[350] Grüsser M, Bott U, Eltermann P, Kronsbein P, Jörgens V. Evaluation of a structured treatment and teaching program for non-insulin-treated type II diabetic outpatients in Germany after introduction of nationwide financing. Diabetes Care 1993; 16: 1268–75.
[351] Lepore M, Pampanelli S, Fanelli C, Porcellati F, Bartocci L, diVincenzo A, Cordoni C, Costa E, Brunetti P, Bolli GB. Pharmakokinetics and pharmacodynamics of subcutaneous injection of long-acting human insulin analog glargine, NPH insulin, and ultralente human insulin and continuous subcutaneous infusion of insulin lispro. Diabetes 2000; 49: 2142–8.
[352] Andersen JH, Brunelle RL, Keohane P, Koivisto VA, Trautmann ME, Vignati L, DiMardi R. Mealtime treatment with insulin analog improves postprandial hyperglycemia and hypoglycemia in patients with non-insulin dependent diabetes mellitus. Arch Intern Med 1997; 157: 1249–55.
[353] Andersen JH, Brunelle RL, Koivisto VA, Trautmann ME, Vignati L, DiMardi R, Multicenter Insulin Lispro Study Group. Improved mealtime treatment of diabetes mellitus using an insulin analogue. Clin Ther 1997; 19: 62–71.
[354] Heinemann L. Hypoglycaemia and insulin analogues: is there a reduction in the incidence? J Diabetes Complications 1999; 13: 105–14.
[355] Renner R, Pfützner A, Trautmann M, Harzer O, Santer K. Landgraf R, on behalf of the German Humalog-CSII Study Group. Use of insulin lispro in continuous subcutaneous insulin infusion treatment: results of a multicenter trial. Diabetes Care 1999; 22: 784–8.
[356] Skyler JS, Cefalu WT, Kourides IA, Landschulz WH, Balagtas CC, Cheng S-L. Gelfand RA, for the Inhaled Insulin Phase II Study Group: Efficacy of inhaled human insulin in type 1 diabetes mellitus: a randomised proof-of-concept study. Lancet 2001; 357: 331–5.
[357] Cefalu WT, Skyler JS, Kourides IA, Landschulz WH, Balagtas CC, Cheng S-L, Galfand RA, for the Inhaled Insulin Study Group. Inhaled human insulin treatment in patients with type 2 diabetes mellitus. Ann Intern Med 2001; 134: 203–7.
[358] Gale EAM. Two cheers for inhaled insulin. Lancet 2001; 357: 324–5.
[359] Nathan DM. Inhaled insulin for type 2 diabetes: solution or distraction? Ann Intern Med 2001; 134: 242–4.
[360] Hansen BF, Danielsen GM, Drejer K, Sörensen AR, Wiberg FC, Klein HH, Lundemore AG. Sustained signalling from the insulin receptor after stimulation with insulin analogues exhibiting increased mitogenic potency. Biochem J 1996; 315: 271–9.
[361] Slieker LJ, Brooke GS, DiMarchi RD, Flora DB, Green LK, Hoffmann JA, Long HB, Fan L, Shields JE, Sundell KL, Surface PL, Chance RE. Modifications in the B10 and B26- 30 regions of the B chain of human insulin alter affinity for the human IGF-1 receptor more than for the insulin receptor. Diabetologia 1997; 40: S54–61.
[362] Kurtzhals P, Schäffer L, Sörensen A, Kristensen C, Jonassen J, Schmid C, Trüb T. Correlations of receptorbinding and metabolic and mitogenic potencies of insulin analogs designed for clinical use. Diabetes 2000; 49: 999–1005.
[363] Fölsch UR, Ebert R, Creutzfeldt W. Response of serum levels of gastric inhibitory polypeptide and insulin to sucrose ingestion during long-term application of acarbose. Scand J Gastroenterol 1981; 16: 629–32.
[364] Chiasson JL, Josse RG, Leiter LA, Mihic M, Nathan DM, Palmason C, Cohen RM, Wolever TMS. The effect of acarbose on insulin sensitivity in subjects with impaired glucose tolerance. Diabetes Care 1996; 19: 1190–3.
[365] Lebowitz HE. α-Glucosidase inhibitors as agents in the treatment of diabetes. Diabetes Rev 1998; 6: 132–45.
[366] Mertes G. Efficacy and safety of acarbose in the type 2 diabetes: data from a 2-year surveillance study. Diabetes Res Clin Pract 1998; 40: 63–70.
[367] Pinol C, Guardiola E, Soler J, Cano F, Hernandez-Mijares A, Jimenez A, Leiva A de, Arroyo JA. A double blind, randomised, placebo controlled study to assess the maximum insulin dose reduction achieved with acarbose in the

treatment of insulin-requiring type 2 diabetic patients. Diabetes Nutr Metab 1998; 11: 242–8.
[368] Holman RR, Cull CA, Turner RC on behalf of the UK PDS Study Group. A randomized double-blind trial of acarbose in type 2 diabetes shows improved glycemic control over 3 years (UK Prospective Diabetes Study 44). Diabetes Care 1999; 22: 960–4.
[369] DeFronzo RA, Barzilai N, Simonson D. Mechanisms of metformin action in obese and lean non-insulin-dependent diabetic subjects. J Clin Endocrinol Metab 1991; 73: 1294–301.
[370] Stumvoll M, Nurjhan N, Periello G, Dailey G, Geriah JE. Metabolic effects of metformin in non-insulin-dependent diabetes mellitus. N Engl J Med 1995; 333: 550–4.
[371] DeFronzo RA, Goodman AM, the Multicenter Metformin Study Group. Efficacy of metformin in patients with non-insulin-dependent diabetes mellitus. N Engl J Med 1995; 333: 541–9.
[372] Johansen K. Efficacy of metformin in the treatment of NIDDM: metaanalysis. Diabetes Care 1999; 22: 33–7.
[373] Inzucchi SE, Maggs DG, Spollett GR, Page SL, Rife FS, Walton V, Shulman GI. Efficacy and metabolic effects of metformin and troglitazone in type II diabetes mellitus. N Engl J Med 1998; 338: 867–72.
[374] Hirschberg Y, Karara AH, Pietri AO, McLeod JF. Improved control of mealtime glucose excursions with coadministration of nateglinide and metformin: a randomized, placebo controlled crossover study. Diabetes Care 2000; 23: 349–53.
[375] Olsson J, Lindberg G, Gottsäter M, Lindwall K, Sjöstrand A, Tisell A, Melander A. Increased mortality in type 2 diabetic patients using sulfonylurea and metformin in combination: a population based observational study. Diabetologia 2000; 43: 558–60.
[376] Bailey CJ, Grant PJ, Evans M, deFine Olivarius N, Andreasen AH, Fowler PBS, Good CB, Turner RC, Holman R, Stratton I, Kerner W. The UK Prospective Diabetes Study Correspondence. Lancet 1998; 352: 1932–4.
[377] American Diabetes Association. Implications of the United Kingdom Prospective Diabetes Study. Diabetes Care 2000; 23 (suppl 1): S 27–31.
[378] Shapiro ET, Cauter E van, Tillil H, et al. Glyburide enhances the responsiveness of the B-cell to glucose but does not corect the abnormal patterns of insulin secretion in non insulin-dependent diabetes mellitus. J Clin Endocrinol Metab 1989; 69: 571–6.
[379] Groop LC, Ratheiser K, Luzi L. Effect of sulfonylurea on glucose-stimulated insulin secretion in healthy and non-insulin dependent diabetic subjects: a dose response study. Acta Diabetol 1991; 28: 162–8.
[380] Groop L, Neugebauer G. Clinical pharmacology of sulfonylureas. In: Kuhlmann J, Puls W, editors. Oral antidiabetics. Berlin Heidelberg New York: Springer-Verlag; 1996: 199–262.
[381] Lotz N, Bachmann W. Kombinationstherapie. In: Mehnert H, Standl E, Usadel KH, editors. Diabetologie in Klinik und Praxis. Stuttgart New York: Thieme; 1999: 212–18.
[382] S 52 Sulfanylharnstoffe (orale Antidiabetika). In: Rote Liste 2002. Aulendorf: Editio Cantor Verlag 2002: 367–8.
[383] Forth W, Henschler D, Rummel W, Starke K, editors. Pharmakologie und Toxikologie, 7th ed. Berlin Oxford Heidelberg: Spektrum; 1996: 570.
[384] Oliver S, Ahmad S. Pharmacokinetics and bioavailability of repaglinide, a new oral antidiabetic agent for patients with type-2 diabetes [abstract]. Diabetologia 1997; 40 (suppl) A1260.
[385] Weaver ML, Orwig BA, Rodrigues LC, Graham ED, Chin JA, Shapiro MJ, McLeod JF, Mangold JB. Pharmacokinetics and metabolism of nateglinide in humans. Drug Metab Dispos 2001; 29: 415–21.
[386] Fuhlendorf J, Rorsman P, Kofod H, Brand CL, Rolin B, MacKay P, Shymko R, Carr RD. Stimulation of insulin release by repaglinide and glibenclamide involves both common and distinct processes. Diabetes 1998; 47: 345–51.
[387] Hu S, Wang S, Fanelli B, Bell PA, Dunning BE, Geisse S, Schmitz R, Boettcher BR. Pancreatic β-cell K_{ATP} channel activity and membrane-binding studies with nateglinide: a comparison with sulfonylureas and repaglinide. J Pharm Exper Ther 2000; 293: 444–52.
[388] Whitelaw DC, Clark PM, Smith JM, Nattrass M. Effects of the new oral hypoglycaemic agent nateglinide in insulin secretion in type 2 diabetes mellitus. Diabetes Med 2000; 17: 225–9.
[389] Hollander PA, Schwartz SL, Gatlin MR, Haas SJ, Zheng H, Foley JE, Dunning BE. Importance of early insulin secretion. Comparison of nateglinide and glyburide in previous diet-treated patients with type 2 diabetes. Diabetes Care 2001; 24: 983–8.
[390] Massi-Benedetti M, Damsbo P. Pharmacology and clinical experience with repaglinide. Exp Opin Invest Drugs 2000; 9: 885–98.
[391] Horton ES, Clinkingbeard C, Gatlin M, Foley J, Mallows S, Shen S. Nateglinide alone and in combination with metformin improves glycemic control by reducing mealtime glucose levels in type 2 diabetes. Diabetes Care 2000; 23: 1660–5.
[392] Hirschberg Y, Karara AH, Pietri AO, McLeod JF. Improved control of mealtime glucose excursions with coadministration of nateglinide and metformin. Diabetes Care 2000; 23: 349–53.
[393] Moses R, Slobodniuk R, Boyages S, Colagiuri S, Kidson W, Carter J, Donnelly T, Moffitt P, Hopkins H. Effect of repaglinide addition to metformin monotherapy on glycemic control in patients with type 2 diabetes. Diabetes Care 1999; 22: 119–24.
[394] Day C. Thiazolidindiones: a new class of antidiabetic drugs. Diabet Med 1999; 16: 179–92.
[395] Matthaei S, Stumvoll M, Häring HU. Thiazolidindione (Insulinsensitizer): Neue Aspekte in der Therapie des Diabetes mellitus Typ 2. Dtsch Ärztebl 2001; 98: 912–8.
[396] Maegawa H, Tachikawa-Ide R, Ugi S, Iwanishi M, Egawa K, Kikkawa R, Shigeta Y, Kashiwagi A. Pioglitazone ameliorates highly glucose induced desensitation of insulin receptor kinase in rat 1 fibroblasts in culture. Biochem Biophys Res Commun 1993; 197: 1078–82.
[397] Sandouk T, Reda D, Hofmann C. The antidiabetic agent pioglitazone increases expression of glucose transporters in 3T3-F442 A cells by increasing messenger ribonucleic acid transcript stability. Endocrinology 1993; 133: 352–9.
[398] Young PW, Cawthorne MA, Coyle PJ, Holder JC, Holman GD, Kozka IJ, Kirkham DM, Lister CA, Smith SA. Repeat treatment of obese mice with BRL 49653, a new and potent insulin sensitizer, enhances insulin action in white adipocytes: association with increased insulin binding and cell surface GLUT-4 as measured by photoaffinity labeling. Diabetes 1995; 44: 1087–92.
[399] Kawamori R, Matsuhisa M, Kinoshita J, Mochizuki K, Niwa M, Arisaka T, Ikeda M, Kubota M, Wada M, Kanda T, Ikebuchi M, Tohdo R, Yamasaki Y. AD-4833 Clamp-OGL Study Group: Pioglitazone enhances splanchnic glucose uptake as well as peripheral glucose uptake in non-insulin-dependent diabetes mellitus. Diabetes Res Clin Pract 1998; 41: 35–43.
[400] Ikeda T, Fujiyama K. The effect of pioglitazone on glucose metabolism and insulin uptake in the perfused liver and hindquarter of high-fructose-fed rats. Metabolism 1998; 47: 1152–5.
[401] DeVos P, Lefebvre AM, Miller SG, Guerre-Millo M, Wong K, Saladin R, Haman LG, Staels B, Briggs MR, Auwerx J. Thiazolidindiones repress ob gene expression in rodents via activation of peroxisome proliferator-activated receptor gamma. J Clin Invest 1996; 98: 1004–9.
[402] Kallen CB, Lazar MA. Antidiabetic thiazolidindiones inhibit leptin (ob) gene expression in 3T3-L1 adipocytes. Proc Natl Acad Sci USA 1996; 93: 5793–6.
[403] Digby JE, Montague CT, Sewter CP, Sanders L, Wilkison WO, O'Rahilly S, Prins JB. Thiazolidindione exposure increases the expression of uncoupling protein 1 in cultured human preadipocytes. Diabetes 1998; 47: 138–41.
[404] Murase K, Odaka H, Suzuki M, Tayuki N, Ikeda H. Pioglitazone time dependently reduces tumor necrosis factor-α level in muscle and improves metabolic abnormalities in Wistar fatty rats. Diabetologia 1998; 41: 257–64.
[405] Grossmann SL, Lessem J. Mechanism and clinical effects of thiazolidindiones. Expert Opin Invest Drug 1997; 6: 1025–40.

[406] Oakes ND, Kennedy CJ, Jenkins AB, Laybutt DR, Chisholm DJ, Kraegan EW. A new antidiabetic agent, BRL 49653, reduces lipid availability and improves insulin action and glucoregulation in the rat. Diabetes 1994; 43: 1203–10.
[407] Gomi-Berthold J, Berthold HK, Weber AA, Seul C, Vetter H, Sachinidis A. Troglitazone and rosiglitazone inhibit the low density lipoprotein-induced vascular smooth muscle cell growth. Exp Clin Endocrinol Diabetes 2001; 109: 203–9.
[408] Salzman A, Patel J. Rosiglitazone is not associated with hepatotoxicity [abstract]. Diabetes 1999; 48 (suppl 1): A95.
[409] Ferman LM, Simmons DA, Diamond RH. Hepatic failure in a patient taking rosiglitazone. Ann Int Med 2000; 132: 118–21.
[410] Al-Salman J, Arjomand H, Kemp DG, Mittal M. Hepatocellular injury in a patient recieving rosiglitazone: a case report. Ann Intern Med 2000; 132: 121–4.
[411] Freid J, Everitt D, Boscia J. Rosiglitazone and hepatic failure [letter]. Ann Intern Med 2000; 132: 164.
[412] Aronof SH, Rosenblatt S, Braithwaite S, Egan SW, Mathisen AL, Schneider RL, the Pioglitazone 001 Study Group. Pioglitazone hydrochloride monotherapy improves glycemic control in the treatment of patients with type 2 diabetes. Diabetes Care 2000; 23: 1605–11.
[413] Gale EAM. Lessons from the glitazones: a story of drug development. Lancet 2001; 357: 1870–5.
[414] Fonseca V, Rosenstock J, Patwardhau R, Salzman A. Effect of metformin and rosiglitazone combination therapy in patients with type 2 diabetes mellitus—a randomized controlled trial. JAMA 2000; 283: 1695–702.
[415] Wolffenbuttel BHR, Gomis R, Squatrito S, Jones MP, Patwardhan RN. Addition of low-dose rosiglitazone to sulfonylurea therapy improves glycaemic control in type 2 diabetic patients. Diabet Med 2000; 17: 40–7.
[416] Buse JB. Pioglitazone in the treatment of type 2 diabetes mellitus: US clinical experience. Exp Clin Endocrinol Diabetes 2000; 108 (suppl 2): S250–5.
[417] Ghazzi MN, Perez JE, Antonui TK, Driscoll JH, Huang SM, Faja BW, the Troglitazone Study Group, Whitcomb RW. Cardiac and glycemic benefits of troglitazone treatment in NIDDM. Diabetes 1997; 46: 433–9.
[418] Williams G. Management of non-insulin-dependent diabetes mellitus. Lancet 1994; 343: 95–100.
[419] Hayward RA, Manning WG, Kaplan SH, Wagner EH, Greenfield S. Starting insulin therapy in patients with type 2 diabetes: effectiveness, complications, and resource utilization. JAMA 1997; 278: 1663–9.
[420] Chow CC, Tsang LWW, Sörensen JP, Cookram CS. Comparison of insulin with or without combination of oral hypoglycemic agents in the treatment of secondary failure in NIDDM patients. Diabetes Care 1995; 18: 307–14.
[421] Pugh JA, Wagner ML, Sawyer J, Ramirez G, Turley M, Friedberg SJ. Is combination sulfonylurea and insulin therapy useful in NIDDM patients: a metaanalysis. Diabetes Care 1992; 15: 953–9.
[422] Bruns W, Melchert J, Fischer S, Köhler C, Julius U, Gudat U, Pfützner A, Frank M, Hanefeld M. Präprandiale komplementäre Insulintherapie bei übergewichtigen Typ 2 Diabetikern mit Normalinsulin oder schnell wirkenden Insulinanalogen (Lispro-Insulin)? Diabet Stoffw 2000; 9: 219–25.
[423] Yki-Järvinen H, Kauppila M, Kujansuu E, Lahti J, Marjanen T, Niskanen L, Rajala S, Ryysy L, Salo S, Seppälä P, Tulokas T, Viikari J, Karjalainen J, Taskinen M-R. Comparison of insulin regimens in patients with non-insulin-dependent diabetes mellitus. N Engl J Med 1992; 327: 1426–33.
[424] Abraira C, Colwell JA, Nuttall FQ, Sawin CT, Johnson Nagel N, Comstock JP, Emanuele NV, Levin SR, Henderson W, Lee HS, VA CSDM Group. Veterans affairs cooperative study on glycemic control and complications in type II diabetes (VA CSDM). Results of the feasibility trial. Diabetes Care 1995; 18: 1113–23.
[425] Bloomgarden ZT. Non-insulin-dependent diabetes mellitus. Diabetes Care 1995; 18: 1215–9.
[426] Wake N, Hisashige A, Katayama T, Kishikawa H, Ohkubo Y, Sakai M, Araki E, Shichiri M. Cost-effectiveness of intensive insulin therapy for type 2 diabetes: a 10 year follow-up of the Kumamoto study. Diabetes Res Clin Pract 2000; 48: 201–10.
[427] Bailey S, Mezitis NHE. Combination therapy with insulin and sulfonylureas for type II diabetes. Diabetes Care 1990; 13: 687–95.
[428] Lebowitz HE, Pasmantier R. Combination insulin–sulfonylurea therapy. Diabetes Care 1990; 13: 667–75.
[429] Pyörälä K, Pedersen TR, Kjekshus J, Faergeman O, Olsson AG, Thorgeirsson G. Cholesterol lowering with simvastatin improves prognosis of diabetic patients with coronary heart disease. A subgroup analysis of the Scandinavian Simvastatin Survival Study (4S). Diabetes Care 1997; 20: 614–20.
[430] Goldberg RB, Mellies MJ, Sacks FM, Moye LA, Howard BV, Howard WJ, Davis BR, Cole TG, Pfeffer MA, Braunwald E, for the CARE Investigators. Cardiovascular events and their reduction with pravastatin in diabetic and glucose intolerant myocardial infarction survivors with average cholesterol levels. Subgroup analysis in the cholesterol and recurrent event (CARE) trial. Circulation 1998; 98: 2513–9.
[431] Gaede P, Vedel P, Parving HH, Pedersen O. Intensified multifactorial intervention in patients with type 2 diabetes mellitus and microalbuminuria: the Steno type 2 randomized study. Lancet 1999; 353: 617–22.
[432] Panzram G. Mortalität und Lebenserwartung des insulinabhängigen Typ 2 Diabetes. Diabetes Dialog 1992; 1: 1–4.
[433] Martin S, Wolf-Eichbaum D, Duinkerken G, Scherbaum WA, Kolb H, Noordzij JG, Roep BO: Development of type 1 diabetes despite severe hereditary B-cell deficiency. New Engl J Med 345: 1036–1040 (2001)
[434] Klein R, Klein BEK, Moss SE, Cruickshank KJ: The Wisconsin Epidemiologic Study of Diabetic Retinopathy. XIV. Ten-year incidence and progression of diabetic retinopathy. Arch Ophthalmol 1994; 112: 1217–28.

2 Structure and Function of the Nervous System

N. E. Cameron and C. J. Mathias

The Somatic Nervous System

N. E. Cameron

Overview

The somatic nervous system is subdivided into motor and sensory components. The motor division is concerned with control of skeletal muscle contraction, and hence of voluntary movement and of posture and reflexes. The somatosensory division is a collection of receptors, tracts, and nuclei that convey the sensations of light touch, vibration, temperature, and pain (nociception) to the consciousness. It also conveys information about movements and position of the body (proprioception and kinesthesia). Somatosensory receptors are found in the skin, muscles, joints, and viscera. In addition to providing sensation, the somatosensory division has a critical role in motor control, through feedback about muscle length and tension, joint position, velocity of muscle and limb movement, and contact with external surfaces. The basic structure and function of the somatic nervous system has been described in numerous physiology, neurology, and neuroscience texts; the reader is referred to two recent books for further information [1,2]. Diabetes affects both the peripheral and the central nervous system (for discussion of the latter see Chapter 5, pages 205–208), although most clinical and scientific interest has focused on the periphery because of the devastating effect on nerve fiber integrity. This section provides an overview of the substrate of the somatic nervous system, with a greater emphasis on peripheral than on central structures.

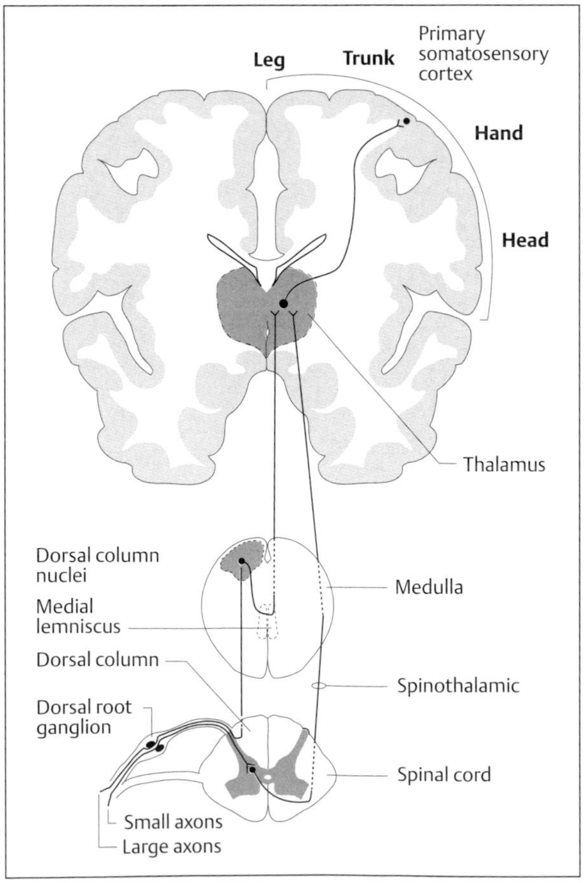

Fig. 2.1 General organization of the somatosensory system, showing the dorsal column–lemniscal system which mediates touch sensation and proprioception, and the spinothalamic system, which deals with temperature and fast pain information

Central Nervous System Pathways

Somatosensory System

There are two major somatosensory pathways running from the spinal cord to the primary sensory area (area 3 or S1) on the postcentral gyrus of the cerebral cortex (Fig. 2.**1**). Information about touch and proprioception is carried in the dorsal column medial lemniscus system, whereas temperature and pain information traverses the spinothalamic pathway [3].

In the touch system, fibers from first-order neurons with cell bodies in the dorsal root ganglia traverse the dorsal columns of the spinal cord (Fig. 2.**1**) to the dorsal column nuclei within the caudal medulla. Of these, the cuneate nucleus receives input from the upper limbs and body whereas the gracile nucleus deals with fibers from the lower limbs. Second-order neurons then project across the midline as the "sensory decussation" and ascend via the medial lemniscus to the ventral posterolateral nucleus of the thalamus. Touch information from the head follows a parallel route, with the first major relay in the principal trigeminal

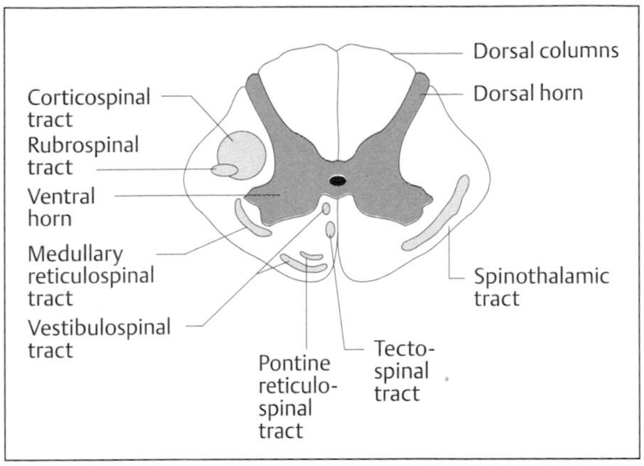

Fig. 2.**2** Schematic cross-section of spinal cord showing the gray matter and white matter containing the major sensory (right) and motor (left) nerve tracts

nucleus of the pons, with mid-pontine decussation to reach the ventral posteromedial nucleus of the thalamus via the ventral trigeminal tract. The inputs from the various regions of the body are segregated and aligned such that the pathway is somatotopically organized. This is reflected by the cortical projection (Fig 2.**1**), where there is an orderly mapping of the contralateral side of the body on the cortical surface.

Information about temperature and pain (particularly the fast component) is transmitted by the spinothalamic tract. Here, the first synaptic relay is in the gray matter of the spinal cord; projection fibers then decussate in the ventral white commissure to form the contralateral spinothalamic (or anterolateral) tract (Fig. 2.**2**). These reach the ventral posterolateral nucleus of the thalamus, and some fibers also project to the small thalamic intralaminar nuclei. Parallel pathways transmit information from the face, via the spinal trigeminal nucleus, to the ventral posteromedial thalamus. The pathway depicted in Figure 2.**1** is also known as the neospinothalamic pathway, and there are other, phylogenetically older pathways transmitting pain information (particularly the slow, poorly localized, long-lasting component). These are the paleospinothalamic and spinoreticulothalamic pathways, which are polysynaptic and ascend through the reticular formation to nonspecific nuclei in the medial thalamus and intralaminar nuclei. They project to widespread regions of cerebral cortex, rather than being associated with the somatotopic organization of the primary sensory cortex: this may contribute to the poor ability to localize slow pain.

Motor System

There are a number of important fiber tracts (Fig. 2.**2**) descending from the brain to control the activity of ventral horn motoneurons supplying the skeletal muscles [2]. These can be divided into lateral and ventromedial groups. The lateral pathway comprises corticospinal and rubrospinal tracts and is primarily involved in voluntary movement, particularly of the distal muscles, under direct cortical control. The ventromedial pathways originate in the brainstem, forming reticulospinal, tectospinal and vestibulospinal tracts, which are involved in the control of posture and locomotion.

The most important component of the lateral pathway is the corticospinal tract, which originates primarily from areas 4 (primary motor cortex or M1) and 6 (supplementary motor area) of the frontal lobe, on the precentral gyrus, located across the central sulcus from the primary somatosensory cortex. The motor cortex is somatotopically organized, and axons pass through the internal capsule and course through the midbrain and pons to form a pyramid-shaped tract running down the ventral surface of the medulla. At the junction with the spinal cord, the pyramidal tract decussates. Thus, as in the somatosensory system, the right motor cortex processes information for the left side of the body and vice versa. The axons from the motor cortex then group to form the lateral corticospinal tract and terminate in the dorsolateral and intermediate gray matter region of the ventral horns, where the motoneurons and interneurons that control the distal muscles are located.

The rubrospinal tract is a much smaller component of the lateral pathway and originates in the red (Latin *ruber*) nucleus of the midbrain. Axons decussate in the pons and join the corticospinal tract in the lateral columns of the spinal cord. The red nucleus itself receives its major input from the motor areas of cerebral cortex, which also give rise to the corticospinal tract. While the rubrospinal tract is important in many mammalian species, in man much of its function has been taken over by the corticospinal pathway.

The ventromedial pathways may be divided functionally into two groups: the tectospinal and vestibulospinal tracts control the posture of head and neck, whereas the pontine and medullary reticulospinal tracts control the posture of the trunk and limb antigravity muscles. The vestibulospinal tract originates in the medullary vestibular nuclei, which are involved with processing sensory activity from the vestibular apparatus of the inner ear. In combination with proprioceptive information about body and neck position, this pathway is importantly involved in maintaining head-body alignment to ensure that the eyes and our image of the world remain stable [4]. The tectospinal tract originates in the superior colliculus of the midbrain. This structure receives direct input from the retina as well as the visual cortex and auditory systems. It is involved with the coordination of head and eye movements and orienting responses towards stimuli [5].

The pontine reticulospinal tract acts to facilitate the antigravity reflexes of the spinal cord to aid the maintenance of a standing posture by promoting extensor activity in the lower limbs and flexor activity in the

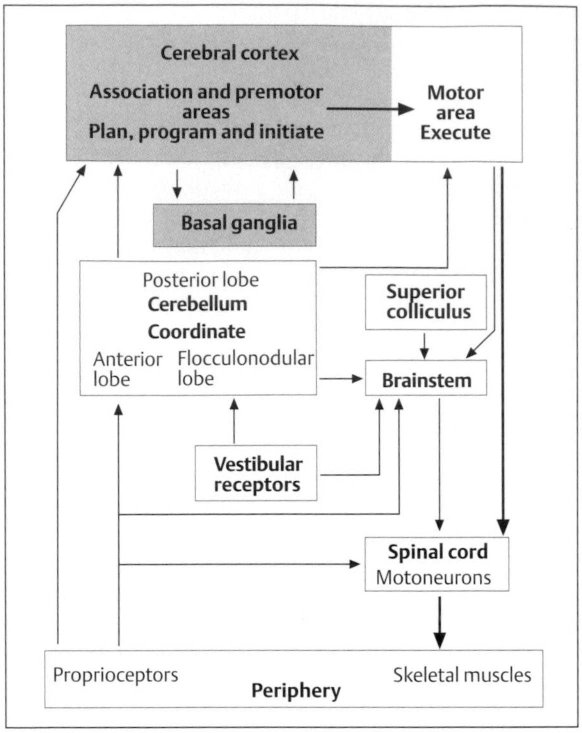

Fig. 2.**3** Schematic of motor control showing the major cortical and subcortical regions of the central nervous system. The association and premotor areas of cerebral cortex, along with the basal ganglia, are responsible for planning and initiating voluntary movements. The motor cortex, and its direct connection with the α-motoneurons in the spinal cord, is responsible for sending the appropriate instructions for execution of the movement by the skeletal muscles. The cerebellum provides information about coordination, sequencing, and timing of complex movements. Brainstem mechanisms, along with the vestibular apparatus, superior colliculus, and older areas of the cerebellum, have a major role in the control of posture and gait

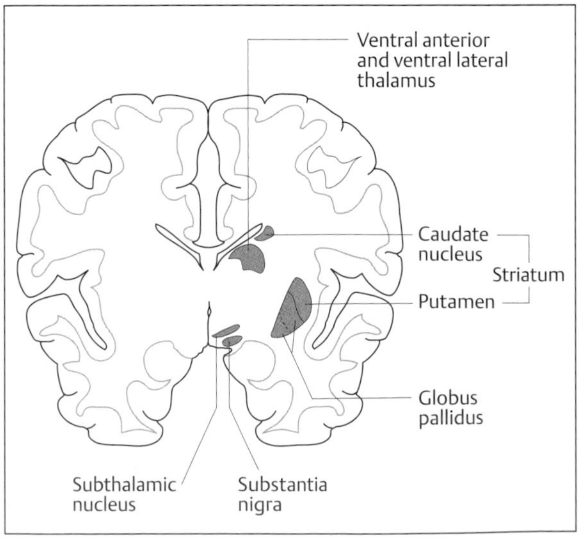

Fig. 2.**4** Cross-section of the brain showing the location of the major nuclei that contribute to basal ganglia function

upper limbs. The medullary reticulospinal tract has an opposite action, to inhibit reflex domination of antigravity muscles, thus allowing greater control by lateral pathways. The balance of activity in these reticulospinal tracts is controlled by descending signals from motor cortex [2].

While cortical areas 4 and 6 comprise the motor cortex, in terms of the control of voluntary movement many other areas of the cerebral cortex are involved as well as important subcortical structures such as the basal ganglia and cerebellum. The overall organization of the motor control system is outlined in Figure 2.**3**. Thus, the processes of planning, programming, and initiating goal-directed movement involve association and premotor cortical areas, including the anterior frontal lobes and regions of the posterior parietal cortex such as area 5, which gets a direct input from somatosensory cortex, and area 7, which receives connections from higher-order visual cortical areas.

The major subcortical input to area 6 of motor cortex arises from the ventral lateral nucleus of the thalamus, which in turn comes from the basal ganglia (Fig. 2.**4**). These comprise the caudate nucleus and the putamen (collectively termed the striatum), the globus pallidus, the subthalamus, and the midbrain substantia nigra. These areas form a complex circuit that funnels or focuses activity from widespread areas of association cortex on to area 6, perhaps supplying basic motor programs for the desired action. This cortex → striatum → globus pallidus → thalamus → motor cortex loop is an integral part of the movement initiation process, and the other structures form side loops that modulate this pathway [6]. Diseases of basal ganglia result in problems with voluntary movement initiation, involving hypokinesia, as in Parkinson's disease, or hyperkinesias, as in Huntington's disease. In addition to their role in initiation, basal ganglia also modulate posture and muscle tone, abnormalities of which are found in basal ganglia disease. The basal ganglia also have a role in nonmotor behaviors, including cognition and mood [7].

The cerebellum is involved with coordination of the sequence of muscle contractions during a movement. In man, there are three important functional subdivisions of the cerebellum. The anterior lobe (paleocerebellum, spinal cerebellum) and its associated deep cerebellar nuclei (fastigial, interposed, and lateral vestibular nuclei) is concerned primarily with processing of information from muscle, joint, and cutaneous mechanoreceptors. It also receives input pertaining to activity in the motor cortex via pontine nuclei and collaterals of corticospinal fibers. The anterior lobe output provides information to modulate the brainstem nuclei from which the reticulospinal tracts originate, and there is a projection to the red nucleus. These circuits are involved in the control of posture and gait.

The flocculonodular lobe (archicerebellum, vestibular cerebellum) and fastigial nucleus are involved with the coordination of the paraxial muscles associated with balance and equilibrium. The major input comes from the vestibular apparatus, and output goes to the vestibular nuclei and then to the vestibulospinal tracts. There is also an important vestibulo-ocular projection to the external ocular muscles.

The posterior lobe (neocerebellum, cerebral cerebellum) and dentate nucleus have massive reciprocal connections with cerebral cortex, including motor, premotor, sensory, and posterior parietal areas. This cerebellar subdivision is involved with coordination of voluntary movement sequences, particularly ballistic movements that are normally too fast to be under feedback proprioceptive control. It is responsible for smooth and accurate execution of movements, and shows evidence of the synaptic plasticity necessary for the learning and refinement of complex motor skills [8].

Peripheral Nerve, Receptors, and Spinal Cord

Peripheral Nerve Fiber Types

Peripheral nerve consists of bundles of nerve fibers, generally mixed sensory and motor. Fiber types have been classified in two ways [2]. The first depends on axon diameter, with categorization into groups A, B, and C. The largest axons, which are myelinated, belong to group A. The smallest fibers, which are unmyelinated, belong to group C. The B group contains myelinated axons from autonomic preganglionic neurons, although this classification is rarely used today. The A group is further classified into the subgroups α, β, δ, and γ.

There is also a second classification system for some of the sensory axons, based primarily on conduction velocity, but also on origin and function. This categorization has numerical classes I–IV in descending order of conduction velocity. Because conduction velocity is directly related to axon diameter for myelinated fibers, the two classification systems can be related as shown in Table 2.**1**. Both terminologies are in common usage, although they were developed independently and do not overlap exactly in terms of fiber categories.

Somatosensory Receptors and Sensation

Somatosensory receptors can be divided into three groups: mechanoreceptors, thermoreceptors, and nociceptors (Table 2.**2**). Mechanoreceptors respond to deformation of their nerve endings, which contain specialized mechanosensitive ion channels whose gating depends on stretching or changes in tension of the surrounding membrane. The nerve endings of mechanoreceptors are usually associated with specialized nonneural structures that govern their detailed response characteristics, so determining the adequate stimulus. Mechanoreceptors mediate the sensations of light touch, pressure, vibration and flutter, and limb position and movement (kinesthesia). Examples of mechanoreceptors in hairy and hairless (glabrous) skin are shown in Figure 2.**5**.

Cutaneous mechanoreceptors [9] have punctate receptive fields whose size is determined by the area of nerve terminal branching and associated nonneural tissue. The information and sensation gleaned from these receptors is governed by their degree of adaptation to a constant stimulus. They may be classified into slowly adapting, moderately rapidly adapting, and very rapidly adapting categories. Slowly adapting receptors respond with an increased frequency of action potentials for the duration of a stimulus. Thus, they are able to accurately signal skin indentation and pressure. Merkel's disk receptors and Ruffini's endings fall into this category. Moderately rapidly adapting receptors respond with a burst of action potentials at stimulus onset and comprise the Meissner's corpuscle of glabrous skin and the hair receptor. They are best at signaling the velocity of movement of a stimulus, and are most sensitive to low-frequency (<50 Hz) repetitive stimulation. In this frequency range, a sinusoidal mechanical stimulus will give rise to the

Table 2.**1** Classification of peripheral nerve afferent and efferent fibers

Source	Myelinated	Diameter range (μm)	Conduction velocity (m/s)	Classification	
				ABC	I–IV
Efferents					
α-Motoneuron to muscle fibers	Y	8–13	44–78	Aα	NA
γ-Motoneuron to muscle spindles	Y	3–8	18–48	Aγ	NA
Afferents					
Limb position and motion	Y	12–20	75–120	Aα	I
Tactile, pressure, vibration	Y	6–12	30–75	Aβ	II
Fast pain, cold	Y	1–6	5–30	Aδ	III
Slow pain, warm	N	<1.5	0.5–2	C	IV

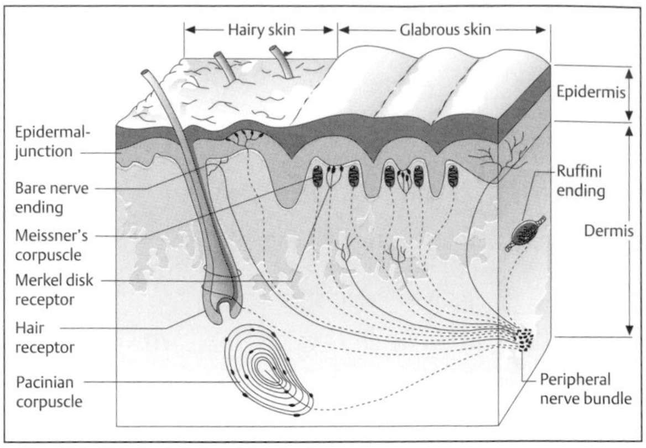

Fig. 2.**5** Schematic of hairy and glabrous (hairless) skin, showing the location of various mechanoreceptors. The receptors in glabrous skin are Meissner's corpuscles and Merkel's disks, located in the dermal papillae, and bare nerve endings. In hairy skin, there are hair receptors around the hair shafts, Merkel's disks, and bare nerve endings. Beneath both types of skin, in the subcutaneous region pacinian corpuscles and Ruffini's endings are found. (From [1], with permission)

sensation of "flutter" where individual waves of the vibration are felt. This contrasts with higher frequencies, which are felt as a true unitary vibration, and this information is transmitted by the most rapidly adapting receptor type, the pacinian corpuscle.

The different receptor types work together along with hand movements and skin patterns such as fingerprints for shape and texture discrimination [10]. Thus, while the discharge of slowly adapting Merkel's disks is best at encoding the spatial characteristics of a stimulus, the more rapidly adapting receptors provide texture information from vibrations set up by the mechanical interaction between surface and fingerprints as the finger tip is moved across a surface.

The sensitivity of the skin to mechanical stimulation varies widely over the body [1], as can be seen from the results of two-point spatial discrimination tests (Fig. 2.**6**). Thus, highest sensitivity is noted for the fingers, lips, nose, and toes, whereas the trunk and upper limbs are relatively insensitive. This is a direct reflection of peripheral innervation density, the number of receptors per unit area of skin, and the average size of individual neural receptive fields, which are correspondingly larger in regions of low sensitivity.

The muscle and skeletal mechanoreceptors comprise muscle spindles, joint receptors, and Golgi tendon organs [11,12]. They are known as proprioceptors because they convey information on the position and movement of the limbs. The major receptor is the muscle spindle (Fig. 2.**7**), formed from specialized skeletal muscle fibers, the intrafusal fibers. Sensory endings contact the midsection of these fibers in an area devoid of contractile machinery. These afferents are stimulated by stretch and signal muscle length and velocity of lengthening. There is also an efferent supply from specialized γ-motoneurons that innervate the contractile ends of the intrafusal fibers. When activated, this causes the ends to contract and in so doing stretches the noncontractile element, including the afferent endings. The function of this efferent system is to regulate the sensitivity of the afferent fibers during active muscle contractions. In the execution of voluntary movements, when activity is supplied to the contractile (extrafusal) fibers of skeletal muscle via the α-motoneurons, there is also modulatory impulse traffic in the γ system – the principle of α-γ coactivation.

Table 2.**2** Classification of peripheral nerve afferent and efferent fibers

Receptor type	Name	Function
Mechanoreceptors		
Muscle and skeletal	Muscle spindle	Limb position and motion
	Golgi tendon organ	Muscle tension
	Joint receptor	Joint tension and angle
Cutaneous and subcutaneous	Ruffini's ending	Pressure
	Merkel's disk	Pressure
	Meissner's corpuscle	Touch velocity (hairless skin), low frequency vibration (flutter)
	Hair receptors	Tactile (hairy skin)
	Pacinian corpuscle	Touch acceleration, high-frequency vibration
Thermoreceptors	C bare nerve endings	Warm
	Aδ myelinated	Cold
Nociceptors	Aδ myelinated	High pressure, thermal and mechanothermal
	C bare nerve endings	Thermal and mechanothermal, polymodal, tissue damage products

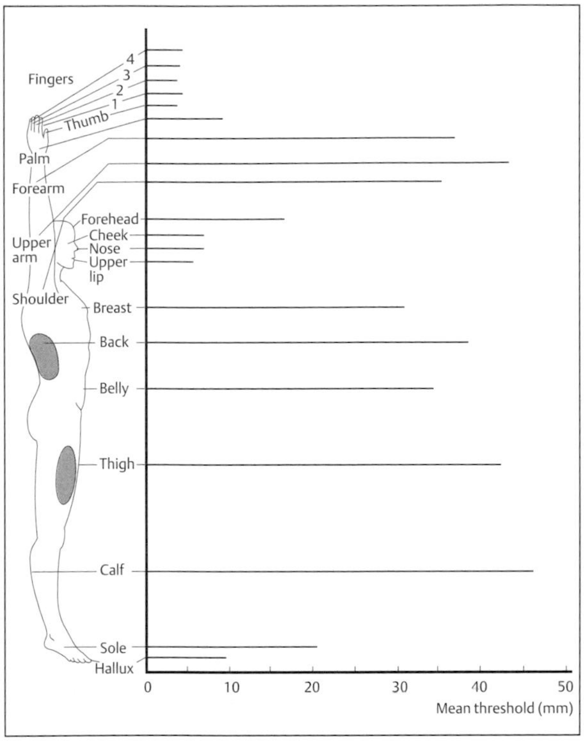

Fig. 2.6 Two-point discrimination thresholds for different regions of the body, measured as the smallest detectable separation distance between the tips of a calibrated compass. Thresholds vary widely over the body, being at their lowest (2 mm) for the finger tips and highest for the forearm, legs, and back (40–50 mm). For selected regions, thresholds are proportional to the diameter of the receptive fields of individual afferents (shown in black). (From [1], with permission)

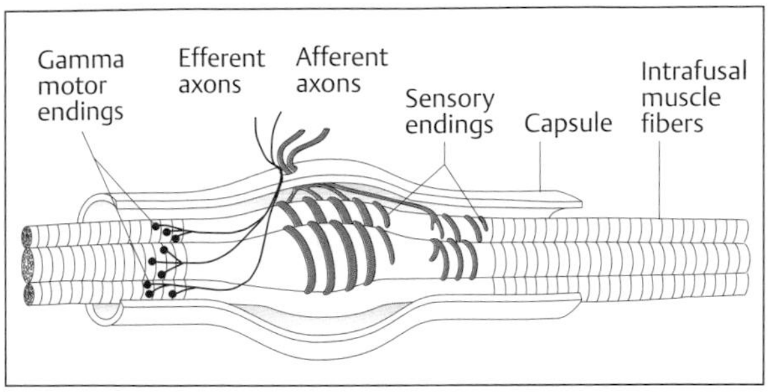

Fig. 2.7 Schematic of the muscle spindle. The main components of the spindle are the intrafusal muscle fibers, sensory afferent endings, and γ-motoneuron efferent fibers. The intrafusal fibers are devoid of contractile apparatus in the region of the afferent endings, although the ends are contractile and are innervated by the γ-motoneurons. The sensory endings are responsive to stretch of the intrafusal fibers. Contraction of the ends of the fibers alters spindle sensitivity. (From [1], with permission)

For the other proprioceptors, joint receptors are located in the connective tissue capsule and they respond to stretch of this tissue to signal joint pressure and angle. Golgi organs are found in the tendons and signal stretch resulting from muscle contraction. In terms of sensation, all these receptor types contribute to the sense of limb position and kinesthesia, along with information from cutaneous mechanoreceptors.

There are separate thermoreceptors for warm or cold stimuli, and like the skin mechanoreceptors they have punctate receptive fields, although they are bare nerve endings rather than encapsulated structures [13]. Warmth is mediated by receptors activated by a range of temperatures between approximately 32 °C and 45 °C, the discharge rate being proportional to temperature. Above 45 °C heat pain, rather than warmth, is perceived, due to the activity of thermal nociceptors, and within this range the discharge of warm receptors actually decreases. Cutaneous cold receptors are activated by temperatures from 1 °C to approximately 20 °C below ambient skin temperature, discharge frequency being roughly proportional to temperature difference. A sensory illusion called paradoxical cold occurs when a 45 °C hot stimulus is selectively applied to a cold fiber receptive field. The stimulus is perceived as cold (rather than warm or painfully hot, which would be the sensation when applied diffusely to the skin), and this coincides with an increased receptor discharge at these high temperatures.

Nociceptors are also bare nerve endings and respond selectively to stimuli that are sufficiently intense that they could damage tissue, and to chemicals released as a result of tissue damage [14]. Thermal nociceptors respond selectively to extreme heat or cold; mechanical nociceptors are activated by strong mechanical stimulation, most effectively by sharp objects. Chemically sensitive, mechanically insensitive nociceptors respond to a variety of agents including K^+, extremes of pH, and neuroactive substances such as histamine, bradykinin, and prostanoids, as well as various irritants. Polymodal nociceptors respond to combinations of mechanical, thermal, and chemical stimulation.

Pain is an unpleasant sensation triggered by tissue damage, real or potential. The high emotive content lends subjectivity to the experience, and simple stimulation of nociceptors does not necessarily lead to pain sensation under all circumstances: there are descending pathways that influence pain transmission. The physiological activation of nociceptors, though, usually gives rise to pricking, burning, aching, and stinging sensations. When the skin is damaged, the initial sensation is conveyed by Aδ fibers. C fibers are more important for the longer-lasting perception that outlives the stimulus. However, pain can also result from neural damage and changes in neural circuitry, and does not necessarily require activation of nociceptors. This is clearly seen in the case of phantom limb pain after surgical limb amputation. Such neuropathic pain following peripheral nerve injury and degeneration/regeneration can be caused by alterations in the balance of inputs to the spinal cord sensory neurons. Thus, large myelinated neurons may regenerate better than C fibers, so that spinal cord neurons that once had predominantly nociceptive input could now be dominated by Aβ touch fibers, although the central connection would remain appropriate for pain transmission. Such a phenomenon may underlie allodynia, where previously innocuous stimuli become severely painful [2,15].

Sensory Input to the Spinal Cord

The cell bodies of sensory neurons are located in the dorsal root ganglia. These bipolar neurons have a relatively long peripheral axon branch, and those in the dorsal column-medial lemniscal pathway also have an extensive central axonal projection. Thus, the cell bodies have a considerable task to supply nutrients and materials to maintain axonal function. This consideration, combined with the potential effects of diabetes on dorsal root ganglion microenvironment, could contribute to a relative vulnerability of sensory neurons, which would affect both peripheral and central projections. Evidence for involvement of central axons is seen in a reduction of spinal cord cross-sectional area, determined by magnetic resonance imaging in diabetic patients with distal symmetrical polyneuropathy [16].

The architecture of the spinal input reflects the segmental organization of embryonic development. As the embryo grows and expands, the developing skin carries its segmentally derived innervation with it. Thus, a single area of skin, a dermatome, is supplied by axons from a single dorsal root ganglion [1,2]. This dermatomal organization is shown in Figure 2.**8**. However, peripheral nerves themselves contain axons from several spinal roots, and different nerves can contain axons from the same root, so the relationship between peripheral nerve trunk and dermatome is complex.

In addition to a central projection, there are also local connections in the spinal cord for neurons that project in the dorsal column-medial lemniscal pathway. Second-order neurons for the spinothalamic projection are also located in the dorsal horn of the spinal cord [17]. The synaptic connections for the different sensory fiber types are made in different layers of the dorsal horn. Thus, Aδ fibers synapse primarily in laminae I and V; C fibers connect mainly in laminae II and I; Aβ input goes to lamina V neurons.

Control of Pain Transmission

Pain transmission from the spinal cord can be modified by nonpainful sensory input as well as by activation of descending pathways from various brain nuclei. Painful sensations evoked by activity of nociceptors (Aδ and C fibers) can be decreased by simultaneous stimulation of low-threshold mechanoreceptors, which may underlie the pain-reducing effects of rubbing of the skin and transcutaneous and dorsal column electrical stimulation. This derives from the gate theory of pain [18], according to which pain results from the balance of activity in nociceptive and nonnociceptive afferent fibers. Thus, nonnociceptive Aβ fiber activity "closes" the central transmission gate whereas nociceptive activity "opens" it. The detailed spinal cord circuitry responsible for this effect is not known, but neurons in lamina V receive convergent input from Aβ, Aδ, and C fiber afferents. Furthermore, Aβ fiber activity can suppress firing of lamina V neurons via inhibitory interneurons in lamina II.

Spinal pain transmission is also modulated by descending inputs [19,20]. Neurons in the periaqueductal gray matter of the midbrain make connections with the cells in the rostroventral medulla, particularly in the nucleus raphe magnus. These in turn project to the spinal cord and make inhibitory connections with neurons in laminae I, II, and IV. Thus, electrical stimulation of periaqueductal gray or raphe nuclei inhibits dorsal horn neurons, including those giving rise to the spinothalamic tract, providing profound analgesia. There are several important neurotransmitter systems involved. The periaqueductal gray area has a very high density of opioid receptors. The raphe nucleus contains many serotonergic neurons. Another descending pathway, from the midbrain locus ceruleus, is noradrenergic. The serotonergic and noradrenergic fibers stimulate dorsal horn interneurons that release the endogenous opiate neurotransmitter enkephalin to pre- and postsynaptically inhibit spinothalamic tract projection neurons.

Motor Output and Sensorimotor Integration in the Spinal Cord

The final common motor pathway to the skeletal muscles is via the motoneurons, whose axons make up a substantial proportion of the myelinated fiber population of peripheral nerve. The major motor output of the spinal cord comes from the α-motoneurons, which directly stimulate skeletal muscle force production by synaptic activation at the motor end plate. The other cord output, from γ-motoneurons, exerts an indirect influence on muscle tension by controlling muscle spindle sensitivity and dynamic range, which consequently affects reflex activation of α-motoneurons.

The basic element of motor control is called the motor unit, which comprises an α-motoneuron together with all of the muscle fibers that it innervates [21]. The collection of α-motoneurons that innervates a single skeletal muscle is termed the motor unit pool of that muscle. The size of the motor units varies greatly. For muscles involved in high-precision movements such as those of the digits or face, the number of muscle fibers may be only 10. For large muscles of the trunk and limbs there may be 3000–4000 fibers per motor unit. These fibers may be distributed over the entire

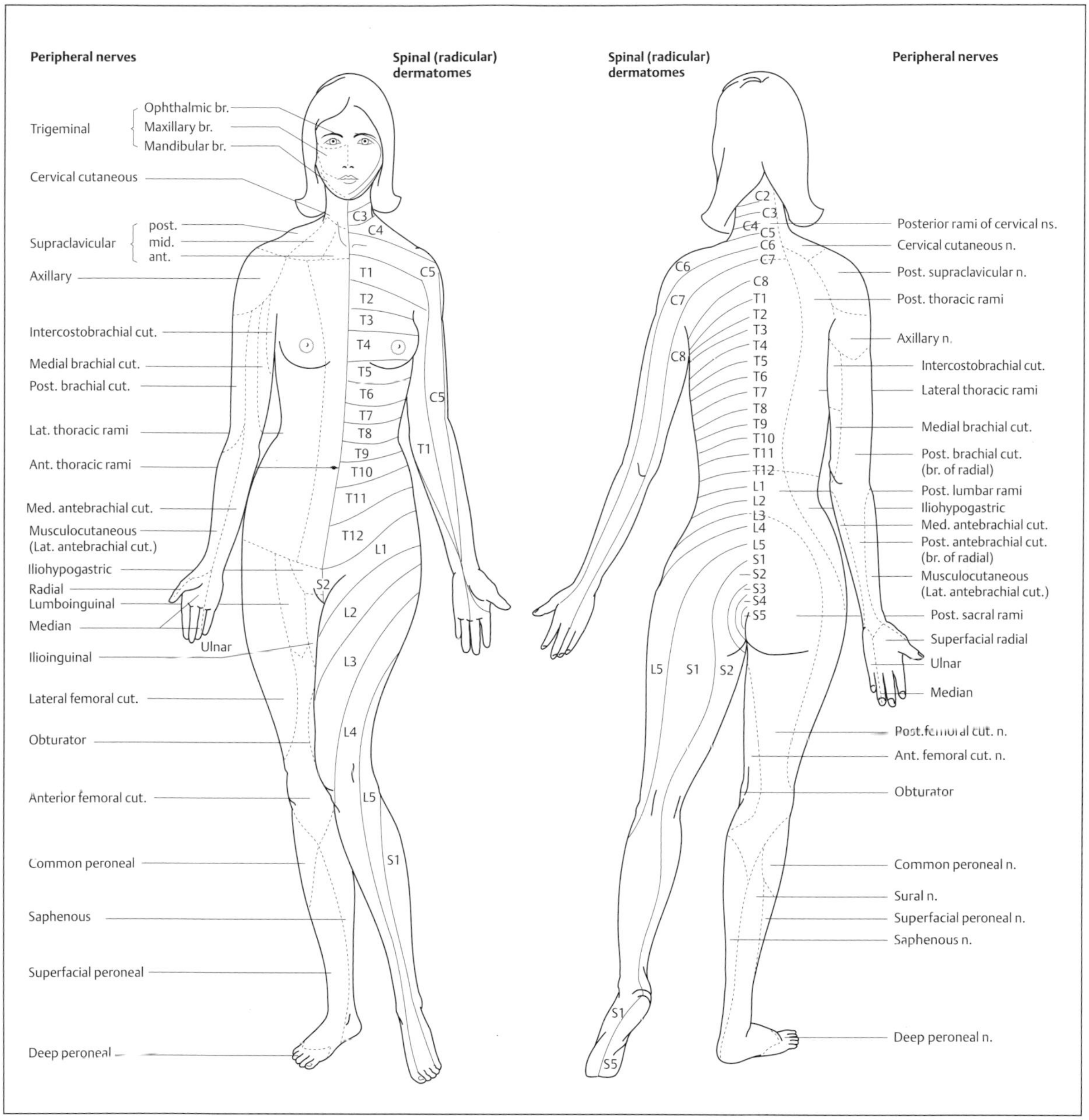

Fig. 2.**8** Distribution of dermatomes and peripheral nerve patterns. Mapping of sensory innervation of the skin by the dorsal roots is shown on the left of the subject: cervical (C1–C7), thoracic (T1–T12), lumbar (L1–L5), and sacral (S1–S5). There is no dorsal root at C1, only a ventral (motor) root. The innervation patterns of peripheral nerves are shown for comparison on the left. Individual peripheral nerves have fibers that arise from several adjacent dorsal roots, leading to rather larger fields of innervation and overlap in the area innervated by each segment. (From [2], with permission)

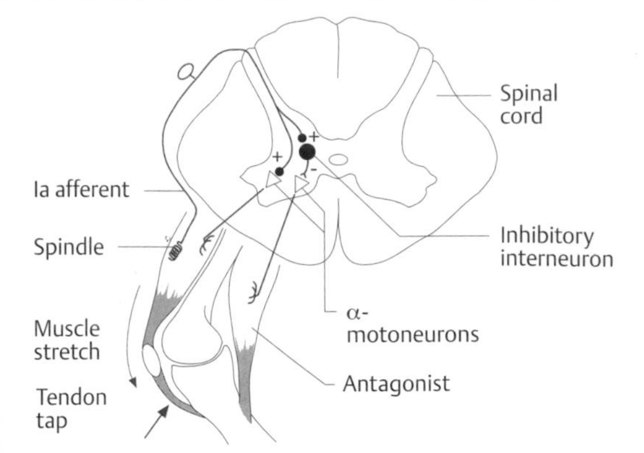

Fig. 2.9 Schematic of the stretch or myotatic spinal reflex circuitry. The essential component is an excitatory (+) monosynaptic connection between muscle spindle Ia afferent fibers and the α-motoneuron pool for that muscle. The reflex may be evoked transiently by tapping the muscle tendon, which stretches the muscle and spindle endings, causing a short reflex contraction. Also shown is a connection via an inhibitory interneuron (–, black cell body), which suppresses activity in the antagonist muscle

area of the muscle, so the territory of a single motor unit may be considerable. All muscle fibers in an individual motor unit are biochemically, histochemically, and physiologically identical, indicating the determination of muscle fiber properties by their innervation. In terms of muscle and contractile properties, there are three motor unit types. Those based on type I muscle fibers are characterized by relatively slow contraction speeds, reliance on aerobic energy metabolism, and a profuse capillary supply-features that confer extreme fatigue resistance. These units are active for much of the time, being involved in postural control, and are preferentially recruited by muscle spindle afferent input to the spinal cord. In contrast, type IIB motor units have fast contraction times, rely on anaerobic metabolism, have relatively poor vascular supply, and fatigue rapidly. They are preferentially recruited for large, fast movements such as limb withdrawal from a painful stimulus. Type IIA units are somewhere in between: the muscle fibers are fast contracting, well supplied with capillaries, have both aerobic and anaerobic energy production, and are moderately fatigue-resistant.

There are two fundamental ways of varying muscle tension production: altering the frequency of action potentials transmitted by an individual α-motoneuron, and altering the range or number of motor units activated in that muscle. This is dependent on the synaptic input to the α-motoneurons, of which there are three sources: muscle spindle afferents, the corticospinal projection, and spinal cord interneurons. The latter category forms a complex control mechanism as it is in turn strongly influenced by both afferent input and all descending motor pathways.

The elegance and simplicity of the spinal cord circuitry involved in sensorimotor integration is apparent for the myotatic or stretch reflex. Thus, Sherrington [22] noted that when a muscle is stretched it tends to contract. This was traced to an excitatory monosynaptic reflex arc between muscle spindle afferents, which are stimulated by the stretch, and the α-motoneurons, which cause that muscle to contract (Fig. 2.**9**). The operation of this circuit is used as a clinical tool, observing the reflex jerk when the tendons are tapped to rapidly stretch muscle. Physiologically, however, this simple circuit acts tonically as a length servo feedback loop, which is crucial for postural stability and has important antigravity functions, for example in the major leg extensors. This circuit is elaborated by interneurons to ensure that antagonistic muscle groups controlling the same joint do not work against each other [23]. Thus, collateral branches of the spindle afferents also synapse on inhibitory interneurons that in turn innervate the motor unit pool of the antagonist muscle.

Another spinal circuit involving proprioceptor input is the reverse myotatic (or clasp knife) reflex arc (Fig. 2.**10**). Golgi tendon organs, which signal muscle tension, are the sensory arm and they innervate inhibitory interneurons that synapse with the α-motoneurons [1,2]. Thus, the reflex is polysynaptic, with increasing muscle tension tending to inhibit further contraction. This may be demonstrated, for example, when a subject is asked to actively resist bending of their knee. At a high level of applied force, the strongly contracted extensors suddenly relax and the resistance disappears. This reflex arc, in extreme circumstances, may function to protect muscles from inappropriately high and potentially damaging tension production. However, the circuitry forms a physiological tension servo feedback mechanism to maintain a particular contracted state of the whole muscle, for example when some fibers weaken or drop out due to fatigue. It also is important for steady tension production required in fine motor control, for example in holding a fragile object. Thus, the tension servo mechanism acts in conjunction with the length servo mechanism provided by the muscle spindles to maintain precise positioning of limbs, postural maintenance, and manipulation of grip.

A third important spinal circuit involves nociceptive input and the complex polysynaptic reflex arc that mediates flexion or withdrawal of a limb from an aversive stimulus [1,2], for example standing on a nail (Fig. 2.**11**). Pain fibers enter the spinal cord and branch profusely to activate excitatory interneurons, which in turn excite α-motoneurons to flexor muscles. The magnitude of the noxious stimulus governs the size of the withdrawal response and the number of flexors responding: a highly painful stimulus will excite all the flexors of the affected limb. Thus, this reflex crosses dermatomal boundaries and involves integration between several spinal segments. As with the myotatic

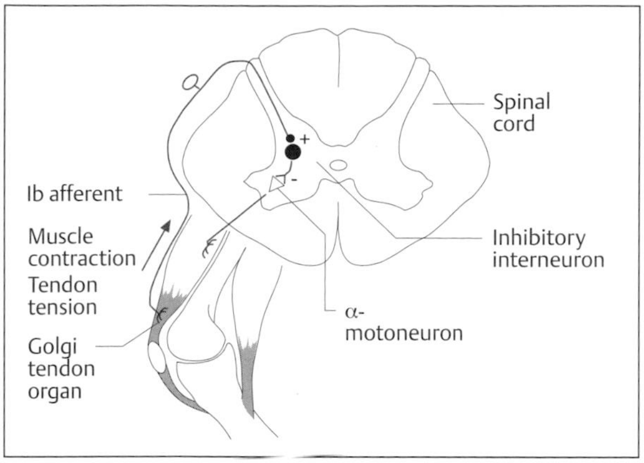

Fig. 2.**10** Circuits for the inverse myotatic or clasp knife spinal reflex. This uses information from the Ib afferents of Golgi tendon organs, which monitor tendon stretch and muscle tension. The reflex may be evoked by attempting to stretch a muscle during an isometric contraction. This causes a rapid increase in tension and a massive volley of action potentials from the tendon organs. Via inhibitory interneurons (–, black cell body), α-motoneuron activity is suppressed and the limb collapses, similar to the closing of a clasp knife blade

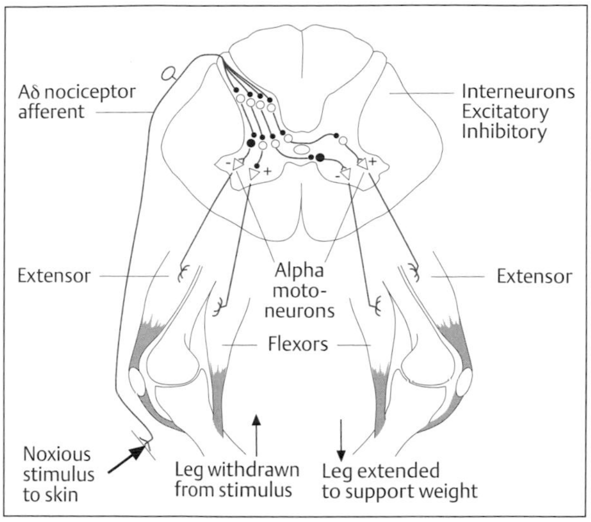

Fig. 2.**11** Circuits for the flexion (withdrawal) and crossed-extension reflexes. These reflexes are mediated by polysynaptic pathways in the spinal cord. Noxious stimulation of Aδ fibers causes excitation of α-motoneurons supplying the ipsilateral flexor muscles, which withdraw the limb from the threat of damage. Excitatory interneurons also connect to the α-motoneurons of the extensors on the contralateral limb, causing contraction to support the weight of the body during limb withdrawal. α-Motoneurons supplying the antagonistic muscles on both sides of the cord are inactivated via inhibitory interneurons during this reflex

reflex, this circuit is elaborated to incorporate reciprocal inhibition of the antagonistic extensor muscles. Furthermore, a postural component is added, the crossed-extensor reflex, to support the weight of the body on the contralateral leg when the foot is withdrawn.

From this brief description, it is clear that the spinal cord carries out the basic steps of sensorimotor integration, which are further elaborated by the brain. However, the spinal cord circuits are not there simply to carry out reflex actions to sensory stimulation. The same circuits are recruited by descending inputs from the brain to simplify voluntary movement and postural adjustment. For example, the crossed-extensor reflex pathway (one leg flexed, the contralateral leg extended, and vice versa) is also an element in the sequencing of walking.

Vascular Supply in the Peripheral Somatic Nervous System

Blood flow to the nervous system is influenced or regulated by a number of factors including local tissue metabolism, oxygen and carbon dioxide tension, pH, circulating vasoactive agents, the intrinsic innervation of the blood vessels, and systemic perfusion pressure. This has been extensively documented for the cerebral circulation (see reviews [24–26]). However, the precise details of vascular regulation differ in the central and peripheral nervous system: moreover, the vascular supply has different characteristics in dorsal root ganglia and nerve trunks of the somatosensory nervous system. Given the importance of impaired blood flow in several peripheral nerve disease states, including diabetic neuropathy (see Chapter 4, pages 115–123), a brief overview of the salient features of the normal vascular supply to the peripheral somatosensory system is appropriate.

Peripheral Nerve Trunk and Spinal Roots

The vasculature of peripheral nerve is relatively unique. Peripheral nerve and its spinal dorsal and ventral roots have a good vascular supply composed of two integrated but independent systems, termed the extrinsic and intrinsic circulations [27–29]. The extrinsic system comprises vessels that arise from local large arteries and veins as well as offshoots from the vessels supplying adjacent muscles and periosteum. These are arranged segmentally and follow the surface along the length of the nerve (Fig. 2.**12**). They form a highly anastomotic plexus within the epi-perineurial layers of nerve sheath, vessels being mainly arterioles, venules, and arteriovenous shunts. This provides numerous connections with the intrinsic circulation. The latter, or vasa nervorum, comprises vessels on the perineurium and in the endoneurial vascular bed. Terminal arterioles from the perineurium penetrate the nerve fascicles and form the endoneurial capillary bed, which consists of a network of intrafascicular capillaries that run longitudi-

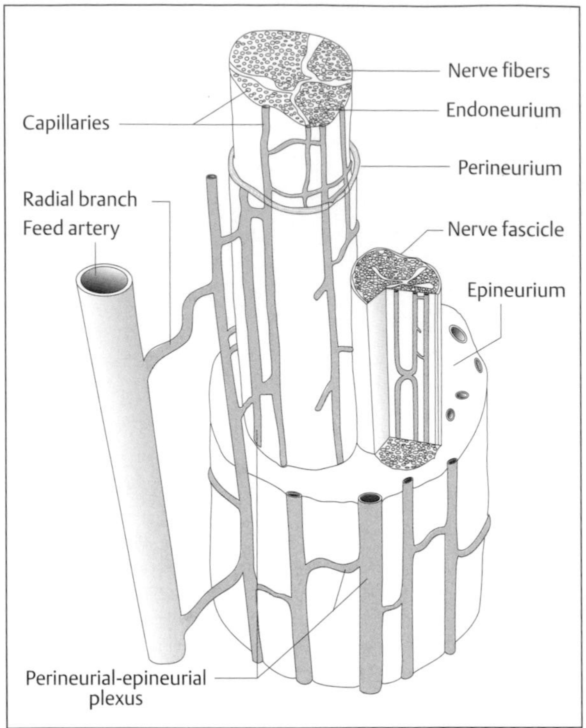

Fig. 2.12 Peripheral nerve gross structure and blood supply. Peripheral nerves are surrounded by a loose connective tissue structure, the epineurium, which contains a plexus of blood vessels supplied by radial branches from multiple feed arteries. Nerves are divided into fascicles by the perineurium, which is a strong connective tissue that isolates the fascicles of nerve fibers physically to form part of the blood–nerve barrier. The other component of the barrier is the tight endothelial lining of the endoneurial capillaries

nally, along with the nerve fibers, throughout the length of the nerve. Endoneurial capillaries are lined by a continuous layer of endothelial cells connected by tight junctions, which forms part of the blood-nerve barrier, analogous to, although somewhat less efficient than, the blood-brain barrier that restricts ingress of blood-borne substances to the central nervous system. The other component of the blood-nerve barrier is the inner layer of the perineurium, which is continuous with the arachnoid membrane of spinal cord [30].

The endoneurial capillaries have a large diameter compared to those in other tissues such as brain and skeletal muscle, and the intercapillary distance is relatively great [31,32]. The latter would tend to render nerve susceptible to ischemic or hypovolemic stresses or nerve edema [33]. However, the extensive anastomotic connections between extrinsic and intrinsic circulatory systems minimize the effect of local disruptions to nerve blood supply, and, coupled with a low metabolic rate, make peripheral nerve relatively resistant to mild ischemia. The intrinsic circulation consists predominantly of capillaries, and there is a paucity of vascular smooth muscle in the endoneurium [32]. Thus, the main neural and humoral control of nerve perfusion is exerted at the level of the epiperineurial arterioles. These vessels are densely innervated by nerve fibers [34,35] containing a number of neurotransmitters, including norepinephrine, serotonin, substance P, neuropeptide Y, vasoactive intestinal peptide, and calcitonin gene-related peptide. By contrast, although nerves containing these neurotransmitters are also found in endoneurium, they are not associated with blood vessels.

The capacity for autoregulation—to match blood flow to local tissue demand—is well established in the central nervous system. Myogenic mechanisms compensate for changes in perfusion pressure to maintain tissue flow. Levels of metabolites such as O_2, CO_2, and pH influence vessels to supply blood to meet metabolic needs. However, in peripheral nerve, pressure autoregulation of endoneurial blood flow is virtually absent, perhaps a reflection of the lack of smooth muscle in endoneurial microvessels. Furthermore, vasa nervorum responses to systemic hypoxia, hypercapnia, or reduced pH are minimal [36]. These factors would make peripheral nerve more vulnerable than many tissues to hypotension-induced ischemia. Conversely, there is some evidence of local metabolite regulation. Following repetitive electrical nerve stimulation, a functional hyperemia is apparent [37]. Moreover, blood flow can be seen to approximately double during maximal but selective electrical stimulation of large myelinated nerve fibers, which do not innervate vasa nervorum [38].

Peripheral Ganglia

Dorsal root (and autonomic) ganglia have blood flow values three to five times greater than the blood flow of peripheral nerve, which reflects the higher metabolic rate of neuronal cell bodies compared to that of nerve fibers [39–41]. The capacity of ganglia to autoregulate their blood supply is considerably better than that of peripheral nerve. Thus, ganglia show excellent flow regulation in the face of changes in systemic blood pressure. However, in common with peripheral nerve and in contrast to brain, there is little response to changes in systemic arterial CO_2 or pH [39].

Although dorsal root ganglia are surrounded by an impermeable perineurium, a proportion of the vessels have a fenestrated endothelial lining. This renders the ganglion-blood barrier weak, and dorsal root ganglion cells are vulnerable to blood-borne toxic substances such as heavy metals, some anticancer drugs, and infectious agents. The reason for this breakdown of the blood-nervous system barrier is not known, but it has been suggested that a subpopulation of ganglion cells may be chemical sensors providing important information on the body's internal milieu [42].

Concluding Remarks

The somatic nervous system, with its motor and sensory divisions, forms the basic output and monitoring capability for all movement, both purposive and reflex. The elaborate organization of proprioceptors and skin mechanoreceptors and their central connections are essential for our sense of body position in space, the control of posture, gait, and accuracy of goal-directed movement. The skin is a particularly important sensory organ, the sentry at the interface of body and environment, monitoring not only mechanical but also thermal and potentially damaging events.

The Autonomic Nervous System

C. J. Mathias

Introduction

The autonomic nervous system innervates every organ in the body and is closely involved in their function (Fig. 2.**13**). Additionally, it plays a key role in integrative function and in maintaining the milieu intérieur, for example through the control of blood pressure, body temperature, and metabolic and fluid balance. This enables optimum functioning in a variety of situations, which at times is essential for survival. It is accomplished by numerous pathways and neurotransmitters, providing considerable flexibility and responsiveness. Dysfunction of the autonomic nervous system may be caused at one or more sites centrally or peripherally (Table 2.**3**). It can be a particular problem in diabetes mellitus, where neural structures can be affected at various sites and their disturbances compounded by target organ involvement. In this section the principles of structure and function of the autonomic nervous system will be described, along with examples pertaining to derangement of function.

Basic Principles

The autonomic nervous system is essentially an efferent system encompassing sympathetic, parasympathetic, and enteric components. The sympathetic efferents emerge from the thoracic and lumbar segments of the spinal cord and ultimately supply all organs and structures. The parasympathetic outflow consists of cranial and sacral efferents. The former accompany cranial nerves III, VII, IX, and X, and supply the eye, lachrymal and salivary glands, heart, lungs, and upper gastrointestinal tract with associated structures down to the level of the colon. The sacral outflow supplies the large bowel, urinary tract, bladder, and reproductive system. The enteric nervous system as originally proposed by Langley in 1898 is effectively the local nervous system of the gut.

There are specific cerebral nucleii, especially in the hypothalamus, midbrain, and brainstem, that influence autonomic activity; an example is the Edinger-Westphal nucleus through the parasympathetic nerves to the iris musculature which controls pupillary constriction. From the brainstem, sympathetic efferent outflow tracts descend through the cervical spinal cord, where axons synapse in the intermediolateral cell mass (Fig. 2.**14**). From the thoracic and upper lumbar spinal segments, myelinated axons emerge and synapse in the paravertebral ganglia, which is some distance from sympathetically innervated target organs. Most parasympathetic ganglia are close to target organs. The major neurotransmitter at ganglia (both parasympathetic and sympathetic) is acetylcholine,

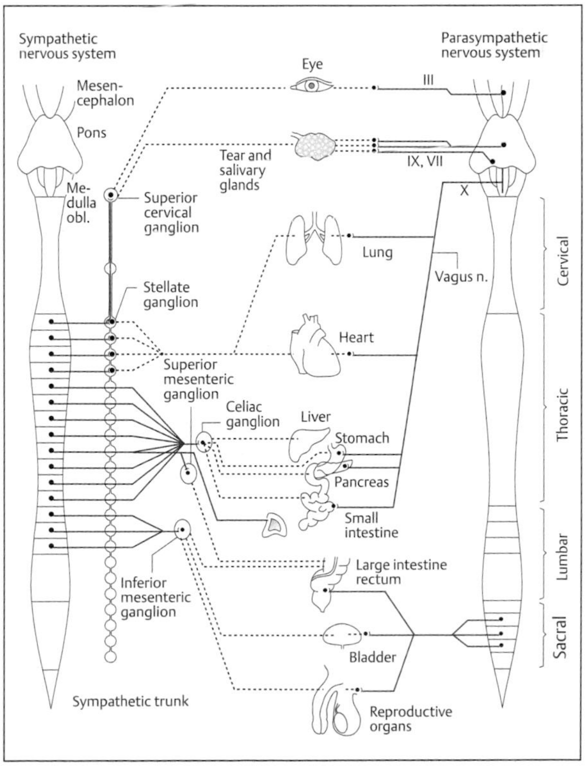

Fig. 2.**13** Parasympathetic and sympathetic innervation of major organs. (From [43], with permission)

Table 2.3 Classification of disorders resulting in autonomic dysfunction[a]

- PRIMARY (Etiology unknown)
  - Acute/subacute dysautonomias
    - Pure cholinergic dysautonomia
    - Pure pandysautonomia
    - Pandysautonomia with neurological features
  - Chronic autonomic failure syndromes
    - Pure autonomic failure
    - Multiple system atrophy (Shy-Drager syndrome)
    - Parkinson's disease with autonomic failure
- SECONDARY
  - Congenital
    - Nerve growth factor deficiency
  - Hereditary
    - Autosomal dominant trait
      - Familial amyloid polyneuropathy
      - Porphyria
  - Autosomal recessive trait
    - Familial dysautonomia (Riley-Day syndrome)
    - Dopamine β-hydroxylase deficiency
    - Aromatic L-amino acid decarboxylase deficiency
  - X-linked recessive
    - Fabry's disease
  - Metabolic diseases
    - Diabetes mellitus
    - Chronic renal failure
    - Chronic liver disease
    - Vitamin B_{12} deficiency
    - Alcohol-induced
  - Inflammatory
    - Guillain-Barré syndrome
    - Transverse myelitis
  - Infections
    - Bacterial: tetanus
    - Viral: human immunodeficiency virus infection
    - Parasitic: *Trypanosoma cruzi* (Chagas' disease)
    - Prion: fatal familial insomnia
  - Neoplasia
    - Brain tumors: especially of third ventricle or posterior fossa
    - Paraneoplastic, to include adenocarcinomas of lung, pancreas, and Lambert-Eaton syndrome
  - Connective tissue disorders
    - Rheumatoid arthritis
    - Systemic lupus erythematosus
    - Mixed connective tissue disease
  - Surgery
    - Regional sympathectomy: upper limb, splanchnic
    - Vagotomy and drainage procedures: "dumping syndrome"
    - Organ transplantation: heart, kidney
  - Trauma
    - Spinal cord transection
- DRUGS, TOXINS and POISONS
    - Direct effects
    - By causing a neuropathy (alcohol)
- NEURALLY MEDIATED SYNCOPE
  - Vasovagal syncope
  - Carotid sinus hypersensitivity
  - Micturition syncope
  - Cough syncope
  - Swallow syncope
  - Associated with glossopharyngeal neuralgia
- POSTURAL TACHYCARDIA SYNDROME

[a] Adapted from [44].

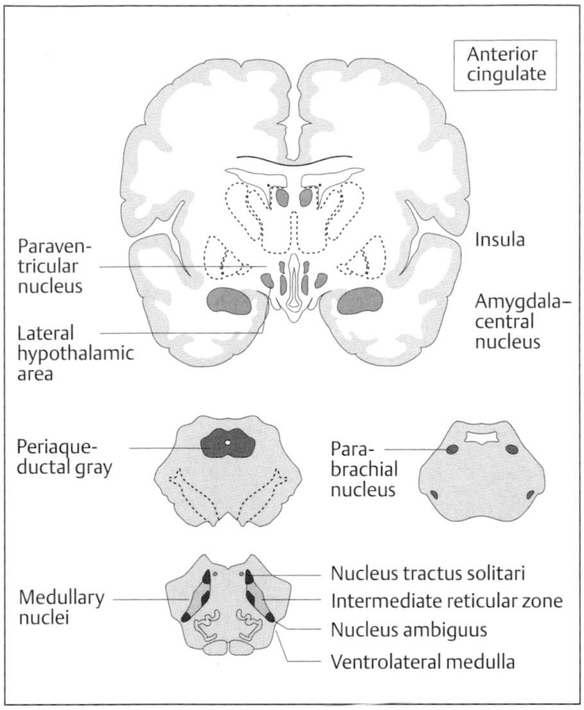

Fig. 2.**14** Anatomic components of the central autonomic network. The diagram of the human brain indicates the areas involved in central autonomic control, as defined by animal studies. The insular cortex is the primary viscerosensory area. The central nucleus of the amygdala is involved in emotional responses. The paraventricular, lateral and other hypothalamic regions are involved in homeostasis and adaptive behavior. The periaqueductal gray integrates autonomic, motor, and antinociceptive receptive responses during stress. The parabrachial region is a viscerosensory relay and participates in cardiovascular and respiratory control. The nucleus of the tractus solitarii (nucleus of the solitary tract) is the primary viscerosensory relay nucleus. The ventrolateral medulla contains sympathoexcitatory, sympathoinhibitory, and respiratory neurons. The nucleus ambiguus contributes innervation to the heart. The intermediate reticular zone of the medulla (shaded area) is critically involved in integration of respiratory, cardiovascular, and other autonomic reflexes. (From [45], with permission)

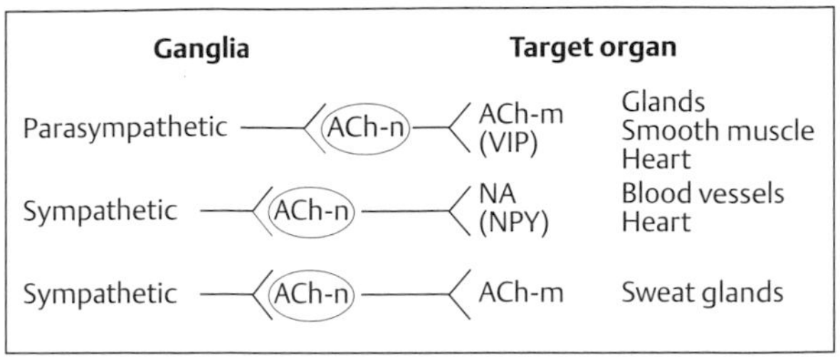

Fig. 2.**15** Outline of the major transmitters at autonomic ganglia and postganglionic sites on target organs supplied by the sympathetic and parasympathetic efferent pathways. The acetylcholine receptor at all ganglia is of the nicotinic subtype (ACh-n). Ganglionic blockers such as hexamethonium thus prevent both parasympathetic and sympathetic activation. Atropine, however, acts only on the muscarinic (ACh-m) receptor at postganglionic parasympathetic and sympathetic cholinergic sites. The cotransmitters along with the primary transmitters are also indicated. NA, norepinephrine (noradrenaline); VIP, vasoactive intestinal polypeptide; NPY, neuropeptide Y. (From [44], with permission)

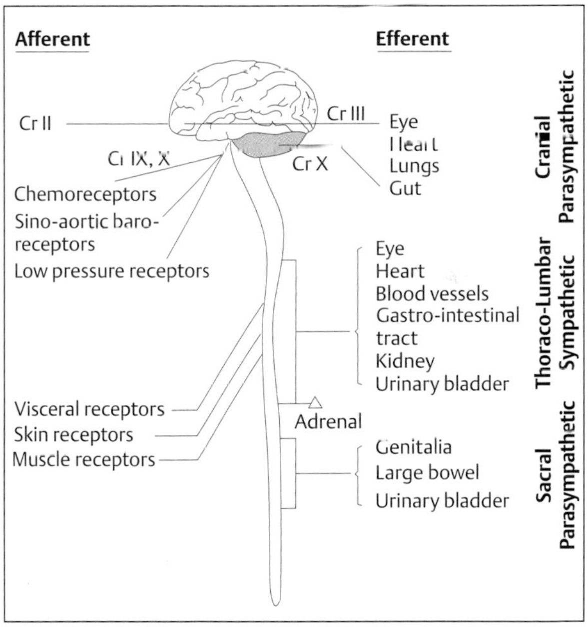

Fig. 2.**16** Schema to indicate the major afferent pathways that influence the major autonomic efferent outflow (the cranial and sacral parasympathetic and the thoracolumbar sympathetic), supplying various organs. Cr = Cranial nerve (From [44], with permission)

which acts on the nicotinic receptor (Fig. 2.**15**). Postganglionic fibers, which are unmyelinated, rejoin the mixed nerves through the gray rami and innervate target organs except for the adrenal medulla, which only has a preganglionic supply. The neurotransmitter at sympathetic postganglionic synapses (as in the heart and blood vessels) is predominantly norepinephrine; sympathetic cholinergic fibers (with acetylcholine as the neurotransmitter that acts on muscarinic receptors) supply sweat glands.

The autonomic nervous system often works as a servo system enabling responsiveness to a variety of local and systemic influences, with interaction and at times control at different levels of the neural axis. Thus, every afferent in the body can influence parasympathetic and sympathetic efferent activity (Fig. 2.**16**). Examples are visual afferents (through cranial nerve II) that influence pupillary function; chemoreceptors, sino-aortic baroreceptors, and low-pressure receptors through cranial nerves IX and X, which regulate cardiac vagal and sympathetic neural control of heart and blood vessels; and visceral, skin, and muscle receptors (through cerebral connections or via the isolated

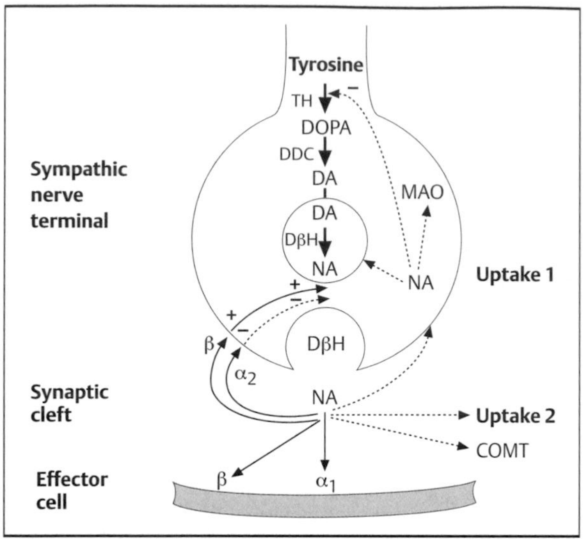

Fig. 2.17 Schema of pathways in the formation, release, and metabolism of norepinephrine from sympathetic nerve terminals. Tyrosine is converted into dihydroxyphenylalanine (DOPA) by tyrosine hydroxylase (TH). DOPA is converted into dopamine (DA) by dopadecarboxylase. In the vesicles DA is converted into norepinephrine (noradrenaline, NA) by dopamine β-hydroxylase (DβH). Nerve impulses release both DβH and NA into the synaptic cleft by exocytosis. NA acts predominantly on α_1-adrenoceptors but has actions on β-adrenoceptors on the effector cell of target organs. It also has presynaptic adrenoceptor effects. Those acting on α_2-adrenoceptors inhibit NA release; those on β-adrenoceptors stimulate NA release. NA may be taken up by a neuronal process (uptake 1) into the cytosol, where it may inhibit further formation of DOPA through the rate-limiting enzyme TH. NA may be taken into vesicles or metabolized by monoamine oxidase (MAO) in the mitochondria. NA may be taken up by a higher-capacity but lower-affinity extraneuronal process (uptake 2) into peripheral tissues, such as vascular and cardiac muscle and certain glands. NA is also metabolized by catechol-*o*-methyl transferase (COMT). NA measured in plasma is the overspill not affected by these numerous processes. (From [44], with permission)

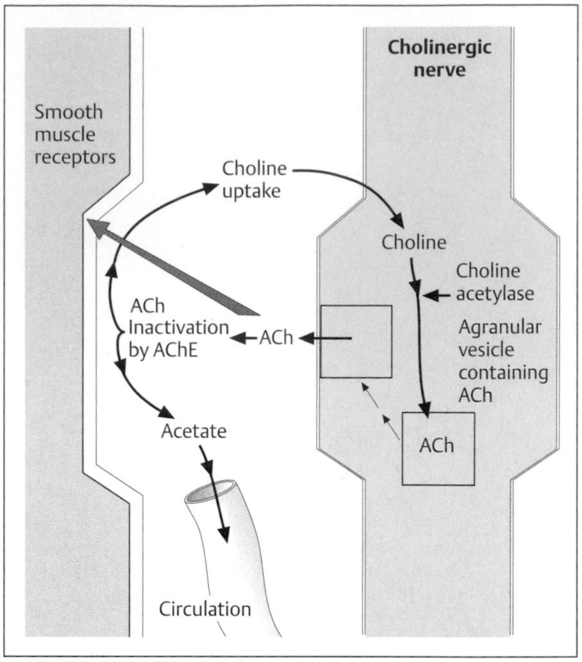

Fig. 2.18 Schema of pathways in the formation from choline of acetylcholine (ACh) and its inactivation by acetylcholine esterase (AChE). (From [46], with permission)

spinal cord as observed in patients with high spinal cord lesions), which influence a wide range of autonomic activity.

There is increasing evidence in humans, resulting from a combination of neuroendocrine and neuroimaging studies, of the role of various cerebral areas that control, influence, and modulate autonomic function. This is in keeping with extensive experimental data of the role of the insular cortex and amygdala in cardiovascular responses, and of hypothalamic nucleii in neuroendocrine control.

In the enteric nervous system, prevertebral ganglia (celiac, superior and inferior mesenteric) have both sympathetic and parasympathetic efferents and a system of neurons and supporting cells within various viscera including the gastrointestinal tract, pancreas, and gall bladder. These innervate the musculature of the alimentary tract (and thus influence gut motility), the secretion of organs (such as the flow of gastric acid), mucosal blood flow, and the intestinal transport of water and electrolytes. There are sensory neurons that monitor factors such as tension in the walls of the intestine or the chemical nature of its content, and associated neurons (interneurons) that link information between enteric and motor neurons and influence smooth muscle contraction, vasodilatation, and transport of water and electrolytes. They interact with sympathetic and parasympathetic pathways and the wide range of enteric endocrine cells, with numerous pancreatic and gut peptides that have roles both locally and elsewhere. Within the enteric nervous system are a number of interconnected networks or plexuses. In the intestines these include the myenteric (Auerbach's) plexus between the external longitudinal and circular muscle coats, and the subserous (Meissner's) plexus in the connective tissue between the serosal mesothelium and external muscle. The major neurotransmitter is acetylcholine, and these plexuses are thus similar to the intrinsic plexuses found in the heart that also are the sites of selective involvement in Chagas' disease following infection with *Trypanosoma cruzi*; dysfunction may result from a specifically targeted immunological process.

The postganglionic autonomic supply to organs and effector cells consists of multiple neurotransmitters with complex machinery relating to their formation, release, interplay with other substances, uptake, and recycling. Schema for the three major neurotransmitters, norepinephrine in adrenergic, acetylcholine in cholinergic, and adenosine triphosphate in purinergic terminals, are provided in Figures 2.**17**–2.**19**. A variety

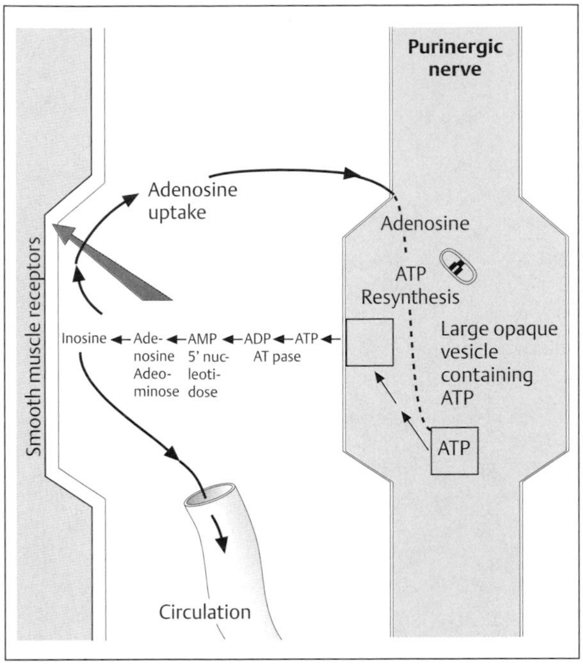

Fig. 2.**19** Purinergic junction: scheme of synthesis, storage, release, and inactivation of autonomic transmitters. (From [47], with permission)

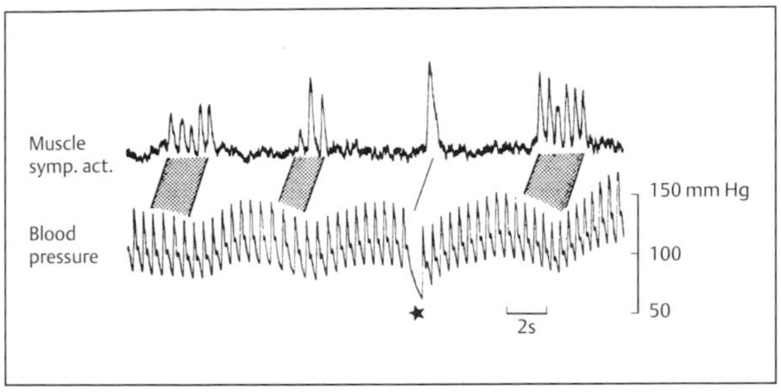

Fig. 2.**20** Relationship between spontaneous fluctuations of blood pressure and muscle nerve sympathetic activity recorded in the right peroneal nerve. Arterial baroreflex activity accounts for the pulse synchrony of nerve activity and the inverse relationship to blood pressure fluctuations. The asterisk indicates a diastolic blood pressure fall due to sudden atrioventricular block. Stippling indicates corresponding sequences of bursts and heart beats. (From [48], with permission)

of other substances may be cosecreted, examples being vasoactive intestinal polypeptide with acetylcholine, and neuropeptide Y with norepinephrine (Fig. 2.**15**). This may explain the inability of specific antagonists to block all the effects of parasympathetic and sympathetic nerve stimulation, as observed with the muscarinic blocker atropine and with α-adrenoceptor blockers, respectively.

Assessing Autonomic Activity

Activity of the autonomic nervous system can be evaluated directly or indirectly. In the sympathetic nervous system this can be performed by electrophysiological (with sympathetic microneurography) or biochemical techniques. The latter include measurement of catecholamines and their metabolites in urine and plasma, spillover techniques using tritiated catecholamines, and use of substances such as metaiodobenzylguanidine (MIBG, a γ-emitter) or 6-[^{18}F] fluorodopamine (a positron emitter) that are taken up by postganglionic sympathetic nerves and detected by appropriate scanning techniques. However, there are limitations to each of these techniques. Sympathetic microneurography is dependent upon insertion of a fine tungsten microelectrode into a peripheral nerve and into a muscle or skin sympathetic fascicle (Fig. 2.**20**). It is an invasive technique, although safe in experienced hands; there are difficulties with electrode placement in autonomic disorders causing underactivity or inactivity. Urinary and plasma catecholamines (Fig. 2.**21**) do not control for small or rapid changes and are affected by metabolism and uptake effects, among other factors. The spillover techniques are invasive and involve direct cannulation of blood vessels, but provide measurement of change in sympathetic activity, especially in key organs such as the heart, kidneys, and brain (Fig. 2.**22**). The imaging techniques using MIBG or fluorodopamine are noninvasive but semiquantitative. These different techniques are used extensively in research but not usually in the routine clinical setting, where tests of function are utilized that are dependent not only on activity of the autonomic nerves but also on the response of target organs.

Investigation of Autonomic Function

An outline of investigational approaches for relevant systems is provided in Table 2.**4**. A detailed history and clinical examination, to include all organs and integrative system function affected by autonomic dysfunction, helps guide the choice of testing. The effects of autonomic underactivity and overactivity should be considered. Cardiovascular autonomic assessment often provides a readily assessable and noninvasive means of screening for dysfunction. A variety of cardiovascular tests are helpful in distinguishing between sympathetic and parasympathetic function (Figs. 2.**23**, 2.**24**). A cardinal feature of sympathetic denervation often is orthostatic (postural) hypotension (Fig. 2.**25**), which will not be detected unless measurements are made in the supine and head-up (sitting or standing) positions. These measurements often are performed when there is clinical suspicion, such as when syncope is reported. However, there can be a variety of

Table 2.**4** Outline of investigations in autonomic failure

Cardiovascular	
Physiological	Head-up tilt (45°); standing; Valsalva maneuver Pressor stimuli: isometric exercise, cold pressor, mental arithmetic Heart rate responses: deep breathing, hyperventilation, standing, head-up tilt, 30:15 ratio Liquid meal challenge Exercise testing Carotid sinus massage
Biochemical	Plasma norepinephrine: supine and head-up tilt or standing; urinary catecholamines; plasma renin activity and aldosterone
Pharmacological	Norepinephrine: α-adrenoceptors, vascular Isoprenaline: β-adrenoceptors, vascular and cardiac Tyramine: pressor and norepinephrine response Edrophonium: norepinephrine response Atropine: parasympathetic cardiac blockade
Sudomotor	Central regulation: thermoregulatory sweat test Sweat gland response: intradermal acetylcholine, quantitative sudomotor axon reflex test (Q-SART), localized sweat test Sympathetic skin response
Gastrointestinal	Barium studies, video-cine-fluoroscopy, endoscopy, gastric emptying studies
Renal function and urinary tract	Day and night urine volumes and sodium/potassium excretion Urodynamic studies, intravenous urography, ultrasound examination, sphincter electromyography
Sexual function	Penile plethysmography Intracavernosal papaverine
Respiratory	Laryngoscopy Sleep studies to assess apnea/oxygen desaturation
Eye	Lachrymal function: Schirmer's test Pupillary function: pharmacological and physiological

Adapted from [49]

symptoms resulting from, or in association with, orthostatic hypotension (Table 2.**5**) that have multiple causes and this may result in failure to consider orthostatic hypotension and thus measure blood pressure before and after postural challenge. Orthostatic hypotension may occur later in the course of disease, as in diabetes mellitus, where cardiac parasympathetic denervation often is an early feature of autonomic neuropathy. When orthostatic hypotension is present, consideration also should be given to a range of causative nonneurogenic factors (Table 2.**6**).

A variety of other tests related to stimuli in daily life need to be considered in relation to diagnosis, understanding pathophysiological mechanisms, and management. Examples include the effects of food and exercise among other factors (Table 2.**7**) that unmask or exaggerate orthostatic hypotension when there is sympathetic vasoconstrictor failure. Food can cause a marked fall in blood pressure because of splanchnic vasodilatation and an inability to compensate in other vascular regions; exercise causes vasodilatation in working muscles. Ambulatory 24-hour blood pressure (Fig. 2.**26**) and heart rate profiles are of value as lack of the expected nocturnal circadian fall indicates autonomic failure; with suitable protocols, orthostatic, postprandial, and exercise-induced hypotension can be evaluated with these ambulatory techniques in the home setting. Spectral analytical techniques provide further information on the differences between sympathetic and parasympathetic control of heart rate and blood pressure, and can assess respiratory influences over heart rate, in particular.

Sudomotor testing should include evaluation of gustatory sweating when relevant. In combination with neurophysiological tests, the sympathetic skin response is of value in determining sympathetic cholinergic activation (Fig. 2.**27**). Details of tests affecting other systems can be obtained from various textbooks [46,52,53].

■ Evaluation of Central Autonomic Activity and Function

The evaluation of central autonomic activity and function is separately described as there are difficulties in accurately making measurements noninvasively. Recently, however, various technological and analytical advances have been utilized to advantage. Neuroimaging using widely available techniques such as brain magnetic resonance imaging is repeatable and reproducible and can determine morphology of even small structures such as the insular cortex, amygdala, and pontine regions; thus, in central autonomic disorders such as multiple system atrophy, discrete

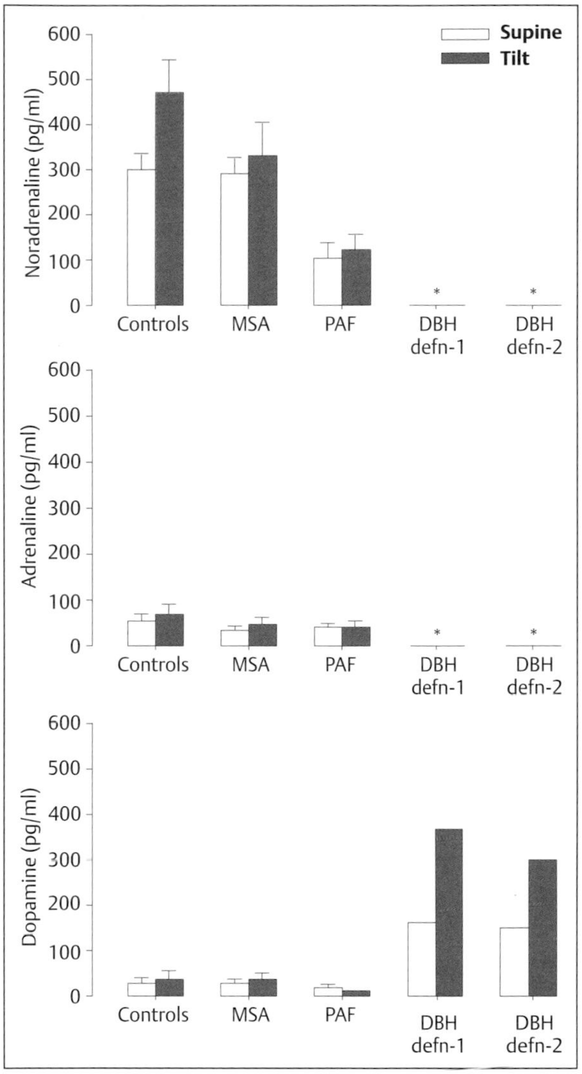

Fig. 2.**21** Plasma norepinephrine, epinephrine, and dopamine levels (measured by high-pressure liquid chromatography) in normal subjects (controls), patients with multiple system atrophy (MSA) or pure autonomic failure (PAF) and two individual patients with dopamine β-hydroxylase deficiency (DBH defn) while supine and after head-up tilt to 45° for 10 minutes. The asterisks indicate levels below the detection limits for the assay, which are less than 5 pg/ml for norepinephrine and epinephrine and less than 20 pg/ml for dopamine. Bars indicate ± SEM. (From [49], with permission)

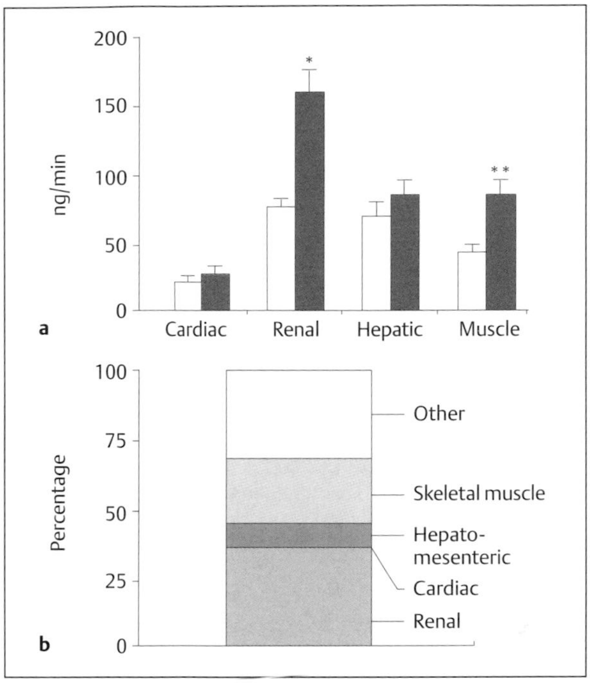

Fig. 2.**22** Pre- and postprandial regional plasma norepinephrine spillover, indicating sympathetic nervous system activation in normal subjects. **a** The open histograms indicate the values while fasting and the filled histograms the postprandial values, in different vascular beds. The percentage changes are indicated in **b**. There is greater activation in the renal and skeletal muscle vasculature than in cardiac or hepatic regions. (From [50], with permission)

Table 2.**5** Some symptoms resulting from orthostatic hypotension and impaired perfusion of various organs

Cerebral hypoperfusion
Dizziness
Visual disturbances
Blurred vision
Tunnel vision
Scotoma
Graying out
Blacking out
Color defects
Loss of consciousness
Impaired cognition
Muscle hypoperfusion
Paracervical and suboccipital ("coathanger") ache
Lower back/buttock ache
Calf claudication
Cardiac hypoperfusion
Angina pectoris
Spinal cord hypoperfusion
Renal hypoperfusion
Oliguria
Nonspecific
Weakness, lethargy, fatigue
Falls

Adapted from [44]

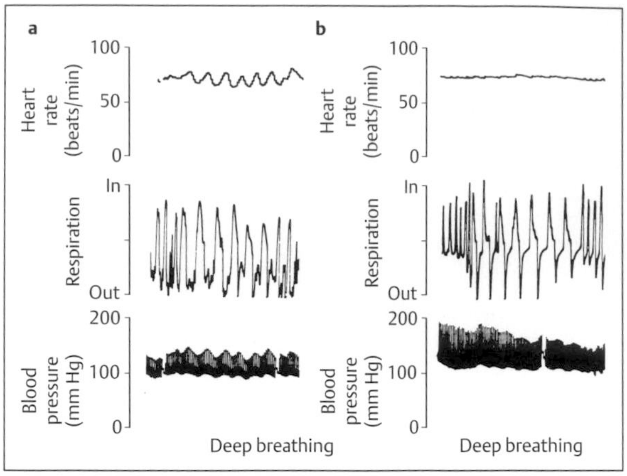

Fig. 2.23 The effect of deep breathing on heart rate and blood pressure in **a** a normal subject and **b** a patient with autonomic failure. There is no sinus arrhythmia in the patient, despite a fall in blood pressure. Respiratory changes are indicated in the middle panel. (From [49], with permission)

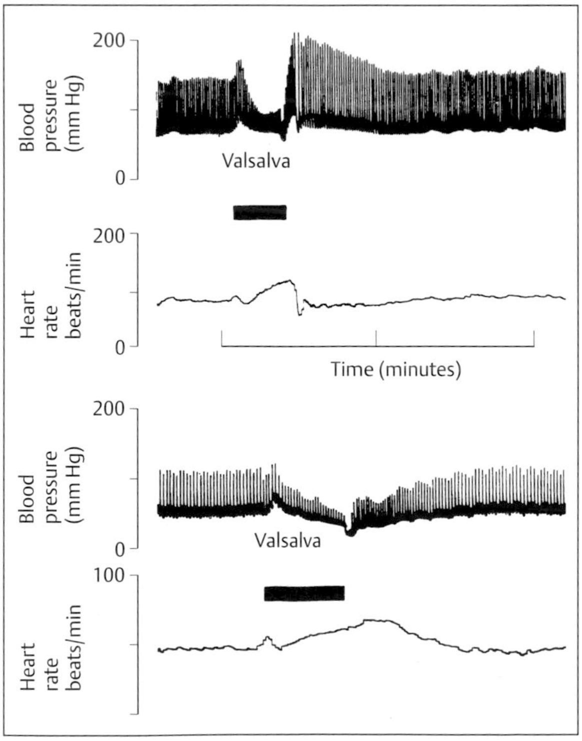

Fig. 2.24 Changes in intra-arterial blood pressure before, during, and after the Valsalva maneuver, when intrathoracic pressure was raised to 40 mmHg in a normal subject (upper trace) and in a patient with autonomic failure (lower trace). In the normal subject, release of intrathoracic pressure was accompanied by an increase in blood pressure and reduction in heart rate below basal levels. In the patient there was a gradual increase in blood pressure, implying impairment of sympathetic vasoconstrictor pathways. The heart rate scale varies in the two subjects. (From [49], with permission)

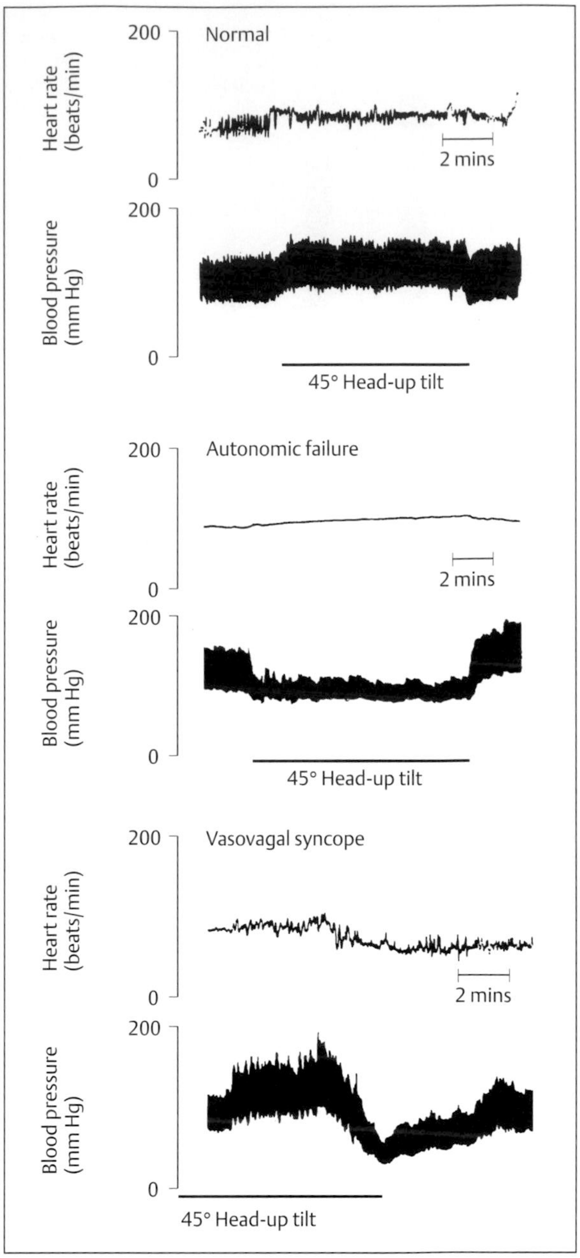

Fig. 2.25 Blood pressure and heart rate before, during, and after head-up tilt in a normal subject (uppermost panel), a patient with autonomic failure (middle panel), and a patient with vasovagal syncope (lowermost panel). In the normal subject there is no fall in blood pressure during head-up tilt, unlike the patient with autonomic failure, in whom blood pressure falls promptly and remains low with a blood pressure overshoot on return to the horizontal. In the patient with autonomic failure there is only a minimal change in heart rate despite the marked blood pressure fall. In the patient with vasovagal syncope there was initially no fall in blood pressure during head-up tilt; in the latter part of tilt, as indicated in the record, blood pressure initially rose and then fell to low levels, so that the patient had to be returned to the horizontal. Heart rate also fell. In each case continuous blood pressure and heart rate was recorded with the Portapress II. (From [49], with permission)

Table 2.6 Nonneurogenic causes of orthostatic hypotension

Low intravascular volume	
Blood/plasma loss	Hemorrhage, burns, hemodialysis
Fluid/electrolyte	Inadequate intake: anorexia nervosa
	Fluid loss: vomiting, diarrhea, losses from ileostomy
	Renal/endocrine: salt-losing neuropathy, adrenal insufficiency (Addison's disease), diabetes insipidus, diuretics
Vasodilatation	
	Drugs: glyceryl trinitrate
	Alcohol
	Heat, pyrexia
	Hyperbradykininism
	Systemic mastocytosis
	Extensive varicose veins
Cardiac impairment	
Myocardial	Myocarditis
Impaired ventricular filling	Atrial myxoma, constrictive pericarditis
Impaired output	Aortic stenosis

Adapted from [49]

abnormalities are discernible in the brainstem. Further amplification of neuronal involvement may be obtained by magnetic resonance spectroscopy, although abnormalities have been described mainly in the basal ganglia. Of importance are the techniques of positron emission tomography (PET) and functional MRI (fMRI) scanning. In normal humans, specific areas may be activated by different stimuli, such as the anterior cingulate gyrus for cardiovascular tasks (Fig. 2.**28**), and the amygdala, with varying hemispheric dominance in response to different emotional stimuli (Fig. 2.**29**). The use of various neuropsychological paradigms to stimulate different brain areas, especially the amygdala, should be of further value in determining the functional anatomy of cerebral autonomic centers in normal humans, and in evaluating disturbances of function in various autonomic disorders.

Another approach to central autonomic evaluation has been the use of neuroendocrine challenge tests, where physiological or pharmacological stimuli in conjunction with measurement of neuroendocrine markers provide, in vivo, an indication of which controlling nucleus, pathway, or even neurotransmitter is involved. This has been demonstrated in multiple system atrophy (MSA), where the lesions are predominantly central, as compared to pure autonomic failure (PAF), where they are peripheral. Thus, the arginine-vasopressin (AVP) response to a physiological stimulus causing baroreceptor activation (with head-up tilt) is abnormal in both MSA and PAF; however, central osmoreceptor stimulation (with hypertonic saline and rise in AVP), is preserved in PAF, but not in MSA. An example of a neuroendocrine test utilizing a neuropharmacological stimulus is based on the α_2-adrenoceptor projection to the hypothalamus, which causes release of human growth hormone releasing factor (HGRF), that then raises growth hormone (GH) levels. In normal subjects, central stimulation with the α_2-agonist clonidine elevates HGRF and GH; this also occurs when there is peripheral autonomic denervation without central involvement, as in PAF (Fig. 2.**30**). However, in MSA, with predominantly central lesions, there is no GH response to clonidine. This lack of rise in GH is not due to an inability of hypothalamic cells to secrete HGRF (and thus stimulate the pituitary), as the GH secretagogue L-dopa, raises both HGRF and GH levels in MSA (Fig. 2.**31**). This favors a specific abnormality in the α_2-adrenoceptor projection to the hypothalamus in MSA, and indicates that the impaired GH response to clonidine is not due to hypothalamic neuronal cell loss or pituitary malfunction. These neuroendocrine mapping approaches therefore help to determine both the central sites and the neurotransmitters involved, especially in autonomic disorders that may selectively affect one or more neuronal systems and pathways.

Table 2.7 Factors influencing orthostatic hypotension

Speed of positional change
Time of day (worse in the morning)
Prolonged recumbency
Warm environment (hot weather, central heating, hot bath)
Raising intrathoracic pressure: micturition, defecation, or coughing
Food and alcohol ingestion
Physical exertion
Physical maneuvers and positions (bending forward, abdominal compression, leg crossing, squatting, activating calf muscle pump)[a]
Drugs with vasoactive properties (including dopaminergic agents)

Adapted from [49]
[a] These maneuvers usually reduce the postural fall in blood pressure, unlike the others.

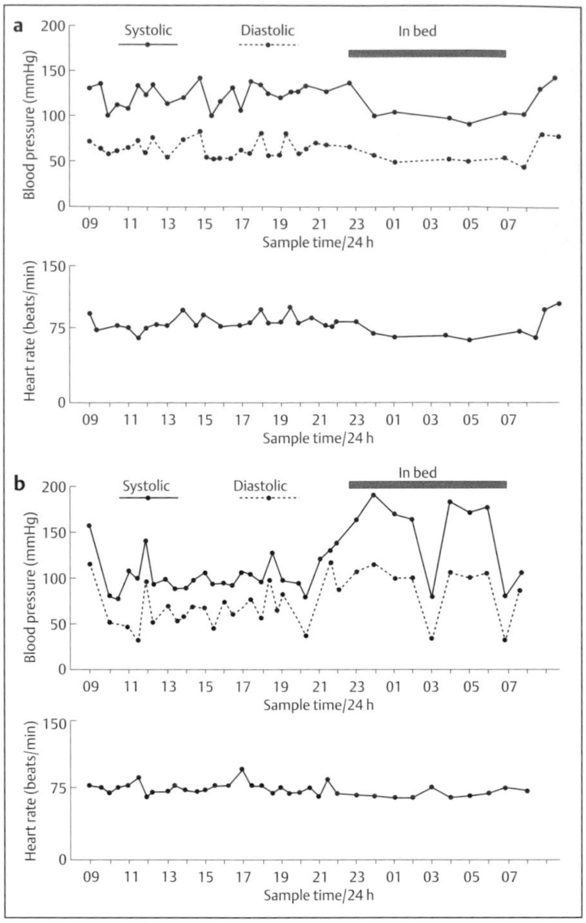

Fig. 2.**26** Twenty-four-hour noninvasive ambulatory blood pressure and heart rate profiles showing systolic (•—•) and diastolic (•···•) blood pressure and heart rate at intervals through the day and night. **a** Changes in a normal subject with no postural fall in blood pressure; there was a fall in blood pressure at night whilst asleep (an expected circadian nocturnal fall), with a rise in blood pressure on wakening. **b** Marked fluctuations in blood pressure in a patient with autonomic failure. The falls in blood pressure are usually the result of postural changes, either sitting or standing. Blood pressure when supine, particularly at night, is elevated. Getting up to micturate causes a marked fall in blood pressure (0300 hours). There is a reversal of the diurnal changes in blood pressure. The changes in heart rate are relatively small, considering the large changes in blood pressure. (From [49], with permission)

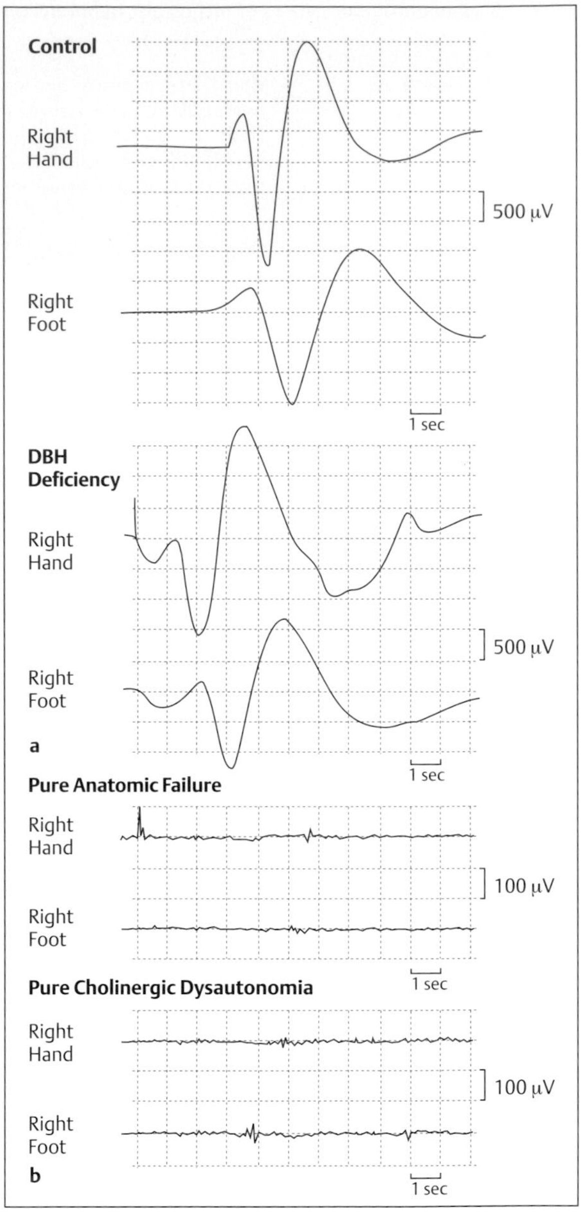

Fig. 2.**27 a** The sympathetic skin response (in microvolts) from the right hand and right foot of a normal subject (control) and a patient with dopamine β-hydroxylase (DBH) deficiency. In pure autonomic failure and pure cholinergic dysautonomia (**b**) the sympathetic skin response could not be recorded. (From [51], with permission)

Additional Nonautonomic Investigations

In clinical practice, evaluation of autonomic function and dysfunction often needs to be combined with other investigations to determine the causative or associated disease (as in secondary autonomic disorders), and whether there are coexistent diseases or complications. This is of particular importance in diabetes mellitus, where multiple systems may be affected.

Thus investigation of both large and small cerebral vessels (to exclude cerebrovascular disease), neurophysiological assessment (to determine the presence and extent of motor and sensory neuropathy), and allied investigations into urinary bladder, gut, and sexual function may be needed to distinguish between neurogenic failure of target organs and other causes of organ dysfunction (see [44,46,52,53]).

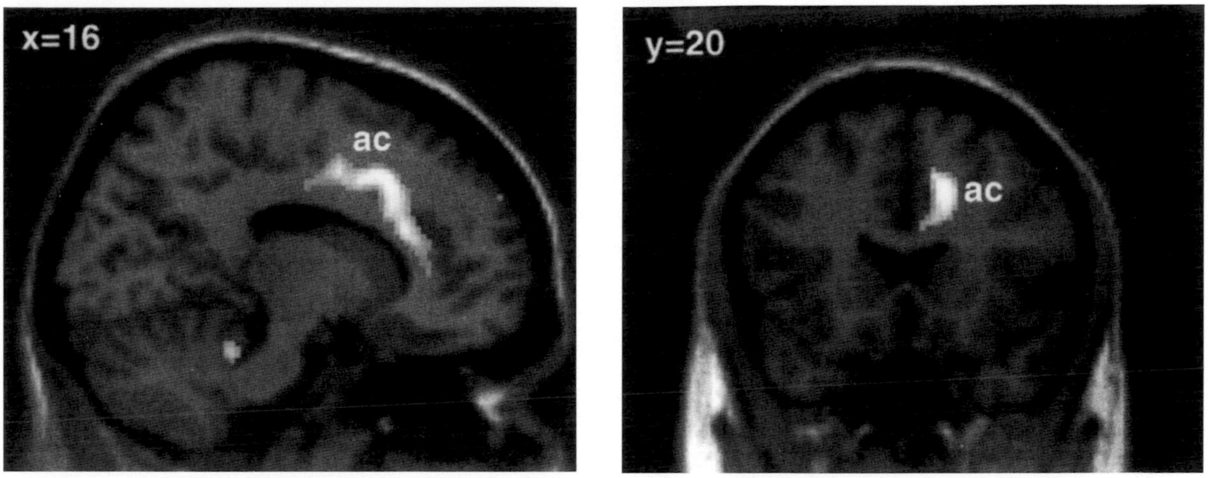

Fig. 2.**28** Right anterior cingulate activity showing positive covariance with mean arterial blood pressure (MAP) during isometric exercise and mental arithmetic tasks. Activity in the right anterior cingulate (ac) covaried significantly with increasing blood pressure. For all subjects, regional activity covarying with MAP was computed for isometric exercise and mental arithmetic tasks. (From [54], with permission)

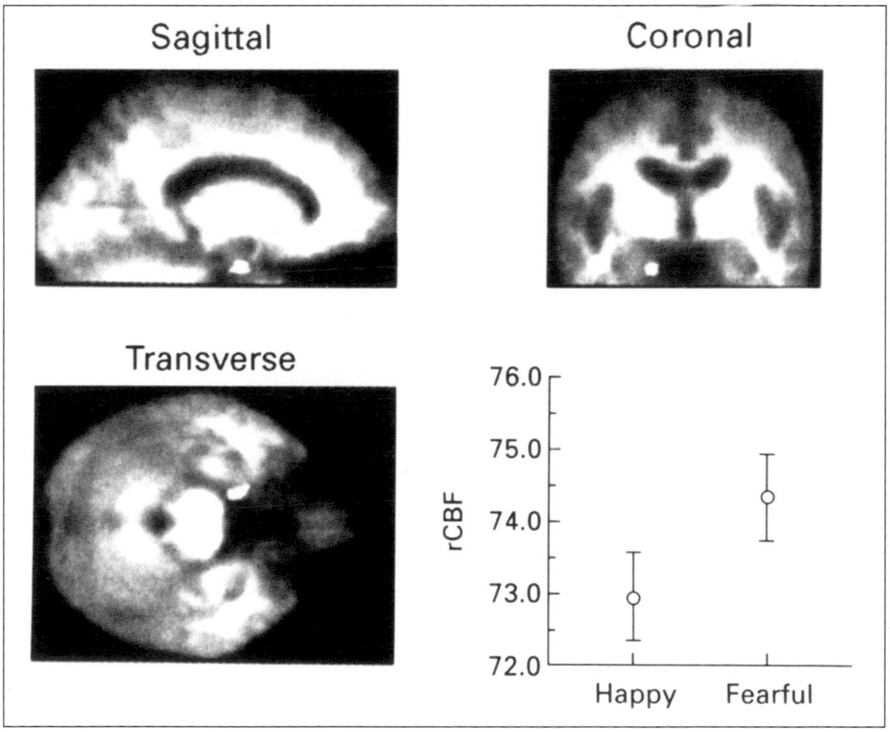

Fig. 2.**29** Views of the brain showing activation of the left amygdala using PET scanning with $H_2{}^{15}O$ superimposed on structural magnetic resonance images, and the construction of a statistical parametric map. This was in response to visual stimuli using photographs showing happy and fearful facial expressions. Regional cerebral blood flow (rCBF) is indicated on the right. Faces with fearful expressions caused greater change in blood flow to the amygdala than happy faces. (From [55], with permission)

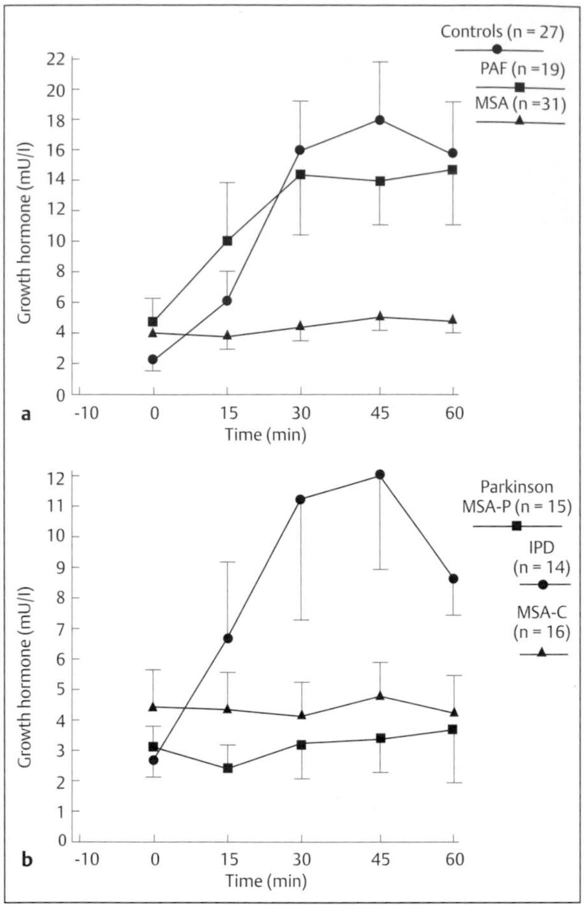

Fig. 2.**30** The upper panel (a) shows mean (SE) serum growth hormone (GH) concentrations before (0) and at 15-minute intervals for 60 minutes after administration of clonidine (2 μg/kg per minute) in normal subjects (controls) and in patients with pure autonomic failure (PAF) and multiple system atrophy (MSA). GH concentrations rise in controls and in patients with PAF with a peripheral lesion; there is no rise in patients with MSA with a central lesion. The lower panel (b) indicates lack of serum GH response to clonidine in the two forms of MSA (the cerebellar form, MSA-C, and the parkinsonian form, MSA-P), in contrast to patients with idiopathic Parkinson's disease (IPD) with no autonomic deficit, in whom there is a significant rise in GH levels. (From [56], with permission)

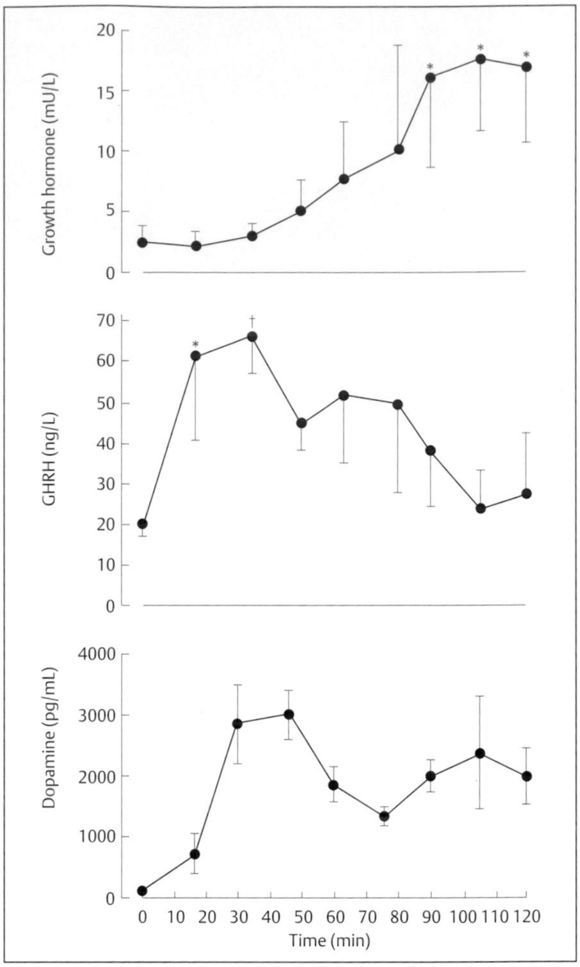

Fig. 2.**31** Mean (SE) serum growth hormone (GH), plasma human growth hormone releasing hormone (GHRH), and dopamine concentrations before and after administration of L-dopa in nine patients with MSA-P. **P* < 0.05 and † *P* < 0.01 vs basal (time 0). (From [56], with permission)

References

[1] Kandel ER, Schwartz JH, Jessell TM, editors. Principles of neural science, 4th ed. New York: McGraw-Hill; 2000.

[2] Kingsley RE. Concise text of neuroscience, 2nd ed. Baltimore: Lippincott, Williams & Wilkins; 2000.

[3] Gardiner EP, Martin JH, Jessell TM. The bodily senses. In: Kandel ER, Schwartz JH, Jessell TM, editors. Principles of neural science, 4th ed. New York: McGraw-Hill; 2000: 430–50.

[4] Keshner EA, Cohen H. Current concepts of the vestibular system reviewed: 1. The role of the vestibulospinal system in postural control. Am J Occup Ther 1989; 43:320–30.

[5] Wurtz RH, Albano JE. Visual-motor function of the primate superior colliculus. Annu Rev Neurosci 1980; 3:189–226.

[6] Brooks DJ. The role of the basal ganglia in motor control: contributions from PET. J Neurol Sci 1995; 128:1–13.

[7] Stocchi F, Brusa L. Cognition and emotion in different stages and subtypes of Parkinson's disease. J Neurol 2000; 247 (Suppl 2):II114–21.

[8] Thach WT. A role for the cerebellum in learning movement coordination. Neurobiol Learning Memory 1998; 70:177–88.

[9] Birder LA, Perl ER. Cutaneous sensory receptors. J Clin Neurophysiol 1994; 11:534–52.

[10] Johnson KO, Hsiao SS. Neural mechanism of tactual form and texture perception. Annu Rev Neurosci 1992; 15:227–50.

[11] Hulliger M. The mammalian muscle spindle and its central control. Rev Physiol Biochem Pharmacol 1984; 101:1–110.

[12] Zimny ML. Mechanoreceptors in articular tissues. Am J Anat 1988; 182:16–32.

[13] Spray DC. Cutaneous temperature receptors. Annu Rev Physiol 1986; 48:625–38.

[14] Cesare P, McNaughton P. Peripheral pain mechanisms. Curr Opinion Neurobiol 1997; 7:493–9.

[15] Baron R. Peripheral neuropathic pain: from mechanisms to symptoms. Clin J Pain 2000; 16 (Suppl):S12–S20.

[16] Eaton SE, Harris ND, Rajbhandari SM, Greenwood P, Wilkinson ID, Ward JD, Griffiths PD, Tesfaye S. Spinal-cord involvement in diabetic peripheral neuropathy. Lancet 2001; 358:35–6.

[17] Fields HL. Pain. New York: McGraw-Hill; 1987.

[18] Melzack R, Wall PD. Pain mechanisms: a new theory. Science 1965; 150:971–9.

[19] Bausbaum AI, Fields HL. Endogenous pain control systems: brainstem spinal pathways and endorphin circuitry. Annu Rev Neurosci 1984; 7:309–38.

[20] Willis WD, Westlund KN. Neuroanatomy of the pain system and of the pathways that modulate pain. J Clin Neurophysiol 1997; 14:2–31.

[21] Burke RE. Motor unit properties and selective involvement in movement. Exerc Sport Sci Rev 1975; 3:31–81.

[22] Liddell EG, Sherrington C. Reflexes in response to stretch (myotatic reflexes). Proc R Soc Lond B Biol Sci 1924; 96:212–42.

[23] Lundberg A. Multisensory control of spinal reflex pathways. Prog Brain Res 1979; 50:11–28.

[24] Paulson OB, Strandgaard S, Edvinsson L. Cerebral autoregulation. Cerebrovasc Brain Metab Rev 1990; 2:161–92

[25] Szabo C. Physiological and pathophysiological roles of nitric oxide in the central nervous system. Brain Res Bull 1996; 41:131–41.

[26] Faraci FM, Heistad DD. Regulation of the cerebral circulation: role of endothelium and potassium channels. Physiol Rev 1998; 78:53–97.

[27] Lundborg G, Branemark PI. Microvascular structure and function of peripheral nerves. Adv Microcirc 1:66–88.

[28] Lundborg G. Intraneural microcirculation. Orthop Clin North Am 1988; 19:1–12.

[29] Petterson CA, Olsson Y. Blood supply of spinal nerve roots. An experimental study in the rat. Acta Neuropathol 1989; 78:455–61.

[30] Olsson Y. Microenvironment of the peripheral nervous system under normal and pathological conditions. Crit Rev Neurobiol 1990; 5:265–311.

[31] Bell MA, Weddell AG. A descriptive study of the blood vessels of the sciatic nerve in the rat, man and other mammals. Brain 1984; 107:871–98.

[32] Bell MA, Weddell AG. A morphometric study of intrafascicular vessels of the mammalian sciatic nerve. Muscle Nerve 1984; 7:524–34.

[33] Low PA, Lagerlund TD, McManis PG. Nerve blood flow and oxygen delivery in normal, diabetic and ischemic neuropathy. Int Rev Neurobiol 1989; 31:355–438.

[34] Appenzeller O, Dhital KK, Cowen T, Burnstock G. The nerves to blood vessels supplying blood to nerves: the innervation of vasa nervosum. Brain Res 1984; 304:383–6.

[35] Rechthand E, Hervonen A, Sato S, Rapoport SI. Distribution of adrenergic innervation of blood vessels in peripheral nerve. Brain Res 1986; 374:185–9.

[36] Low PA, Tuck RR. Effects of changes of blood pressure, respiratory acidosis and hypoxia on blood flow in the sciatic nerve of the rat. J Physiol (Lond) 1984; 347:513–24.

[37] Kihara M, Nickander KK, Low PA. The effect of aging on endoneurial blood flow, hyperaemic response and oxygen free radicals in rat sciatic nerve. Brain Res 1991; 562:1–5.

[38] Cameron NE, Cotter MA, Robertson S, Maxfield EK. Nerve function in experimental diabetes in rats: effects of electrical stimulation. Am J Physiol 1993; 264:E161–6.

[39] McManis PG, Schmelzer JD, Zollman PJ, Low PA. Blood flow and autoregulation in somatic and autonomic ganglia: comparison with sciatic nerve. Brain 1997; 120:445–9.

[40] Sasaki H, Schmelzer JD, Zollman PJ, Low PA. Neuropathology and blood flow of nerve, spinal roots and dorsal root ganglia in longstanding diabetic rats. Acta Neuropathol 1997; 93:118–28.

[41] Cameron NE, Cotter MA. Diabetes causes an early reduction in autonomic ganglion blood flow in rats. J Diabetes Complications 2001; 15:198–202.

[42] Devor M. Unexplained peculiarities of the dorsal root ganglion. Pain 1999; Suppl 6:S27–35.

[43] Janig W. Autonomic nervous system. In: Schmidt RF, Thews G, editors. Human physiology, 2nd ed. Berlin: Springer-Verlag; 1987: 333–70.

[44] Mathias CJ. Disorders of the autonomic nervous system. In: Bradley WG, Daroff RB, Fenichel GM, Marsden CD, editors. Neurology in clinical practice, 3rd ed. Boston: Butterworth-Heinemann; 2000: 2131–65.

[45] Westmoreland BF, Benarroch EE, Daube JR, et al. Medical neurosciences: an approach to anatomy, pathology and physiology by systems and levels, 3rd ed. Boston: Little, Brown and Co; 1994.

[46] Appenzeller O, Oribe E. The autonomic nervous system, 5th ed. Amsterdam: Elsevier; 1997.

[47] Burnstock G. Autonomic neuroeffector functions – reflex vasodilatation of the skin. J Invest Derm 1997; 69:47–57.

[48] Wallin BG, Linblad L-E. Baroreflex mechanisms controlling sympathetic outflow to muscles. In: Sleight P, editor. Arterial baroreceptors and hypertension. Oxford: Oxford University Press 1980:101.

[49] Mathias CJ, Bannister R. Investigation of autonomic disorders. In: Mathias CJ, Bannister R, editors. Autonomic failure: a textbook of clinical disorders of the autonomic nervous system, 4th ed. Oxford: Oxford University Press; 1999: 169–95.

[50] Vaz M, Cox HS, Kaye DM, Turner AG, Jennings GL, Esler MD. Fallibility of plasma noradrenaline measurements in studying postprandial sympathetic nervous responses. J Auton Nerv Syst 1995; 56: 97–104.

[51] Magnifico F, Misra VP, Murray NMF, Mathias CJ. The sympathetic skin response in peripheral autonomic failure-evaluation in pure autonomic failure, pure cholinergic dysautonomia and dopamine beta-hydroxylase deficiency. Clin Auton Res 1998; 8: 133–38.

[52] Low PA., editor. Clinical autonomic disorders, 2nd ed. Philadelphia: Lippincott-Raven; 1997.

[53] Mathias CJ, Bannister R, editors. Autonomic failure: a textbook of clinical disorders of the autonomic nervous system, 4th ed. Oxford: Oxford University Press; 1999.

[54] Critchley HD, Corfield DR, Chandler MP, Mathias CJ, Dolan RJ. Cerebral correlates of autonomic cardiovascular arousal: a functional neuroimaging investigation in humans. J Physiol 2000; 523: 259–70.

[55] Morris JS, Frith CD, Perreth DI, et al. A differential neural response in the human amygdala to fearful and happy facial expressions. Nature 1996; 383: 812–5.

[56] Kimber JR, Watson L, Mathias CJ. Distinction of idiopathic Parkinson's disease from multiple system atrophy by stimulation of growth hormone release with clonidine. Lancet 1997; 349: 1877–81.

3 Epidemiology of Diabetic Neuropathy

J. E. Shaw, P. Z. Zimmet, F. A. Gries, and D. Ziegler

Introduction

The epidemiology of a disease primarily describes the frequency with which it occurs, and determines the risk factors associated with it. The former informs the clinician about the likelihood that the patient in front of him or her has the condition and the public health authorities about the potential overall burden relating to the condition. The latter sheds light on etiological processes, although the associations described by epidemiological studies cannot alone be taken as proof of causality.

In order to understand the epidemiology of a disease properly, it is important to have well-validated diagnostic tests that can be used by a variety of investigators assessing different populations in a similar manner. Furthermore, it is important that the populations studied are representative of the total population being considered, and have not been subjected to significant selection biases. However, the study of the epidemiology of diabetic neuropathy has been beset by numerous problems relating both to diagnostic tests and to population selection.

Testing for Peripheral Neuropathy

Diabetic peripheral neuropathy is a complex disorder in which the disease process may affect different sets of nerve fibers to different degrees in different individuals. Thus, one individual may have an abnormality of large-fiber sensory function, which could be detected by measuring the vibration perception threshold (VPT), whilst another may have a predominantly small-fiber neuropathy that can only be detected by measuring the thermal perception threshold (TPT). This feature of neuropathy can cause problems in the selection of a single test with which to screen a population. The issue of measurement of neurological function is further complicated by the nature of the tests. Many are psychophysical tests, in which the subject is required to interpret the nature of an external stimulus (usually applied to the foot). This subjectivity can lead to relatively poor reproducibility of tests such as VPT, in which the subject has to differentiate light touch from vibratory sensation.

This lack of certainty over the value of individual tests for the assessment of diabetic neuropathy has led to recommendations that several different tests should be performed, and that diabetic neuropathy should only be diagnosed when more than one is abnormal [1]. Whilst this may make the diagnostic process more rigorous in any individual or in an individual study, it can make comparisons between studies more difficult. Such recommendations have been only patchily adopted, and where they have been put into practice, the selection of tests has not been uniform. Thus, we are faced with having to compare the prevalence when neuropathy is determined by a single test with the prevalence when neuropathy is diagnosed when any two out of perhaps three to five tests are abnormal. Increasing the number of tests that are performed will automatically increase the number of individuals in whom an abnormality is found, while requiring that more than one abnormality is present will then tend to decrease the prevalence. The overall effect is thus complex. The impact of varying the diagnostic testing procedure can be seen in the Diabetes Control and Complications Trial (DCCT) data (Table 3.**1**), where the prevalence of distal symmetrical polyneuropathy (DSP) at baseline in the conventional therapy cohort varied from 0.3 % (abnormalities of reflexes, sensory examination, and neuropathic symptoms) to 21.8 % (abnormal nerve conduction in at least two nerves) [2]. Confirmed clinical neuropathy (abnormal history or examination, confirmed by abnormal nerve conduction or autonomic function) was the gold standard for the study, and was found in 2.1 % of this cohort. This 73-fold difference in the prevalence of DSP, between the two extremes, but within a single population, highlights the difficulties of comparing studies with differing diagnostic criteria.

The influence of test selection on the understanding of etiological factors associated with neuropathy is likely to be considerably smaller than that on prevalence. As long as each diagnostic process is indeed measuring some aspect (or aspects) of neuropathy, it is likely that those who are rated as having neuropathy are genuinely more severely affected than those who are not so rated. Thus, associations with factors such as age or glycemic control may be easier to compare across different studies than are prevalences, which are highly dependent not only on the test (or tests) selected, but also on the diagnostic threshold that is used. For example, the groups selected either by absent ankle reflexes or by elevated VPT are both likely to be older and have poorer glycemic control than the groups who are normal on these respective tests. However, unless loss of ankle reflexes represents the same degree of neuropathy as does an abnormal VPT

Table 3.1 Prevalence of polyneuropathy within the DCCT conventional therapy primary prevention cohort, according to diagnostic test

Diagnostic criteria[a]	Neuropathy prevalence (%)
Sensory examination, reflexes, and symptoms	0.3
Symptoms and reflexes	0.5
Sensory examination and symptoms	1.1
Symptoms or sensory examination, confirmed by abnormal nerve conduction or autonomic function[b]	2.1
Sensory examination and reflexes	2.1
Abnormal autonomic function	2.4
Symptoms alone	3.7
Any two out of symptoms, sensory examination, reflexes	4.5
Reflexes alone	5.8
Sensory examination alone	12.2
Nerve conduction (abnormal in at least 2 nerves)	21.8

Data adapted from [2]

[a] Abnormalities required in the fields listed
[b] Gold standard measure of neuropathy for the study

(according to the threshold selected – see below), the prevalences generated from the same population by these two tests could be quite different.

Even when the same test has been used, the methods and the selection of thresholds have not been uniform. VPT is widely used, but some studies use age-related thresholds (based on UK normal data) [3], while others have ignored age and used a single cutoff [4]. More recently, locally derived normal ranges have been applied, although in one study these were derived separately for different age groups [5], while another compared all diabetic subjects to a young nondiabetic population [6].

It is obvious from the discussion above that there is a long way to go in finding a definition of neuropathy that can be widely used, although it is clearly needed for accurate epidemiological study. This definition needs to be appropriate for the clinical forms that the disease may take (e.g., small fiber or large fiber involvement), related to hard endpoints, such as foot ulceration, agreed upon widely, and useful for a range of both clinical and research purposes. Multiple testing of different neurological functions, although recommended as the gold standard [1], can be difficult and expensive, especially in large field studies. Furthermore, recent data suggest complex patterns of sensation in DSP with decreased VPT (hypoesthesia) and heat stimulus-induced hyperesthesia (low thresholds), both being characteristic of mild DSP as they correlate with neuropathic symptoms and deficits, whereas panmodality hypoesthesia is typical of severe DSP [7]. The only studies that relate measures of neurological function (in a prospective manner) with subsequent foot ulceration and amputation have used simple quantitative sensory tests, such as VPT or monofilament sensitivity [8,9].

Population Selection

The second important obstacle in determining the prevalence of neuropathy is the selection of people who are going to be tested. Hospital clinic-based studies will usually be biased towards those with more serious problems, and are likely to overestimate the prevalence of neuropathy in the general diabetic population. Nevertheless, the value of hospital-based prevalence studies should not be underestimated. Whilst they do not directly address the issue of what the general risk of having neuropathy is in a person with diabetes, they precisely answer the question of how common neuropathy is amongst hospital clinic patients. This in itself may be a very important and valuable issue. The problem, however, is that one hospital-based population may not be the same as another – an issue that can be partially overcome with multicenter studies [10]. Another problem is that temporal trends in referral patterns from primary care can make today's hospital population quite different to tomorrow's.

Studies using registers of people with diabetes that are derived from primary care will overcome the hospital-based biases, and not surprisingly have reported lower prevalences [11]. However, this selection methodology remains dependent on the proportion of people with diabetes who are actually diagnosed. Since approximately 50% of all of those with diabetes are undiagnosed [12], this method also has flaws. Population-based epidemiological surveys, in which a high proportion of a representative sample of the general population is directly tested for diabetes (by blood glucose testing), and then those found to have diabetes (previously diagnosed and newly diagnosed) are screened for neuropathy, represent an alternative approach. This should be a more reliable and reproducible way of determining the prevalence of diabetic neuropathy, but only two such studies have been reported [5,6].

One drawback of this approach is that the group with "newly diagnosed" diabetes (i.e., diagnosed as part of the study by blood glucose testing) is usually identified by an abnormal glucose value measured on a single day. Since the diagnosis of diabetes requires verification of this on another day [13], it is likely that the group identified includes a number of individuals who would have a nondiabetic glucose value on repeat testing, and therefore do not actually have diabetes. Assuming that these people do not have neuropathy (since they do not have diabetes), their inclusion would dilute the sample and lead to an underestimate of the prevalence of neuropathy in the newly diagnosed group. Nevertheless, neuropathy prevalence estimates derived from population-based samples that include all of those people who have diabetes (both diagnosed and undiagnosed) should be the most accurate and reproducible approach.

How Common Is Diabetic Neuropathy?

Distal Symmetrical Polyneuropathy

Prevalence in Diabetes

Taking into account the issues discussed above, it is difficult to determine with any precision the prevalence of diabetic neuropathy. Several large studies have examined the prevalence in hospital-based populations. A number of these are in fairly close agreement, and reveal prevalences of DSP at approximately 30 %, amongst both European and African populations [8,14–16]. However, other hospital-based studies have produced figures closer to 20 % [3], and a prevalence of 50 % was reported from a US veterans population [17]. The higher figure in this last study may relate to the age of the participants, and to the fact that they were almost all male.

Studies which have used primary care registers of people with diabetes, or which report the prevalence in people with previously diagnosed diabetes derived from population-based surveys, have mainly reported lower prevalences than those given in hospital-based studies. Some studies report prevalences of around 20 % [6,11,18–20], although a figure as high as 54 % in type 1 and 45 % in type 2 diabetic patients was reported from a population based sample from Rochester [21], and 42 % of a sample of 811 type 2 diabetic subjects drawn from 37 UK general practices were found to be neuropathic [22]. The Rochester study used electrophysiology as part of the neurological assessment. This is frequently abnormal in diabetes, even within a short time of diagnosis of type 1 diabetes, and has not been validated as a predictor of foot ulceration. The prevalence rates of DSP in type 1 and type 2 diabetic patients are summarized in Table 3.**2**.

When general populations are screened by glucose tolerance testing, and those identified as having diabetes are assessed for peripheral neuropathy, the prevalence has been relatively low (Table 3.**3**). In our own study from the Indian Ocean island of Mauritius (in which 70 % of the population originates from India) the data showed the lowest prevalence of DSP yet reported [5]. The overall prevalence in the total diabetic population was 8.3 %, i.e., 12.7 % in subjects with known diabetes and just 3.6 % among those with newly diagnosed diabetes. Consistent with the low neuropathy prevalence was a low prevalence of lower limb amputation – a finding that has been reported elsewhere for people who originate from the Indian subcontinent [36]. Neuropathy was based on VPT measurements, using locally derived age specific normal ranges. In the only similar study, from Egypt [6], 14 % of the newly diagnosed diabetic population were found to have DSP. However, the reference range used for VPT in that study related to healthy adults under the age of 45, and therefore probably did not account for the normal age related rise in VPT. Thus, since the majority of those with diabetes were over the age of 45, the neuropathy prevalence in that study may be an overestimate. In two Native American populations, which are regularly screened for diabetes with glucose tolerance testing, the prevalence of DSP in the whole diabetic population was 19 % [4,9].

The prevalence of diabetic neuropathy in general populations was evaluated in two door-to-door surveys that were restricted to a questionnaire which represents the most crude and simple screening instrument [37,38]. However, since no screening for diabetes had been performed, the exact prevalence of diabetes in these populations was unknown.

It can be seen from Tables 3.**2** and 3.**3** that diagnostic methodology is far from uniform. Indeed, there are hardly any two studies that have used identical methods. Nevertheless, a pattern can be discerned in these studies. The prevalence in hospital-based populations is probably around 30 %, falling to about 20 % when people with established diabetes are selected from a community base. Amongst the complete diabetic

Table 3.2 Prevalence of distal symmetric polyneuropathy in subjects with established type 1 or type 2 diabetes

Study site	Neuropathy diagnosis	Population selection			
		Hospital-based		Primary care or population screening	
		Type 1	Type 2	Type 1	Type 2
Australia, 1986 [23]	Reduced pin-prick			8	17
USA, 1987 [24]	NCV				46
USA, 1989 [25]	Symptoms, signs			34	
USA, 1990 [20]	Signs				26
USA, 1993 [21]	Symptoms, signs, QST, NCV, HRV (deep breathing)			54	45
USA, 1993 [26]	Symptoms			30	38
USA, 1997 [17]	Monofilament		50		
Tanzania, 1997 [16]	Symptoms and signs		28		
Egypt, 1998 [6]	VPT[a]				22
Mauritius, 1998 [5]	VPT[b]				13
Saudi Arabia, 1998 [27]	Absent pin-prick or vibration		20		
Europe, 1996 [14]	Symptoms, signs, VPT[c], AFTs		28		
Netherlands, 1991 [28]	Symptoms				18
Netherlands, 1996 [29]	Absent VPT (big toe/ malleolus)		50/8		
Germany, 1993 [30]	VPT			25	27
Germany, Austria, Switzerland, 1993 [31]	Symptoms and signs	17	35		
Italy, 1993 [32]	Symptoms and signs			28	
Italy, 1997 [15]	Signs		32		
Italy, 1997 [18]	Symptoms and signs				19
UK, 1992 [11]	Symptoms and signs			13	17
UK, 1993 [10]	Symptoms, signs	23	32		
UK, 1994 [22]	Signs				42
Spain, 1998 [19]	Symptoms and signs	13	24		
France, 1998 [3]	VPT[c]		20		
Sweden, 1998 [27]	Absent pin-prick or vibration		19		

Data shown are percentages
AFTs, autonomic function tests; HRV, heart rate variability; NCV, nerve conduction velocity; QST, quantitative sensory testing; VPT, vibration perception threshold
[a] Compared to locally derived values for healthy young adults
[b] Compared to locally derived age-specific normal values
[c] Adjusted for age, sex, and height

population, including both diagnosed and undiagnosed diabetes, the prevalence of DSP is probably less than 20%.

Prevalence in Impaired Glucose Tolerance

Although the development of diabetic polyneuropathy is typically insidious over several years, it may occasionally be the presenting feature in type 2 diabetic patients [39]. It is not known whether this "early" nerve alteration has developed during a period of unrecognized diabetes or evolves gradually during a state of impaired glucose tolerance (IGT) prior to the transition to overt diabetes. In this context, it is unclear whether there is a glycemic threshold beyond which nerve dysfunction develops. If IGT constitutes such a threshold which needs to be passed, subjects with IGT should not have a degree of neuropathy higher than

Table 3.**3** Prevalence of distal symmetric polyneuropathy in subjects with newly diagnosed diabetes

Study	Neuropathy diagnosis	Population selection	
		Clinically diagnosed	OGTT screening
Egypt, 1998 [6]	VPT[a]		14
Mauritius, 1998 [5]	VPT[b]		4
Finland, 1995 [33]	Symptoms and NCV	8	
Germany, 1991 [34]	Symptoms and signs		6
Netherlands, 1996 [29]	VPT (big toe/malleolus)		39/7
	Ankle/knee reflexes		29/3
Hong Kong, 1998 [35]	VPT	13	
USA, 1988 [4]	VPT >20 V		19[c]
USA, 1992 [9]	Monofilament		19[c]

Data shown are percentages
OGTT, oral glucose tolerance test
[a] Compared to locally derived values for healthy young adults
[b] Compared to locally derived age-specific normal values
[c] These figures relate to the total diabetic population including both diagnosed and undiagnosed diabetes

Table 3.**4** Prevalence of polyneuropathy in subjects with impaired glucose tolerance (IGT)

Study site	Neuropathy diagnosis	Population selection			
		Hospital-based		Primary care of population screening	
		IGT	Control	IGT	Control
USA, 1987 [24]	NCV			3	5
USA, 1990 [20]	Signs			11	4
USA, 1992 [41]	VPT, TPT hallux	No difference			
Sweden, 1994 [40]	NCV, VPT, TPT	No difference			
	Abnormal E/I ratio	29	8		
Sweden, 2000 [42]	Sural nerve morphology	No difference			
Netherlands, 1996 [29]	Absent VPT at malleolus/big toe			5/27	5/28
	Absent knee/ankle reflexes			3/26	2/16

NCV, nerve conduction velocity; VPT, vibration perception threshold; TPT, thermal perception threshold; E/I, expiration/inspiration

that of nondiabetic subjects [40]. The results of several studies comparing the prevalence of nerve dysfunction in patients with IGT and normal glucose tolerance (NGT) are summarized in Table 3.**4**. The hospital-based studies could not demonstrate a difference in peripheral nerve function and structure between patients with IGT and NGT, except for an abnormal expiration/inhalation ratio, a marker of cardiovascular autonomic neuropathy (CAN), which was found to be more frequent in IGT than in NGT [40]. In one population-based study ankle reflexes were detected less frequently in patients with IGT than in those with NGT [29]. Thus, there is preliminary evidence suggesting that peripheral neuropathy may be slightly more frequent in IGT than in NGT, but further studies are needed to confirm these findings.

Incidence and Natural History

Most of the data describing the frequency of diabetic neuropathy relate to prevalence. The long-term natural history and progression of diabetic neuropathy has been difficult to study owing to the following problems: (1) various nerve fiber populations may be affected at different rates, (2) expected changes may take place over several years, (3) minor changes may not be detected due to a low reproducibility of some methods, (4) measures of nerve function such as nerve conduction velocity (NCV) may deteriorate with age in nondiabetic subjects, and (5) glycemic control or risk factor profile may change and nerve dysfunction may be reversible over time. It has been emphasized that inception cohorts followed from the diagnosis onward are needed to determine the impact of diabetic neuropathy, because prevalence rates consider only the surviving cases and therefore might underestimate the true risk of acquiring the disease [43].

A long-term clinic-based study carried out in a large group of type 1 and type 2 diabetic patients, designed to investigate the relationship between the duration and degree of hyperglycemia and the prevalence of clinically overt neuropathy from the onset of diabetes, was performed by Pirart [44] over a period of 25 years. He defined neuropathy as a loss of Achilles and/or patellar reflexes combined with a reduced vibration sensation or presence of "a more dramatic polyneuropathy or mono- or multi-neuropathy." The prevalence of neuropathy increased from about 8% among the 1900 patients evaluated at the time of diagnosis to about 50% among 100 patients reassessed after a follow-up of 25 years. The incidence of neuropathy increased from three cases per 100 unaffected patients per year to about 19 cases per 100 patients after 25 years. However, Pirart's study had several drawbacks: it was not population-based, no standardized diagnostic measures were employed, the various forms of neuropathy were not differentiated, control subjects were not assessed, and the types of diabetes were not evaluated separately.

In a study focusing on 133 Finnish patients with newly diagnosed (following clinical presentation) type 2 diabetes, the 10-year incidence of DSP among those who were free of neuropathy at baseline was 17–20% depending on whether electrophysiological or clinical parameters were used [33]. This gives an annual incidence of approximately 2%. However, the development of DSP and CAN was divergent in that approximately the same proportions of patients with and without peripheral neuropathy developed CAN, either with predominant parasympathetic or sympathetic involvement or both [45]. To explain this finding different underlying mechanisms involved in the evolution of peripheral neuropathy and CAN have been suggested: while hypoinsulinemia predicted the development of DSP, it was hyperinsulinemia that predicted the development of CAN [45].

Over the first 12 years of the UK Prospective Diabetes Study (UKPDS), which similarly studied people newly presenting with type 2 diabetes, neuropathy (as judged by a VPT >25 V) developed in approximately 20% of subjects irrespective of treatment arm, giving an annual incidence of just under 2% [46]. In the American San Luis Valley study [47], DSP was determined by a combination of symptoms and clinical signs. Over nearly five years, its average annual incidence was 6.1% (6.1 per 100 person-years). A study of US veterans reported neuropathy (monofilament insensitivity) developing in 20% of subjects over approximately 2.5 years [17]. The higher incidence in the last two studies was probably due to the fact they only included people with established diabetes, who, consequent on their longer disease duration, would have had a higher baseline risk than the subjects with newly diagnosed diabetes who were included in the other two studies.

In the Rochester Diabetic Neuropathy Study (RDNS), after two years the Neuropathy Impairment Score (NIS) was unchanged in 81%, worse in 10%, and better in 9% of the patients and the Neuropathy Symptom Score (NSS) was unchanged in 92% and worse or better in 4% of the patients, respectively. The most prominent monotone (consistent) worsening over two years was found for a composite score combining neuropathic deficits and quantitative measures of DSP (NIS[lower limbs] + 7 tests), which worsened on average by 0.34 points per year in the entire cohort and by 0.85 points per year in patients with DSP [48].

The Epidemiology of Diabetes Complications Study (EDCS) reported on a six-year follow-up of 453 type 1 diabetic patients who were free of DSP at baseline, 15% of whom developed DSP in six years, giving an incidence of 2.8 per 100 person-years and a cumulative probability of 0.29 [49]. DSP was defined as the presence of two or more of the following: symptoms, sensory and/or motor signs, and/or absent (or present only with reinforcement) tendon reflexes. In the DCCT, which included groups of highly selected individuals with type 1 diabetes, polyneuropathy (abnormal history or examination, confirmed by abnormal nerve conduction or autonomic function) developed in 9.6% of those who were conventionally treated, and in 2.8% of those in the intensively treated group, over five years [2].

Comparing to the data for type 2 diabetes, it appears that the incidence of neuropathy in type 1 diabetes (using the data from the conventionally treated group – approximately 2% per year) is similar to that in newly diagnosed type 2 diabetes, but less than that in previously diagnosed type 2 diabetes. However, age is an important factor in diabetic neuropathy (see below), and the considerably younger age of the subjects in the DCCT probably accounts for the differences seen. Indeed, when age has been corrected for, the prevalence of neuropathy does not differ between type 1 and type 2 diabetes [8,11].

In the EURODIAB Prospective Complications Study, which included 986 type 1 diabetic subjects without DSP at baseline, the cumulative prevalence after an average follow-up of 7.3 years was 25% [50].

Several clinic-based prospective studies examined the relationship between the natural history of abnormalities in nerve function tests and the degree of long-term glycemic control. Hillson et al [51]. followed 71 patients who showed a slight deterioration in mean pedal VPT during the first five years after diagnosis of type 2 diabetes, which correlated significantly with increased mean fasting blood glucose. A more pronounced deterioration in sensory nerve function assessed by thermal, vibration, and pressure perception thresholds has been observed over 1–3.5 years and two years in newly diagnosed and longer-term type 2 diabetic patients, respectively [35,52]. There was a correlation between the changes in the various sensory thresholds [52], suggesting that small and large nerve fiber dysfunction may develop in parallel in type 2 diabetic patients.

Young et al. [53,54] studied 75 type 1 diabetic patients aged 16–19 years over an average of 2.4 years, 70 of whom were reassessed again after six years. During the first study period the deterioration in motor and sensory NCV was associated with poor glycemic control, but no patient had symptoms and only seven had minor signs of neuropathy [53]. After six years 16 patients had symptoms, 12 had "major signs," 15 had "minor signs", and 27 showed no symptoms of neuropathy. Baseline HbA_1 was significantly higher in patients who developed symptoms or major signs compared with those showing minor signs or no symptoms. In addition, peroneal motor NCV (MNCV) deteriorated in the symptomatic but not in the asymptomatic group [54]. On the other hand, it has been demonstrated that neuropathic pain may improve and resolve completely within three to four years of follow-up despite persistent poor glycemic control, but thermal perception thresholds continue to deteriorate [55]. Thus, small-fiber function tests do not seem to predict the evolution of painful symptoms.

Regarding the magnitude of changes in the quantitative measures of DSP, we have shown that over the first decade of type 1 diabetes the mean difference between poorly controlled and well-controlled patients in the annual rate of slowing of peroneal MNCV is 0.6 m/s per year and that of sural sensory NCV (SNCV) is 0.7 m/s per year. After 12 years from the diagnosis of type 1 diabetes, none of the well-controlled patients but 60% of those with long-term poor control developed polyneuropathy [56]. Macleod et al. [57] estimated the annual rate of change for the VPT on the great toe to be 0.4 V in healthy subjects and 2.5 V in those with diabetic neuropathy.

In a mixed cohort of type 1 and type 2 diabetic subjects followed over 9–16 years (mean 10 years) peroneal MNCV was progressively reduced with increasing duration of diabetes, but it stabilized once it reached a "plateau" between 36 and 38 m/s [58].

Focal and Multifocal Neuropathies

Prevalence

In the Rochester Diabetic Neuropathy Study the prevalence of neuropathies other than DSP was low: symptomatic carpal tunnel syndrome in 9% of type 1 and 4% of type 2 patients, proximal asymmetric neuropathy in 1% each of type 1 and type 2 patients, ulnar neuropathy in 2% each of type 1 and type 2 patients, peroneal neuropathy in one type 2 patient, lateral femoral cutaneous neuropathy of the thigh (meralgia paresthetica) in 1% each of type 1 and type 2 patients. Cranial neuropathy or truncal neuropathy was not present in any of the patients at the time of examination. Approximately 10% of diabetic patients had neurological deficits attributable to nondiabetic causes [21].

In a Japanese survey among 1961 diabetic patients, 19 (1%) had cranial nerve palsies: 19 facial nerve, 6 oculomotor nerve, and 2 abducent nerve palsies. Among 3841 nondiabetic subjects only 5 (0.1%) showed cranial nerve palsies, all of which were facial palsies. Only 1 out of 9 patients with facial palsy compared to 7 out of 10 patients with ophthalmoplegia had diabetic complications, suggesting that ophthalmoplegia rather than facial palsy is related to diabetes [59].

Natural History

Proximal motor neuropathy (femoral neuropathy, diabetic amyotrophy) is characterized by pain with or without wasting in one thigh, or, more often, both thighs. It develops over several weeks, and recovery is the rule. The worst pain resolves within 6–12 months, while the remaining discomfort disappears within three years. Function recovers completely, although slight wasting may persist [39].

The onset of cranial nerve palsies is abrupt and oculomotor nerve involvement may be accompanied by supraorbital pain. Cranial nerve palsies resolve completely in three to six months, and relapses are infrequent [39].

Diabetic polyradiculopathy most commonly affects the trunk, where it causes unilateral or bilateral truncal pain and abdominal muscle bulging. It may be accompanied by profound weight loss. Spontaneous recovery within 4–30 months is the rule, but relapses may occur [60].

For the natural history of painful neuropathies see Chapter 5, pages 212–213.

Cardiovascular Autonomic Neuropathy

Prevalence

Although the impact of autonomic neuropathy is increasingly being recognized, little information exists as to its incidence in representative diabetic populations. The difficulties encountered in epidemiological studies of diabetic neuropathy particularly affect the evaluation of autonomic dysfunction, which involves an even greater variety of nonspecific clinical manifestations that can be explored by numerous diagnostic approaches. Of the manifestations of diabetic autonomic neuropathy, cardiovascular autonomic neuropathy (CAN) has attracted most attention, because it is easily detected at subclinical stages by noninvasive cardiovascular autonomic function tests (AFTs) based on heart rate variability (HRV) and blood pressure responses, before the late sequelae such as resting tachy-cardia or orthostatic hypotension develop.

To date there have been two population-based studies that assessed the prevalence of autonomic dysfunction in diabetic patients. The Oxford Community Diabetes Study [61] included 29 873 adults aged at least 20 years, 412 of whom were known diabetic patients. Autonomic function was assessed in 43 type 1 and 202 type 2 diabetic patients using the standard deviation of HRV at rest, expiration/inhalation (E/I) ratio from a single deep breath, and Valsalva ratio. The overall prevalence of abnormal results in one or more of the three tests was 20.9% in type 1 patients and 15.8% in type 2 patients. Since this study did not include control subjects, the reported prevalence of autonomic dysfunction is difficult to interpret. The definition of one abnormality (<2.5th percentile of normal range) among three tests might yield one abnormal test result in up to 7.5% of a control population. Hence, the specificity of the test battery and the prevalence of CAN in that study were relatively low.

In the Pittsburgh Epidemiology of Diabetes Complications Study [62] autonomic neuropathy was evaluated in 168 type 1 diabetic subjects aged 25–34 years, representing 71% of those who were eligible. Cardiovascular autonomic function tests included the E/I ratio and mean circular resultant (MCR) to deep breathing, 30:15 ratio to standing, and Valsalva ratio. The results of the E/I ratio and MCR were significantly associated with the hypertension status, LDL and HDL cholesterol, and gender. The prevalence of autonomic symptoms, ranging from 0 to 8%, was relatively low except for hypoglycemia unawareness, which was present in 26% of the patients. However, this study neither reported the prevalence of abnormal test results nor did it take into account treatment with drugs that potentially influence autonomic function. Orthostatic hypotension, defined as a systolic blood pressure fall of at least 30 mmHg, was noted in 3.4% of the patients.

In a clinic-based multicenter study (DiaCAN) we have found prevalence rates of borderline CAN (2 out of 7 indices abnormal) or definite CAN (≥3 out of 7 indices abnormal) of 8.5% and 16.8% respectively among 647 unselected type 1 diabetic patients, and 12.2% and 22.1% respectively in 524 type 2 diabetic patients [31]. The percentage of type 1 diabetic patients with definite CAN was identical with the 16.6% rate observed in 506 patients randomly selected from four hospital diabetic clinics in Bristol [63]. In that study CAN was diagnosed by HRV responses during rest and in response to a single deep breath, Valsalva maneuver, and standing, and was defined by abnormal test results in at least two of these four tests. In the EURODIAB IDDM Complications Study [64], among the total of 3250 patients studied, 19.3% (range among centers: 7.8–51.8%) had abnormal HRV and 5.9% (range: 0–14.5%) had postural hypotension. In a Japanese clinic-based cohort of 886 type 2 diabetic patients the prevalence of orthostatic hypotension was 7% [65].

Since particularly in type 2 diabetes the actual onset of the disease may often be preceded by a long period of unrecognized metabolic abnormality, it appears likely that neural dysfunction can be detected at the time of diagnosis of diabetes. Two studies have reported the frequency of neuropathy in type 2 diabetic patients who were examined within four weeks following the diagnosis of the disease. Lehtinen et al. [66] evaluated 132 patients aged 45–64 years in the district of Kuopio University Central Hospital and 142 controls randomly selected from the population registers. The rates of abnormal E/I ratio were 6.3% and 1.4%, respectively. A similar study was performed by Ratzmann et al. [34] in 95 newly diagnosed type 2 diabetic patients who were representative of the East Berlin community. The prevalence of abnormal maximum/minimum heart rate during deep breathing was 7.3%.

In a clinic-based study we determined the prevalence of CAN in 120 healthy subjects and 130 newly diagnosed type 1 diabetic patients within 3–49 days after the initiation of insulin treatment with stable mean blood glucose levels. The prevalence of CAN defined by the strict criterion of at least three abnormal tests out of six was 7.7% in the patients and 0 in the controls. Two abnormal tests out of six were found in an additional 9.2% of the patients but in only 1.7% of the controls [67].

Thus, CAN cannot be generally regarded as a late complication of diabetes, but it should be borne in mind that subclinical cardiovascular autonomic dysfunction may be detected even in newly diagnosed type 1 diabetic patients if sensitive indices of spectral analysis are applied in conjunction with tests based on standard analysis of HRV.

Incidence and Natural History

Only a few studies have evaluated the natural history of CAN in inception cohorts. Töyry et al. [68] followed 133 newly diagnosed type 2 diabetic patients and 144 control subjects over 10 years in Kuopio, Finland. CAN was assessed by the E/I ratio as an index of parasympathetic activity and the systolic blood pressure drop on standing as a measure of sympathetic activity. The prevalence of "parasympathetic neuropathy" rose from 5% in diabetic patients vs 2% in controls at baseline to 65% vs 28% after 10 years, while the prevalence of "sympathetic neuropathy" increased from 7% vs 6% at five years to 24% vs 9% after 10 years. Poor glycemic control and high insulin levels were significant predictors of the development of CAN [68]. Moreover, the presence of CAN at five years was an independent risk factor for the development of stroke after 10 years [69]. Clinic-based studies in patients with variable duration of type 2 diabetes showed a gradual increase in the prevalence of AFT score abnormalities from 41% at baseline to 64% after four years [70], and worsening of the AFT score in 57% of the patients after five years of follow-up [71].

There are no population-based studies including inception cohorts at the time of diagnosis of type 1 diabetes. In a clinic-based study we have shown that the natural evolution of abnormal HRV during the first five years following diagnosis of type 1 diabetes is clearly related to the degree of glycemic control [72]. The rates of abnormalities in HRV at five years were 5% in well-controlled patients and 23% in those who were poorly controlled. In type 1 diabetic children the prevalence of abnormal HRV at rest increased from 27% at the time of diagnosis to 56% after 10 years, but abnormal HRV during deep breathing changed only from 12% to 14% [73].

In longer-term teenage type 1 diabetic patients Young et al. [53] found an increase in the rates of abnormal HRV from 19% to 28% within 20–35 months in poorly controlled type 1 diabetic teenagers. Sampson and colleagues [74] noted a relatively slow decline in HRV of about 1 beat/min per year, approximately three times faster than in healthy subjects [39], over a decade in patients with initially normal HRV. Postural hypotension was persistent, but did not deteriorate in the majority of patients. In contrast, a six-year study has reported the relatively rapid development of postural hypotension in a small group of long-term diabetic patients, which was preceded by a decrease in E/I ratio [75]. In two recent studies in type 1 diabetic patients, AFTs and autonomic symptoms and signs had not changed after 5 and 9 years, respectively [76,77]. In a prospective study over 10–11 years, CAN has been shown to predict future deterioration in glomerular filtration rate in type 1 diabetic patients. It has been hypothesized that nocturnal rise in intraglomerular pressure could be one possible link between CAN and the observed deterioration in glomerular filtration rate [78].

Gastrointestinal Neuropathy

There are no population-based studies reporting the prevalence or incidence of gastrointestinal symptoms or motor abnormalities in diabetic patients. A number of clinic-based studies reported relatively high rates of delayed gastric emptying in diabetic subjects, but most of these included small samples of highly selected populations subject to referral bias. Thus, the true prevalence of delayed gastric emptying is not known. Using the ^{13}C-octanoic acid breath test, delayed gastric emptying has been shown in 16% of type 1 diabetic subjects without gastrointestinal symptoms, while the rate increased to 43% in those with these symptoms [79]. Several clinic-based studies reported the prevalence of gastrointestinal symptoms in diabetic and nondiabetic subjects [80–82] (Table 3.5). In type 1 diabetic patients only nausea, vomiting, early satiety, and fullness after meals occurred significantly more frequently than in the nondiabetic subjects in some studies. In type 2 diabetic patients nausea, early satiety, fullness after meals, diarrhea, and constipation were significantly more frequent than in the nondiabetic subjects. The prevalence of gastrointestinal symptoms such as dysphagia, heartburn, or bloating was comparable to that seen in nondiabetic subjects. However, there were considerable differences between the studies regarding the prevalence of the individual symptoms. For example, diarrhea was observed in 35% of the type 2 patients studied in Hong Kong vs 7% of those studied in Germany [80–82].

The gallbladder may become atonic in association with autonomic neuropathy, which increases the gallbladder volume by retention of bile. It is unknown whether these changes result in symptoms. It may be that biliary stasis explains the increased risk of gallstones shown by recent epidemiological data. In a population-based study from Tivoli, Rome, the prevalence of diabetes in subjects affected by gallstone disease was significantly higher than in controls matched for sex, age, and body mass index (12% vs 5%) [83].

"Gustatory sweating" refers to sweating over the face and scalp (and sometimes upper trunk), often accompanied by a flush, that follows the ingestion of food or drink. Diabetic gustatory sweating has been reported in a clinic-based study to occur in 69% of patients with nephropathy, 36% with peripheral neuropathy, and 4% of those without either complication [84]. Diabetic gustatory sweating is believed to be triggered by the taste buds as it is not evoked by chewing inert substances, thinking of food, smelling food or by placing food or alcohol in the stomach by a gastric tube. The tongue is the most sensitive area, and even cocainization fails to inhibit gustatory sweating completely. The etiology of diabetic gustatory sweating is uncertain. The hypothesis that it results from aberrant regrowth of parasympathetic fibers leading to a connection between salivation centers and facial sweat glands seems to have been disproved by a series of case reports of immediate cessation of gustatory sweating after renal transplantation [84].

Erectile Dysfunction

Prevalence

Male erectile dysfunction, defined as "the inability to achieve or maintain an erection sufficient for sexual intercourse" [85], is one of the most common sexual dysfunctions in men. Erectile dysfunction is more common with advancing age, and since the aged

Table 3.**5** Prevalence of gastrointestinal symptoms in diabetic and control subjects

Symptom	Study site	Type 1	Control 1	Type 2	Control 2
Dysphagia	Germany, 1994 [80]	3	7	4	2
	Sweden, 1996 [81]	6	1		
	Hong Kong, 1999 [82]			4	0
Heartburn	Germany, 1994 [80]	13	15	16	10
	Sweden, 1996 [81]	27	23		
Nausea	Germany, 1994 [80]	13	12	12*	3
	Sweden, 1996 [81]	23*	9		
Vomiting	Germany, 1994 [80]	7	3	9	4
	Sweden, 1996 [81]	12*	3		
Early satiety	Sweden, 1996 [81]	27*	6		
	Hong Kong, 1999 [82]			7*	1
Fullness after meals	Sweden, 1996 [81]	19*	9		
	Hong Kong, 1999 [82]			17*	1
Bloating	Germany, 1994 [80]	15	13	21	16
	Hong Kong, 1999 [82]			22	13
Diarrhea	Germany, 1994 [80]	7	12	7	4
	Sweden, 1996 [81]	19	13		
	Hong Kong, 1999 [82]			35*	5
Constipation	Germany, 1994 [80]	5	3	22*	10
	Sweden, 1996 [81]	14	10		
	Hong Kong, 1999 [82]			28*	7
Fecal incontinence	Germany, 1994 [80]	1	1	2	2
	Hong Kong, 1999 [82]			3	0

Data shown are percentages; $^*P < 0.05$ vs control

population is increasing, its prevalence will continue to rise [86]. Diabetes mellitus is the most frequent organic cause of erectile dysfunction. In the population-based Massachusetts Male Aging Study (MMAS), the age-adjusted prevalence of complete erectile dysfunction was 28% in men with treated diabetes. Minimal, moderate, and complete erectile dysfunction together had a prevalence of 64% in men with treated diabetes [87]. In a recent clinic-based survey in Italy involving 9868 men with diabetes, 45.5% of those aged over 59 years reported erectile dysfunction [88]. Table 3.**6** shows that erectile dysfunction is encountered in 20–52% of type 1 and 36–54% of type 2 diabetic patients [61,87–93]. Once erectile dysfunction has developed, it is likely to persist in most patients. Risk factors and clinical correlates include duration of diabetes, glycemic control, each of the chronic diabetic complications, and smoking [88].

Incidence

The MMAS recently reported the incidence of erectile dysfunction after an average follow-up of 8.8 years in a population-based cohort of 847 men aged 40–69 years without erectile dysfunction at baseline. The crude incidence of erectile dysfunction was 26 cases per 1000 man-years (95% CI: 23–30) and increased with age, lower education, diabetes, heart disease, and hypertension. In diabetic patients the incidence of erectile dysfunction was twice as high, 51 cases per 1000 man-years. Population projections for men aged 40–69 years suggest that 617 715 new cases of erectile dysfunction in the USA (white males only) are expected annually, a considerable proportion of whom will be diabetic subjects [94].

Etiological Factors Related to Diabetic Neuropathy

Whilst debate continues about the precise nature of the pathophysiological changes that eventually result in diabetic neuropathy, there is some agreement over the risk factors associated with its development. The risk factors and risk indicators for DSP and the relative degrees of their association with it are listed in Table 3.**7**.

Table 3.**6** Prevalence of erectile dysfunction in diabetic men

<table>
<tr><th rowspan="3">Study site</th><th rowspan="3">n</th><th rowspan="3">Age range in years (mean)</th><th colspan="4">Population selection</th></tr>
<tr><th colspan="2">Hospital-based</th><th colspan="2">Primary care or population screening</th></tr>
<tr><th>Type 1</th><th>Type 2</th><th>Type 1</th><th>Type 2</th></tr>
<tr><td>USA, 1974 [89]</td><td>175</td><td>>18 (49)</td><td colspan="2">49</td><td></td><td></td></tr>
<tr><td>USA, 1994 [87]</td><td>88</td><td>40–70</td><td></td><td></td><td colspan="2">57</td></tr>
<tr><td>USA, 1996 [90]</td><td>365</td><td>21–76 (38), DD ≥10 years</td><td></td><td></td><td>20</td><td></td></tr>
<tr><td>Italy, 1998 [88]</td><td>9868</td><td>20–69</td><td>26</td><td>37</td><td></td><td></td></tr>
<tr><td>UK, 1980 [91]</td><td>541</td><td>20–59</td><td>35</td><td>36</td><td></td><td></td></tr>
<tr><td>UK, 1987 [92]</td><td>292</td><td>20–59 (44)</td><td colspan="2">23</td><td></td><td></td></tr>
<tr><td>UK 1989 [61]</td><td>245</td><td>≥20</td><td></td><td></td><td colspan="2">41</td></tr>
<tr><td>UK, 1995 [93]</td><td>250</td><td>18–75</td><td></td><td></td><td>52</td><td>54</td></tr>
</table>

Data shown are percentages
DD, duration of diabetes

Table 3.**7** Risk factors and markers of diabetic polyneuropathy

	Type 1 diabetes	Type 2 diabetes
Age	+	+
Sex	–	–
Height	+	(+)
Weight	–	(+)
Hyperglycemia	++	++
Hypoinsulinemia	n.a.	+
Duration of diabetes	++	++
Smoking	+	(+)
Alcohol	(+)	(+)
Hyperlipidemia	(+)	(+)
Hypertension	++	(+)
Nephropathy	++	+
Retinopathy	++	+
CAN	++	++
Macroangiopathy	(+)	(+)

Association strong, ++; moderate, +; disputed, (+); not found, –; CAN, cardiovascular autonomic neuropathy; n.a., not applicable

■ Hyperglycemia

The central role of hyperglycemia has been demonstrated in a range of studies. Mean HbA_{1c} was approximately 1% higher in men with newly diagnosed type 2 diabetes who went on to develop DSP 10 years later, than in those who did not [33]. The risk of developing DSP (as measured by the odds ratio) has been calculated to rise by approximately 10–15% for every 1 mmol/l rise in fasting plasma glucose or every 1% rise in HbA_{1c} [6,17]. The importance of hyperglycemia has of course been confirmed in interventional studies. The DCCT demonstrated that intensive glycemic control led to a 64% reduction in the five-year risk of developing DSP [2] in patients with type 1 diabetes. In the similar but smaller Stockholm Diabetes Intervention Study, symptoms of DSP developed in only 14% of those who were intensively treated, compared to 32% in the conventional treatment arm [95]. The effect of glucose lowering in type 2 diabetes is less clear. In the large UKPDS study, strict glycemic control had no significant impact on the development of DSP over the first 12 years [46]. Among the relatively small number of subjects who were followed to 15 years, a significant risk reduction was apparent, but only in those in the main study. Amongst the overweight subjects, whose intensive therapy was primarily with metformin, there was no impact of intensive therapy at all on DSP [96].

In the Rochester Diabetic Neuropathy Study, mean HbA_1, severity of diabetic retinopathy, and a term calculated mean ln (24-hour proteinuria multiplied by duration of diabetes) were the main covariates for severity of DSP at the 7-year follow-up [97].

Thus, the etiological link between hyperglycemia and DSP seems sound, but while it is clear that glucose lowering protects against the development of neuropathy in type 1 diabetes, the case is not yet proven in type 2 diabetes.

■ Diabetes Duration

DSP, like the other specific diabetic complications, is rare at the outset of type 1 diabetes. It is more common amongst people with established type 2 diabetes than among those with newly diagnosed diabetes [5,6]. This association between disease duration and the risk of diabetes is strong, has been confirmed in a variety of studies in both type 1 and type 2 diabetes, and remains after adjustment for age [5,14,17,49]. In a UK study, the prevalence of DSP rose from 21% in those with a diabetes duration of less than five years to 37% in people with a duration of over 10 years [8]. In a Spanish study, the prevalence rose from 14% at under five years' duration to 44% at a duration of more than 30 years [19]. Interestingly, in one study the association between DSP and duration of diabetes was not seen in those over the age of 54, but was strong in those aged under 54 [3]. This, however, has not been reported elsewhere.

Age

Advancing age has been widely reported to increase the risk of DSP. In a large sample (6487 subjects) of UK diabetic hospital outpatients, the prevalence of DSP rose from 5% in the 20- to 29-year age group to 44% in the 70- to 79-year age group [8]. Amongst a population-based sample from Egypt, DSP was detected in 8% of those aged 20–44, and in 23% of those aged 45 years or over [6]. In this study, the risk of DSP independently attributed to age approximately doubled for every 10 year increment in age. A number of other studies have also documented age as an independent risk factor for DSP neuropathy [11,14,17,20]. However, the influence of age may not be straightforward. Neurological function, especially vibration perception threshold (VPT), deteriorates with advancing age even in the normal, nondiabetic population [98,99]. Whilst some studies have adjusted for the effects of age on VPT, this is not universal. Furthermore, diagnostic criteria for DSP often include other parameters, such as clinical signs, monofilament sensitivity and electrophysiology, which are not adjusted for age. Interestingly, in a study from France, where VPT was adjusted for age, height, and gender, there was no relationship between neuropathy and age [3]. Data from Mauritius confirmed the increase in VPT with age in both diabetic and nondiabetic subjects [5]. However, when neuropathy was defined as having a VPT above the normal range (mean plus 2 standard deviations in the nondiabetic population) defined separately in each of three age categories, there was no relationship between age and neuropathy in either cross-sectional or prospective analyses [5]. Thus, the influence of age may have been overestimated in some studies.

Hypertension

Hypertension is attractive as an etiological factor in DSP, as it could be viewed as lending weight to the vascular theory of the pathophysiology of DSP. Hypertension has been associated with DSP in several studies, most notably in the data from the Pittsburgh cohort of type 1 diabetes [49]. In this study, hypertension was the single strongest predictor of DSP, and was associated with an approximately four-fold risk of developing DSP over six years. In the EURODIAB Prospective Complications Study, systolic blood pressure was shown to be one of the predictors of the development of DSP after adjustment for age, duration of diabetes, and HbA_{1c} [50]. Reports in type 2 diabetes, however, have been conflicting [17,20,33,61,100], but mainly have not confirmed this association. In a small interventional study (including subjects with both type 1 and type 2 diabetes), treatment with the ACE inhibitor trandolapril reduced progression of electrophysiological parameters of DSP, and also lowered systolic blood pressure [101]. However, the UKPDS reported that intensive blood pressure lowering with a variety of agents had no effect in ameliorating the progression to DSP [102].

Hypoinsulinemia

Partanen et al. [33] have suggested a link between hypoinsulinemia and DSP, which they believed resulted from the possible beneficial effects of insulin and C-peptide on neuronal metabolism and function [103]. They found that baseline fasting and 2-hour insulin levels were lower in newly diagnosed Finnish male subjects with type 2 diabetes who developed DSP 10 years later than in those who remained free of DSP. In the San Luis Valley Study [47], these findings were also evident (using C-peptide), but this univariate association disappeared when diabetes duration was taken into account. Our own data from Mauritius [5] also suggested a similar association with hypoinsulinemia, but, perhaps because of the low prevalence of DSP in that study, the association was not apparent in all analyses.

Diabetes duration almost certainly has an important confounding effect on the assessment of this potential relationship, since it might be expected both to increase the prevalence of DSP and to reduce insulin levels. It is difficult to account for duration in type 2 diabetes, as the date of disease onset is not usually known. Only a study in a population in which the time of onset of type 2 diabetes can be accurately estimated will allow better insight into the role of hypoinsulinemia.

Hyperinsulinemia

Several population-based studies suggest that high insulin levels are associated with disturbed autonomic nervous system activity. High insulin levels were significant predictors of the development of CAN 10 years after the diagnosis of type 2 diabetes, irrespective of obesity and glycemia [68]. In the Atherosclerosis Risk in Communities (ARIC) Study patients with the metabolic syndrome (hypertension, type 2 diabetes, and/or dyslipidemia) showed significantly lower HRV indices than did those without these disorders. An increase in fasting insulin of 1 SD was associated with 88% higher odds of having lower HRV [104]. In nondiabetic individuals an inverse association was observed between serum fasting insulin and parasympathetic activity [105]. In the Zutphen Elderly Study fasting C-peptide and glucose tolerance were associated with a QTc prolongation which itself is related to CAN [106].

Other Risk Factors

Cigarette smoking has been identified as an independent risk factor for DSP in two different studies of type 1 diabetes, in which it was associated with an approximate doubling of the risk of DSP [14,49]. Smoking was also found to carry an independent risk in the San Luis Valley study of type 2 diabetes [47], but was actually associated with a protective effect in US veterans [17], and had only a weak (and not independent) association in the study from Mauritius [5].

Alcohol consumption has been associated with DSP on a number of occasions [17], but it may be difficult, at least in epidemiological studies, to differentiate between diabetic neuropathy in which alcohol is a risk factor, and alcoholic neuropathy in a person with diabetes.

DSP, like other metabolic, nutritional, and toxic neuropathies, is a distal disease which is first manifest in the feet. It is therefore, clearly a length-dependent process, although the pathophysiology underpinning this phenomenon is not understood. It seems logical, therefore, that height, as a surrogate measure of the length of the longest nerves, might be associated with DSP. This hypothesis has been borne out in a number of different cross-sectional and prospective studies [5,14,17,49].

There are no consistent findings that would indicate a relationship between gender and the risk of DSP.

High total cholesterol [6] and elevated triglycerides [14] have been reported as independent risk factors for DSP (after adjustment for HbA_{1c}, age, and other potential confounders). Elevated LDL was also found to predict neuropathy in a study of type 1 diabetes, but the association was lost after adjustment for other risk factors [49]. In the EURODIAB Prospective Complications Study BMI, albuminuria, triglycerides, cholesterol, and systolic blood pressure were shown to be significant predictors of the development of DSP after adjustment for age, duration of diabetes, and HbA_{1c} [50]. In type 2 diabetic patients the link between DSP and dyslipidemia must, however, remain tentative at this stage, as several studies have failed to observe such a relationship [5,33].

Physiological factors for which an inverse relationship to HRV has been described include age, heart rate, female gender, body mass index, sitting or standing body position, blood pressure, and pregnancy. Pathophysiological correlates unfavorably affecting HRV include the duration of diabetes, any of the chronic diabetic complications, metabolic syndrome, peripheral vasomotor abnormalities, medial arterial calcification, peripheral edema, reduced muscle sympathetic nerve activity (MSNA), cardiovascular risk factors such as high LDL cholesterol and smoking, as well as various drugs [107]. The population-based Hoorn Study, including subjects with NGT, IGT, and type 2 diabetes, recently reported that the strongest determinants of cardiovascular autonomic function were age and use of antihypertensive drugs in subjects with NGT, insulin levels in those with type 2 diabetes [108], and albuminuria in subjects with IGT or type 2 diabetes [109].

Genetic Factors

Striking ethnic and racial differences in the prevalence of nephropathy and macroangiopathy have been reported, but no such effects have been observed in the population-based surveys of diabetic neuropathy [20,26]. Although hyperglycemia and duration of diabetes are generally accepted to represent major contributory factors to the prevalence of diabetic neuropathy, many diabetologists have come across patients who do not develop neuropathy despite long-term poor glycemic control. Whole-genome screening and candidate gene strategies can be applied to the genetics of type 1 diabetes complications [110]. The most significant results were obtained regarding a role for polymorphisms of the renin-angiotensin system in diabetic nephropathy [110]. In diabetic polyneuropathy, reduced Na^+/K^+-ATPase activity and increased aldose reductase activity have been suggested to play an important pathogenetic role. Na^+/K^+-ATPase is encoded by various genes, of which the ATP1 A1 gene is expressed predominantly in peripheral nerves and erythrocytes. A case-control study found that type 1 diabetic patients bearing a restriction fragment length polymorphism (RFLP) of the ATP1 A1 gene carried a 6.5-fold (95% CI: 3.3–13) increased risk of peripheral neuropathy. Moreover, these patients showed reduced erythrocyte Na^+/K^+-ATPase activity [111]. Another case-control study showed increased susceptibility to peripheral neuropathy in type 1 diabetic patients who had a polymorphism at the 5′ end of the aldose reductase (ALR2) gene [112]. In contrast, a study in Japanese type 2 diabetic patients found an association of the ALR2 gene polymorphism in the 5′ region with retinopathy but not peripheral and autonomic neuropathy or nephropathy [113].

Thus, at present only a low level of evidence for a role of these candidate genes obtained from case-control studies is available. Only prospective controlled trials using strata selected along a candidate gene would clarify whether polymorphisms might have therapeutic relevance in future.

Prognosis

Distal Symmetrical Polyneuropathy

Available information on the mortality associated with DSP is sparse. In a cohort of 134 type 2 diabetic patients randomly selected from the register of the Helsinki Diabetes Association followed prospectively over 9 years, neuropathy as assessed by NCV was identified as an independent predictor of mortality after adjusting for macroangiopathy, albumin excretion rate, and HbA_{1c} [114]. In the Stockholm Diabetes Intervention Study 7.5-year mortality was predicted not only by albuminuria but also by sural sensory nerve action potential amplitude and sympathetic nerve function [115]. In a university hospital setting a 14-year observational study including 794 patients demonstrated that reduced VPT was the most significant predictor of mortality. Proteinuria and type 1 diabetes, but not HbA_{1c} and smoking, were other important risk factors [116]. In a clinic-based cohort of 583 type 1 diabetic patients who were followed over 1–11.5 years, both abnormal NCV and abnormal AFTs were associated with an increased risk of mortality. Mortality rates after 10 years in the groups with normal and highly abnormal NCV were 10% and 50% respectively, while the corresponding percentages were 10% and 43% respectively for the AFTs. Combining NCV and AFTs into a total neuropathy score resulted in an even stronger predictor of mortality than each of the two measures alone [117]. Thus, there is accumulating evidence to suggest that not only surrogate markers of microangiopathy, such as albuminuria, but also those used for polyneuropathy, such as NCV and VPT, may predict mortality in diabetic patients, but clearly further studies are needed to assess the prognostic role of polyneuropathy in diabetes. In diabetic patients with ultimate clinical endpoints of neuropathy such as foot ulcers the risk of death was increased to 12 per 100 person-years of follow-up, compared to 5 per 100 person-years in those without foot ulcers [118].

Cardiovascular Autonomic Neuropathy

A number of largely clinic-based prospective studies have demonstrated increased mortality among diabetic patients with symptomatic CAN or those with abnormal cardiovascular reflex tests. Their major findings are summarized in Table 3.**8** [68,74,117,119–128]. The overall mortality rates over periods up to 10 years were about 26% in diabetic patients with CAN compared with 4% in those without evidence of CAN. However, it must be kept in mind that autonomic dysfunction may also be found in the absence of diabetes as a consequence of common cardiovascular diseases such as coronary artery disease, myocardial infarction, and heart failure. It has been shown that reduced HRV is an independent indicator of poor prognosis in these patients [129]. Since cardiovascular diseases represent the major cause of death in diabetic patients [130], the impact of diabetes and, for example, coronary sclerosis on the autonomic nervous system may overlap in a number of patients to such a degree that CAN may at least not be the only factor responsible for the increased mortality [127]. On the other hand, there is evidence that CAN contributes to the poor prognosis in diabetic patients as an independent factor [122].

The mechanisms by which CAN leads to the increased mortality remain a matter of debate, but two hypotheses have been suggested [123,131]. A number of studies have shown an association between CAN and QT interval prolongation, and a recent meta-analysis revealed a 2.3-fold increased risk of CAN in diabetic patients showing a prolonged QT interval [132], leading to the speculation that, in analogy to the QT prolongation encountered in the idiopathic long QT syndrome, which is characterized by recurrent episodes of syncope or cardiac arrest due to torsades de pointes [133], CAN might also predispose patients to malignant ventricular arrhythmias and sudden death. A recent five-year study from Italy showed a considerably increased risk of mortality in type 1 diabetic patients with QTc prolongation (odds ratio: 24.6 [95% CI: 6.5-92.9]) which requires further confirmation [128]. Although the studies listed in Table 3.**8** were not sufficiently large to allow unequivocal conclusions regarding an increased incidence of sudden death in CAN, recent evidence indicates an important role of the autonomic nervous system in triggering sudden death in both nondiabetic and diabetic subjects with low HRV. A marked decrease in HRV in nondiabetic patients with coronary artery disease was present immediately before the onset of the ST shift precipitating ischemic sudden death, suggesting that sympathovagal imbalance may trigger fatal arrhythmias during acute myocardial ischemia [134]. HRV was also diminished in nondiabetic survivors of sudden death not associated with coronary artery disease, indicating that abnormal autonomic activity may trigger malignant arrhythmia independently of coronary artery disease [135]. In subjects with inducible ventricular tachycardia (VT), 42% of whom were diabetic, HRV was

Table 3.**8** Mortality in diabetic patients with (CAN+) and without cardiac autonomic neuropathy (CAN−)

Reference	Follow-up (years)	Number of tests	Mortality				*P* value
			CAN+		CAN−		
			n	%	*n*	%	
Ewing et al., 1980 [119]	5	3+S	21/40	53	5/33	15	<0.05
Hasslacher et al., 1983 [120]	5	1	3/16	19	3/42	7	NS
Navarro et al., 1990 [121]	3.3 (1–7.3)	2	41/175	23	2/57	4	<0.05
Sampson et al., 1990 [74]	10	1+S	18/49	37	4/38	11	<0.05
O'Brien et al., 1991 [122]	5	4	23/84	27	21/422	5	<0.05
Ewing et al., 1991 [123]	3	5+QTc	10/32	31	3/39	8	<0.05
Jermendy et al., 1991 [124]	5	4+QTc	12/30	40	1/23	4	<0.05
Rathmann et al., 1993 [125]	8	2+QTc	8/35	23	1/35	3	<0.05
Luft et al., 1993 [126]	8 (6–10)	4	7/34	21	1/19	5	NS
Navarro et al., 1996 [117]	1–11.5	2	101/359	28	6/128	5	<0.05
Orchard et al., 1996 [127]	2	1	8/88	9	9/399	2	<0.05
Töyry et al., 1996 [68]	10	1	3/23	13	3/99	3	<0.05
Veglio et al., 2000 [128]	5	2+QTc	10/76	13	10/240	4	<0.05
Total	Median: 5	–	265/1041	25	69/1574	4	–

NS, not significant; QTc, corrected QT interval; S, autonomic symptoms

markedly lower than in those without evidence of VT [136]. In unselected patients a 2.6-fold higher relative risk of sudden death within two years (after adjustment for age, left ventricular dysfunction, and history of myocardial infarction) was observed among patients with reduced HRV than in those with normal HRV. Among the subjects who died suddenly, 9.3% were diabetic, whereas only 3.5% of the patients who survived had diabetes [137]. The Zutphen Study [138] recently showed that low HRV predicts mortality from all causes in the general population. The population-based Honolulu Heart Program demonstrated that orthostatic hypotension defined as a drop in systolic blood pressure of at least 20 mmHg or in diastolic blood pressure of at least 10 mmHg predicts four-year all-cause mortality in a cohort of 3522 elderly Japanese-American men aged 71–93. Four-year age-adjusted mortality rates were 57 and 39 per 1000 person-years in men with and without orthostatic hypotension, respectively [139].

The second hypothesis for the explanation of the increased mortality in CAN suggests that impaired central control of respiration rather than abnormal cardiovascular reflexes contributes to the poor prognosis [131]. This view is supported by studies reporting an increased prevalence of sleep apnea and nocturnal oxygen desaturation in diabetic patients with CAN [140,141]. Several studies have demonstrated impaired ventilatory responses to progressive hypercapnia or hypoxemia in CAN [142–144]. This impairment is not due to peripheral factors such as abnormal lung function or diaphragmatic muscle alterations, but to defective central control of respiration. This last suggestion is supported by the finding that naloxone, a specific opioid antagonist, produced no increase in CO_2 response in diabetic patients with CAN, in contrast to healthy subjects. However, a lack of effect of naloxone on CO_2 response was also observed in diabetic patients without CAN [143]. Hence, the question remains open as to whether the altered central control of respiration is specific to CAN or is rather a feature of diabetes itself. To complicate matters even more, an increased hypercapnic drive, indicating an exaggerated response of the central drive due to removal of the sympathetic inhibition, was recently found in patients with CAN and orthostatic hypotension [144].

There is little information available on the prognostic significance of the other manifestations of autonomic neuropathy. Diabetic gastroparesis diagnosed by scintigraphy was not associated with a poor prognosis in two studies performed over 3–5 and 9–14 years, respectively [145,146].

Conclusions

The study of the epidemiology of diabetic neuropathy remains clouded by lack of agreement over diagnostic criteria and variation in subject selection methods. It is essential that agreement is reached over diagnosis, although it is hard at the present time to see how this is going to come about. One issue that may be relevant in this context is the basis on which the diagnosis should be made. Is diabetic neuropathy a condition which predisposes to clinical endpoints such as foot ulceration and amputation, in which case quantitative sensory testing should suffice, or is it a condition in which neurological function differs from that in a healthy population, in which case diagnosis may require a more detailed assessment?

The available data indicate that DSP is present in approximately 30% of hospital clinic patients, 20% of patients in primary care, and 10% of the total diabetic population, including both diagnosed and undiagnosed diabetes. The major confirmed risk factors are poor glycemic control, diabetes duration and height, with possible roles for hypertension (probably only in type 1 diabetes), age, smoking, hypoinsulinemia, and dyslipidemia.

There are as yet relatively few epidemiological data on the various manifestations of autonomic neuropathy from representative cohorts of diabetic patients, except for erectile dysfunction. Estimates from the available studies suggest that CAN is encountered one of every 4-6 men and ED is observed in one of every 2-3 men. Symptomatic orthostatic hypotension is relatively uncommon. Gastrointestinal symptoms are common in both diabetic and nondiabetic subjects, suggesting that a considerable proportion of these symptoms in diabetic patients is due to causes other than autonomic neuropathy

Clinic-based data suggest that particularly CAN but possibly also DSP are associated with increased mortality in diabetic patients, but prospective population-based studies are required to confirm these findings.

References

[1] Statement C. Report and recommendations of the San Antonio Conference on diabetic neuropathy. Diabetes Care 1988; 37: 1000–4.

[2] The Diabetes Control and Complications Trial Research Group. The effect of intensive diabetes therapy on the development and progression of diabetic neuropathy. Ann Intern Med 1995; 122: 561–8.

[3] Delcourt C, Vauzelle-Kervroedan F, Cathelineau G, Papoz L. Low prevalence of long-term complications in non-insulin-dependent diabetes mellitus in France: a multicenter study. J Diabetes Complications 1998; 12: 88–95.

[4] Nelson RG, Gohdes DM, Everhart JE, Hartner JA, Zwemer FL, Pettitt DJ, Knowler WC. Lower-extremity amputations in NIDDM: 12-yr follow-up study in Pima Indians. Diabetes Care 1988; 11: 8–16.

[5] Shaw JE, Hodge AM, Courten M de, Dowse GK, Gareeboo H, Tuomilehto J, Alberti KGMM, Zimmet PZ. Diabetic neuropathy in Mauritius: prevalence and risk factors. Diabetes Res Clin Pract 1998; 42: 131–9.

[6] Herman WH, Aubert RE, Engelgau MM, Thompson TJ, Ali MA, Sous ES, Hegazy M, Badran A, Kenny SJ, Gunter EW, Malarcher AM, Brechner RJ, Wetterhall SF, DeStefano F, Smith PJ, Habib M, abd el Shakour S, Ibrahim AS, el Behairy EM. Diabetes mellitus in Egypt: glycaemic control and microvascular and neuropathic complications. Diabet Med 1998; 15: 1045–51.

[7] Dyck PJ, Dyck PJB, Velosa JA, Larson TS, O'Brien PC, the Nerve Growth Factor Study Group. Patterns of quantitative sensation testing of hypoesthesia and hyperalgesia are predictive of diabetic polyneuropathy. A study of three cohorts. Diabetes Care 2000; 23: 510–7.

[8] Young MJ, Breddy JL, Veves A, Boulton AJM. The prediction of diabetic neuropathic foot ulceration using vibration perception thresholds. A prospective study. Diabetes Care 1994; 17: 557–60.

[9] Rith-Najarian SJ, Stolusky T, Gohdes DM. Identifying diabetic patients at high risk for lower-extremity amputation in a primary health care setting. A prospective evaluation of simple screening criteria. Diabetes Care 1992; 15: 1386–9.

[10] Young MJ, Boulton AJ, MacLeod AF, Williams DR, Sonksen PH. A multicentre study of the prevalence of diabetic peripheral neuropathy in the United Kingdom hospital clinic population. Diabetologia 1993; 36: 150–4.

[11] Walters DP, Gatting W, Mullee MA, Hill RD. The prevalence of diabetic distal sensory neuropathy in an English community. Diabet Med 1992; 9: 349–53.

[12] Harris MI. Classification, diagnostic criteria, and screening for diabetes. In: National Diabetes Data Group, editors. Diabetes in America, 2nd ed. Bethesda Md: National Institutes of Health and Digestive and Kidney Diseases; 199NIH publ 1995; 95–1468: 15–36.

[13] American Diabetes Association. Report of the expert committee on the diagnosis and classification of diabetes mellitus. Diabetes Care 1997; 20: 1183–97.

[14] Tesfaye S, Stevens LK, Stephenson JM, Fuller JH, Plater M, Ionescu-Tirgoviste C, Nuber A, Pozza G, Ward JD. Prevalence of diabetic peripheral neuropathy and its relation to glycaemic control and potential risk factors: the EURODIAB IDDM Complications Study. Diabetologia 1996; 39: 1377–84.

[15] Fedele D, Comi G, Coscelli C, Cucinotta D, Feldman EL, Ghirlanda G, Greene DA, Negrin P, Santeusanio F. A multicenter study on the prevalence of diabetic neuropathy in Italy. Italian Diabetic Neuropathy Committee. Diabetes Care 1997; 20: 836–43.

[16] Wikblad K, Smide B, Bergstrom A, Kessi J, Mugusi F. Outcome of clinical foot examination in relation to self-perceived health and glycaemic control in a group of urban Tanzanian diabetic patients. Diabetes Res Clin Pract 1997; 37: 185–92.

[17] Adler AI, Boyko EJ, Ahroni JH, Stensel V, Forsberg RC, Smith DG. Risk factors for diabetic peripheral sensory neuropathy. Results of the Seattle Prospective Diabetic Foot Study. Diabetes Care 1997; 20: 1162–7.

[18] Beghi E, Monticelli ML. Diabetic polyneuropathy in the elderly. Prevalence and risk factors in two geographic areas of Italy. Italian General Practitioner Study Group (IGPSG). Acta Neurol Scand 1997; 96: 223–8.

[19] Cabezas-Cerrato J. The prevalence of clinical diabetic polyneuropathy in Spain: a study in primary care and hospital clinic groups. Neuropathy Spanish Study Group of the Spanish Diabetes Society (SDS). Diabetologia 1998; 41: 1263–9.

[20] Franklin GM, Shetterly SM, Cohen JA, Baxter J, Hamman RF. Risk factors for distal symmetric neuropathy in NIDDM. San Luis Val Diabetes Study. Diabetes Care 1994; 17: 1172–7.

[21] Dyck PJ, Kratz KM, Karnes JL, Litchy WJ, Klein R, Pach JM, Wilson DM, O'Brien PC. Melton LJ 3d, Service FJ. The prevalence by staged severity of various types of diabetic neuropathy, retinopathy, and nephropathy in a population-based cohort: the Rochester Diabetic Neuropathy Study. Neurology 1993; 43: 817–24.

[22] Kumar S, Ashe HA, Parnell LN, Fernando DJ, Tsigos C, Young RJ, Ward JD, Boulton AJM. The prevalence of foot ulceration and its correlates in type 2 diabetic patients: a population-based study. Diabet Med 1994; 11: 480–4.

[23] Knuiman MW, Welborn TA, McCann VJ, Stanton KG, Constable IJ. Prevalence of diabetic complications in relation to risk factors. Diabetes 1986; 35: 1332–9.

[24] Fujimoto WY, Leonetti DL, Kinyoun JL, Shuman WP, Stolov WC, Wahl PW. Prevalence of complications among second-generation Japanese-American men with diabetes, impaired glucose tolerance, or normal glucose tolerance. Diabetes 1987; 36: 730–9.

[25] Maser RE, Steenkiste AR, Dorman JS, Kamp Nielsen V, Bass EB, Manjoo Q, Drash AL, Becker DJ, Kuller LH, Greene DA, Orchard TJ. Epidemiological correlates of diabetic neuropathy. Report from Pittsburgh Epidemiology of Diabetes Complications Study. Diabetes 1989; 38: 1456–61.

[26] Harris M, Eastman R, Cowie C. Symptoms of sensory neuropathy in adults with NIDDM in the US population. Diabetes Care 1993; 16: 1446–52.

[27] Nielsen JV. Peripheral neuropathy, hypertension, foot ulcers and amputations among Saudi Arabian patients with type 2 diabetes. Diabetes Res Clin Pract 1998; 41: 63–9.

[28] Verhoeven S, Ballegooie E van, Casparie AF. Impact of late complications in type 2 diabetes in a Dutch population. Diabet Med 1991; 8: 435–8.

[29] Neeling JND De, Beks PJ, Bertelsmann FW, Heine RJ, Bouter LM. Peripheral somatic nerve function in relation to glucose tolerance in an elderly Caucasian population: the Hoorn Study. Diabet Med 1996; 13: 960–6.

[30] Müller UA, Ross IS, Klinger H. Häufigkeit der Hypopallästhesie bei insulinspritzenden Diabetikern in einer unausgewählten Stadtpopulation. Diab Stoffw 1993; 2: 439–42.

[31] Ziegler D, Gries FA, Mühlen H, Rathmann W, Spüler M, Lessmann F, the DiaCAN Multicenter Study Group. Prevalence and clinical correlates of cardiovascular autonomic and peripheral diabetic neuropathy in patients attending diabetes centers. Diab Metab 1993; 19: 143–51.

[32] Veglio M, Sivieri R. Prevalence of neuropathy in IDDM patients in Piemonte, Italy. The Neuropathy Study Group of the Italian Society for the Study of Diabetes, Piemonte Affiliate. Diabetes Care 1993; 16: 456–61.

[33] Partanen J, Niskanen L, Lehtinen J, Mervaala E, Siitonen O, Uusitupa M. Natural history of peripheral neuropathy in patients with non-insulin-dependent diabetes mellitus. N Engl J Med 1995; 333: 89–94.

[34] Ratzmann KP, Raschke M, Gander B, Schimke P. Prevalence of peripheral and autonomic neuropathy in newly diagnosed type II (noninsulin dependent) diabetes. J Diab Complications 1991; 5: 1–5.

[35] Wang WQ, Ip TP, Lam KS. Changing prevalence of retinopathy in newly diagnosed non-insulin dependent diabetes mellitus patients in Hong Kong. Diabetes Res Clin Pract 1998; 39: 185–91.

[36] Gujral JS, McNally PG, O'Malley BP, Burden AC. Ethnic differences in the incidence of lower extremity amputation secondary to diabetes mellitus. Diabet Med 1993; 10: 271–4.

[37] Bharucha NE, Bharucha AE, Bharucha EP. Prevalence of peripheral neuropathy in the Parsi community of Bombay. Neurology 1991; 41: 1315–7.

[38] Savettieri G, Rocca WA, Salemi G, Meneghini F, Grigoletto F, Morgante L, Reggio A, Costa V, Coraci MA, Di Perri R. Prevalence of diabetic neuropathy with somatic symptoms: a door-to-door survey in two Sicilian municipalities. Neurology 1993; 43: 1115–20.

[39] Watkins PJ. The natural history of the diabetic neuropathies. Q J Med 1990; 77: 1209–18.

[40] Eriksson KF, Nilsson H, Lindgärde F, Österlin S, Dahlin LB, Lilja B, Rosen I, Sundkvist G. Diabetes mellitus but not impaired glucose tolerance is associated with dysfunction of peripheral nerves. Diabet Med 1994; 11: 279–85.

[41] Sosenko JM, Kato M, Soto R, Goldberg RB. Sensory function at diagnosis and in early stages of NIDDM in patients detected through screening. Diabetes Care 1992; 15: 847–52.

[42] Sundkvist G, Dahlin L-B, Nilsson H, Eriksson K-F, Lindgärde F, Rosen I, Lattimer SA, Sima AAF, Sullivan K, Greene DA. Sorbitol and myo-inositol levels and morphology of sural nerve in relation to peripheral nerve function and clinical neuropathy in men with diabetic, impaired, and normal glucose tolerance. Diabet Med 2000; 17: 259–68.

[43] Melton III LJ, Dyck PJ. Epidemiology. In: Dyck PJ, Thomas PK, Asbury AK, Winegrad AI, Porte D Jr, editors. Diabetic neuropathy. Philadelphia, Pa: W. B. Saunders; 1987: 27–35.

[44] Pirart J. Diabetes mellitus and its degenerative complications: a prospective study of 4,400 patients observed between 1947 and 197Diabetes Care 1978; 252: 168–88.

[45] Töyry JP, Partanen JVS, Niskanen LK, Länsimies EA, Uusitupa MIJ. Divergent development of autonomic and peripheral somatic neuropathies in NIDDM. Diabetologia 1997; 40: 953–8.

[46] UK Prospective Diabetes Study (UKPDS) Group. Intensive blood-glucose control with sulphonylureas or insulin compared with conventional treatment and risk of complications in patients with type 2 diabetes (UKPDS 33). Lancet 1998; 352: 837–53.

[47] Sands ML, Shetterly SM, Franklin GM, Hamman RF. Incidence of distal symmetric (sensory) neuropathy in NIDDM. San Luis Val Diabetes Study. Diabetes Care 1997; 20: 322–9.

[48] Dyck PJ, Davies JL, Litchy WJ, O'Brien PC. Longitudinal assessment of diabetic polyneuropathy using a composite score in the Rochester Diabetic Neuropathy Study cohort. Neurology 1997; 49: 229–39.

[49] Forrest KY, Maser RE, Pambianco G, Becker DJ, Orchard TJ. Hypertension as a risk factor for diabetic neuropathy: a prospective study. Diabetes 1997; 46: 665–70.

[50] Tesfaye S, Chaturvedi N, Eaton SEM, Ward JD, Fuller JH. Cardiovascular risk factors predict the development of diabetic peripheral neuropathy. Diabetes 2000; 49 (Suppl 1): A34.

[51] Hillson RM, Hockaday TDR, Newton DJ. Hyperglycaemia is one correlate of deterioration in vibration sense during the 5 years after diagnosis of type 2 (non-insulin-dependent) diabetes. Diabetologia 1984; 26: 122–6.

[52] Sosenko JM, Kato M, Soto R, Bild DE. A prospective study of sensory function in patients with type 2 diabetes. Diabet Med 1993; 10: 110–4.

[53] Young RJ, Macintyre CCA, Martyn CN, Prescott RJ, Ewing DJ, Smith AF, Viberti G, Clarke BF. Progression of subclinical polyneuropathy in young patients with type 1 (insulin-dependent) diabetes: associations with glycaemic control and microangiopathy (microvascular complications). Diabetologia 1986; 29: 156–61.

[54] Young RJ, Macintyre CCA, Ewing DJ, Prescott RJ. Prediction of neuropathy over 5 years in young insulin-dependent diabetic patients. Diabet Med 1988; 5: 7.

[55] Benbow SJ, Chan AW, Bowsher D, MacFarlane IA, Williams G. A prospective study of painful symptoms, small-fibre function and peripheral vascular disease in chronic painful diabetic neuropathy. Diabet Med 1994; 11: 17–21.

[56] Ziegler D, Piolot R. Prevention of diabetic neuropathy by near-normoglycemia. A 12-year prospective study from the diagnosis of IDDM. Diabetes 1998; 47 (Suppl 1): A63.

[57] Macleod AF, Till S, Sönksen PHS. Discussion of the clinical trials of the aldose reductase inhibitor tolrestat. Int Proc J 1991; 4: 17–24.

[58] Negrin P, Zara G. Conduction studies as prognostic parameters in the natural history of diabetic neuropathy: a long-term follow-up of 114 patients. Electromyogr Clin Neurophysiol 1995; 35: 341–50.

[59] Watanabe K, Hagura R, Akanuma Y, Takasu T, Kajinuma H, Kuzuya N, Irie M. Characteristics of cranial nerve palsies in diabetic patients. Diabetes Res Clin Pract 1990; 10: 19–27.

[60] Longstreth GF. Diabetic thoracic polyradiculopathy: ten patients with abdominal pain. Am J Gastroenterol 1997; 92: 502–5.

[61] Neil HA, Thompson AV, John S, McCarthy ST, Mann JI. Diabetic autonomic neuropathy: the prevalence of impaired heart rate variability in a geographically defined population. Diabet Med 1989; 6: 20–4.

[62] Maser RE, Pfeifer MA, Dorman JS, Kuller LH, Becker DJ, Orchard TJ. Diabetic autonomic neuropathy and cardiovascular risk. Pittsburgh Epidemiology of Diabetes Complications Study III. Arch Intern Med 1990; 150: 1218–22.
[63] O'Brien IAD, O'Hare JP, Lewin IG, Corrall RJM. The prevalence of autonomic neuropathy in insulin-dependent diabetes mellitus: a controlled study based on heart rate variability. Q J Med 1986; 61: 957–67.
[64] Stephenson J, Fuller JH, and EURODIAB IDDM Complications Study Group. Microvascular and acute complications in IDDM patients: the EURODIAB IDDM Complications Study. Diabetologia 1994; 37: 278–85.
[65] Tsutsu N, Nunoi K, Yokomizo Y, Kikuchi M, Fujishima M. Relationship between glycemic control and orthostatic hypotension in type 2 diabetes mellitus—a survey by the Fukuoka Diabetes Clinic Group. Diabetes Res Clin Pract 1990; 8: 115–23.
[66] Ziegler D, Dannehl K, Spüler M, Mühlen H, Gries FA. Prevalence of cardiovascular autonomic nerve dysfunction assessed by spectral analysis and standard tests of heart rate variation in newly diagnosed IDDM patients. Diabetes Care 1992; 15: 908–11.
[67] Lehtinen JM, Uusitupa M, Siitonen O, Pyörälä K. Prevalence of neuropathy in newly diagnosed NIDDM and nondiabetic control subjects. Diabetes 1989; 38: 1307–13.
[68] Töyry JP, Niskanen LK, Mäntysaari MJ, Länsimies EA, Uusitupa MIJ. Occurrence, predictors, and clinical significance of autonomic neuropathy in NIDDM. Ten-year follow-up from the diagnosis. Diabetes 1996; 45: 308–15.
[69] Töyry JP, Niskanen LK, Lansimies EA, Partanen KPL, Uusitupa MLJ. Autonomic neuropathy predicts the development of stroke in patients with non-insulin-dependent diabetes mellitus. Stroke 1996; 27: 1316–8.
[70] Mustonen J, Uusitupa M, Mäntysaari M, Länsimies E, Pyörälä K, Laakso M. Changes in autonomic nervous function during the 4-year follow-up in middle-aged diabetic and nondiabetic subjects initially free of coronary heart disease. J Intern Med 1997; 241: 227–35.
[71] Quadri R, Ponzani P, Zanone M, Maule S, Grotta A La, Papotti G, Valentini M, Matteoda C, Chiandussi L, Fonzo D. Changes in autonomic nervous function over a 5-year period in non-insulin-dependent diabetic patients. Diabet Med 1993; 10: 916–9.
[72] Ziegler D, Mayer P, Mühlen H, Gries FA. The natural history of somatosensory and autonomic nerve dysfunction in relation to glycaemic control during the first 5 years after diagnosis of type 1 (insulin-dependent) diabetes mellitus. Diabetologia 1991; 34: 822–9.
[73] Solders G, Thalme B, Aguirre-Aquino M, Brandt L, Berg U, Persson A. Nerve conduction and autonomic nerve function in diabetic children. Acta Paediatr 1997; 86: 361–6.
[74] Sampson MJ, Wilson S, Karagiannis P, Edmonds M, Watkins PJ. Progression of diabetic autonomic neuropathy over a decade in insulin-dependent diabetics. Q J Med 1990; 75: 635–46.
[75] Sundkvist G, Lilja B. Autonomic neuropathy in diabetes mellitus: a follow-up study. Diabetes Care 1985; 8: 129–33.
[76] Donaghue KC, Fung ATW, Fairchild JM, Howard NJ, Silink M. Prospective assessment of autonomic and peripheral nerve function in adolescents with diabetes. Diabet Med 1996; 13: 65–71.
[77] Levitt NS, Stansberry KB, Wynchank S, Vinik AI. The natural progression of autonomic neuropathy aund autonomic function tests in a cohort of people with IDDM. Diabetes Care 1996; 19: 751–4.
[78] Sundkvist G, Lilja B. Autonomic neuropathy predicts deterioration in glomerular filtration rate in patients with IDDM. Diabetes Care 1993; 16: 773–9.
[79] Ziegler D, Piolot R, Pour Mirza A, Karallus M, Feng B, Schommartz B, Schadewaldt P. ^{13}C-octanoic acid breath test to assess diabetic gastroparesis: patterns of gastric emptying in newly diagnosed and long-term type 1 and type 2 diabetic patients. Clin Auton Res 1997; 7: 246.
[80] Enck P, Rathmann W, Spiekermann M, Czerner D, Tschöpe D, Ziegler D, Strohmeyer G, Gries FA. Prevalence of gastrointestinal symptoms in diabetic patients and non-diabetic subjects. Z Gastroenterol 1994; 32: 637–41.
[81] Schvarcz E, Palmer M, Ingberg CM, Aman J, Berne C. Increased prevalence of upper gastrointestinal symptoms in long-term type 1 diabetes mellitus. Diabet Med 1996; 13: 478–81.
[82] Ko GTC, Chan W-B, Chan JCN, Tsang LWW, Cockram CS. Gastrointestinal symptoms in Chinese patients with type 2 diabetes mellitus. Diabet Med 1999; 16: 670–4.
[83] Santis A De, Attili AF, Corradini SG, Scafato E, Cantagalli A, Luca C De, Pinto G, Lisi D, Capocaccia L. Gallstones and diabetes: a case-control study in a free-living population sample. Hepatology 1997; 25: 787–90.
[84] Shaw JE, Parker R, Hollis S, Gokal R, Boulton AJM. Gustatory sweating in diabetes mellitus. Diabet Med 1996; 13: 1033–7.
[85] NIH consensus development panel on impotence. Impotence. JAMA 1993; 270: 83–90.
[86] Wagner G, Saenz de Tejada I. Update on male erectile dysfunction. BMJ 1998; 316: 678–82.
[87] Feldman HA, Goldstein I, Hatzichristou DG, Krane RJ, McKinlay JB. Impotence and its medical and psychosocial correlates: results of the Massachusetts male ageing study. J Urol 1994; 151: 54–61.
[88] Fedele D, Coscelli C, Santeusanio F, Bortolotti A, Chatenoud L, Colli E, Landoni M, Parazzini F. Erectile dysfunction in diabetic subjects in Italy. Diabetes Care 1998; 21: 1973–7.
[89] Kolodny RC, Kahn CB, Goldstein HH, Barnett DM. Sexual dysfunction in diabetic men. Diabetes 1974; 23: 306–9.
[90] Klein R, Klein BEK, Lee KE, Moss SE, Cruickshanks KJ. Prevalence of self-reported erectile dysfunction in people with long-term IDDM. Diabetes Care 1996; 19: 135–41.
[91] McCulloch DK, Campbell IW, Wu FC, Prescott RJ, Clarke BF. The prevalence of diabetic impotence. Diabetologia 1980; 18: 279–83.
[92] Cavan DA, Barnett AH, Leatherdale BA. Diabetic impotence: risk factors in a clinic population. Diabetes Res 1987; 5: 145–8.
[93] Hackett GI. Impotence—the most neglected complication of diabetes. Diabetes Care 1995; 28: 75–83.
[94] Johannes CB, Araujo AB, Feldman HA, Derby CA, Kleinman KP, McKinlay JB. Incidence of erectile dysfunction in men 40 to 69 years old: longitudinal results from the Massachusetts male aging study. J Urol 2000; 163: 460–3.
[95] Reichard P, Pihl M, Rosenqvist U, Sule J. Complications in IDDM are caused by elevated blood glucose level: the Stockholm Diabetes Intervention Study (SDIS) at 10-year follow up. Diabetologia 1996; 39: 1483–8.
[96] UK Prospective Diabetes Study (UKPDS) Group. Effect of intensive blood-glucose control with metformin on complications in overweight patients with type 2 diabetes (UKPDS 34). Lancet 1998; 352: 854–65.
[97] Dyck PJ, Davies JL, Wilson DM, Service JF, Melton III. LJ, O'Brien PC. Risk factors for severity of diabetic polyneuropathy. Diabetes Care 1999; 22: 1479–86.
[98] Wiles PG, Pearce SM, Rice PJ, Mitchell JM. Vibration perception threshold: influence of age, height, sex, and smoking, and calculation of accurate centile values. Diabet Med 1991; 8: 157–61.
[99] Bloom S, Till S, Sonksen P, Smith S. Use of a biothesiometer to measure individual vibration thresholds and their variation in 519 non-diabetic subjects. Br Med J (Clin Res Ed) 1984; 288: 1793–5.
[100] Savage S, Estacio RO, Jeffers B, Schrier RW. Urinary albumin excretion as a predictor of diabetic retinopathy, neuropathy, and cardiovascular disease in NIDDM. Diabetes Care 1996; 19: 1243–8.
[101] Malik RA, Williamson S, Abbott C, Carrington AL, Iqbal J, Schady W, Boulton AJ. Effect of angiotensin-converting-enzyme (ACE) inhibitor trandolapril on human diabetic neuropathy: randomised double-blind controlled trial. Lancet 1998; 352: 1978–81.
[102] UK Prospective Diabetes Study Group. Tight blood pressure control and risk of macrovascular and microvascular complications in type 2 diabetes. UKPDS 3BMJ 1998; 317: 703–13.
[103] Ido Y, Vindigni A, Chang K, Stramm L, Chance R, Heath WF, DiMarchi RD, Di Cera E, Williamson JR. Prevention of vascular and neural dysfunction in diabetic rats by C-peptide. Science 1997; 277: 563–6.
[104] Liao D, Sloan RP, Cascio WE, Folsom AR, Liese AD, Evans GW, Cai J, Sharrett AR. Multiple metabolic syndrome is associated

with lower heart rate variability. The Atherosclerosis Risk in Communities Study. Diabetes Care 1998; 21: 2116–22.
[105] Liao D, Cai J, Brancati FL, Folsom A, Barnes RW, Tyroler HA, Heiss G. Association of vagal tone with serum insulin, glucose, and diabetes mellitus—the ARIC Study. Diabetes Res Clin Pract 1995; 30: 211–21.
[106] Dekker JM, Feskens EJM, Schouten EG, Klootwijk P, Pool J, Kromhout D. QTc duration is associated with levels of insulin and glucose tolerance. Zutphen Elderly Study. Diabetes 1996; 45: 376–80.
[107] 10Ziegler D. Diabetic cardiovascular autonomic neuropathy: prognosis, diagnosis, and treatment. Diabetes Metab Rev 1994; 10: 339–83.
[108] Gerritsen J, Dekker JM, TenVoorde BJ, Bertelsmann FW, Kostense PJ, Stehouwer CDA, Heine RJ, Nijpels G, Heethaar RM, Bouter LM. Glucose tolerance and other determinants of cardiovascular autonomic function: the Hoorn Study. Diabetologia 2000; 43: 561–70.
[109] Smulders YM, Jager A, Gerritsen J, Dekker JM, Nijpels G, Heine RJ, Bouter LM, Stehouwer CDA. Cardiovascular autonomic function is associated with (micro-)albuminuria in elderly caucasian subjects with impaired glucose tolerance or type 2 diabetes. Hoorn Study. Diabetes Care 2000; 23: 1369–74.
[110] Marre M. Genetics and the prediction of complications in type 1 diabetes. Diabetes Care 1999; 22 (Suppl 2): B53–58.
[111] Vague P, Dufayet D, Coste T, Moriscot C, Jannot MF, Raccah D. Association of diabetic neuropathy with NA/K-ATPase gene polymorphism. Diabetologia 1997; 40: 506–11.
[112] Heesom AE, Millward A, Demaine AG. Susceptibility to diabetic neuropathy in patients with insulin dependent diabetes mellitus is associated with a polymorphism at the 5′ end of the aldose reductase gene. J Neurol Neurosurg Psychiatry 1998; 64: 213–6.
[113] Ichikawa F, Yamada K, Ishiyama-Shigemoto S, Yuan X, Nonaka K. Association of an (A-C)n dinucleotide repeat polymorphic marker at the 5′-region of the aldose reductase gene with retinopathy but not with nephropathy or neuropathy in Japanese patients with type 2 diabetes mellitus. Diabet Med 1999; 16: 744–8.
[114] Forsblom CM, Sane T, Groop P-H, Tötterman KJ, Kallio M, Saloranta C, Laasonen L, Summanen P, Lepäntalo M, Laatikainen L, Matikainen E, Teppo A-M, Koskimies S, Groop L. Risk factors for mortality in type II (non-insulin-dependent) diabetes: evidence of a role for neuropathy and a protective effect of HLA-DRDiabetologia 1998; 41: 1253–62.
[115] Reichard P, Pihl M. Mortality and treatment side-effects during long-term intensified conventional insulin treatment in the Stockholm Diabetes Intervention Study. Diabetes 1994; 43: 313–7.
[116] Coppini DV, Bowtell PA, Weng C, Young PJ, Sönksen PH. Showing neuropathy is related to increased mortality in diabetic patients – a survival analysis using an accelerated failure time model. J Clin Epidemiol 2000; 53: 519–23.
[117] Navarro X, Kennedy WR, Aeppli D, Sutherland DER. Neuropathy and mortality in diabetes: influence of pancreas transplantation. Muscle Nerve 1996; 19: 1009–16.
[118] Boyko EJ, Ahroni JH, Smith DG, Davignon D. Increased mortality associated with diabetic foot ulcer. Diabet Med 1996; 13: 967–72.
[119] Ewing DJ, Campbell IW, Clarke BF. The natural history of diabetic autonomic neuropathy. Q J Med 1980; 49: 95–108.
[120] Hasslacher C, Bässler G. Prognose der kardialen autonomen Neuropathie bei Diabetikern. Münch Med Wochenschr 1983; 125: 375–7.
[121] Navarro X, Kennedy WR, Loewenson RB, Sutherland DER. Influence of pancreas transplantation on cardiorespiratory reflexes, nerve conduction, and mortality in diabetes. Diabetes 1990; 39: 802–6.
[122] O'Brien IA, McFadden JP, Corral RJM. The influence of autonomic neuropathy on mortality in insulin-dependent diabetes. Q J Med 1991; 79: 495–502.
[123] Ewing DJ, Boland O, Neilson JMM, Cho CG, Clarke BF. Autonomic neuropathy, QT interval lengthening, and unexpected deaths in male diabetic patients. Diabetologia 1991; 34: 182–5.
[124] Jermendy G, Toth L, Vörös P, Koltai MZ, Pogatsa G. Cardiac autonomic neuropathy and QT interval length. A follow-up study in diabetic patients. Acta Cardiol 1991; 46: 189–200.
[125] Rathmann W, Ziegler D, Jahnke M, Haastert B, Gries FA. Mortality in diabetic patients with cardiovascular autonomic neuropathy. Diabet Med 1993; 10: 820–4.
[126] Luft D, Rak R, Renn W, Konz K, Eggstein M. Diabetische autonome Neuropathie: Verlauf und prognostische Bedeutung kardiovaskulärer Reflexteste. Diab Stoffw 1993; 2: 239–44.
[127] Orchard TJ, Lloyd CE, Maser RE, Kuller LH. Why does diabetic autonomic neuropathy predict IDDM mortality? An analysis from the Pittsburgh Epidemiology of Diabetes Complications Study. Diabetes Res Clin Pract 1996; 34 (Suppl): S165–171.
[128] Veglio M, Sivieri R, Chinaglia A, Scaglione L, Cavallo-Perin P. QT interval prolongation and mortality in type 1 diabetic patients: a 5-year cohort prospective study. Neuropathy Study Group of the Italian Society of the Study of Diabetes, Piemonte Affiliate. Diabetes Care 2000; 23:1381–3.
[129] Task Force of the European Society of Cardiology and the North American Society of Pacing and Electrophysiology. Heart rate variability, standards of measurement, physiological interpretation, and clinical use. Circulation 1996; 93: 1043–65.
[130] Jacobi RM, Nesto RW. Acute myocardial infarction in the diabetic patient: pathophysiology, clinical course and prognosis. J Am Coll Cardiol 1992; 20: 736–44.
[131] Page MMcB, Watkins PJ. Cardiorespiratory arrest and diabetic autonomic neuropathy. Lancet 1978; i: 14–6.
[132] Whitsel EA, Boyko EJ, Siscovick DS. Reassessing the role of QTc in the diagnosis of autonomic failure among patients with diabetes. A meta-analysis. Diabetes Care 2000; 23: 241–7.
[133] Anonymous. Neural mechanisms in sudden cardiac death: insights from long QT syndrome. Lancet 1991; 338: 1181–2.
[134] Pozzati A, Pancaldi LG, Di Pasquale G, Pinelli G, Bugiardini R. Transient sympathovagal imbalance triggers "ischemic" sudden death in patients undergoing electrocardiographic Holter monitoring. J Am Coll Cardiol 1996; 27: 847–52.
[135] Fei L, Anderson MH, Katritsis D, Sneddon J, Statters DJ, Malik M, Camm AJ. Decreased heart rate variability in survivors of sudden cardiac death not associated with coronary artery disease. Br Heart J 1994; 71: 16–21.
[136] Bikkina M, Alpert MA, Mukerji R, Mulekar M, Cheng B-Y, Mukerji V. Diminished short-term heart rate variability predicts inducible ventricular tachycardia. Chest 1998; 113: 312–6.
[137] Algra A, Tijssen JGP, Roelandt JRTC, Pool J, Lubsen J. Heart rate variability from 24-hour electrocardiography and the 2-year risk for sudden death. Circulation 1993; 88: 180–5.
[138] Dekker JM, Schouten EG, Klootwijk P, Pool J, Swenne CA, Kromhout D. Heart rate variability from short electrocardiographic recordings predicts mortality from all causes in middle-aged and elderly men. Zutphen Study. Am J Epidemiol 1997; 145: 899–908.
[139] Masaki KH, Schatz IJ, Burchfiel CM, Sharp DS, Chiu D, Foley D, Curb JD. Orthostatic hypotension predicts mortality in elderly men: the Honolulu Heart Program. Circulation 1998; 98: 2290–5.
[140] Rees PJ, Cochrane GM, Prior JG, Clark TJH. Sleep apnea in diabetic patients with autonomic neuropathy. J R Soc Med 1981; 74: 192–5.
[141] Neumann C, Martinez D, Schmid H. Nocturnal oxygen desaturation in diabetic patients with severe autonomic neuropathy. Diabetes Res Clin Pract 1995; 28: 97–102.
[142] Sobotka PA, Liss HP, Vinik AI. Impaired hypoxic ventilatory drive in diabetic patients with autonomic neuropathy. J Clin Endocrinol Metab 1986; 62: 658–63.
[143] Wanke T, Abrahamian H, Lahrmann H, Formanek D, Merkle M, Auinger M, Zwick H, Irsigler K. No effect of naloxone on ventilatory response to progressive hypercapnia in IDDM patients. Diabetes 1993; 42: 282–7.
[144] Tantucci C, Scionti L, Bottini P, Dottorini ML, Puxeddu E, Casucci G, Sorbini CA. Influence of autonomic neuropathy of different severities on the hypercapnic drive to breathing in diabetic patients. Chest 1997; 112: 145–53.
[145] Chaudhuri TK, Fink S. Prognostic implications of gastroparesis in patients with diabetes mellitus. Clin Auton Res 1992; 2: 221–4.
[146] Kong M-F, Horowitz M, Jones KL, Wishart JM, Harding PE. Natural history of diabetic gastroparesis. Diabetes Care 1999; 22: 503–7.

4 Pathogenesis and Pathology of Diabetic Neuropathy

Histopathology

Diabetic Peripheral Neuropathy

A.P. Mizisin and H.C. Powell

The frequent occurrence of neurologic complications of diabetes has long been recognized and no doubt contributed to the erroneous belief of nineteenth-century physicians that diabetes mellitus was a disease of the nervous system. While disturbances in the central nervous system related to insulin deficiency are recognized, the major neurologic complication is the peripheral neuropathy occurring in both insulin-dependent and insulin-independent forms of diabetes mellitus. Although conventional medical treatment prolongs life span and attenuates neurologic complications of diabetes, hyperglycemic control is not sufficient to prevent the development of neuropathy. The peripheral nerve disorders related to diabetes mellitus are clinically heterogeneous and often subdivided into symmetric polyneuropathies and focal or multifocal neuropathies.

The pathology of diabetic neuropathy and its interpretation have been a continuing source of controversy. Points of contention have ranged from whether peripheral nerve injury is primary or secondary to neuronal degeneration to whether demyelination or axonal loss is the primary or main lesion. The pathogenesis of diabetic neuropathy has also been contentious and variously described as having a metabolic or ischemic etiology. Despite disagreement about the primary role of a particular lesion or the etiology of diabetic neuropathy, it is clear that diabetes mellitus has the potential to induce pathologic changes in most cellular and noncellular components of the peripheral nerve. This chapter will consider first the histopathologic changes induced by hyperglycemia in the peripheral nerve and then the relationship of this pathology to the type of diabetic neuropathy.

Hyperglycemia-Induced Histopathology

Myelinated Nerve Fibers

Loss of myelinated nerve fibers has been repeatedly documented. While fiber loss is most prominent distally, it may also be apparent in spinal roots, particularly in dorsal roots. Some have suggested that proximal multifocal fiber loss in the sciatic nerve summates to produce diffuse distal lesions in the peroneal, tibial, and sural nerves [1]. Although marginal fiber loss is difficult to assess qualitatively, moderate to gross loss has been extensively illustrated (Fig. 4.**1a**), often with considerable variation between adjacent fascicles. A diabetes-induced decrease in the density and occupancy of myelinated fibers represents quantitative evidence of loss affecting both large and small fibers [2–4].

Changes noted prior to the axoplasmic dissolution that constitutes axonal degeneration include accumulation of glycogen and dystrophic accumulation of vesicular and cytoskeletal elements [5,6]. Demyelination secondary to axonal degeneration has been observed [7]. Characteristic of axonal degeneration of the Wallerian type, osmiophilic lipid droplets can be observed within otherwise vacant neurilemmal tubes in teased fiber preparations (Fig. 4.**2a**). The Schwann cell basal laminae that form neurilemmal tubes are frequently circular, as if failing to collapse, and assume the corrugated profile seen in typical Wallerian degeneration [8]. In earlier stages of diabetic neuropathy, axonal regeneration has been reported to be robust and greater than that in control subjects [2]. Regenerative clusters appear in plastic sections as a group of myelinated sprouts within a residual, circular basal lamina [5,8].

In human diabetic neuropathy, the existence of axonal atrophy or the diminution of axonal caliber without myelin or axonal degeneration is disputed. Axonal atrophy was suggested by an early report of teased fibers with long internodes and inappropriately small diameters [9]. However, despite qualitative descriptions [5] and quantitative evidence employing multiple parameters [4,10,11], axonal atrophy has not been observed in other studies [12,13], including one involving a large sample size and claiming an improved morphometric method for detecting this change [14].

Segmental demyelination has long been described as a pathologic change occurring in diabetic neuropathy [2,9,15,17]. It is recognized in teased fibers as an internode lacking myelin or with an inappropriately thin myelin sheath compared to the myelin surrounding the adjacent internodes (Fig. 4.**2b**). In plastic section, demyelination was described as splitting of myelin sheaths with accumulation of granular and

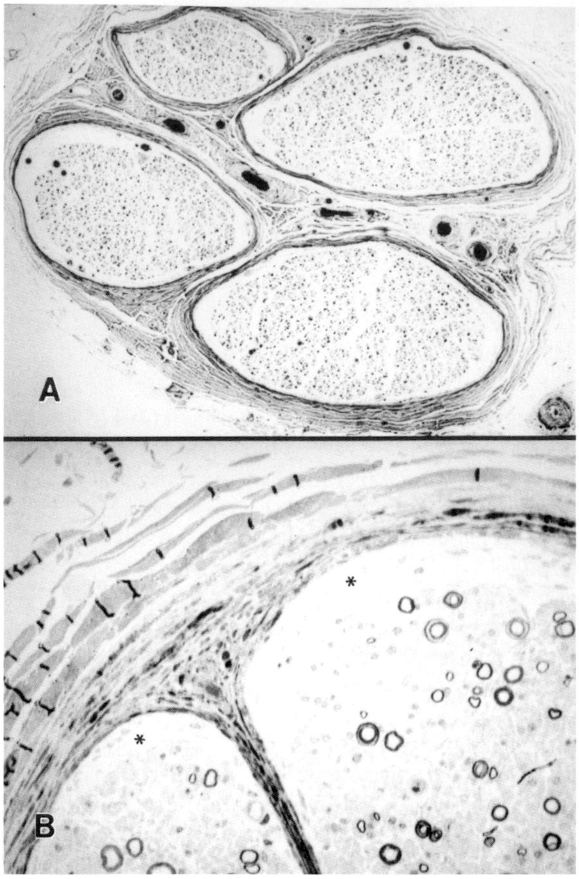

Fig. 4.1 Myelinated fiber loss in chronic human diabetic neuropathy. **A** A sural nerve biopsy shows fascicles with severe fiber loss. Several fascicles also show increased subperineurial structureless space, consistent with endoneurial edema. **B** Higher magnification view of a plastic section from a sural nerve showing subperineurial edema (asterisks) and myelinated fiber loss

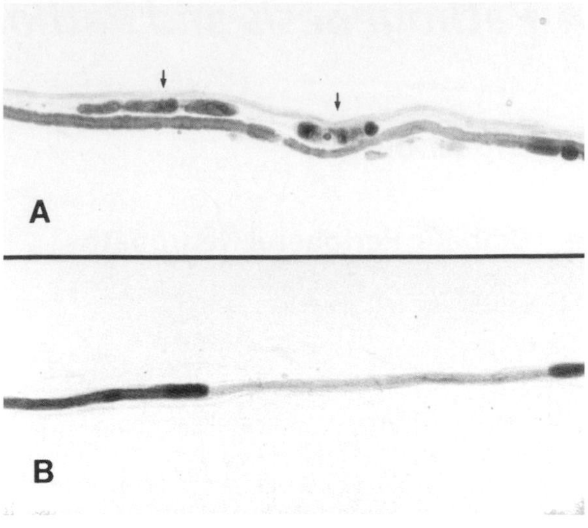

Fig. 4.2 Pathological abnormalities of teased nerve fibers from sural nerve biopsies in human diabetic neuropathy. **A** Wallerian degeneration, characterized by nerve fiber breakdown and consequent formation of myelin ovoids (arrows), is seen above an intact myelinated fiber. **B** A teased fiber from another biopsy shows an internode with severe myelin loss, consistent with either segmental demyelination or early remyelination. (Micrographs kindly provided by Nigel A. Calcutt, PhD)

vesicular debris [5]. Early reports of segmental demyelination without prominent axonal degeneration no doubt contributed to the view that demyelination is the primary lesion of diabetes-induced nerve injury. However, some investigators [9] noted that certain clinical features of diabetic neuropathy were best explained as resulting from a combination of segmental demyelination and axonal degeneration. Indeed, both primary segmental demyelination and demyelination secondary to axonal degeneration have been documented in the same nerve biopsy [7].

Schwann cell changes that appear to precede the dissolution of the myelin sheath have been observed in human diabetic neuropathy by several investigators [5,6,18]. Nonspecific, reactive changes include: accumulation of lipid droplets, paracrystalline inclusions (Pi granules of Reich) and glycogen granules; increased numbers of plasmalemmal vesicles; and cytoplasmic expansion and capping (Fig. 4.**3a**). Enlarged mitochondria with effaced cristae and disintegration of abaxonal and adaxonal cytoplasm and organelles have been described as degenerative Schwann cell changes (Fig. 4.**3b**). Thickening and reduplication of the Schwann cell basal lamina of myelinated fibers have also been illustrated [6].

Remyelination following segmental demyelination has been observed in diabetic neuropathy and is recognized in teased fiber preparations [9,16] and plastic section [12,18,19] by axons with inappropriately thin myelin sheaths. In some but not all nerve biopsies, proliferative Schwann cell changes are evident as clusters of Schwann cells in a concentric arrangement (Fig. 4.**4**) [5,9,20]. These concentric arrangements resemble small "onion bulbs," a nonspecific hypertrophic change consisting of supernumerary Schwann cell processes surrounding individual axons. "Onion bulbs" are thought to result from recurrent segmental demyelination and remyelination [20].

Paranodal abnormalities described in diabetic neuropathy include demyelination, paranodal swelling and axo-glial dysjunction. Several investigators [4,9,10] have emphasized the occurrence of restricted paranodal demyelination (Fig. 4.**5a**), which may be resolved with selective remyelination by surviving Schwann cells or with the formation of an intercalated internode as noted in teased fibers [2]. Paranodal swelling has been suggested to precede paranodal demyelination and is thought to be associated with axo-glial dysjunction, the loss of the gap-junction-like connections of terminal Schwann cell loops to the axolemma on either side of the node of Ranvier [4]. The

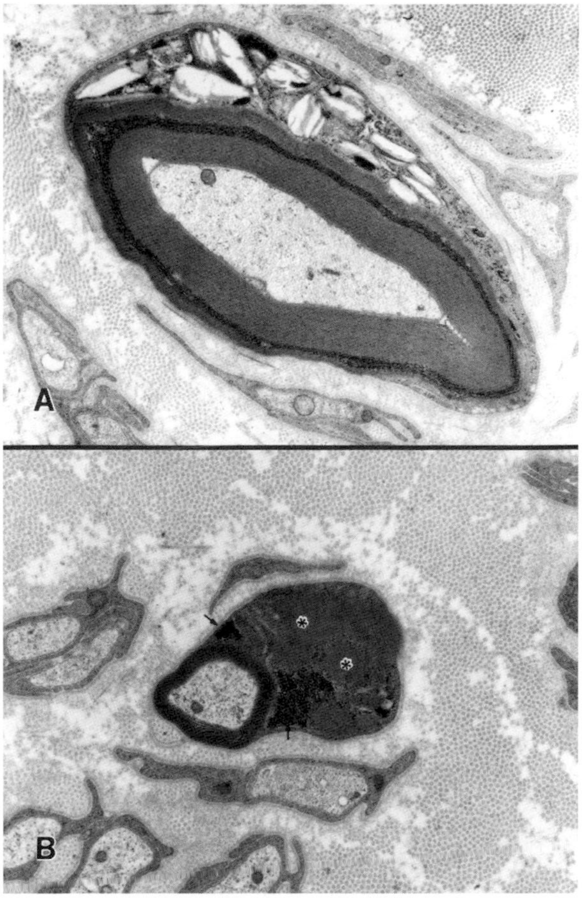

Fig. 4.3 Reactive and degenerative Schwann cell changes in poorly controlled human diabetic neuropathy. **A** Lysosomal inclusions (Pi granules of Reich), a nonspecific reactive change characteristic of chronic neuropathies with extensive myelinated fiber loss, are evident in an internodal band of Schwann cell cytoplasm in this myelinated fiber. **B** A small myelinated fiber with degenerative changes shows conspicuous Schwann cell cytoplasmic enlargement with glycogen accumulation (arrows) and darkened profiles of giant mitochondria with effaced cristae (asterisks)

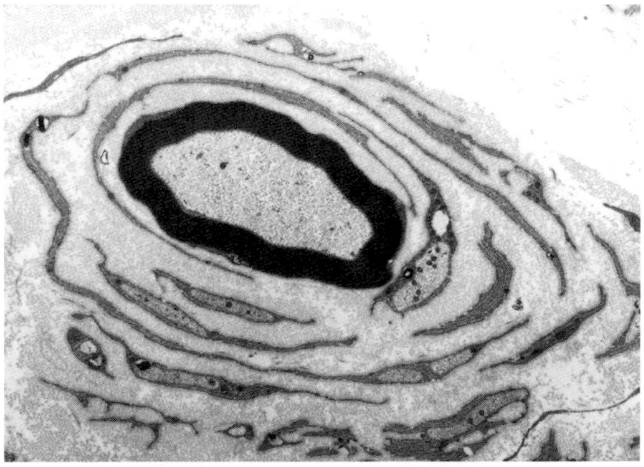

Fig. 4.4 Proliferative Schwann cell changes in chronic human diabetic neuropathy. Concentric arrays of supernumerary Schwann cells form an "onion bulb" around a myelinated fiber

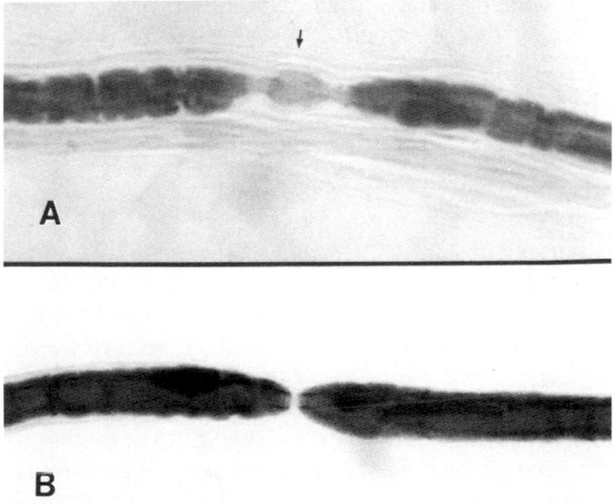

Fig. 4.5 Paranodal demyelination of a teased nerve fiber in human diabetic neuropathy. **A** The paranodal region (arrow) of this teased fiber is incompletely ensheathed by myelin, resulting in an exaggeration of the length of the node of Ranvier. **B** A normal-appearing node of Ranvier in a teased fiber is shown for comparison. (Micrographs kindly provided by Nigel A. Calcutt, PhD)

existence of paranodal swelling and axo-glial dysjunction is a contentious issue. Although repeatedly documented by some in experimental and human diabetic neuropathy [4,10], others [21] have not detected these abnormalities.

Unmyelinated Nerve Fibers

Early electron microscopic studies of diabetic neuropathy noted a distinct loss of unmyelinated fibers [6]. Characteristic degenerative changes of these fibers include shrinkage of axons, accumulation of enlarged vesicular elements, and deterioration of tubular and filamentous elements of the cytoskeleton. Edematous Schwann cell cytoplasm has also been observed, as well as hyperplasia of surrounding basal lamina [6]. Complete degeneration results in empty or denervated Schwann cell subunits surrounded by a basal lamina. It is thought that eventually the Schwann cells degenerate, leaving the basal lamina that persists before disappearing. In the sural nerve of a patient dying with diabetes mellitus, unmyelinated fiber density was only a third of that observed in control patients [3]. Although unmyelinated fiber density is a quantitative reflection of fiber loss, empty Schwann cell subunits are considered by some to be a better indicator of such loss [22].

Vasa Nervorum

The blood supply of peripheral nerve trunks, the vasa nervorum, consists of intrinsic endoneurial vessels and extrinsic vessels of the epineurium and perineurium. In diabetes mellitus, histopathologic changes have been described in all components of this vasculature. In the endoneurium, vessels with thickened walls and reduced luminal caliber were documented in an early report [23]. Subsequent qualitative and quantitative work has demonstrated endothelial cell hypertrophy and hyperplasia with a reduction in luminal size [11,24–29]. Fenestrated endothelial cells, a feature normally present only in epineurial vessels, have been observed in endoneurial vessels [26], as has endothelial cell dysjunction or the loss of junctional contacts between cells [29]. Desquamation of endothelial cells [30] and degeneration of pericytes have also been described [31]. Reduplication of the basal lamina of endoneurial microvessels, although a feature of other chronic neuropathies, appears to be more pronounced in diabetic neuropathy (Fig. 4.**6a**). Luminal occlusion resulting from endothelial hyperplasia or fibrin plugs has been documented [30,32,33] but not confirmed in subsequent studies [24,28,29].

With respect to the extrinsic circulation, epineurial capillary abnormalities include endothelial cell hyperplasia and thickening of the basal lamina [25]. The intima of epineurial arterioles is increased in diabetic neuropathy [34]. However, in spite of these changes, endoneurial microvessels show significantly more pathology than epineurial microvessels with respect to basal lamina thickening, endothelial cell hypertrophy, and luminal narrowing [25]. Similar findings are reported for the transperineurial circulation, with hypertrophy and hyperplasia of endothelial cells and reduced luminal area [35]. Diabetic patients exhibit a greater degree of abnormal innervation of the epineurial and transperineurial circulation in that there appears to be a reduction in the vessels with perivascular axons and an increase in vessels with denervated Schwann cell units [36]. In the media of denervated arterioles, structural changes, such as an increase in glycogen, edematous smooth muscle cells, accumulation of cellular debris, and collagenous scarring, have been reported.

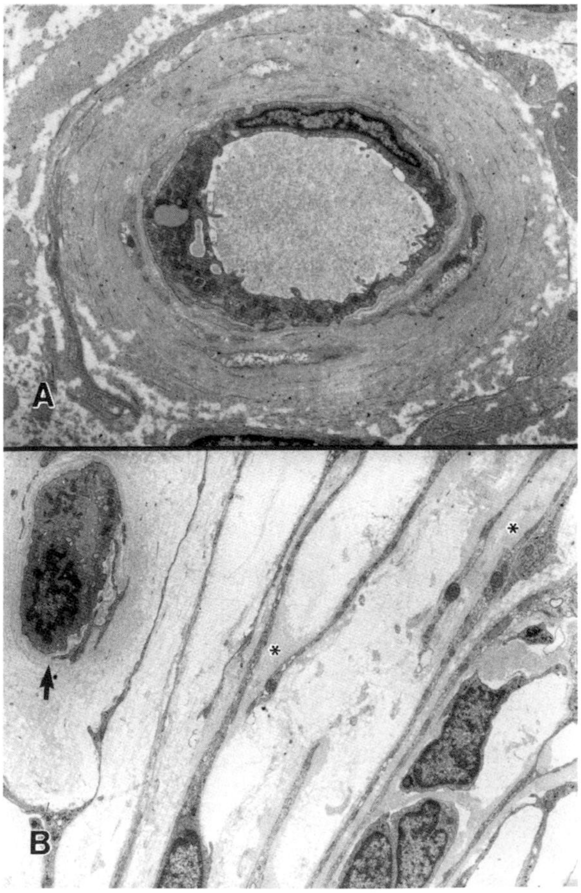

Fig. 4.**6** Vascular and perineurial abnormalities in chronic human diabetic neuropathy. **A** Markedly thickened and reduplicated basal lamina is evident surrounding an endoneurial microvessel. **B** The perineurial sheath is shown with focal basal laminar thickening (asterisks). A subperineurial capillary (arrow) shows a reduplicated basal lamina

Connective Tissue

Where substantial loss of myelinated fibers was apparent in diabetic neuropathy, early workers noted fibrosis and probable increase in endoneurial collagen and, in one instance, an accumulation of fibrillar material in an enlarged endoneurial interstitium [9]. Recent work points to extensive deposition of endoneurial collagen in nerves from diabetic patients, predominantly involving collagen types I and III [37]. Type VI collagen is increased in the endoneurium surrounding groups of Schwann cells, with types IV, V, and VI increased around endoneurial microvessels. The diameter of endoneurial collagen fibrils is increased in diabetic nerves. The hyperplasia and reduplication of basal laminae surrounding Schwann cells and microvessels have been noted above.

An increase in endoneurial area in diabetic neuropathy has been observed in plastic section [2,18,24,38] and considered by some to represent endoneurial edema (Fig.4.**1b**). In several studies using noninvasive magnetic resonance spectroscopy [39,40], hydration was increased in nerves from both asymptomatic and symptomatic diabetic patients but not in those receiving treatment with aldose reductase inhibitors. Edematous nerves appear to be an inconstant feature of diabetic neuropathy.

In diabetic patients, there are several abnormalities in the perineurium, the lamellar cellular ensheathment of individual fascicles of peripheral nerves. Thickening of the basal lamina surrounding cells of each layer of the perineurium has been documented (Fig. 4.**6b**) [8,41–43]. Reduplication as seen in basal laminae of Schwann cells and endoneurial microvessels is not present [43]. Calcification of the extracellular matrix of the perineurium has also been documented in diabetic neuropathy and is thought to result from deposition on matrix vesicles or lipid droplets derived from perineurial cells [44].

Relationship of Histopathology to Type of Diabetic Neuropathy

Because most cellular and noncellular components of peripheral nerves are affected in diabetes mellitus, it is difficult to ascribe a corresponding set of pathologic changes to any clinical presentation. Nevertheless, the topic has received sufficient attention in the literature to warrant consideration.

Symmetric Polyneuropathy

Among the various clinical presentations of diabetic neuropathy, distal symmetrical polyneuropathy with a "glove and stocking" distribution is the most typical. While causation remains uncertain, hyperglycemia underlies other putative mechanisms and there are some differences in patterns of structural injury in treated versus untreated patients. In treated diabetic patients with chronic neuropathy, fibers undergoing axonal degeneration predominate [45]. In contrast, in untreated diabetics with symptomatic neuropathy, both segmental demyelination and axonal degeneration are evident. Segmental demyelination appears to precede axonal degeneration and is in some instances accompanied by proliferative changes of Schwann cells including "onion bulbs" [12,18,46].

Although the most severe neuropathies are associated with profound loss of myelinated and unmyelinated axons, disturbances of lesser severity do not lend themselves to ready morphologic distinction. It appears that even in mild neuropathy, there is significant loss of myelinated fibers [19]. Although axonal regeneration may be more vigorous in milder cases of diabetic sensory neuropathy [12], it is diminished in proportion to the amount of myelinated nerve fiber loss [47]. In addition to proliferative changes of Schwann cells, marked thickening of vessel walls including thickening and reduplication of basal lamina has been found in asymptomatic patients with minimal or no signs of neuropathy [46].

Studies of painful diabetic neuropathy have investigated possible morphologic correlates of pain in patients with differing presentations of pain-related symptoms [11]. Axonal degeneration and reductions in fiber density were present in both patients with chronic neuropathy and those with diabetic pain of recent onset. In another study of patients with active acute painful neuropathy and patients with recently remitted pain [48], the occurrence of nerve fiber degeneration and regeneration was not sufficient to account fully for diabetic neuropathic pain. However, certain stages of the pathologic process of Wallerian degeneration may be linked to painful symptoms [48]. Another large clinicopathologic study also failed to establish a correlation between axonal degeneration or regeneration and painful neuropathy [12].

In severe diabetic neuropathy, autonomic disturbances are prominent but the disease is often painless. In such cases, nerve fiber loss may be profound [12]. Recurrent foot ulcers are most likely to occur in this group [11]. In the most severe neuropathies, sometimes presenting in untreated patients, demyelination and remyelination are prominent. An increase in capillary wall thickness was most pronounced in patients in whom neuropathy was painless, the degree of thickening in patients with painful neuropathy being less exaggerated [11]. With respect to capillary mural thickening, similar findings have been reported in asymptomatic patients [46].

Asymmetric Neuropathy

Focal neuropathic disorders in patients with diabetes mellitus are not symmetric in distribution and may involve cranial nerves or spinal roots. With respect to cranial nerves, the most frequently cited examples describe lesions involving the oculomotor nerve [49–51], although the trochlear and abducens nerves may be affected. Neuropathies affecting these cranial nerves are characterized by relatively sudden onset, focal distribution, and limited course [51]. Early published reports linked these neuropathies to ischemic events, and evidence of centrofascicular degeneration observed in postmortem studies reinforces this view. Nerve fiber atrophy and microfasciculation have also been documented in oculomotor nerves [51].

Proximal diabetic neuropathy is a severe form of asymmetric neuropathy that has been subject to confusing terminology and incomplete pathologic information. The clinical presentation typically involves one leg or thigh with eventual spreading to the buttock and opposite lower limb. In contrast to symmetrical polyneuropathy, this disorder appears to have an inflammatory basis [52–54]. Centrofascicular axonal loss in association with vasculitis [53] and evidence of epineurial vasculitis [54] support an ischemic causation. Occlusive vascular disease has also been detected in proximal diabetic neuropathy [53]. The presence of both axonal degeneration and demyelination attests to the role of ischemia in producing these changes in association with the inflammatory process [54].

Diabetic Autonomic Neuropathy

R.E. Schmidt

Neuropathology of Clinical Diabetic Autonomic Neuropathy

The neuropathology of diabetic autonomic neuropathy has, until recently, been largely unstudied despite its substantial clinical importance and wealth of pathophysiologic characterization of autonomic function in humans.

Sympathetic Ganglia

Degenerative changes culminating in the significant loss of sympathetic neurons have been claimed and disputed in classical nonquantitative studies [55–57]. Quantitative, although nonstereologic, analysis of neuronal density (expressed as number/mm^2) in the diabetic paravertebral superior cervical (SCG) and prevertebral superior mesenteric ganglia (SMG) in one large series [58] showed only a small (14 %), although statistically significant, decrease in neuronal density in diabetic subjects and did not identify significant numbers of actively degenerating neurons. The size and plexiform anatomy of human prevertebral ganglia and the existence of preferentially targeted subpopulations of sympathetic neurons may even complicate nonbiased stereologic analysis. Chromatolytic neurons or nodules of Nageotte (i.e., collections of satellite cell nuclei at sites of neuronal dropout) were not more common in diabetic human ganglia than in age-matched nondiabetics [59]. One often-quoted study by Duchen and colleagues [55] involved the detailed histopathologic characterization of the sympathetic ganglia of five patients with symptomatic diabetic autonomic neuropathy and reported a variety of apparently pathologic findings including neuronal necrosis, an inflammatory infiltrate, neuronal gigantism, dilated perikaryal endoplasmic reticulum, vacuolated neurons, and neuroaxonal dystrophy (NAD). Unfortunately, no controls were included in the study. In a large controlled study of NAD (Fig. 4.**7**), the distinctive and marked enlargement of distal preterminal axons and synapses, also represented the most striking histologic alteration in diabetic sympathetic ganglia. Dystrophic swellings consisted either of disorganized neurofilamentous aggregates (Fig. 4.**7**) or collections of mitochondria, dense bodies, lucent proteinaceous material, and tubulovesicular elements [59]. Quantitative studies demonstrated a progressive increase in the frequency of dystrophic axons as a function of age, diabetes, and gender (males more affected than females). Diabetic patients developed lesions (immunohistochemically and ultrastructurally identical to those in aged subjects) earlier and in greater numbers than age-matched control subjects, suggesting possible shared pathogenetic mechanisms in aging and diabetes. Perikarya of diabetic principal sympathetic neurons, although compressed and distorted by presynaptic NAD, were otherwise unremarkable.

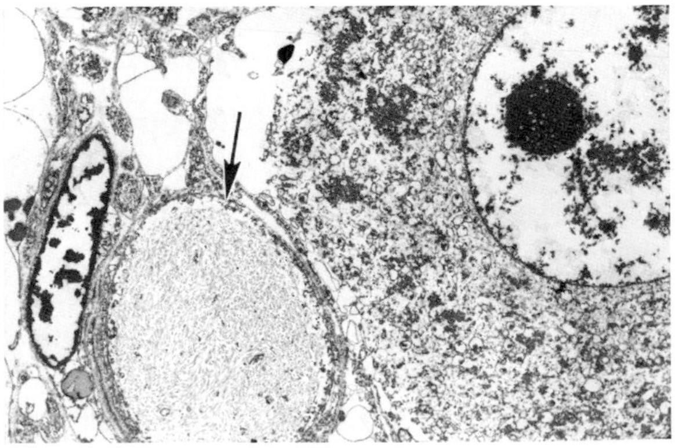

Fig. 4.**7** A swollen dystrophic axon (arrow) filled with neurofilaments distorts the contours of an adjacent principal sympathetic neuron in diabetic human sympathetic SMG (magnification 3000×)

Not all sympathetic ganglia are equally affected in human diabetics. The frequency of NAD in prevertebral SMG and celiac ganglia was more than 10-fold that of the paravertebral SCG. We have reexamined (R.E. Schmidt, unpublished data) multiple prevertebral and paravertebral chain ganglia of one of Duchen's original patients [55] who had symptomatic diabetic autonomic neuropathy with prominent alimentary dysfunction. Although the prevertebral celiac ganglia and paravertebral SCG were extensively and minimally involved, respectively, in that case the paravertebral lumbar sympathetic chain ganglia showed a frequency of NAD intermediate between those of the SCG and celiac ganglia. Prominent NAD in the celiac ganglia of the relatively young diabetics with symptomatic alimentary autonomic neuropathy [55] suggests possible pathophysiologic significance.

Lymphocytic infiltrates in postmortem sympathetic diabetic ganglia [55] have been interpreted as evidence of an autoimmune pathogenesis [60]; however, similar infiltrates were present in nearly half of all examined SCG and SMG in a large series [59] and their presence failed to correlate statistically with age, gender, or diabetes. Although the presence of antibodies against sympathetic ganglia and vagus nerve has also been reported to correlate [60] with autonomic dysfunction in diabetics, other studies have failed to show such a relationship [61].

Studies of prevertebral sympathetic ganglia in man and experimental animals have demonstrated the complexity and importance of function of prevertebral ganglion neurons in the integration of visceral reflexes [62]. Nerve terminals in the SMG reflect the contribution of neurons originating in the spinal cord intermediolateral nucleus, dorsal root ganglia, parasympathetic nervous system, other sympathetic ganglia or intraganglionic projections from neighboring principal sympathetic neurons, and from myenteric neurons projecting retrogradely. Dystrophic terminals in diabetic human SMG [58] were immunoreactive for neuropeptide Y (NPY), tyrosine hydroxylase, dopamine-β-hydroxylase, trkA (the cognate receptor for NGF), and p75; however, adjacent substance P, vasoactive intestinal peptide (VIP), gastrin-releasing polypeptide (GRP)/bombesin, and met-enkephalin terminals were spared. In some cases, ganglia contained increased numbers of delicate NPY processes, thought to represent axonal sprouts. This immunophenotype is consistent with origination of dystrophic axons from a subpopulation of NPY-containing noradrenergic neurons, most likely originating within the sympathetic nervous system, either intrinsic or extrinsic to the SMG, and, possibly, as locally recurrent collaterals. The neurofilaments (NF) which accumulated in diabetic and aged dystrophic sympathetic nerve terminals consisted almost exclusively of extensively phosphorylated 200-kDa NF-H epitopes [63]. Antisera directed against NF-L, NF-M, and nonphosphorylated epitopes of 200-kDa NF-H as well as MAP-2 preferentially labeled sympathetic neuronal perikarya and principal dendrites and did not label dystrophic axons. Peripherin, a 58-kDa cytoskeletal element distinct from any NF subunit which is present in subpopulations of sympathetic and DRG neurons, was colocalized with highly phosphorylated NF-H in many dystrophic elements [63], suggesting the possibility of a shared degradative pathogenetic mechanism, rather than altered synthesis, as a target of diabetes.

Although the development of neuroaxonal dystrophy represents unambiguous and compelling pathology in the sympathetic ganglia of diabetic humans, early studies described axon loss in preganglionic sympathetic communicating ("white") rami and greater splanchnic [57,64,65] nerves. Loss of preganglionic sympathetic innervation may, together with NAD, result in diminished numbers of normal presynaptic elements innervating principal sympathetic neurons.

Autonomic Axons in Somatic Nerves

Autonomic axons, particularly small unmyelinated axons, may be lost in somatic nerves as part of symmetrical sensorimotor neuropathy [66], which is thought to have an ischemic basis, resulting in local, distally accentuated autonomic symptoms. The loss of autonomic innervation of the vasa nervorum of somatic nerves, thought to affect blood flow to the nerve trunk, may significantly contribute to nerve ischemia described in somatic sensory polyneuropathy [67].

Diabetic Parasympathetic Nervous System

Although significant loss of vagal axons and active axonal degeneration have been described in various studies of diabetic autonomic neuropathy [68,69], the number of patients examined has typically been small. In one case of diabetic gastroparesis, dramatic axon loss in the abdominal vagus nerve was described [70]; however, a similar study failed to identify morphological abnormalities in the gastric wall or abdominal vagus nerve [71]. Immunofluorescence studies of diabetic human penis have shown preferential loss of VIP-containing axons in the corpora cavernosa [72,73].

Miscellaneous

Neuropeptide immunolocalization techniques have described decreased substance P content of human rectal mucosa in diabetic patients compared to nondiabetic controls [74]. The involvement of distal axons innervating diabetic bladder [75], skin, and penile corpora [76] has been proposed. Meissner's and Auerbach's plexuses in patients with diabetic diarrhea have failed to demonstrate reproducible histopathology [77], although one ultrastructural study has claimed the demonstration of marked axonal swellings within intramural ganglia [78]. PET scanning techniques have demonstrated the loss of sympathetic innervation in the distal myocardium in diabetic patients with autonomic neuropathy, although proximal segments were hyperinnervated, perhaps reflecting disorganized axonal sprouting and reinnervation [79].

Experimental Diabetic Autonomic Neuropathy

Animal models of diabetic autonomic neuropathy have been sought to provide insight into the pathogenetic mechanisms of the latter and to develop rational forms of therapy.

Sympathetic Nervous System

An unequivocal neuropathy of the alimentary tract of the streptozotocin (STZ)-diabetic and genetically diabetic BB rat and Chinese hamster has been characterized in detail [80–82]. The regular occurrence of degenerating, regenerating, and pathologically distinctive dystrophic axons has been demonstrated in: (1) preterminal axons and synapses within the prevertebral celiac and superior mesenteric sympathetic ganglia (Figs. 4.**8**–4.**10**), and (2) noradrenergic axons contained in ileal mesenteric nerves innervating the distal alimentary tract (Fig. 4.**11**) in rats with chronic long-term STZ-induced diabetes. As in diabetic humans, NAD again developed in the prevertebral superior mesenteric and celiac ganglia but not comparably in the paravertebral superior cervical ganglia. Dystrophic swellings involved postganglionic sympathetic noradrenergic distal ileal paravascular mesenteric nerve axons and their terminals on intramural myenteric and submucosal ganglia; however, the equally lengthy noradrenergic axons which innervate the adjacent mesenteric vasculature consistently failed to develop NAD. The time course over several months of the development of NAD, its anatomical distribution (chiefly alimentary and distal), relationship to axonal length, and its response to islet cell transplantation, short- or long-term insulin therapy, aldose reductase inhibitors, and several other novel therapeutic agents (administered in a preventive or reversal mode) have been reported. A recent study [83] has demonstrated the ability of the neurotrophic substance IGF-I to reverse established neuroaxonal dystrophy in STZ-diabetic rats without correction of the metabolic severity of the diabetic state, which may reflect the known ability of IGF-I to affect axonal regeneration, collateral sprouting, or synaptic plasticity [84].

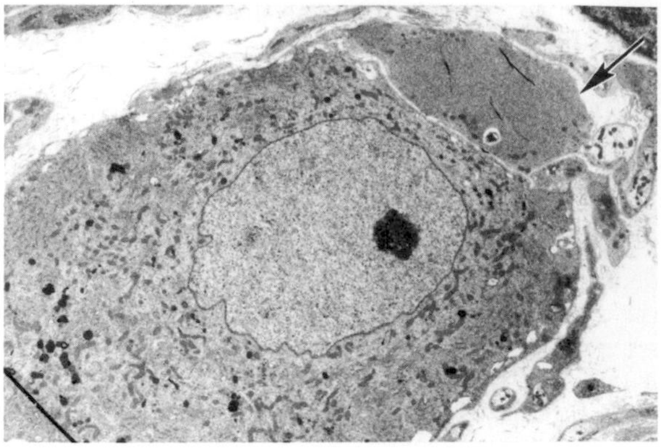

Fig. 4.8 A dystrophic axon (arrow) in the diabetic rat SMG is located within the satellite cell sheath (magnification 3000×)

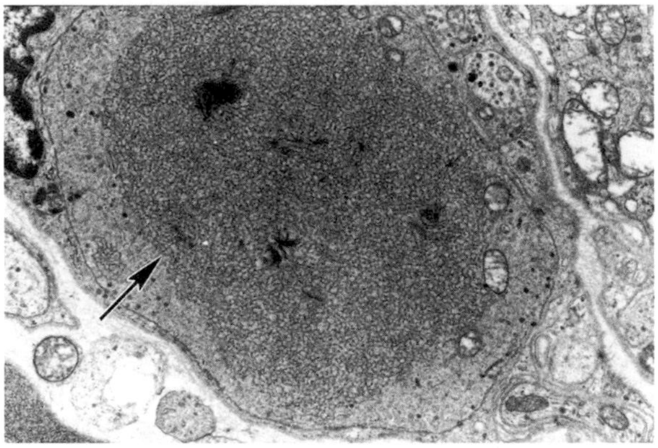

Fig. 4.9 Typically, dystrophic axons in diabetic rat SMG contain large numbers of anastomosing tubulovesicular elements (arrow; magnification 10 000×)

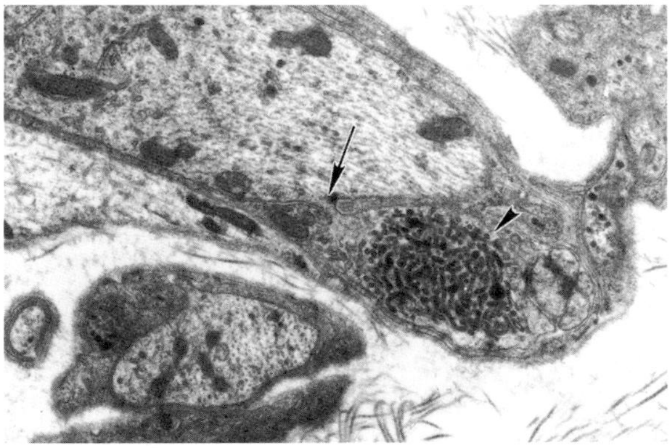

Fig. 4.10 Occasional swellings containing coarse tubulovesicular elements (arrowhead) appear to arise from projections from the adjacent perikaryon or principal dendrites, visible in this electron micrograph as a narrow cytoplasmic bridge (arrow; magnification 15 000×)

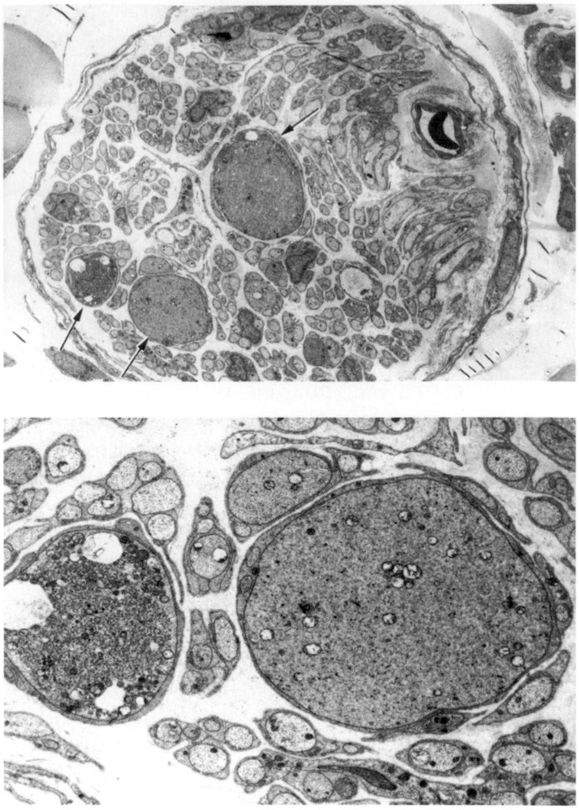

a

b

Fig. 4.11 Dystrophic axons (arrows, **a**), which may dominate the histologic appearance of the ileal mesenteric nerves of chronically diabetic rats, contain aggregates of tubulovesicular elements, mitochondria, and synaptic vesicles (seen better at higher magnification in **b**) (magnification: **a** 1200×; **b** 5000×)

Investigation of the effect of diabetes on postsynaptic dendritic structure has demonstrated dystrophic dendritic lesions (and involvement of dendritic spines in particular, Fig. 4.**10**) in diabetic rat prevertebral sympathetic ganglia [80,81].

The effect of diabetes on the STZ-induced diabetic rat gastrointestinal system has been further defined using electrophysiologic, immunohistologic, biochemical, and ultrastructural techniques. Degenerative changes, but not NAD, have also been described in the alimentary tract of eight-week STZ-diabetic rats, involving subpopulations of axons containing VIP [85] and calcitonin-gene-related peptide (CGRP) [86] but not substance P. Measurement of neuropeptides in diabetic rat ileum has demonstrated increased VIP and decreased substance P content [87], although changes may vary with duration of diabetes [88]. In addition, VIP and CGRP in the diabetic gut wall are not released appropriately in response to electrical stimuli [89].

Changes in neuropeptidergic and noradrenergic innervation of the diabetic rodent bowel may underlie changes in gut electrophysiology. Delayed small intestine transit time has been reported in STZ-diabetic rats

[90] and in chronically diabetic Chinese hamsters [91]. Other electrophysiologic studies of the alimentary tract in experimental diabetes have also established deficiencies of cholinergic transmission [92] and muscarinic signal transduction [93], prejunctional impairment of ileal sympathetic nerve function, as well as abnormal transmucosal ionic flux apparently mediated by abnormalities in noradrenergic innervation [94].

Extra-alimentary Endorgans

Recent studies have examined the effect of diabetes on innervation of the vasa nervorum [67], heart [95] and cardiac valves, urinary bladder [96], pancreatic islets [97], and the penile corpora [98]. These studies have consistently reported decreased innervation of diabetic endorgans. However, the sympathetic innervation of the iris of long-term diabetic rats is relatively spared [99].

Parasympathetic Nervous System

Unmyelinated and myelinated axons in the vagus nerve of chronically diabetic rats [100] and Chinese hamsters [82] are reported to show axonal atrophy (but not axon loss) and regenerative changes, respectively, which may underlie changes in the variability of cardiac rhythm [100] and altered alimentary motility. Axonal atrophy and degenerative changes have also been reported in parasympathetic innervation of the diabetic rat penis, distal myenteric nerves, and urinary bladder [101,102].

Immunofluorescence studies of STZ-diabetic rat penis have shown preferential loss of VIP-containing axons in the corpora cavernosa [73] and selective degeneration of nitrergic nerves [103].

Pathogenetic Mechanisms

The terminal aspects of autonomic axons appear to be preferentially targeted in diabetes. Ganglionic neuroaxonal dystrophy may represent an abnormal outcome of synaptic turnover, which may normally subserve synaptic plasticity, or the synaptic detachment/reattachment process that follows postganglionic sympathetic axotomy [104]. Other possible pathogenetic mechanisms have been previously described in detail [105].

Pathobiochemistry and Pathophysiology

■ Glycemic Control

D. Ziegler

Introduction

It was as early as in 1864 when Marchal de Calvi established that neurologic symptoms reflect the consequence rather than the cause of diabetes mellitus [106]. However, one of the most intriguing questions in clinical research in diabetes during the past decades was whether long-term near-normoglycemia may retard or improve the chronic diabetic complications, including diabetic neuropathy [107,108]. The recent publications of the two largest and longest studies in the history of diabetes research, the Diabetes Control and Complications Trial (DCCT), conducted in type 1 diabetic patients, and the United Kingdom Prospective Diabetes Study (UKPDS), performed in type 2 diabetic patients, have been interpreted as providing evidence of the benefit of intensive diabetes therapy on the development and progression of the chronic diabetic complications [109–111]. However, while in both studies the effects of improved glycemic control on the microvascular endpoints were unanimously considered as being favorable [107,112], the effects on macrovascular endpoints in the UKPDS have also been interpreted as showing a clinically important benefit on macrovascular endpoints only in patients treated with metformin, but not those treated with sulfonylureas or insulin. Because metformin provided blood glucose levels similar to those of sulfonylureas or insulin, the benefit from metformin appeared to be independent of its blood-glucose-lowering effect [113]. Moreover, in both studies microvascular or macrovascular rather than neuropathic endpoints were used as the primary outcome measures.

Numerous previous short-term studies have shown that neuropathic symptoms or abnormal nerve function tests occurring during periods of metabolic derangement can be ameliorated within several days or weeks following improvement of blood glucose control [114–122]. However, possible long-term effects have been difficult to study due to the following problems: (1) the progression of diabetic polyneuropathy is relatively slow, so that expected changes may take place over several years, (2) the various nerve fiber populations might be affected at different rates, (3) minor changes may not be detected due to a low reproducibility of some methods, (4) glycemic control or the risk factor profile may fluctuate over time, and (5) even with the modern intensive diabetes therapy regimens, long-term near-normoglycemia is difficult to achieve in some patients. These problems may in part account for the conflicting findings in the earlier reports, with some showing improvement of peripheral nerve function [123–125], while others have failed to demonstrate any changes [126,127].

Rapidly Reversible Nerve Dysfunction After Correction of Metabolic Derangement

Untreated, newly diagnosed type 1 diabetic patients show slight reduction in motor nerve conduction velocity (NCV), which has been shown to improve significantly as soon as one week following the elimination of ketosis and hyperglycemia by insulin treatment [116–118]. Similarly, other findings of neural dysfunction, such as increased resistance to ischemia in the diabetic nerve [118] or impaired retinal neurophysiologic function [119] were rapidly reversible within one to three weeks of improved glycemic control after the diagnosis of type 1 diabetes. In hyperglycemic patients with various durations of diabetes, who were treated with an artificial endocrine pancreas, H-reflex conduction velocity or motor and sensory conduction increased significantly during two or three days of normoglycemia [120,121]. Metabolic derangement resulting in diabetic ketoacidosis is often associated with nerve conduction slowing which has been shown to be reversible following insulin treatment for three months or less [122].

The aforementioned studies suggest that the acutely reversible changes in nerve function observed after improvement in glycemic control are attributable to functional rather than structural alterations in the diabetic nerve during episodes of metabolic derangement. Experimental studies have shown a marked reduction of the compound nerve action potential in isolated dorsal rat spinal roots incubated in 25-mM extracellular glucose and transiently exposed to hypoxia. This electrophysiologic alteration appeared to be caused by acidosis, because it was prevented when bicarbonate-containing solutions were used [128].

Although the rapidly reversible abnormalities in nerve function are related to restoring near-normoglycemia, acute painful neuropathy associated with the initiation of tight glycemic control has been reported in some patients [129]. Caravati [130] first described this rare phenomenon, which he called "insulin neuritis," in 1933 (see Chapter 5, pages 306–309). This effect has been observed in poorly controlled patients with markedly raised HbA_1 levels and occurred within several weeks of lowering of blood glucose by intensive insulin treatment but without evidence for frequent hypoglycemic episodes. Continuation of insulin treatment and maintenance of good glycemic control leads to a recovery from the painful symptoms after periods of up to six months. Sural nerve biopsy in one case during the acute phase revealed predominant small-fiber loss and regenerating axon sprouts [129].

Role of Intensive Diabetes Therapy in Treatment and Prevention of Diabetic Neuropathy

Earlier Small Trials in Type 1 Diabetic Patients

Earlier uncontrolled short-term studies including relatively small numbers of patients with diabetic neuropathy have reported that neuropathic symptoms or abnormal nerve function tests seen during hyperglycemic conditions may be more or less ameliorated following improvement of glycemic control [131–134]. Previous randomized controlled studies have assessed the influence of improved glycemic control on peripheral nerve function for periods of up to two years. However, several shortcomings are apparent in these studies: (1) two studies have used retinopathy as the primary selection criterion for entry and provided no information as to the prevalence and severity of clinical neuropathy [123,127], (2) only one study used reliable and clinically meaningful criteria for the diagnosis of neuropathy [126], (3) three studies did not measure nerve conduction [123,125,127], which is thought to be the most objective, sensitive, and reliable test in the evaluation of diabetic neuropathy [135], and (4) intensified insulin treatment did not lower the elevated HbA_1 values to the normal range. In addition, in most of these studies the differences in mean HbA_1 between the conventionally and intensively treated patients were relatively rather small to result in meaningful differences in peripheral nerve function. According to Dyck and O'Brien [136], the following degrees of changes in motor and sensory NCV that are associated with a change in the Neuropathy Impairment Score (NIS) of two points can be regarded as meaningful in controlled clinical trials: median motor NCV: 2.5 m/s, ulnar motor NCV: 4.6 m/s, peroneal motor NCV: 2.2 m/s, median sensory NCV: 1.9 m/s, and sural sensory NCV: 5.6 m/s. A change in NIS of two points corresponds to, e. g., bilateral change in dorsiflexor muscle strength of 25%, or change in ankle reflexes, or pin-prick perception from normal to decreased and vice versa.

Ziegler et al. [137] conducted a prospective study in 55 initially poorly controlled type 1 diabetic patients who were treated with continuous subcutaneous insulin infusion (CSII) or intensive conventional therapy (ICT) for four years. Patients were divided into three groups according to their mean HbA_1 levels during the study. Group 1 ($n = 19$) had mean HbA_1 during months 3–48 in the normal range of less than 7.8% (near-normoglycemic control), group 2 ($n = 18$) showed moderately elevated mean HbA_1 between 7.8% and 8.5% (satisfactory control), and group 3 ($n = 18$) had clearly elevated mean HbA_1 of 8.6% or above (poor control). In the three groups studied, the changes in median and peroneal motor NCV over baseline as well as median and ulnar sensory NCV after four years were inversely related to the mean HbA_1 levels of months 3–48

($P<0.05$). No significant associations with mean HbA_1 were noted for ulnar motor NCV, sural sensory NCV, and heart rate variability (HRV) as an index of autonomic dysfunction. Thus, near-normoglycemia maintained for four years in type 1 diabetic patients was associated with an increase in NCV in the upper limbs but not sensory NCV in the lower limbs and HRV. These results indicate that the susceptibility of different nerve fiber populations to long-term improvement in blood glucose control may be variable.

Long-Term Trials in Type 1 Diabetic Patients

Three pivotal long-term prospective studies that included type 1 diabetic patients either with mild retinopathy or without evidence of diabetic complications have been published (Table 4.**1**). The results of the Stockholm Diabetes Intervention Study (SDIS) over 10 years [138], the Oslo Study over eight years [139], and the DCCT over five years [140] demonstrate that long-term near-normoglycemia retards the deterioration in motor and sensory NCV. In the DCCT, intensive insulin therapy reduced the appearance of nerve conduction deficits after five years by approximately 50%. The risk for the development of clinical neuropathy was reduced by 64% within five years (5% vs 13% for the intensive therapy [IT] vs the conventional therapy [CT] group) [109]. Most attributes of nerve conduction remained stable or showed modest improvement in patients on IT, whereas they generally deteriorated in those on CT. Among patients in the primary prevention cohort (for retinopathy) without neuropathy at baseline, the IT group had significantly higher NCVs at five years compared with the CT group, the most prominent difference being noted for the peroneal motor NCV, which was 4.1 m/s faster [140]. A comparable effect was observed in the subgroup of patients with possible or definite neuropathy at baseline and in the secondary intervention cohort. Thus, the magnitude of treatment effect was relatively independent of the presence or absence of clinical neuropathy at baseline. Abnormal R-R interval variation at deep breathing as a measure of cardiovascular autonomic neuropathy (CAN) was significantly more frequent in the CT group than the IT group (14.8% vs 7.6%) in the secondary intervention cohort at 5–6 years [141]. The corresponding percentages for any abnormality among R-R interval variation, Valsalva ratio, and postural testing in the secondary intervention cohort at 5–6 years were 16.2% and 8.2%, respectively. These differences were considerably smaller and did not reach statistical significance in the primary prevention cohort. Overall, less than 3% of the DCCT subjects reported symptoms consistent with autonomic dysfunction. Thus, intensive therapy can slow the progression and development of autonomic dysfunction in type 1 diabetic patients with retinopathy.

The Epidemiology of Diabetes Interventions and Complications (EDIC) study, a long-term observational continuation of the DCCT in which the CT patients were offered IT, showed that the reduction in the risk of progressive retinopathy and nephropathy resulting from IT persists for four years, despite a narrowing in the difference in mean HbA_{1c} between the groups, which decreased from 9.1% to 8.2% in the original CT group and increased from 7.2.% to 7.9% in the IT group [142]. However, no data were reported for neuropathy.

Table 4.**1** Effects of randomized clinical trials of intensive diabetes therapy in prevention and treatment of diabetic somatosensory and cardiovascular autonomic neuropathy

Trial	*n*	Duration (years)	HbA_{1c} [%] CT vs IT	Neuropathy outcome			
				Clinical	NCV	VPT	HRV
Type 1 diabetes							
DCCT [140]	1441	up to 9	9.1 vs 7.2	+	+	n. a.	+
SDIS [138]	91	10	8.3 vs 7.2	+	+	n. a.	n. a.
Oslo study [139]	45	8	n. a.	n. a.	+	n. a.	n. a.
Type 2 diabetes							
UKPDS [110]	3867	up to 15	7.9 vs 7.0	–	n. a.	+ [a]	–
Kumamoto study [143]	110	6	9.4 vs 7.1	n. a.	+ [b]	+ [c]	–
Steno Type 2 study [145]	160	3.8	9.0 vs 7.6	n. a.	n. a.	–	+ [d]
VA CSDM [146]	153	2	9.5 vs 7.4	–	n. a.	–	–

n. a., not available; +, benefit; –, no effect; CT, conventional treatment; IT, intensive treatment; NCV, nerve conduction velocity; VPT, vibration perception threshold; HRV, heart rate variability

[a] Only 217 patients available after 15 years, out of 3836 at baseline
[b] NCV available only for the upper, not the lower limbs
[c] Significant difference between CT and IT for VPT on the hand but not the foot
[d] Effects of ACE inhibitors, antioxidants, and statins not discernible from those of glycemic control

Table 4.2 Randomized clinical trials of intensive diabetes therapy: adverse effects

Trial	*n*	Weight gain IT vs CT	Severe hypoglycemia CT vs IT
Type 1 diabetes			
DCCT [140]	1441	4.6 kg/5 years	19 vs 62/100 pat-yr*
SDIS [138]	91	n. a.	0.47 vs 1.06/pat/yr*
Oslo study [139]	45	n. a.	n. a.
Type 2 diabetes			
UKPDS [110]	3867	2.9 kg/10 years	0.7 vs 1.0–1.8/pat/yr*+
Kumamoto study [143]	110	1.1 BMI/6 years	0
Steno Type 2 study [145]	160	0.9 BMI/3.8 years	3 vs 2 patients
VA CSDM [146]	153	n. a.	n. a.

n. a., not available; pat-yr, patient-years; *$P < 0.05$ for CT vs IT; + diet vs sulfonylurea/insulin

In the Oslo Study, a difference in HbA_1 of 1% was associated with changes in peroneal motor NCV of 1.2 m/s, in tibial motor NCV of 1.3 m/s, and in sural sensory NCV of 1.4 m/s during the eight-year follow-up period [139]. In the SDIS the mean differences in NCV between the IT and CT groups after 10 years were 5.1 m/s for the peroneal nerve, 6.0 m/s for the tibial nerve, and 8.9 m/s for the sural nerve. Pin-prick sensitivity deteriorated significantly in the CT vs the IT groups, and the rates of neuropathic symptoms were 14% vs 32% after 10 years for IT vs CT, respectively [138]. However, these studies do not provide information about the reversibility of established nerve conduction deficits. Fur-thermore, in the Oslo Study the original randomization to the three treatment groups was abolished, and the patients were retrospectively allocated to new groups according to their mean HbA_1 over eight years. A certain degree of deterioration and development of deficits in NCV was also observed in the well-controlled groups, suggesting that, using the current methods of intensive insulin therapy, complete prevention of neuropathy is difficult to achieve. Moreover, in the DCCT, intensive therapy was associated with a three-fold increased risk of severe hypoglycemia and mean weight gain of 4.6 kg within five years. In the SDIS, a two-fold increased risk of severe hypoglycemia was observed for intensive therapy (Table 4.**2**).

Long-term Trials In Type 2 Diabetic Patients

The UKPDS showed a lower rate of impaired vibration perception threshold (VPT>25 V) after 15 years for IT with a sulfonylurea or insulin vs CT with diet (31% vs 52%). However, only 217 patients were available for assessment of VPT after 15 years, out of 3836 available at baseline. Thus, a bias due to the small sample size may have influenced this result. Moreover, the only additional time point at which VPT reached a significant difference between IT and CT was the nine-year follow-up, whereas the results after three, six, and 12 years did not differ between the groups. Likewise, the rates of absent knee and ankle reflexes as well as the heart rate responses to deep breathing did not differ between the groups. IT was associated with an increased risk of weight gain and hypoglycemia [110] (Table 4.**2**).

In the Kumamoto Study of insulin-treated type 2 diabetic patients, after six years NCV in the median motor and sensory nerves was significantly slower in patients given conventional insulin injection therapy (CT) compared with those given multiple insulin injections (IT), but unfortunately NCV was not measured in the lower limbs, where it would be more likely to reflect an effect on polyneuropathy. This is particularly important in view of the fact that VPT in the upper but not the lower limbs was significantly improved in IT as compared with CT. Similar to the findings of the UKPDS, HRV at rest and during deep breathing and posture-related change in blood pressure did not differ between the groups after six years [143]. The 10-year follow-up of the Kumamoto Study showed a relative risk reduction in the progression of clinical neuropathy by 64% in the IT group compared to the CT group. Moreover, IT prolonged the period in which patients were free of clinical neuropathy by 2.2 years, and was more cost-effective, mainly because of reduced costs for management of diabetic complications [144].

In the Steno type 2 Study, intensified multifactorial intervention including the use of intensive diabetes treatment, ACE inhibitors, antioxidants, statins, aspirin, and smoking cessation in patients with microalbuminuria had no effect on the progression of polyneuropathy after 3.8 years. By contrast, a positive effect of this approach was seen on HRV. It cannot be deduced from this study that this effect was due to improved glycemic control, because any of the other interventions, particularly the administration of ACE inhibitors and antioxidants, or even smoking cessation, may have been responsible for this result [145].

In the Veterans Administration Cooperative Study on type 2 diabetes mellitus (VA CSDM), no significant effect of IT (four-step plan of multiple insulin injections) compared to CT (one morning insulin injection per day) on peripheral neuropathy, abnormal Valsalva ratio and/or R-R interval variation, or erectile dysfunction could be demonstrated after two years, despite a difference in HbA_{1c} between the groups comparable with those in the above studies [146].

In conclusion, these trials have shown heterogeneous effects of intensive diabetes therapy on the progression of distal symmetric polyneuropathy and autonomic neuropathy. It cannot be concluded unequivocally from these results that improved glycemic control prevents the development or retards the progression of polyneuropathy in type 2 diabetic patients treated for periods of 2–15 years. In the UKPDS intensive therapy was associated with an increased risk of weight gain and mild or severe hypoglycemia.

Pancreas Transplantation in Type 1 Diabetic Patients

Pancreas transplantation is the most effective method of achieving long-term normoglycemia in type 1 diabetic patients, but is usually limited to patients with end-stage diabetic nephropathy in combination with a renal graft. Other indications have been questioned [147]. Several long-term studies in patients with established diabetic polyneuropathy who underwent successful pancreatic transplantation have been published (Table 4.**3**). Kennedy et al. [148] have shown that 42 months after transplantation the neuropathy was only slightly improved, but a significant difference was seen in the mean motor and sensory nerve conduction in the transplanted group compared with a control group who did not have a functioning graft after 42 months. Improvement was more pronounced when only mild dysfunction was present initially.

Solders et al. [149] have demonstrated beneficial effects of combined pancreatic and renal transplantation on NCV after four years of normoglycemia. The initial improvement in motor NCV observed in these patients was also noted in diabetic patients receiving a renal transplant only, and was most likely due to the elimination of uremia. However, further improvement was seen only in the euglycemic pancreas graft recipients. Müller-Felber et al. [150] have shown modest improvement in neuropathic symptoms and increase in motor but not sensory NCV after three years in patients who underwent successful pancreas and kidney transplantation as compared to those with early pancreas rejection and functioning kidney graft. None of the beneficial effects described in these three studies were demonstrable after two years, and none of these studies could demonstrate an effect on HRV as an index of cardiovascular autonomic dysfunction, while the effects on clinical measures were variable (Table 4.**3**). These findings are confirmed in the more recent studies shown in the last three columns of Table 4.**3** [151–153]. Thus, periods of normoglycemia of more than two years following pancreas transplantation retard the further progression of deficits in motor and sensory NCV, but no such clear effect is noted for neuropathic symptoms and deficits, while no beneficial effect is seen on cardiovascular autonomic dysfunction. The reasons for this divergent effect are not known but may be due to a different susceptibility of the autonomic nerves to metabolic changes or to methodological factors.

Table 4.**3** Effects of pancreatic transplantation on diabetic neuropathy

	Kennedy et al. [148]	**Solders et al. [149]**	**Müller-Felber et al. [150]**	**Navarro et al. [151]**	**Allen et al. [152]**	**Martinenghi et al. [153]**
Study design	PTx vs awaiting/ failure PTx	PTx + KTx vs KTx	PTx + KTx vs rejection+ KTx	PTx vs awaiting/ failure PTx	PTx + KTx vs KTx+PTx failure	PTx + KTx vs PTx failure+ KTx
Number	11 vs 12	13 vs 15	27 vs 14	115 vs 92	44 vs 9	5
Follow-up (years)	3.5	4	3	10	0.5–8	2 + 2 sequential
Mean HbA_{1c} (%)	7.5 vs 10	5.2 vs 9.7	6.9 vs 8.5	n. a.	n. a.	6.6 vs 8.0
MNCV index	Improvement	Improvement	Improvement	Improvement	Improvement	Improvement
SNCV index	Improvement	No effect	No effect	Improvement	Improvement	Improvement
Clinical measures	NDS: −14→ −11 vs −16→ −27 (NS)	Not reported	NSS: 1.7→0.6* vs 1.6→1.6	Improvement	No effect	n. a.
Autonomic function	No effect	No effect	No effect	No effect	n. a.	n. a.

PTx, pancreas transplantation; KTx, kidney transplantation; NDS, Neuropathy Disability Score; MNCV, motor nerve conduction velocity; SNCV, sensory nerve conduction velocity; NS, not significant
* $P < 0.05$ vs baseline

Is There a Glycemic Threshold for the Risk of Diabetic Complications?

Two retrospective studies suggested the existence of a glycemic threshold at a HbA_{1c} level of approximately 8% for microalbuminuria and retinopathy, below which there is no further reduction in risk [154,155]. This would imply that improving glycemic control below this level is unnecessary, thereby potentially reducing the risk of hypoglycemia in some type 1 diabetic patients [156]. In contrast, the DCCT could not identify such a HbA_{1c} threshold. The risks of retinopathy progression and of developing microalbuminuria and neuropathy were found to be continuous but nonlinear over the entire range of HbA_{1c} values. As HbA_{1c} was reduced below 8% there were continuing relative reductions in the risk of diabetic complications, whereas the rate of increase in the risk of hypoglycemia was slower [157,158]. Likewise, in the Pittsburgh Epidemiology of Diabetes Complications Study no definitive threshold was found after six years for any complication in type 1 diabetic subjects [159].

Conclusions

1. The large randomized long-term clinical trials such as the DCCT and UKPDS were not designed to evaluate the effects of intensive diabetes therapy on diabetic polyneuropathy, but rather to study the influence of such treatment on the development and progression of the chronic diabetic complications. Thus, only a minority of the patients enrolled in these studies had symptomatic polyneuropathy at entry. In type 1 diabetic patients these studies show that intensive diabetes therapy retards but does not completely prevent the development of polyneuropathy and autonomic neuropathy. In contrast, in type 2 diabetic patients, who represent the vast majority of people with diabetes, the results were variable. Intensive diabetes therapy either had no effect or only partially slowed the progression of polyneuropathy, and the effect on autonomic neuropathy was largely lacking. Moreover, improved glycemic control was achieved at the expense of increased risk of hypoglycemia and weight gain.
2. Only a few small studies have evaluated the effects of intensive diabetes therapy on established polyneuropathy in type 1 diabetic patients. They indicate that improved glycemic control may improve some aspects of diabetic neuropathy, but imperfect study designs and methodology hamper the validity of most of these small trials. At more advanced stages improvement is still possible for some measures of nerve function such as motor NCV, but is less likely for autonomic dysfunction. This may be due to the fact that true normoglycemia could not be achieved in many patients. No large, randomized, controlled trial has been performed specifically to show favorable effects of intensive diabetes therapy on diabetic polyneuropathy.
3. In type 1 diabetic patients with the most advanced stages of peripheral neuropathy, progression of nerve conduction deficits is halted after three to four years of normoglycemia following pancreas transplantation, but no effect is seen in autonomic neuropathy. However, successful pancreas transplantation results in long-term normoglycemia. Hence, the effect on nerve function that can be achieved with this method cannot be extrapolated to the widely used current methods of intensive diabetes therapy, since for various reasons the majority of diabetic patients in whom these methods are used do not achieve sustained normoglycemia.
4. Although observational studies suggested a glycemic threshold for the development and progression of long-term complications in type 1 diabetes, the DCCT data do not support such an assumption. Thus, attempts to achieve optimal glycemic control should not aim at a particular HbA_{1c} threshold within the diabetic range, but should follow "the goal of achieving normal glycemia as early as possible in as many IDDM patients as is safely possible" [158].

Metabolic Alterations in Experimental Models

A.A.F. Sima and C.R. Pierson

Introduction

Glycemic control is the treatment goal of managing diabetic patients. The Diabetes Control and Complications Trial (DCCT) demonstrated that intensive insulin treatment to control serum glucose reduces the onset of clinical neuropathy at five years by 57% [109]. Epidemiologic data show that only 50% of diabetic subjects experience clinical manifestations of diabetic neuropathy [160], suggesting that other metabolic and genetic factors may be at play. However, hyperglycemia is probably the most important initiator of diabetic neuropathy, by activating the polyol pathway, affecting nonenzymatic glycation, nerve blood flow, and leading to the generation of reactive oxygen species (ROS). All of these metabolic factors contribute to the development of diabetic neuropathy and will be dealt with in more detail elsewhere in this volume. The fact that, despite intensive insulin therapy and near-normal glycemic control, diabetic neuropathy still occurred in the DCCT cohort suggests that additional factors may be of pathogenic significance in diabetic neuropathy. Such factors include insulin and/or C-peptide deficiencies in type 1 diabetes and hyperinsulinemia in type 2 diabetes and genetic susceptibility [161,162]. Support for a role of insulin and/or C-peptide deficiencies stems from the differences in severity of the neuropathy encountered in type 1 and type 2 diabetes. Studies have demonstrated that in human diabetic neuropathy, type 1 diabetes is a prominent risk factor for the severity of diabetic neuropathy [163]. More severe structural and functional alterations are evident in animal models of type 1 neuropathy than in type 2 neuropathy despite comparable levels of hyperglycemia [164–167]. Insulin and C-peptide deficiencies characterize type 1 diabetes, whereas these hormones are unchanged or increased in type 2 diabetes. Therefore, do insulin and C-peptide possess neuroprotective effects, and could their deficiencies in type 1 diabetes account for its association with more severe diabetic neuropathy than that of type 2 diabetes? In this section we will explore the role of both hyperglycemia and hypoglycemia, and the potential contribution of insulin and C-peptide deficiencies to the development of diabetic neuropathy.

How the metabolic alterations of diabetes contribute to the pathogenesis of neuropathy has been the subject of extensive research during the last 20–30 years. Available data indicate that the metabolic causes of diabetic neuropathy are multifactorial, interrelated, and mutually perpetuating, and have until recently been ascribed solely to hyperglycemia [168]. The metabolic alterations involved include the activation of the polyol pathway, nonenzymatic glycation, impaired nerve blood flow, and generation of ROS. Each of these mechanisms appears to be most prominent during a certain phase of diabetic neuropathy, but they are interrelated and mutually perpetuating (Fig. 4.**12**). The accumulation of sorbitol from increased polyol pathway flux is an early event in experimental [169] and human diabetic neuropathy [170] and increased sorbitol content is not evident in chronically diabetic human nerve [171]. Studies in BB/W rats show that sorbitol accumulation, *myo*-inositol depletion, and impaired Na^+,K^+-ATPase activity wane as the neuropathy progresses and additional metabolic pathways become more prominent [169]. By contrast, the reduction in the expression of neurotrophic factors [172] develops later in the course of the disease.

The Polyol Pathway and the Na^+, K^+-ATPase Defect

Hyperglycemia enhances flux through the polyol pathway resulting in glucose being converted by the high-Km enzyme aldose reductase into sorbitol and to fructose by sorbitol dehydrogenase [173]. Immunohistochemical studies have localized polyol pathway enzymes to a variety of sites including the nodes of Ranvier of myelinated fibers and the endoneurial vasculature [174,175]. Sorbitol is an organic osmolyte and its accumulation leads to a compensatory

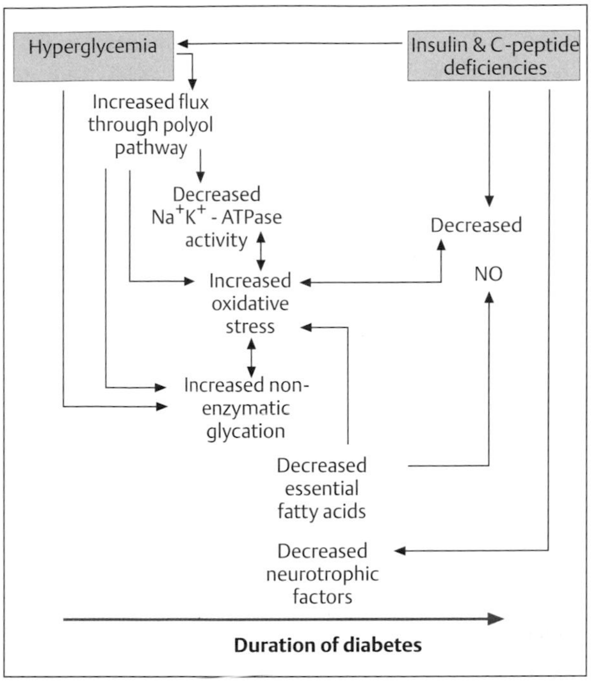

Fig. 4.**12** Metabolic alterations caused by hyperglycemia and/or insulin and C-peptide deficiencies. The individual metabolic abnormalities occur sequentially and are often mutually perpetuating

depletion of other osmolytes such as *myo*-inositol and taurine [176]. As an example of the intricacy of these metabolic alterations, taurine is also an antioxidant and promoter of nerve regeneration, and hence contributes to these pathogenic processes [177,178]. The loss of *myo*-inositol leads to alterations in phosphoinositide metabolism, with decreased availability of diacylglycerol [173], which contributes to the reduction in neural Na^+,K^+-ATPase activity. Perturbed Na^+,K^+-ATPase activity leads to intra-axonal Na^+ accumulation and decreased nodal Na^+ equilibrium potential, resulting in the early reversible nerve conduction velocity (NCV) defect [179–181]. These relationships account for the beneficial effects of aldose reductase inhibition and *myo*-inositol supplementation on Na^+,K^+-ATPase activity and NCV in experimental models of acute diabetes [179].

Na^+,K^+-ATPase activity can be modulated by means other than the polyol pathway, such as impaired nitric oxide synthesis [173], pseudohypoxia [182], and prostacyclin deficiency [183]. The normalizing effect on neural Na^+,K^+-ATPase activity can be achieved by prostacyclin analogues [184], acetyl-L-carnitine [185], and C-peptide [164,167]. The Na^+,K^+-ATPase deficit is therefore linked to multiple metabolic alterations, not just those resulting from altered flux through the polyol pathway. Acetyl-L-carnitine, which has no effect on the polyol pathway, has been shown to correct nerve Na^+,K^+-ATPase activity [169,186], blood flow [187, 188], levels of vasoactive prostaglandins, and NCV

[169]. C-peptide also normalizes Na^+,K^+-ATPase activity believed to occur via a Ca^{2+}-mediated pathway [164,189]. Taken together, these data indicate that the alterations in Na^+,K^+-ATPase activity are the result of several metabolic alterations.

The activation of the polyol pathway by hyperglycemia leads to increased oxidative stress, and aldose reductase inhibitor (ARI) treatment has been shown to decrease oxidative stress in the sciatic nerve of diabetic rats [190]. NADPH is used as a cofactor not only for aldose reductase, but also for the glutathione cycle and nitric oxide synthase (NOS). Therefore, activation of the polyol pathway due to hyperglycemia depletes NADPH, limiting the amount of NADPH available for the recycling of reduced glutathione (GSH) from its oxidized form, GSSG, and nitric oxide synthesis. In the second step of the polyol pathway, sorbitol is oxidized to fructose, which increases the $NADH/NAD^+$ and the lactate/pyruvate ratio. This state has been termed "pseudohypoxia" by Williamson et al. [182] and was improved by sorbitol dehydrogenase inhibition [191]. However, Cameron et al. [192] and Schmidt et al. [193] were unable to reproduce these results.

The relative lack of structural changes in the peripheral nerve such as demyelination or fiber degeneration, coincident with the acute slowing of NCV, suggests underlying biochemical mechanisms [194]. The association between acute metabolic alterations, slowing of NCV, and decreased Na^+,K^+-ATPase activity is confirmed by direct measurements of Na^+,K^+-ATPase activity accompanied by decreased NCV. Structurally, the diminished Na^+,K^+-ATPase activity manifests as early paranodal swellings due to intra-axonal accumulation of Na^+ [181,194]. These changes are correctable by insulin treatment [181], *myo*-inositol supplementation [179,180], ARI treatment [180], acetyl-L-carnitine administration [169], and C-peptide treatment [164,167].

Experimental models of type 1 diabetic neuropathy demonstrate that increased flux through the polyol pathway is a critical component in the early pathogenesis of diabetic neuropathy. Activation of the polyol pathway also impacts secondarily by promoting generation of ROS and nonenzymatic glycation and perturbing nitric oxide synthesis and blood flow [173]. Despite the prominence of the early polyol pathway activation in human and rat diabetic neuropathy, it may not be an absolute requirement for the development of diabetic neuropathy. Diabetic mice, which show no or low polyol pathway activity, still exhibit functional and structural diabetic neuropathy similar to that seen in rat models [195,196].

Role of Nonenzymatic Glycation

Nonenzymatic glycation is enhanced in the peripheral nerve in both experimental animal models and human diabetic subjects [197,198]. In this process, reducing monosaccharides combine with free amino groups on proteins or other cellular molecules forming early reversible products, known as Schiff bases or ketamines or Amadori adducts. In the Wolff pathway, glycoxidative products form and contribute to cellular oxidative stress [199]. Advanced glycation end products (AGE) form through critical intermediates such as 3-deoxyglucosone (3DG) from fructose-lysine and glyoxal, and methylglyoxal (MGO), from Amadori compounds, Schiff bases, or by the direct oxidation of monosaccharides [200–202]. Subsequent chemical rearrangements, dehydration, fragmentation, and cross-linking occur, forming irreversible AGEs.

A number of compounds participate in the glycation process, including glucose, glucose-6-phosphate, galactose, pentose phosphate pathway compounds, various trioses, and fructose generated via the polyol pathway [203]. Fructose is a potent glycator and its activity far exceeds that of glucose [203]. Fructose can be metabolized to fructose-6-phosphate and triose phosphate and these intermediates are sources of 3DG and MGO, both of which induce oxidative stress via cross-link formation [204]. Interestingly, the activity of sorbitol dehydrogenase decreases following its glycation [205]. Hence accumulation of fructose from the increased polyol pathway flux may contribute to inhibition of sorbitol dehydrogenase, providing a negative feedback mechanism [168]. Aldose reductase inhibition in humans and experimental animals results in a reduction of glycated protein content in various tissues; however, the levels in peripheral nerve have not been ascertained [206].

AGEs accumulate in specific tissue constituents of peripheral nerve including certain myelin components such as P_0, myelin basic protein, and proteolipid protein [197,207]. This raises the possibility that AGE-modified myelin proteins may contribute to segmental demyelination in diabetes via their recognition by AGE-specific receptors on macrophages, resulting in myelin breakdown and phagocytosis [198]. The receptor for AGE (RAGE) has been characterized and is considered a member of the immunoglobulin superfamily of cell adhesion molecules, with considerable homology to the neural cell adhesion molecule (NCAM) [208,209]. The RAGE-ligand interaction generates intracellular oxidative stress and activates NF-κB, a redox sensitive transcription factor [210,211].

Axonal cytoskeletal proteins such as tubulin, neurofilament, and actin are glycated, resulting in abnormalities in axonal structure, slow transport, atrophy, and degeneration [198,212]. It is suggested that glycation of these cytoskeletal components hampers their polymerization and phosphorylation and, ultimately, their exportation from the perikaryon. Glycation of extracellular matrix proteins may compromise nerve regeneration ability in diabetic neuropathy. Glycation of laminin, a molecule that serves as guidance for the axonal growth cone, may impact upon both initiation and sustaining of nerve regeneration [213].

AGEs are capable of generating cellular oxidative stress. Two compounds, N^{ε}-[carboxymethyl]-lysine (CML) and pentosidine, result from glycation and oxidation reactions and are considered markers of glycative and oxidative stress [214]. CML immmunolocalizes to perineural basal laminae, axons, Schwann cells, and endoneurial microvessels in human nerve. The immunoreactivity increases significantly with diabetes and correlates with fiber loss [215]. Glycation may perpetuate oxidative stress by inactivation of protective enzymes such as Cu-Zn-superoxide dismutase [216]. AGEs binding to RAGE on macrophages generate oxidative stress as GSH and vitamin C depletion results, which is accompanied by nuclear factor-κB (NF-κB) induction [217]. Treatment with α-lipoic acid, an antioxidant, prevents the induction of NF-κB in this scenario [217].

Aminoguanidine inhibits the formation of AGE by preventing cross-linking, and has a beneficial effect on neuropathy, nephropathy, and retinopathy in diabetic rats. In peripheral nerve aminoguanidine improves NCV and morphometric parameters after long-term treatment, as its beneficial effects become apparent only after a lag period. Nerve blood flow improves in diabetic animals after aminoguanidine treatment; however, no effect on free radical activity could be detected [218,219]. When administered short-term, aminoguanidine improves NCV and the Na^+,K^+-ATPase defect; however, long-term administration is required before structural improvements of the endoneurial vasculature are evident [220,221].

Role of Oxidative Stress and Alterations in Blood Flow

Diabetes is a state of increased oxidative stress characterized by both an increased production of ROS and impaired ability to scavenge ROS; however, the precise mechanisms responsible for these phenomena are not completely understood and are probably multifactorial [214,222,223]. Superoxide, hydrogen peroxide, and hydroxyl radicals are toxic products derived from the chemical reduction of molecular oxygen via the Haber-Weiss reaction [224]. ROS promote the autoxidation of cellular molecules such as glucose, thiols, and catecholamines, and the rate of this reaction can be accelerated by transition metals such as copper and iron [224]. Polyunsaturated fatty acids are especially vulnerable to peroxidation by ROS, and this reaction can initiate an autocatalytic chain reaction which peroxidizes other fatty acids [225]. Other targets of ROS peroxidation include proteins and DNA.

Cells are not defenseless against ROS; superoxide dismutase scavenges superoxide in both cytoplasm and mitochondria. Glutathione peroxidase destroys lipid hydroperoxides and hydrogen peroxide. Most of the scavenging mechanisms are not due to enzymatic activity but rather to a variety of compounds that interact with ROS. These compounds can be placed into two groups based upon their chemistry, those that are hydrophobic, such as vitamin E (α-tocopherol), ubiquinone, and carotenoids, and can inactivate hydrophobic ROS, and those that are hydrophilic and capable of inactivating hydrophilic ROS, such as ascorbic acid and cystine [225].

The vascular system bears a considerable burden from the pro-oxidant activity in the diabetic state. Oxidative stress underlies the propensity to develop microvascular complications and atherosclerosis. The microvascular complications are pertinent to the development of neuropathy in diabetes and include alterations in the function of endothelial cells and vascular reactivity, which in turn leads to impaired endoneural blood flow and oxygenation.

Endothelial cell function and gene expression are altered by the pro-oxidant state. The resulting altered gene expression favors endothelial-mediated vasoconstriction, which compromises nerve blood flow. Serum levels of angiotensin-converting enzyme are increased in both diabetic human and rat models [22], and the renin-angiotensin system is up-regulated in the vasa nervorum [227]. The increase in serum angiotensin-converting enzyme is prevented by administration of the antioxidant probucol in experimental models [185]. Oxidative stress leads to an increase in the expression of endothelin-1 (ET-1), a potent vasoconstrictor. NF-κB probably serves as the mediator of ET-1 transcription as NF-κB consensus binding sites are present in the ET-1 promoter [228]. BQ123 and BM5 182874 are ET_A receptor antagonists, and when administered to experimental animal models they restore blood flow and NCV [229]. Basentan is an ET_A/ET_B antagonist, and when it is used to treat diabetic rats a smaller effect on nerve blood flow and NCV is observed [230]. This is probably due to the fact that ET_B stimulation produces nitric oxide (NO) and prostacyclin, and the activity of these vasodilators probably counters the vasoconstrictive activity of ET_A stimulation [229]. Superoxide dismutase generates peroxynitrite from NO, which is toxic to endothelial cells, and further illustrates the need for a proper balance between antioxidative factors and oxidative stress [231]. Increased leukocyte adhesion to endothelial cells also results from NF-κB activity, and this may explain a component of the increased propensity to thrombus formation in diabetics [232]. Antioxidant therapy with α-tocopherol and probucol prevents leukocyte adhesion [233].

Nonspecific and β-specific protein kinase C (PKC) inhibitors normalize NCV and sciatic nerve blood flow in the streptozotocin (STZ)-induced diabetic rat [234,235]. α-Lipoic acid is an antioxidant and has been shown to correct *myo*-inositol depletion, perhaps by augmenting Na^+,K^+-ATPase activity or increasing energy production by normalizing blood nerve blood flow [236]. Vasodilators such as niceritol and β-specific PKC inhibitors have comparable effects, which may be exerted by similar mechanisms [237].

Acute hyperglycemia alters endothelial-mediated vascular relaxation. In aortic rings incubated in high-glucose medium a reduction in acetylcholine-mediated endothelial relaxation is elicited, and this change can be prevented by probucol or superoxide dismutase administration [238, 239]. Acetylcysteine, another antioxidant, has also been shown to improve nerve blood flow and NCV [240]. Acetylcysteine and α-tocopherol mitigate axonal atrophy and enhance nerve fiber regeneration in experimental diabetic neuropathy, further supporting the role of oxidative stress [241,242].

Transition metals are probably important for the generation of oxidative stress in diabetic peripheral nerve. Transition metals catalyze the autoxidation of glucose, fructose, and other monosaccharides and AGEs to ROS. Diabetic rats treated with metal chelators show a correction of nerve blood flow and NCV [225].

Assessment of the expression and activity of nitric oxide synthase (NOS), which produces the critical vasodilator NO, in 12-month STZ-diabetic rat dorsal root ganglia (DRGs) revealed increased enzyme activity but no increase in NOS expression. In the same study, at two months of diabetes endothelial NOS (eNOS) immunoreactivity acquired a novel pattern, with perineural staining of sciatic nerve and capsular staining of DRGs, which was not evident in long-standing diabetes. Therefore, since increases in NO production were not associated with increases in NOS expression, it may be that enhanced efficiency of NOS enzymatic activity, rather than increased expression, accounts for the increase of NOS activity in diabetes [243]. One intriguing finding is that C-peptide mediates vasodilatation of muscle vascular beds by a mechanism that incorporates NO [244]. The potential pathogenic roles of NO and C-peptide in diabetic neuropathy remain unexplored.

Role of Essential Fatty Acids

Diabetes leads to alterations in the levels of essential fatty acids. The synthesis of prostanoids, which possess critical vasoactive properties, is markedly decreased in diabetes [225]. This can be attributed to impaired desaturation at the Δ-6 step in the synthetic pathway and additional deficits in ω-6 essential fatty acids. Hepatocyte desaturation activity is likely due to hyperglycemia, hypoinsulinemia, and oxidative stress [245]. Deficient Δ-6 desaturation reduces tissue and plasma levels of γ-linoleic acid and arachidonic acid, so a dearth of products normally generated by cyclo-oxygenase catalytic activity results. These products include prostaglandins with vasodilatory and antiplatelet effects [226], so increased vascular tone and diminished nerve blood flow follow. Treating diabetic rats with evening primrose oil replenishes PGI_2 and PGE_2 levels in sciatic nerve by increasing arachidonic acid levels [169] and restores blood flow, preventing nerve hypoxia and normalizing the NCV [246,247]. Vascularization of the endoneurium is augmented by extended treatment with evening primrose oil [248]. Cyclooxygenase inhibitors block this effect, showing the importance of prostaglandins in this process [225]. It seems from these studies that deficiency in fatty acid synthesis exerts its main effect on the endoneural vasculature. The resulting increase in blood flow arising from the correction of essential fatty acid levels is potentiated by subsequent prostanoid synthesis and NO release.

L-Carnitine levels are also reduced in experimental models of diabetes, and replenishment averts the development of diabetic neuropathy [169,249]. L-Carnitine has numerous physiologic effects, but how it specifically prevents diabetic neuropathy is unknown. L-Carnitine assists cellular energy metabolism by facilitating mitochondrial transport of long-chain fatty acids for β-oxidation. Other functions of L-carnitine include restoring Na^+,K^+-ATPase activity, improving NO synthesis, normalizing prostaglandin levels [169,186], and improving nerve blood flow [178], as well as having possible antioxidant properties [205].

The role of essential fatty acid metabolism and vasoactive prostanoids in the pathogenesis of diabetic neuropathy is important. However, deficits in essential fatty acid probably act together with other metabolic pathways such as the polyol pathway, nonenzymatic glycation, and possibly C-peptide deficiency to compromise vascular and nerve function.

Role of Neurotrophic Factors

Perturbations in the synthesis and function of a variety of neurotrophic factors have been implicated in the development of diabetic neuropathy [250]. Neurotrophins are synthesized by the target cells of particular axons and transported by retrograde transport to the neuronal soma, where they regulate the expression of a variety of proteins. The neurotrophin family includes nerve growth factor (NGF), which is the most widely studied member, but also neurotrophin-3 (NT-3), neurotrophin-4/5 (NT-4/5), and brain-derived neurotrophic factor (BDNF). It appears that each neurotrophic factor may be responsible for maintaining a particular population of neurons within the peripheral nervous system [251]. In the case of NGF, it is synthesized by muscle and skin, then retrogradely transported to DRGs and sympathetic neurons. After transport it can bind one of two receptors, the high-affinity trkA or the low-affinity p75 [251,252]. Diabetic rats experience decreased NGF levels as a result of decreased synthesis in axonal target tissues and decreased axonal transport [253,254]. Furthermore, the expression of both NGF receptors is down-regulated, reflected by decreased trkA levels in DRG and decreased levels of p75 in sciatic nerve [255]. Importantly, these changes do not take place acutely but occur slowly over weeks to months in diabetic rats [250,254].

NGF is responsible for maintaining the production of medium- and low-molecular-weight neurofilaments, and NGF treatment in axotomized DRG up-regulates the mRNA of these structural proteins [256,257]. Insulin has also been shown to up-regulate neurofilament synthesis [258]. The deficiencies in neurotrophic factors are likely to contribute to the characteristic axonal atrophy of diabetic neuropathy, since neurofilaments are the chief determinant of axonal size [259]. Substance P is another protein under the influence of NGF, which may explain the hyperalgesia and allodynia experienced by patients around the injection site of NGF [260,261].

During nerve fiber regeneration the connection of the nerve fiber to its target tissue is lost and NGF support is then provided by Schwann cells and fibroblasts at the site of injury. This response is probably mediated by *c-fos* and *c-jun* [250]. NGF elaborated from Schwann cells and fibroblasts is believed to induce interleukin-1 from macrophages that are recruited to the site of injury, and which in turn maintain sustained production of NGF by Schwann cells and fibroblasts [262]. The delayed initiation and the decrease in the sustaining of nerve fiber regeneration in diabetic neuropathy can be attributed to derangement in immediate gene responses, such as the IGF system and *c-fos* and the markedly decreased local levels of NGF and trkA mRNAs [250]. Other factors leading to inefficient or inadequate nerve fiber regeneration in diabetic neuropathy include decreased induction of growth-associated protein 43 [263]. Far fewer data are available as to the roles of other neurotrophins in diabetic neuropathy. NT-3 may be particularly useful in treating sensory symptoms, and one study showed improvement in sensory NCV in diabetic rats after four weeks of NT-3 treatment [250].

Circulating peptides such as insulin-like growth factor-1 (IGF-1), insulin and C-peptide have neuroprotective effects on peripheral nerve. The majority of IGF-1 is synthesized by hepatocytes, but IGF-1 is also elaborated by Schwann cells of peripheral nerve, where it has autocrine and paracrine functions. Both hepatic and peripheral nerve IGF-1 levels show gradual and progressive declines that can be profound by eight weeks of diabetes in experimental models [172]. In type 1 diabetes, insulin and C-peptide are markedly deficient, whereas in type 2 diabetes normal or even increased serum levels of these hormones occurs. This may explain, at least in part, the tendency for type 1 diabetic neuropathy to be more severe than the neuropathy associated with type 2 diabetes [163]. This concept will be further explored later in this chapter. IGF-1, insulin, and C-peptide all possess neurotrophic actions on sensory, autonomic, and motor neurons [167,264]. It has been suggested that IGF-1 synthesis may be compromised by insulin deficiency [264].

The IGF-1 receptor (IGF-1R) is expressed on neuronal somata, neurites, and Schwann cells of peripheral nerve, while the insulin receptor (IR) immunolocalizes to paranodal Schwann cells and paranodal axolemma [265]. A C-peptide receptor has not been conclusively identified, but specific binding of C-peptide to cell membranes has been demonstrated by fluorescence correlation spectroscopy [266]. Studies in our laboratory demonstrate that C-peptide possesses insulinomimetic effects and enhances IR phosphorylation and activity [267]. IGF-1 has been shown to enhance the synthesis of low- and medium-molecular-weight neurofilaments, and insulin assists in their phosphorylation, which is critical for their polymerization and exportation to the neurites [264]. Insulin, IGF-1, and NGF have been shown to stabilize α- and β-tubulin mRNAs in vivo [258,268]. IGF-1 also enhances the motility of neural growth cones by activating focal adhesion kinases and reorganizing actin [269]. ARI-treated type 1 diabetic rats show a six-fold up-regulation of IGF-1 mRNA, linking an early metabolic alteration in diabetic neuropathy to the change in neurotrophic factors, which is considered a late change [255].

Neuropathy Associated with Hyperinsulinemia and Hypoglycemia

Some authors suggest that frequent hypoglycemic episodes may play a role in the pathogenesis of diabetic neuropathy [270,271]. Insulinoma patients experience a distal axonopathy that affects both sensory and motor nerves [272]. In transgenic mice with insulinoma a predominantly motor axonopathy ensues [273], while STZ rats harboring an insulinoma develop severe axonal atrophy, degeneration, regeneration, and demyelination that involves both sensory and motor nerve fibers [274]. Severe hypoglycemia has also been associated with demyelination and anterior horn cell pathology [168,275]. Mohseni et al. examined hypo- and euglycemic type 1 BB/W rats and found mild changes in plantar skin innervation but structurally normal DRGs. In contrast, the ventral roots at L5 showed pathologic alterations, supporting the notion that hypoglycemic neuropathy tends to affect motor neurons [276]. Mohseni et al. also contend that hypoglycemia preferentially affects the nerve trunk, but this is controversial, and the proximal spread of the changes may be variable depending on the severity or duration of hypoglycemic events [277].

It is well documented that strict glycemic control with insulin can precipitate painful neuropathy in diabetic subjects. Painful idiopathic neuropathy is common in patients with impaired glucose tolerance. These observations are consistent with the finding of a small fiber neuropathy in long-term glucose-intolerant GK rats [277a]. In sural nerve biopsies from diabetics with acute painful neuropathy, fluorescein angiography demonstrated epineurial vessel proliferation, increased vascular permeability, and arteriovenous shunting-changes comparable to those of diabetic retinopathy [278]. Vascular endothelial growth factor (VEGF) expression is stimulated in the retina by insulin and is considered an important endothelial cell mitogen, angiogenic factor, and enhancer of vascular permeability. The role of VEGF in diabetic neuropathy has not been tested, but, in rats with insulinoma, insulin levels correlate directly with microvascular density of the endoneurium [279]. These findings tend to suggest a pathogenic role for hyperinsulinemia, particularly in type 2 diabetic neuropathy, which in many respects is distinct from that of type 1 [280,281].

Physiologic Role of Proinsulin C-Peptide

Historically, proinsulin C-peptide was thought to possess no biological function besides that of insulin biosynthesis. However, recent studies compromise the veracity of this claim. The technique of fluorescence correlation microscopy has demonstrated that C-peptide binds to cell membranes in a specific fashion and has an affinity binding constant of 3×10^9 M^{-1} [266]. This means that physiologic concentrations of C-peptide (0.9 nM) saturate the receptor. The nature of the C-peptide receptor remains to be elucidated, but the C-terminal pentapeptide segment of C-peptide appears to be essential for binding and may be the biologically active portion of the molecule [266]. Early reports regarding C-peptide activity showed that an increase in intracellular [Ca^{2+}] occurred followed by activation of Ca^{2+}-dependent protein phosphatase IIB, which activates Na^+,K^+-ATPase by dephosphorylation [282]. Renal tubular cell, sciatic nerve, and erythrocyte Na^+,K^+-ATPase might be activated in this manner. The rise in intracellular [Ca^{2+}] also activates eNOS [283]. Recent studies in our laboratory show that C-peptide has insulinomimetic effects including up-regulation of glycogen synthesis and amino acid uptake. In rat L6 myoblasts and human neuroblastoma cells (SH-SY5Y), physiologic levels of C-peptide autophosphorylates the insulin receptor, promoting tyrosine kinase activity, IRS-1 phosphorylation, PI3K activity, MAPK phosphorylation, GSK-3 phosphorylation, and p90Rsk activity [267]. Importantly, an additive effect results from physiologic C-peptide concentrations and submaximal insulin concentrations, but if C-peptide is added in the face of maximal insulin levels it blunts insulin activity [267].

Physiologic roles for C-peptide have been described in a number of tissues. In type 1 BB/W rats, sciatic nerve Na^+,K^+-ATPase activity was restored by C-peptide replacement [167], which in turn corrected the acute defect in NCV and paranodal swelling that occurs secondarily to a rise in intra-axonal [Na^+], the consequences of which will be discussed below (see p 104). Nitric oxide release from bovine aortic endothelial cells is augmented by C-peptide in a concentration-dependent manner [284]. This metabolic effect may underlie the increase in forearm blood flow by C-peptide treatment in type 1 patients and C-peptide-dependent dilation of rat skeletal muscle arterioles [244,285]. The functions of C-peptide are probably intertwined with those of other hormones. The effect of C-peptide on Na^+,K^+-ATPase activity is potentiated with subthreshold concentrations of neuropeptide Y [282]. Insulin-mediated glycogen synthesis and amino acid uptake are potentiated in vitro within a narrow concentration range by C-peptide (0.1–1.0 nM) [267].

Human data regarding the effect of C-peptide are limited, but some studies in type 1 diabetic subjects have been conducted. C-peptide improves erythrocyte deformabilty in type 1 diabetic patients, possibly via enhancing Na^+,K^+-ATPase function [283]. A 25% increase in glucose utilization is observed in type 1 diabetics under euglycemic clamp when C-peptide levels are normalized [286]. This is congruent with the finding of increased glucose uptake in forearm muscle [287] and muscle strips in vitro from diabetic subjects [288]. Evidence is mounting that C-peptide may be important in the development of some diabetic complications. In type 1 diabetic subjects normalization of C-peptide level is associated with decreased glomerular filtration rate and increased renal plasma flow [286]. When C-peptide was provided continuously by a subcutaneous pump, a decrease in glomerular filtration rate and a marked reduction in urinary albumin resulted [289]. The function of the autonomic nervous system, as assessed by heart rate variability, improved after C-peptide administration [165] and in patients given C-peptide for three months [290]. None of these effects were apparent when insulin was administered alone. No studies have been performed to examine the effect of C-peptide replacement on type 1 diabetic retinopathy.

In the insulin and C-peptide deficient type 1 BB/W rat IR and IGF-1R mRNA are up-regulated in peripheral nerve, but down-regulated in the hippocampus. C-peptide administration to these animals normalizes IR and IGF-1R mRNA levels in peripheral nerve and the central nervous system [265,291]. In addition, hippocampal apoptosis in the type 1 BB/W rat is prevented by C-peptide, and this may be mediated by up-regulation of hippocampal IGF-1R [291].

How these metabolic effects lead to correction of the structural changes of the peripheral nerve in type 1 diabetic neuropathy is an evolving field of investigation. At this point, we will turn towards describing the structural changes present in experimental diabetic neuropathy and compare the structural changes in type 1 and type 2 animal models.

Relationships Between Metabolic Alterations and Structural Pathology in Type 1 and Type 2 Diabetic Neuropathy

Mounting clinical and experimental evidence indicates that the neuropathy associated with type 1 diabetes is more severe than that associated with type 2 diabetes (Table 4.4) [163,166,292]. Briefly, type 1 diabetic neuropathy is typified by severe axonal atrophy, diffuse fiber loss, axoglial dysjunction, and nodal and paranodal changes. The structural changes of type 2

Table 4.**4** Comparisons between metabolic, functional, and structural changes in experimental models of type 1 and type 2 diabetic neuropathy

	Type 1 diabetes	**Type 2 diabetes**
Metabolic alterations		
Hyperglycemia	+	+
Insulin/ C-peptide deficiencies	+	–
Decreased nitric oxide	+	?
Polyol pathway activation	+ (Early phase)	+ (Protracted)
Decreased Na^+,K^+-ATPase activity	+ (Early phase)	+ (Protracted)
Increased oxidative stress	+	?
Increased nonenzymatic glycation	+	+
Deficient neurotrophic factors	+	?
Decreased essential fatty acids	+	?
Functional alterations		
Decreased NCV	+ (Rapid acute decrease which levels off with duration)	+ (Slowly progressive during the course of diabetes)
Decreased blood flow	+	?
Structural changes		
Axonal atrophy	+ (Severe)	+ (Mild)
Nodal changes	+	–
Segmental demyelination	+ (Mild)	+ (Moderate)
Impaired nerve fiber regeneration	+	?
Increased neuronal apoptosis	+/–	?

diabetic neuropathy are characteristically less severe and manifest as mild axonal atrophy, focal fiber loss, segmental demyelination, and Wallerian degeneration. In the past, controversy reigned regarding the nature of diabetic neuropathy, with one camp supporting an underlying axonal disorder and another in favor of a Schwann cell disorder with segmental demyelination as the primary alteration. It now appears that those favoring a primary axonal disorder were describing the changes of type 1 diabetic neuropathy while those supporting a primary Schwann cells disorder were studying the changes of type 2 diabetes [4,15,293].

Experimental models, mostly rodent models, have been indispensable in categorizing the changes of diabetic neuropathy, but have also led to discrepancies between studies. These discrepancies are probably due to the variety of diabetic animals studied and even the age at which diabetes is induced [294]. The STZ-induced diabetic rat is considered a model of type 1 diabetes despite the fact that it does not require insulin supplementation. The biochemical and functional abnormalities of the STZ rat are analogous to those of human type 1 diabetic neuropathy [295]. On the other hand, the morphologic changes in the peripheral nerve are mild and not well developed in this model; even after a long duration of diabetes the animal fails to show fiber loss and severe nerve fiber degeneration [295]. Nonetheless, nodal swelling, and paranodal and segmental demyelination occur in a small percentage of fibers after about one year of diabetes [257, 291, 296]. Other studies have demonstrated alterations in the axoglial interaction with accompanying paranodal demyelination [291,297]. Nerve fiber atrophy with a distinct proximal-distal gradient is evident in STZ rats [298,299]. Some authors have postulated that the axonal atrophy in STZ rats is due either to osmotic shrinkage [300] or to failure of axonal maturation [301], but neither explanation seems satisfactory to explain this phenomenon. The axoplasmic organelles are not condensed, as would be expected in the case of osmotic shrinkage [166], and ARI treatment has no effect on rat somatic development, but axonal size recovers [296]. A progressive defect in axonal transport and synthesis of neurofilaments may explain the distal atrophy and proximal swelling of axons in STZ rats after eight weeks of diabetes [298]. The proximal portion of the axon may also undergo atrophy as the disease progresses [259]. The onset of proximal axonal atrophy coincides with evolving defects in NGF and IGF-1, which hampers the synthesis of structural proteins within the nerve somata [253]. Structural alterations involving the neuronal cell soma have been described in STZ rats. In long-standing STZ diabetes anterior horn cells are reduced in number and DRGs develop a reduction in cell volume [302,303]. The decrease in IGF-1 that occurs in the diabetic state may contribute to these changes in the neuronal soma by weakening neuronal resistance to apoptosis [304].

The BB/W rat spontaneously develops diabetes at about 70 days of age due to an autoimmune-mediated destruction of pancreatic β-cells [305]; these animals need exogenous insulin on a regular basis to sustain life. We have extensively used this model of type 1 diabetic neuropathy in our laboratory as it is probably the best rodent model of human type 1 diabetes. Unlike the STZ rat, the BB/W rat develops severe structural alterations in somatic sensory, motor, and autonomic nerves [102,306].

An abrupt 20% decrease in NCV and evoked potential amplitudes is noted shortly after onset of diabetes in the BB/W rat [297]. This decrease levels off, but by four months' duration of diabetes the decline in NCV continues in a progressive manner [297]. This second decline in NCV correlates with progressive axoglial dysjunction during which paranodal axonal and Schwann cell contacts are disrupted. Morphometrically, these irreversible alterations succeed the early nodal and paranodal axonal swellings. The nodal swellings are associated with increased axonal [Na^+] that is due to increased inactivation of nodal Na^+ channels and the Na^+,K^+-ATPase defect described above [170,194,307]. These early neuropathic changes in the BB/W rat are reversible by insulin (presumably by correcting hyperglycemia), ARI treatment, *myo*-inositol supplementation, or C-peptide replacement [167,170,194,307].

The irreversible axoglial dysjunction leads to impaired Na^+ permeability, which is probably due to the lateralization of Na^+ channels from the node into the paranodal and internodal axolemma [308]. The axonal GLUT-3 transporter is also redistributed in this manner [309]. An analogous phenomenon involving the lateralization of GLUT-1 occurs in Schwann cells following axoglial dysjunction [309]. The electrophysiologic consequence of Na^+ channel redistribution is a slowing of the initial inward Na^+ current of the evoked potential, which generates a block in the conduction of the action potential and manifests as a slowing of NCV.

The molecular abnormalities underlying axoglial dysjunction and the lateralization of nodal molecules are topics of ongoing investigation. Earlier studies using ELISA have shown an up-regulation in NCAM, tenascin, and N-cadherin at six months in BB/W rats, whereas substrate-adhesive molecules showed little change except for polysialic acid [310]. Additional candidates to explain the molecular pathology of the nodal alterations include Caspr and paranodin, an axonal protein localized to the paranode [311,312]. Caspr is closely related to neurexin IV, which is required for the development of septate junctions in *Drosophila* that are structural homologues of vertebrate axoglial junctions [313]. Caspr has an SH3 domain, which interacts in vitro with p85, the regulatory subunit of PI3K, and a critical signal mediator in the insulin signaling cascade [314]. The identification of the high-affinity insulin receptor and Caspr in the paranode [281] creates the potential for cross-talk between molecules responsible for maintaining the axoglial junction and the insulin signaling system. In support of this idea, the direct application of insulin to the sciatic nerve of diabetic rats improves NCV and myelinated fiber number, and C-peptide replacement prevents axoglial dysjunction, presumably via its insulinomimetic effect [167,267,315].

Alterations in the expression or function of ankyrin$_G$ may contribute to the pathology of diabetic neuropathy. Ankyrin$_G$ has multiple binding sites for Na^+ channels, Na^+,K^+-ATPase, and various cell adhesion molecules, promoting their sequestration to the node of Ranvier [316-318]. Perturbations in ankyrin$_G$ may be responsible for the lateralization of Na^+ channels from the node during diabetic neuropathy, which in turn may explain the decrease in NCV. In diabetic neuropathy the lateral displacement of Na^+ channels from the node leads to a diffuse inward Na^+ current rather than the highly localized and intense current required to depolarize the axolemma and propagate the action potential.

The BB/W rat, like the STZ rat, develops a neuropathy characterized by a progressive distal axonal atrophy of both myelinated and unmyelinated fibers; however, these changes are far more severe in the BB/W rat [319]. A loss of up to 33% of the myelinated fibers in the sural nerve may occur at one year of diabetes in the BB/W rat [194,293].

Nerve regeneration is impaired in the BB/W rat, probably due to alterations in the expression of neurotrophic factors such as IGF-1, NGF, and their respective receptors [255]. Apart from a numerical impairment in regenerating fibers, defects in nerve fiber maturity may take place in fibers that do regenerate. Evidence for this phenomenon comes from studies in which ARI-treated axotomized rats showed an increased number of regenerating fibers that did not acquire structural and functional maturity even 220 days after axotomy [320]. The paranodal axoglial junction failed to mature properly in regenerated fibers of ARI-treated and nontreated BB/W rats, which may explain the inability of regenerating nerves to normalize NCV and evoked potential amplitudes [255,320]. It is possible that these failures may be ascribed to insulin/C-peptide deficiencies.

A variety of rodent models of type 2 diabetes have been described; in our laboratory we employ the BB/Z rat. The BB/Z rat develops diabetes spontaneously at about 70 days of age. This model mimics the typical clinical picture of human type 2 diabetes in that diabetes is preceded by obesity and accompanied by peripheral insulin resistance with hyperglycemia, hyperinsulinemia, hyperlipidemia, hypercholesterolemia, and hypertension [166,255]. The BB/Z rat is a relatively new rodent model and its characterization is only beginning. Nonetheless, the structural and functional changes of the diabetic neuropathy encountered in the BB/Z rat are less severe and different from those in the BB/W rat. A relatively mild structural neuropathy develops in the BB/Z rat despite 14 months of hyperglycemia [166]. Compared to the BB/W rat, the hyperinsulinemic BB/Z rats have a propensity to develop focal areas of nerve fiber loss, in keeping with a more prominent vascular component of the diabetic neuropathy. At 14 months BB/Z rats show only mild nerve fiber loss, but segmental demyelination and Wallerian degeneration are more prominent than those seen in the BB/W rat [166]. The defect in NCV evolves slowly, and the initial abrupt decrease evident in the BB/W rat is absent [166]. Interestingly, the polyol pathway undergoes a significant increase in flux, with sorbitol accumulation in the face of rather insignificant *myo*-inositol depletion at six months of diabetes [166]. However, *myo*-inositol levels increase in long-standing diabetes, indicating that other osmoregulatory mechanisms may be operative at this stage [166,176]. Glucose concentrations in sciatic nerve were significantly lower at 14 months of diabetes than at six months, despite similar sorbitol concentrations, indicating that aldose reductase activity increases over time in the BB/Z rat. These data suggest that the dynamics of the polyol pathway differ between the BB/Z and the BB/W rat.

Comparative studies of diabetic neuropathy occurring in the type 1 BB/W and the type 2 BB/Z rat can be performed as both models develop spontaneous diabetes at the same age and experience similar levels of hyperglycemia. The BB/Z rat lacks paranodal alterations; in fact, axoglial dysjunction and the resulting paranodal demyelination characteristic of BB/W rats are not present in BB/Z rats even at 14 months [166]. The chronic NCV defect is milder in the type 2 BB/Z rat, which is probably due to the fact that it lacks the chronic nodal changes. These differences in nodal functions and pathology between the two models may point to the pathogenic influences of insulin and C-peptide levels in diabetic neuropathy.

Future Directions

Future directions of research into the metabolic alterations of diabetic neuropathy will revolve around eliminating or decreasing the impact of biologically relevant pathogenic mechanisms. The next generation of clinical trials will need to take into account that certain metabolic pathways in the pathogenesis of diabetic neuropathy are more responsive at certain time points in its course and that targeting these pathways at appropriate times is likely to maximize the therapeutic benefit. This may explain the relative lack of success, given the initial enthusiasm caused by the ARI clinical studies. Furthermore, the differences in the pathogenic mechanisms underlying type 1 and type 2 diabetic neuropathy need to be fully explored and considered in future clinical trials. Research into the role played by additional metabolic alterations such as mitochondrial dysfunction, oxidative stress, and neuronal apoptosis are now evolving [321,322]. C-peptide has been shown to provide benefit to many of the chronic complications of type 1 diabetes [189], including neuropathy [167], and novel uses of some agents such as ACE inhibitors have promise [323]. Exploration of the possibility that potential genetic factors may predispose individuals to develop diabetic neuropathy is an exciting avenue of research. This prospect could have tremendous potential given the advances in functional genomics and the recent sequencing of the human genome. The development of transgenic animals could be an asset in the study of diabetic complications [324]. Finally, studies aiming at identifying molecules responsible for specific structural and functional alterations of type 1 and type 2 diabetic neuropathy are likely to provide additional therapeutic targets in the more distant future.

Summary

It is becoming increasingly clear that diabetic neuropathy is a multifactorial disorder, with sequential pathogenic components that may be mutually perpetuating, causing an intricate, complex, and dynamic disease process. To add to this complexity, it is also increasingly clear that the complications—in this case, diabetic neuropathy—appear in part to be pathogenically different in the two major forms of diabetes. These differences may be accounted for by factors in addition to hyperglycemia, such as hyper- or hypoinsulinemia and C-peptidemia. The contributions of these aberrations have only recently been recognized and need to be fully explored in order to design biologically meaningful paradigms for the prevention and treatment of this common complication.

Glycation and Advanced Glycation Reactions

J.W. Baynes

Introduction

The glycation or Maillard hypothesis offers a chemical rather than a metabolic perspective on the pathogenesis of diabetic complications. It proposes that glucose and other carbohydrates react continuously and nonenzymatically with proteins in the body and that the resultant chemical modifications and cross-links contribute to the deterioration in protein structure and function with age. Neuropathy and other complications of diabetes are seen as a direct consequence of acceleration of Maillard reactions during hyperglycemia [325,326]. The Maillard hypothesis is an extension of food science into biological systems. It views the human body as a low temperature (37° C) oven with a long (~75-year) cooking cycle. Mixtures of proteins and sugars brown and caramelize in real ovens during baking, and similar reactions proceed spontaneously, albeit much more slowly, in blood and body fluids.

The Maillard hypothesis provides a rational explanation for the similarities in complications in type 1 and type 2 diabetes. Despite significant differences in etiology, both diseases are characterized by high blood glucose concentration. In both diseases, complications develop in tissues, such as the kidney, nerve, retina, and vascular wall, in which cells are freely permeable to glucose and in which glucose transport is largely independent of insulin. These tissues are also rich in long-lived proteins, such as collagens and elastin in the extracellular matrix (ECM) and myelin in nerve. Chronic, cumulative damage to collagen and elastin is a possible cause of the decreased elasticity, altered turnover, and changes in the permeability of the vascular wall in diabetes. Chemical changes in the structure of collagen might explain not only the origin of diabetic vascular disease, but also the loss of pericytes from retinal capillaries, leading to retinopathy, and changes in the thickness and filtration properties of the glomerular basement membrane, leading to nephropathy. Similar changes in the endoneurial vasculature may underlie ischemia and hypoxia in the diabetic nerve. While much of the research on the Maillard reaction in biological systems has focused on cumulative damage to long-lived proteins, there is also growing evidence that intracellular proteins, including tubulin and actin in nerve tissue, are also modified by Maillard reactions, possibly affecting axonal transport processes.

Although the Maillard hypothesis is now about 20 years old, its role in diabetic complications, especially neuropathy, is still controversial. This text therefore addresses a number of alternative hypotheses in successive sections. The uncertainty about the origin of complications results from the fact that there may be multiple mechanisms, tissue-specific mechanisms, or an as yet undefined unifying mechanism of pathogenesis. It is clear, regardless of the outcome, that the current hypotheses are not freestanding entities—they all intersect with one another and with the alterations in intermediary metabolism in diabetes. As discussed below, changes in metabolism affect the level of Maillard reaction precursors, metabolic intermediates may participate in Maillard reactions, and Maillard products are a source of oxidative stress.

This section provides an introduction to the complex nature of the Maillard reaction and its hypothesized role in diabetes and its complications, followed by discussion of the relevance of this reaction to the pathogenesis of diabetic neuropathy. Most of the references in the section on the Maillard reaction are to review articles that provide a more chemical or a broader clinical perspective on the Maillard reaction in aging and disease, while those in the neuropathy section focus on original research.

Maillard Reaction Products

Advanced Glycation Endproducts

The first step in the Maillard reaction, the reaction of glucose with amino groups in protein, is known as nonenzymatic glycosylation or, more commonly, glycation (Fig. 4.**13**). The primary product of glycation is known as fructoselysine (FL) (Fig. 4.**13**). Glycation of protein is a nonoxidative, reversible reaction, and there is limited evidence that this reaction is damaging per se. In contrast, postglycation reactions, leading to formation of advanced glycation endproducts (AGEs), contribute to permanent, cumulative chemical modification of proteins. AGEs are considered the damaging species, and over a dozen AGE adducts and crosslinks have now been identified in tissue proteins (Fig. 4.**14**); all of these compounds can be found in baked goods such as bread and pretzels, especially in the crust.

There are two AGEs that are most often measured as indices of Maillard reaction damage to protein. These compounds are commonly measured in skin collagen, because of its accessibility, with the underlying assumption that the Maillard reaction damage is systemic and that events occurring in skin collagen reflect similar processes occurring in collagen and in proteins throughout the body. N^{ε}-(carboxymethyl) lysine (CML) (Fig. 4.**14**) was the first structurally characterized AGE identified in skin collagen and is quantitatively the major AGE in tissue proteins. It is a nonfluorescent adduct, formed from glycated protein by sequential glycation and oxidation (glycoxidation) reactions [204]. Pentosidine was the first fluorescent AGE and cross-link identified in skin collagen (Fig. 4.**14**); it is also a glycoxidation product. Accurate measurement of CML, pentosidine, and other AGEs requires specific and sensitive techniques, such as gradient HPLC analysis or gas or liquid chromatography-mass spectrometry. Polyclonal and monoclonal anti-AGE antibodies are also commercially available for use in enzyme-linked immunosorbent assays (ELISA) and immunohistochemistry, although most laboratories still use polyclonal antibodies that are largely specific for CML.

In contrast to FL, which remains relatively constant with age, levels of CML and pentosidine increase with age in skin collagen, and their accumulation is accelerated in diabetes. Importantly, the increase in age-adjusted levels of CML and pentosidine in diabetic collagen is more pronounced in patients with advanced stages of complications, including neuropathy [327]. These associations are statistically significant, even after adjustment for the increase in glycated hemoglobin, a long-term index of mean blood glucose concentration. It is not clear whether Maillard reactions or AGEs cause the complications, or are merely secondary manifestations of pathology resulting from other mechanisms. Several laboratories are evaluating the usefulness of measuring AGEs as risk factors for predicting the development of complications.

Role of Oxidation in the Maillard Reaction

The term "glycoxidation product" refers to AGEs that require both glycation and oxidation for their formation from glucose. Because CML and pentosidine were

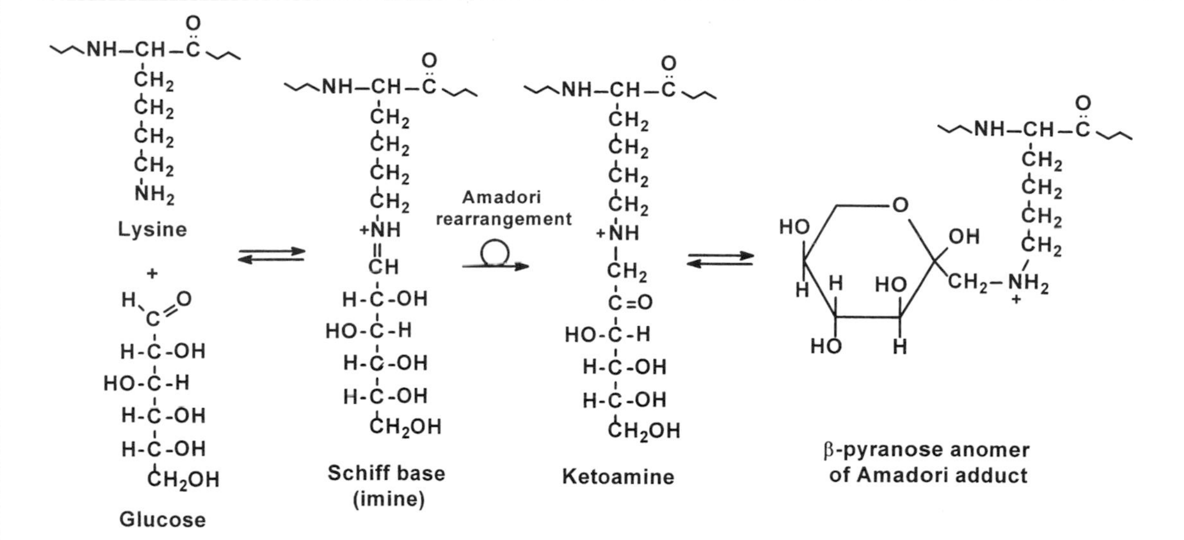

Fig. 4.**13** Pathway of nonenzymatic glycation of protein. Glucose reacts with the ε-amino group of a lysine residue in protein. A labile Schiff base (imine) intermediate is formed, which undergoes an Amadori rearrangement to yield a stable ketoamine adduct, fructoselysine

the first Maillard products known to accumulate irreversibly in tissue proteins with age and both are glycoxidation products, oxidation was described as a fixative of irreversible Maillard reaction damage to protein [204]. Studies on glycation of collagen in vitro demonstrated that oxidation, catalyzed by transition metal ions such as iron and copper, was required not only for formation of glycoxidation products, but also for the cross-linking and browning of collagen by glucose. Chelators, reducing agents, and antioxidants were potent inhibitors of these reactions. The association between oxidation and protein damage was confirmed by the observation that hydrogen peroxide was produced during Maillard reactions in vitro and that glycoxidized proteins contained oxidized amino acids, including *ortho*-tyrosine and methionine sulfoxide. Thus, AGEs are not the only products of modification of protein formed during the Maillard reaction.

Glycoxidation reactions proceed through a complex array of intermediates, known as reactive carbonyl compounds, that react with protein to form AGEs. These intermediates may be formed by oxidation of the sugar or Schiff base or Amadori adducts to protein (Fig. 4.**13**); some may be released free into solution, while others remain chemically bound to protein. The formation of CML from glucose, for example, may involve glycation and oxidative cleavage of the Amadori adduct between C-2 and C-3 of the carbohydrate chain, or oxidative cleavage of glucose to glyoxal, which then reacts with protein to form CML. CML may also be formed from fructose and sugar phosphate intermediates in glycolysis, and even from ascorbate, so that it is impossible to identify the precise mechanism of formation or even the source of CML measured in tissue proteins. Similar uncertainties apply to the mechanism and source of pentosidine and other AGEs in tissue proteins.

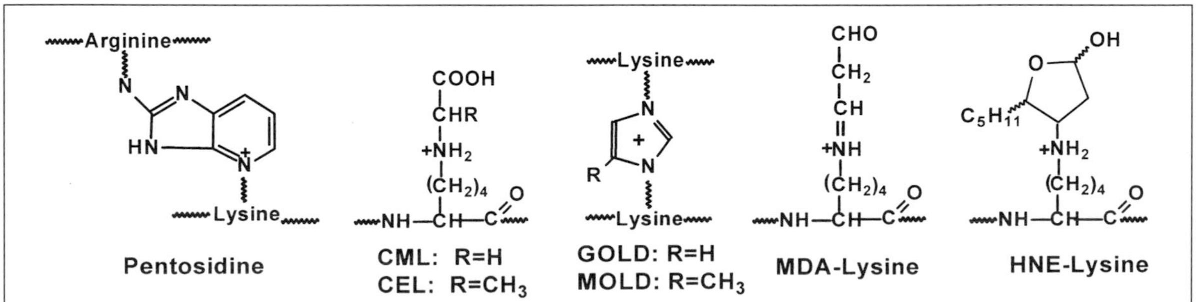

Fig. 4.**14** Structures of characteristic AGEs/ALEs (advanced lipoxidation endproducts) in tissue proteins. Pentosidine is a fluorescent AGE. CML, CEL, GOLD and MOLD are AGE/ALEs, while MDA-lysine and HNE-lysine are ALEs. Hydroxynonenal also forms adducts with cysteine and histidine. Pentosidine and the AGE/ALEs increase with age in tissue proteins and at an increased rate in diabetes. MDA-lysine and HNE-lysine do not accumulate with age in proteins, but are increased in concert with AGE/ALEs in tissues at sites of inflammation and in atherosclerotic plaque

In addition to involvement of oxidation in the formation of some AGEs, there is evidence that AGE proteins may also be sources of oxidative stress. AGE proteins catalyze lipid peroxidation reactions in vitro, and AGE-mediated catalysis of lipoprotein oxidation in the aortic wall may contribute to the development of macrovascular disease in diabetes [328]. AGE proteins also chelate transition metal ions in redox active form and may promote metal-catalyzed oxidation reactions in tissues [329]. Interaction of AGE proteins with receptors for AGEs also induces oxidative damage to the receptor-bearing cells [330]. The best-characterized among the AGE receptors are RAGE (receptor for AGE), the macrophage scavenger receptor, and galectin-3. Each of these receptors recognizes a range of AGE-modified, but not native proteins, and mediates their endocytic uptake and lysosomal degradation. Binding of AGE proteins to RAGE appears to induce oxidative stress to the RAGE-bearing cells—the AGEs are considered the source of the oxidative stress. Binding and uptake of oxidized lipoproteins by scavenger receptors also causes oxidative stress to macrophages bearing scavenger receptors. Thus, there is some risk to the cell involved in recognition and catabolism of AGEs, and chronic increases in AGE-induced oxidative stress have been invoked as a source of damage to endothelial cells during development of diabetic vascular disease and nephropathy.

Despite growing interest in the oxidative chemistry of the Maillard reaction, browning of proteins by sugars smaller than hexoses occurs efficiently under nonoxidative conditions. The reactive dicarbonyl compound, methylglyoxal (MGO), for example, is formed in vivo primarily by anaerobic decomposition of triose phosphate intermediates in *anaerobic* glycolysis [331]. Triose phosphates and MGO brown and cross-link proteins and form AGEs, such as N^{ε}-(carboxyethyl)lysine (CEL), and methylglyoxal-lysine dimer (MOLD) (Fig. 4.**14**) under anaerobic conditions. As with other AGEs, however, the actual source of the increase in CEL and MOLD in tissue proteins is not known. MGO may also be formed by oxidation of ascorbate or sugar adducts to protein and may be derived from lipoxidation reactions (see below).

In contrast to uncertainty about the origin of MGO and MGO-derived AGEs, 3-deoxyglucosone (3DG), another dicarbonyl intermediate in AGE formation, is clearly not a product of oxidation of glucose. 3DG is formed by rearrangement and hydrolysis of FL, or by spontaneous decomposition of fructose-3-phosphate, an intermediate in glucose metabolism via the polyol pathway. Although formation of CML and pentosidine from 3DG requires oxygen, 3DG browns and cross-links proteins rapidly under nonoxidative conditions. The concentrations of 3DG and the 3DG-protein adducts pyrraline and 3DG-arginine imidazolone [326] are increased in blood proteins in diabetes. There is no evidence that these nonoxidative AGEs accumulate in tissue proteins with age, but the detection of 3DG and its adducts in tissue proteins and the ability of 3DG to cross-link proteins in the absence of oxygen illustrate clearly that oxidation is not essential for AGE formation.

Glycoxidation Versus Lipoxidation

Diabetes is not a disease of carbohydrate metabolism alone. It is also characterized by derangements in fat and protein metabolism, and hyperlipidemia and dyslipidemia occur commonly in diabetic patients. Polyunsaturated fatty acids (PUFAs), such as linoleate and arachidonate in triglycerides and phospholipids, are much more susceptible to oxidation than sugars. Thus, it is reasonable to ask whether chemical modification of proteins by lipids, like nonenzymatic glycation of protein, might also be increased in diabetes. Oxidation of PUFAs leads to formation of a spectrum of reactive carbonyl intermediates that yield products analogous to AGEs, known as advanced lipoxidation endproducts (ALEs). The best studied among these carbonyl intermediates are malondialdehyde (MDA) and 4-hydroxynonenal (HNE) and their adducts to lysine (MDA-Lys and HNE-Lys) (Fig. 4.**14**). CML and MDA-Lys appear together in atherosclerotic plaque and in LDL isolated from diabetic patients, and their levels correlate with one another. The interface between glycoxidation and lipoxidation is blurred by the observation that both CML and CEL are formed during metal-catalyzed oxidation of LDL in vitro and that they are derived from lipids, rather than from Amadori adducts, on the protein. Thus, the CML in atherosclerotic plaque of nondiabetic, normoglycemic individuals is most likely to be an ALE, rather than an AGE. Measurement of pentosidine in atherosclerotic plaque and plasma lipoproteins (or of some other compound that is derived exclusively from carbohydrates) would be helpful in determining the relative roles of glycoxidation and lipoxidation in modification of lipoproteins in diabetes.

CML and CEL, and probably also glyoxal-lysine dimer (GOLD) and MOLD (Fig. 4.**14**), should be viewed as common products of oxidative modification of proteins by carbohydrates and/or lipids. Because of the uncertainty regarding their origin, they are termed "AGE/ALEs." AGEs and ALEs colocalize in tissues and most anti-AGE antibodies recognize the AGE/ALE CML. Thus, the scope of Maillard reaction damage to tissue proteins should be expanded to include lipid-derived products, an analogy to the fact that browning reactions of foods during cooking are derived from reactions of proteins with both carbohydrates and lipids.

Intracellular AGE/ALE Formation

Phosphorylated sugars and metabolic intermediates in the hexose monophosphate pathway and glycolysis are much more reactive with proteins than glucose. The low intracellular concentration of these sugars, combined with substrate channeling between enzymes, is probably important for protection against intracellular damage from the Maillard reaction. However, increased intracellular concentrations of fructose and phosphorylated sugars in diabetes could lead to increased rates of chemical modification of intracellular proteins. CML and CEL have been identified in intracellular proteins, including nuclear proteins, cytoskeletal proteins, and growth factors. Interestingly, these classes of proteins may have relatively long half-lives, nuclear proteins in the nucleus, cytoskeletal proteins in the cytoplasm, and growth factors in secretory granules. Research on intracellular glycation and AGE formation is still in its infancy, but it is possible that the increase in metabolic intermediates in diabetes may be a more significant and acute source of AGEs than the increase in blood glucose or glycated proteins.

Quantitative Issues Regarding the Role of AGEs in Diabetic Complications

The known AGEs (Fig. 4.**14**) are only trace components of proteins in vivo. Even in skin collagen and lens proteins of elderly diabetic patients, CML and CEL, the predominant AGEs, are present at only 1–2% of total lysine residues. Cross-link structures, such as pentosidine, GOLD, and MOLD, are present at 10% or less of the concentrations of CML and CEL [328], so that they are unlikely to have a significant effect on the overall structural properties of protein. It is difficult to argue on quantitative grounds that AGEs have a major role in the chemical modification of proteins, and thus in diabetic complications. It is important to recognize, however, that the AGEs that can be measured today represent only a fraction of the AGEs that may be formed. This is the "tip of the iceberg" corollary to the AGE hypothesis. It based on the observation that known AGEs represent only a fraction of the total chemical modifications and cross-links in AGE proteins prepared in vitro. Thus, the sum of all AGEs, identified and unidentified, in tissue proteins may be quantitatively significant and could have a direct role in the pathogenesis of complications. The number of structurally characterized AGEs has increased at the rate of 1 – 2 per year for the past decade. There is a general consensus that there are many more AGEs that are heterogeneous in structure and labile to the acid, base, or enzymatic hydrolysis used for their isolation. Recent developments in tandem mass spectrometry instrumentation for proteomics research should accelerate the characterization of new AGEs in protein.

Diabetic Neuropathy

Because the polyol pathway and oxidative stress are treated elsewhere in this volume, the following discussion will focus on structural and biochemical changes in the peripheral nerve that might be caused by AGE/ALE formation. Diabetic peripheral neuropathy is characterized by a decrease in blood flow to the nerve, alterations in nerve conduction velocity, and structural changes that are consistent with hypoxic and ischemic damage. As summarized in Table 4.**5**, there are a number of mechanisms by which AGE/ALE formation could contribute to these changes, leading not only to alterations in nerve function, but also loss of neurons resulting from deficiencies in neuronal regeneration. Inhibitors of AGE formation, discussed below, may therefore act on a number of possible targets to limit the progression of diabetic neuropathy.

Nerve Proteins

Myelin was one of the earliest long-lived proteins considered as a target for nonenzymatic modification by glucose [332]. The extent of glycation of myelin, like other proteins in the body, is increased in proportion to the increase in mean blood glucose in diabetes. A four- to 10-fold increase in IgG and IgM was detected by ELISA of peripheral nerve myelin from diabetic versus nondiabetic patients and was attributed to the entrapment of immunoglobulins by AGEs, secondary

Table 4.**5** Possible mechanisms by which AGE/ALEs may contribute to diabetic neuropathy

Process	Effect
Formation of AGEs on myelin	Attraction and activation of macrophages, demyelination
Covalent entrapment of plasma proteins (albumin and immunoglobulins) in the ECM	Alterations in immunogenicity, cell attachment, and permeability of the ECM
Cross-linkage of basement membrane proteins	Alterations in elasticity, inhibition of turnover, and thickening of basement membranes
Interference with action of nitric oxide and other vasomodulators	Alterations in vascular tone and autoregulation
Source of oxidative stress	Alterations in vascular tone, inflammation, increased protein turnover
Glycation and AGE formation on intracellular proteins, actin and tubulin	Alterations in axonal transport

to increased glycation of myelin. The increase in IgM and IgG in peripheral myelin, but not in brain myelin, despite similar increases in glycation in both tissues, was attributed to limited transport of immunoglobulins across the blood-brain barrier. Although these observations were consistent with a role for AGE/ALEs in the trapping of immunoglobulins and with in vitro studies demonstrating covalent trapping of plasma protein by glycated versus control collagen [333], the covalent linkage between myelin and immunoglobulins was not confirmed. Further, despite the increase in glycosylation of peripheral nerve myelin from diabetic rats, there was no direct evidence for increased levels of specific AGE/ALEs or cross-links in the myelin protein. In other studies, however, glycation and AGE formation induced the uptake of myelin by macrophages in vitro, consistent with a three- to five-fold increase in macrophage uptake of peripheral nerve myelin from diabetic versus control donors [334]. Control experiments were performed, demonstrating competition for uptake between myelin glycated in vitro and myelin from diabetic versus nondiabetic donors, arguing that the increase in uptake of myelin from diabetic versus control patients was not mediated by bound immunoglobulins. These observations are consistent with a role for glycation as a mediator of the increased entrapment of plasma proteins and macrophage-mediated degradation of myelin, setting the stage for segmental demyelination and axonal degeneration in peripheral nerves in diabetes.

More recent studies have focused on the chemical modification of intracellular axonal proteins as a possible mechanism underlying impaired axonal transport in diabetes. Immunohistochemical staining with anti-AGE/ALE antibody (largely CML-specific) revealed increased deposition of both intracellular and extracellular AGE/ALEs in perineurial, endoneurial, and microvascular cells in diabetic peripheral nerve [335]. The AGE/ALEs were associated with electron-dense intracellular aggregates, possibly composed of tubular and neurofilament proteins. AGE/ALE deposition also correlated with a reduction in myelinated fiber density, but was not directly associated with degenerative changes in nerve fibers. The increased AGE/ALEs in spinal and sciatic nerve appeared to be reversible in the diabetic rat, since islet transplantation into streptozotocin (STZ)-diabetic rats (STZ-DR) led to a significant decrease in AGE formation within four months [336]. In these studies, AGE/ALEs, measured by ELISA, were increased two- to four-fold over control values in both spinal cord and sciatic nerve of rats after four months of diabetes. However, levels of AGE/ALEs did not increase further in either the control or the diabetic rats between the fourth and the eighth month of diabetes. The lack of a change in AGE/ALEs with age or duration of diabetes, and the method used for preparation of proteins for the ELISA, suggest that the AGE/ALEs measured in these studies were in shorter-lived, largely intracellular proteins, rather than long-lived ECM proteins. Islet transplantation after either four or eight months of diabetes also led to near-normalization of AGEs, i.e. return to nondiabetic levels within four months. These changes were associated with significant but only partial recovery of nerve function in the diabetic animals [337,338], which may have resulted from continuing, active growth of nerve in the young animals used in the study. Levels of AGEs in ECM proteins in nerve were not measured in these studies, and although AGEs in tail collagen decreased in response to islet transplantation, these changes might also be attributed to growth and turnover of tail collagen during the course of the study. Unfortunately, the structural and functional changes in these experiments were measured only at four months after islet transplantation, so that it is possible that changes in function may have preceded changes in structure, e. g., in response to restoration of normoglycemia. Based on the above studies, it is clear that AGE/ALEs accumulate in both intracellular and ECM proteins in the diabetic peripheral nerve, but the relationship between altered structure (AGE/ALE formation) and altered function (neuropathy) is at this point only correlative, at best.

Effects of AGE Inhibitors

The ultimate test of the Maillard hypothesis is the demonstration that inhibition of AGE/ALE formation in the presence of hyperglycemia and/or hyperlipidemia protects against diabetic neuropathy. To this end, a number of AGE inhibitors have been evaluated in experimental models of diabetes, primarily the diabetic rodent. The best characterized of these inhibitors, aminoguanidine [339], pyridoxamine [340], and OPB-9195 [341], are known to inhibit both glycoxidative and lipoxidative modification of proteins [342–344] so that they are properly described as AGE/ALE inhibitors. These and other AGE/ALE inhibitors are nonspecific nucleophilic traps that scavenge reactive carbonyl intermediates in AGE/ALE formation. They have a broad range of effects on the development of long-term diabetic complications [339–344].

Aminoguanidine has been studied in greatest detail with respect to diabetic neuropathy. Treatment with aminoguanidine inhibited changes in nerve blood flow and conduction velocity in sciatic-tibial and caudal nerves of STZ-DR [219]. Effects on blood flow were maximal at lower doses of aminoguanidine, while effects on conduction velocity were dose-dependent and were almost normalized at the higher dose (50 mg/kg per day, intraperitoneal injection). In a later study, aminoguanidine inhibited the decrease in both motor (sciatic) and sensory (saphenous) nerve conduction velocity [345]. In both cases, the nerve functional parameters were measured after only a short (eight-week) duration of diabetes in STZ-DR. Levels of AGEs were not measured, nor did the authors evaluate the effects of intervention with aminoguanidine after established or chronic neuropathy, i.e., longer than eight weeks.

In other studies [346,347], aminoguanidine inhibited the decline in motor (sural) nerve conduction velocity and the increase in myelinated fiber size and axonal atrophy in STZ-DR after 16 weeks of diabetes. Aminoguanidine also preserved myelin density and prevented atrophy in optic nerve fibers of the STZ-DR [348]. Although there were no changes in sural nerve basement membrane thickening at 16 weeks, aminoguanidine did inhibit the accumulation of AGEs, measured by fluorescence, in nerve tissues. Fluorescence is a nonspecific assay for AGEs, but these results suggest that aminoguanidine may inhibit AGE/ALE formation in diabetic nerve. In a similar study [349], aminoguanidine inhibited the decline in sciatic nerve conduction velocity, but not morphological changes, in STZ-DR. AGE/ALEs, measured by ELISA, were increased in the renal cortex of diabetic rats, and this increase was inhibited 40% by aminoguanidine. The correlation between renal AGE/ALEs and sciatic nerve conduction velocity in aminoguanidine-treated rats was interpreted as evidence that aminoguanidine may inhibit AGE formation in peripheral tissues.

There are several studies indicating that aminoguanidine may not be effective in treatment of diabetic peripheral neuropathy. Aminoguanidine did not affect the loss of relaxant response to NO in STZ-DR anococcygeus nerve, and, in fact, further exacerbated the loss of the nerve's response to nitrergic stimulation [350]. This and most of the other studies cited above may be criticized because they focus on early, acute changes in very poorly controlled animals, rather than on chronic neuropathy. Changes in AGE/ALEs are not documented in most of these studies, but it is unlikely that they would be significant, particularly within eight weeks, so that any conclusions regarding the effects of aminoguanidine as an AGE/ALE inhibitor in these studies should be viewed with caution.

In two long-term studies, aminoguanidine has shown less promise. Treatment with aminoguanidine for seven to 10 months failed to affect the progression of sympathetic autonomic neuropathy in STZ-DR [351], and in a recent study aminoguanidine failed to inhibit the progression of long-term neuropathy in diabetic baboons (approx. five years' duration of diabetes and three years of aminoguanidine therapy) [352]. Although aminoguanidine did not affect the progression of neuropathy, measured by the decline in motor (sciatic) and sensory (sural) nerve conduction velocity in the diabetic baboons, the study was somewhat compromised by the low level of aminoguanidine used (10 mg/kg) and the once daily subcutaneous injection. The maximum and mean daily plasma aminoguanidine concentrations were 100 and 50 nM, respectively, which is low for a chemical agent designed to trap reactive carbonyl compounds. Typical plasma concentrations in the rat are in the 50- to 100-μM range and are frequently maintained at this level by providing the aminoguanidine continuously in drinking water. A slow-release form of aminoguanidine might be more appropriate for long-term, chronic studies. The effects of diabetes and aminoguanidine therapy on levels of AGEs in the baboon tissues has not yet been reported.

Aside from aminoguanidine, the guanidino compound metformin is the only other drug commonly used in therapy for diabetes that is known to function as a carbonyl trap and inhibitor of AGE formation in vitro [353,354]. At high doses, metformin caused a decrease in the concentration of MGO, a dicarbonyl AGE/ALE precursor, in plasma of diabetic patients. Because this effect was independent of effects of metformin on glycemia, the observations suggest that, in addition to its effects on glycemic control, metformin may also inhibit AGE/ALE formation in vivo. Unfortunately, levels of AGEs were not measured in these experiments, and effects on neuropathy were not reported [355]. In the STZ-DR, however, metformin caused a 50% correction of the decrease in sciatic nerve conduction velocity after 10 weeks of diabetes [356]. There was a corresponding approximately 25% decrease in AGEs in sciatic nerve, measured by ELISA, but this was associated with a similar decrease in glycemia and glycated hemoglobin. In this model, the STZ-DR had some residual pancreatic β-cell function since plasma insulin concentration was about 5% of normal values, and the insulin concentration also tended to be higher in the metformin-treated animals. The lower glucose and higher insulin concentration in the metformin-treated rats makes it uncertain whether the effects of metformin should be attributed to AGE inhibition, as opposed to its effects on glycemic control.

Alternative Mechanisms of Action of AGE Inhibitors

Like metformin, few drugs have a single mechanism of action. Aminoguanidine, for example, is a potent inhibitor of monoamine oxidase and NO synthase (NOS), which may affect vascular and neural tone, independent of effects on AGE/ALEs. Pyridoxamine also inhibits benzylamine and semicarbazide-sensitive amine oxidases, and OPB-9195 is a potent chelator of transition metal ions. Under these circumstances, it is difficult to tease out the mechanism of action of the drug. In one study aminoguanidine, but not the NOS inhibitor L-NAME, significantly improved nerve blood flow and conduction velocity in STZ-DR after four weeks of diabetes [357]. However, the duration of diabetes was short and half-maximal effects were observed within six days, arguing against a role for AGEs in neuropathy in this model. In a long-term study (32 weeks), aminoguanidine, but not L-NAME, also inhibited the loss of neurons from the retina of STZ-DR [358]. The implication of this study was that loss of neurons from the retina and peripheral nerves might affect vascular tone and autoregulation of blood flow, contributing to ischemic damage. These and other studies suggest that the aminoguanidine protection against diabetic neuropathy is not the result of its NOS inhibitory activity, although other effects on NO signaling pathways cannot be excluded. AGE/ALE inhibitors, including both aminoguanidine and pyridoxamine, also have lipid-lowering effects [358a] and protect against the development of nephropathy in diabetic rats. Hyperlipidemia and/or dyslipidemia are major risk factors for the development of renal and vascular disease in diabetes, but their role in pathogenesis of neuropathy is less certain.

Conclusions

In summary, the evidence for the role of AGE/ALEs in development of diabetic neuropathy is less convincing, for example, than the evidence linking AGE/ALEs to diabetic renal and vascular disease. The lack of experimental data on nerve is, in part, the result of the limited mass of tissue available and the difficulty in its isolation in comparison to kidney, aorta, or skin. For this reason, there are few published reports of quantitative measurements of AGE/ALEs in either intracellular or extracellular proteins in the nerve in diabetes or in response to AGE/ALE inhibitors. Though untested, or at least not rigorously tested, the Maillard hypothesis still presents a reasonable explanation for many of the neuronal deficits associated with diabetic neuropathy (Table 4.**5**).

■ Polyolpathway: Aldose Reductase Inhibitors—Hope for the Future?

E.L. Feldman, K.A. Sullivan, and M.J. Stevens

Introduction

Diabetic peripheral neuropathy is a common complication of types 1 and 2 diabetes [359]. It occurs in approximately half of all patients after 25 years of diabetes [160], and in more than 40% of patients with diabetes between the ages of 70 and 79 [360]. Thirty-nine percent of healthy type 1 patients screened for entry into the Diabetes Control and Complications Trial (DCCT) met the diagnostic criteria of diabetic peripheral neuropathy [361,362]. While peripheral neuropathy represents the most common complication of diabetes, the pathways underlying glucose-mediated damage to the nervous system remain unknown. Despite the fact that the DCCT [361,362] and the United Kingdom Prospective Diabetes Study [363] established that hyperglycemia mediates the onset and progression of peripheral neuropathy in diabetes, the nature and cellular localization of the underlying vascular and metabolic insults remain speculative and a source of active investigation [364–366]. An understanding of exactly how glucose alters nerve metabolism, blood flow, and function is essential for the development of rational mechanism-based therapies.

The aldose reductase pathway represents one of most intensively investigated metabolic pathways in the field of diabetic neuropathy [364,365]. Evidence accumulated over the last 20 years reveals a role for the aldose reductase pathway in a wide variety of metabolic and vascular defects critical to the development of diabetic peripheral neuropathy [366–375]. These defects appear to be multifactorial with the potential to injure specific cellular components of the nerve, such as nerve cell bodies, axons, or Schwann cells. In parallel, essential supporting elements, such as the nerve vasculature and the extracellular matrix, are also adversely affected by events occurring in the aldose reductase pathway [173,376]. The cross-talk between the aldose reductase pathway and other key metabolic pathways suggests that disruption of one aspect of cellular metabolism adversely affects many interdependent essential cellular functions (Fig. 4.**15**). A combination of individual therapies aimed at distinct pathways altered or disrupted by hyperglycemia may afford beneficial synergistic effects in the treatment of peripheral neuropathy. Certainly, the use to date of single agents in clinical trials has lead to modest improvements at best. Our belief is that an increased understanding of the mechanism(s) underlying diabetic peripheral neuropathy is critical for the development of new therapies aimed at preventing both the onset and the progression of nerve dysfunction and loss.

Pathophysiology

Role of Aldose Reductase in Experimental Diabetic Neuropathy

Glucose is reduced to sorbitol by aldose reductase in a concentration-dependent manner, independent of glucose phosphorylation. Sorbitol, in turn, is oxidized by sorbitol dehydrogenase (SDH), the second enzyme in the aldose reductase pathway, to fructose. Both aldose reductase and SDH are highly expressed in complication-prone tissue like nerve, kidney, and eye [173]. Because glucose uptake into these tissues is essentially insulin-independent, the aldose reductase pathway is activated by the mass action of glucose entry. NADPH is used by aldose reductase to reduce glucose to sorbitol, while SDH depends on NAD^+ to oxidize sorbitol to fructose. Sorbitol accumulation leads to an osmotic imbalance and a compensatory loss of cellular taurine and *myo*-inositol. Osmolyte imbalance impairs cellular function and may augment the negative impact of several other cellular consequences of aldose reductase pathway activity, including changes in the cytoplasmic redox state and the balance of NADPH and NAD^+ in the cell. Aldose reductase pathway production of fructose is responsible for

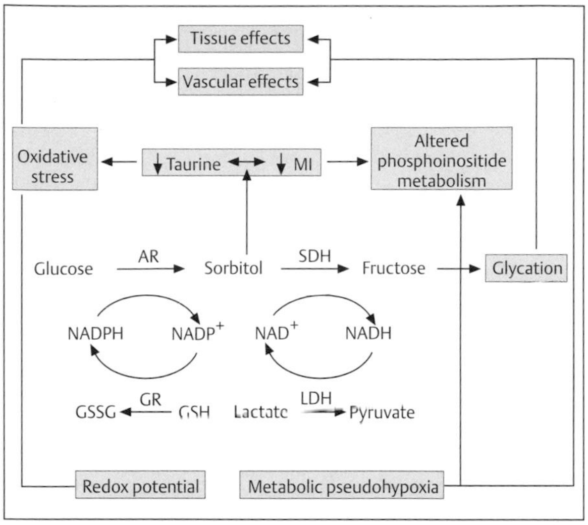

Fig. 4.**15** Pathogenesis of diabetic neuropathy: unification of metabolic and vascular theories. AR, aldose reductase; MI, *myo*-inositol; LDH, lactate dehydrogenase; GSSG, oxidized glutathione; GR, glutathione reductase; GSH, reduced glutathione. (From [911], with permission)

nonenzymatic glycation/glycoxidation of cellular proteins and lipids, leading to further cellular dysfunction.

The aldose reductase pathway has been extensively studied in the streptozotocin diabetic rat model of experimental diabetic neuropathy. Several different investigators report that blocking aldose reductase activity with an aldose reductase inhibitor (ARI) improves one or more of the metabolic, vascular, or physiologic defects that are the hallmark of experimental diabetic neuropathy. Treatment with ARIs normalizes nerve conduction velocities in diabetic rodents and restores normal rates of axonal transport [377,378]. ARI therapy blocks several crucial and probably interdependent metabolic defects present in diabetic nerve, including decreased neurotrophism [374,375], nerve osmolyte depletion [367,368], increased oxidative stress and cellular redox imbalance [368,372,379], increased activity of protein kinase C [370,371], decreased activity of nerve Na^+,K^+-ATPase [173,380], loss of nerve vasoreactivity [373], and decreases in nerve blood flow with resultant nerve ischemia [373,381].

Aldose Reductase Expression and Diabetic Complications

Around 10 years ago several groups reported a link between increased aldose reductase pathway activity and the presence of diabetic complications [382,383] including severe neuropathy [384]. Studies suggested an association between increased aldose reductase enzymatic activity and/or protein measured in neutrophils [382] and erythrocytes [385] and the presence of microvascular complications [382,383]. These ideas are upheld by the more recent work of Shah and colleagues, who report increased aldose reductase gene expression in the peripheral blood mononuclear cells in diabetic patients with nephropathy [386]. In support of these ideas, Maeda and colleagues found increases in aldose reductase protein levels in red blood cells harvested from Japanese patients with type 2 diabetes and nephropathy [387]. The aldose reductase gene is transcriptionally up-regulated [388] (but not apparently down-regulated [380]) by tonicity elements in the 5′ flanking sequence [388]. There is definite variability of aldose reductase gene and protein expression among individuals. For example, human retinal pigment epithelial cell lines harvested from unrelated patients undergoing ophthalmologic surgery express heterogeneous basal levels of aldose reductase gene expression and activity [390–392]. Aldose reductase transcription parallels aldose reductase mRNA and activity, suggesting that transcription of the aldose reductase gene is the basis of high levels of aldose reductase expression in complication-prone tissues [393].

The identification of polymorphisms at the 5′ end of the aldose reductase gene supports the idea that those individuals with diabetes who are prone to developing microvascular complications may have higher aberrant levels of aldose reductase pathway activity. An area in the $(A-C)_n$ dinucleotide repeat in the aldose reductase gene basal promoter is present in patients with diabetic nephropathy [161,386]. The same polymorphism occurs in high frequency in individuals with diabetic retinopathy [162,394–396] and neuropathy [397]. A second polymorphism, a C(–106)T substitution in the aldose reductase gene basal promoter, is also present in certain diabetic subjects with nephropathy [398] and retinopathy [162]. Polymorphisms in the aldose reductase promoter correlate with increased aldose reductase gene expression [399], strengthening the argument for the existence of a genetic predisposition to microvascular complications in patients with polymorphisms at the 5′ end of the aldose reductase gene. Recently, this idea has been questioned, particularly in patients with nephropathy [387,398–401]. There are many possible reasons for differences between the patient studies, including the ethnic background of the different study populations and the type of diabetes. More studies are needed to confirm or refute the idea that polymorphisms in the aldose reductase promoter increase an individual's susceptibility to the microvascular complications of diabetes.

Therapy

Therapeutic Efficacy of ARIs in Clinical Trials

Several large-scale clinical trials have been undertaken to test the therapeutic role of ARI therapy in diabetic peripheral neuropathy. Collectively, approximately 60% of patients in these studies have shown improvement in one or more measurement(s) of peripheral neuropathy, most commonly either in the subjective assessment of symptoms or the more objective assessment of nerve conduction velocities [402]. For example, in Japan, the ARI epalrestat had a significant effect on improving symptoms and restoring nerve conductions towards normal levels in patients with peripheral neuropathy [403,404].

Many factors have contributed to the well-documented variability between the large-scale ARI trials. The pharmacokinetics and toxicity of the different ARIs vary widely and toxicity has frequently been dose-limiting. The ARIs have different abilities to penetrate the nerve, and lack of penetration has been cited as the reason for one failed trial. Because diabetic peripheral neuropathy progresses slowly, many investigators believe previous therapeutic trials have been too short. This is coupled with the fact that the severity of neuropathy has differed in individual ARI trials, as have the clinical and electrophysiologic measures used to establish the diagnosis of diabetic peripheral neuropathy and to monitor disease progression.

For an ARI to be clinically useful, the drug must effectively inhibit the aldose reductase pathway in complication-prone tissues at doses that are tolerated by diabetic patients. Zopolrestat is a potent ARI. Three hundred and seventy-eight patients with painful diabetic peripheral neuropathy entered a double-blind placebo-controlled phase II study, receiving either placebo or 1000 mg/day zopolrestat for 12 weeks. Compared to the placebo group, the patients who received zopolrestat had clear statistical improvements in neuroelectrophysiologic measurements of nerve function. There were concerns, however, about dose-related zopolrestat toxicity. Some patients receiving 1000 mg/day zopolrestat experienced hepatic transaminase elevations and mild decreases in hematocrit, hemoglobin, and red blood cell count. In an attempt to eliminate these drug-related toxicities, the pivotal phase III clinical studies employed lower dosages, 250 and 500 mg once daily. Unfortunately, these lower doses were clinically ineffective.

Another ARI, zenarestat, was used in a 52-week phase IIB dose-finding study; like previous ARI trials, this study had a randomized placebo-controlled design and enrolled patients with mild to moderate diabetic peripheral neuropathy. Two objective clinical endpoints were examined in this study. Nerve conduction velocities were measured at onset and at the end of the study. Each patient also underwent a sural nerve biopsy at the beginning and end of the study. Sural nerves were examined in two ways: for aldose reductase pathway intermediates, and for myelinated nerve fiber density and evidence of fiber degeneration and regeneration. Doses of zenarestat that lowered sural nerve sorbitol content by 80–85% also reversed the loss of myelinated sensory nerve fibers in sural nerve (expressed as the density of myelinated nerve fibers per square millimeter of cross-sectional area) [405]. The main increase in fiber density occurred in small diameter (<5 μM) myelinated fibers. In parallel, there was a loss of myelinated nerve fiber density in untreated diabetic patients. The improvement within 12 months in both nerve conduction velocities and density of small myelinated nerve fibers, especially when taken in the context of the observed loss in untreated patients, suggested that zenarestat therapy was effective in ameliorating the progression of diabetic peripheral neuropathy [405]. Zenarestat at doses of 600 mg twice a day had a similar toxicity profile to zopolrestat, with a nonprogressive decrease in patient hemoglobin and red blood cell count. In addition, zenarestat produced a dose-dependent uricosuria and increase in serum creatinine and serum β_2-microglobulin [405]. A large phase III study was begun but subsequently terminated this year due to concerns about zenarestat toxicity. The results with both zopolrestat and zenarestat suggest the potential efficacy of ARI therapy but also underscore the need for development of ARIs with an improved safety profile.

ARI Therapy and Autonomic Neuropathy

Recent work suggests that ARIs may have a role in the treatment of diabetic autonomic neuropathy. Quantitative scintigraphic assessment of the sympathetic innervation of the heart is currently in use using radiolabeled analogues of norepinephrine [79,406]. Norepinephrine is actively taken up by the sympathetic terminals in the heart. Using either single photon emission computed tomography (SPECT) [407] or positron emission tomography (PET) [79], the uptake of norepinephrine can be monitored and provides a quantitative assessment of cardiac autonomic function. Deficits in left ventricular function in type 1 diabetic patients [79,406,407] and type 2 patients [95] have been identified using SPECT and PET. Compared to conventional bedside autonomic function testing, SPECT and PET are more sensitive and reveal earlier cardiac abnormalities [79]. The observed changes begin distally in the left ventricle, spread in a circumferential pattern, and travel more proximally. The anterior, inferior, and lateral ventricular walls are all involved [79].

A recent study using SPECT revealed that type 1 patients with poor glycemic control had progressive left ventricular dysfunction which could be prevented by good glycemic control [408]. Similar results have been reported using PET as a means of visualizing cardiac autonomic functioning [409]. A preliminary study using SPECT reports a beneficial effect of ARI therapy on left ventricular function [410]. These results have prompted the initiation of a two-year randomized, blinded, placebo-controlled study in type 1 diabetic patients with cardiovascular autonomic neuropathy, using PET as the surrogate marker of sympathetic function.

Summary

In summary, there are several lines of evidence to support the concept that the aldose reductase pathway plays a critical role in the development of diabetic microvascular complications. The interdependent nature of the aldose reductase pathway with other key metabolic cellular functions suggests that aldose reductase expression and activity is instrumental in the developmental of complications. This tenet is further supported by our understanding of the association of aldose reductase gene promoter polymorphisms with the development of chronic diabetic complications. Recent trials using ARI therapy in diabetic peripheral neuropathy prove the clinical efficacy of ARIs but also point up the current drug safety issues. The future challenge lies in the development of ARIs that retain clinical efficacy at doses that are not toxic to patients. Developing these drugs, and using them in well-designed trials with reproducible and meaningful clinical endpoints, will answer the question that has been asked for the last 20 years: Can ARI therapy ameliorate the progression of diabetic peripheral neuropathy?

Nerve Blood Flow

M.A. Cotter, A. Veves, S. Tesfaye, and N.E. Cameron

Introduction

Diabetes mellitus has widespread deleterious effects on the vascular endothelium, leading to damage to both small and large blood vessels in type 1 and type 2 subjects. While microvascular disease is accepted as an important causative factor in the development of the major clinical complications of retinopathy and nephropathy, it is also increasingly recognized as centrally important in the etiology of diabetic neuropathy.

The relation between glycemic control and development of diabetic microangiopathy has been convincingly established in type 1 diabetic patients by the Diabetes Control and Complications Trial [361] and in type 2 diabetic subjects by the United Kingdom Prospective Diabetes Study [411], as well as a large Pima Indian study [412]. Many of the risk factors for development of diabetic complications, including neuropathy, are the same as those for cardiovascular disease, including age, body weight, reduced HDL cholesterol, elevated serum triglycerides, hypertension, and smoking [413–417].

The risk of developing diabetic maculopathy was closely associated with neuropathy and nephropathy as well as with several atherosclerotic risk factors in a large mixed cohort of over 3000 patients with type 1 and type 2 diabetes [418]. The assessment of nerve function involved thermal and vibration sensory tests as well as multiple estimates of autonomic function. In the EURODIAB prospective study, (502 type 1 subjects), nerve conduction velocities in ulnar and sural sensory nerves and the peroneal motor nerve were negatively related to severity of both retinopathy and nephropathy. The authors concluded that even with no clinically detectable diabetic neuropathy, abnormalities in nerve function were strongly correlated with other manifestations of diabetic microvascular disease [419].

While there is no doubt that it is the metabolic disturbances of hyperglycemia (and dyslipidemia) that are the initiating insults, the primary target is the endothelial cell, and thus the manifestations of complications are primarily vascular. The occurrence of vascular changes is detectable very early in the disease process. For type 2 diabetes, reactivity in the skin microcirculation is already diminished at the stage of impaired glucose tolerance before overt diabetes develops [420]. Indeed, it is also evident in the first-degree relatives of type 2 diabetics, even though they have normal glucose tolerance [421]. Elevated plasma levels of von Willebrand factor, a marker of vascular endothelium dysfunction, predict the subsequent development and progression of nephropathy [422] and diabetic neuropathy [423]. A recent study [424] found evidence of increased von Willebrand factor associated with prolonged retinal circulation time and reduced retinal blood flow in type 1 diabetic patients with minimal or no retinopathy. Elevated von Willebrand factor is also a risk factor for macrovascular mortality in type 2 diabetes [425]. Endothelin-1, a potent vasoconstrictor and another marker of endothelial cell activation, was also shown to be increased in first-degree relatives and individuals with impaired glucose tolerance as well as type 2 patients [421].

In the case of large-vessel disease, partial surgical restoration of perfusion, increasing peripheral transcutaneous oxygen, resulted in improved nerve function as assessed by nerve conduction velocity in diabetic patients with no evidence of gangrene as well as in nondiabetic subjects [426,427]. Moreover, in nondiabetic subjects with chronic hypoxemia [428], functional abnormalities such as reduced nerve conduction velocity and increased resistance to ischemic conduction failure were found as well as neurodegenerative changes characteristic of mild diabetic neuropathy.

Thus there is increasingly compelling evidence that diabetic neuropathy should be viewed as another manifestation of the vasculopathy that is most likely the primary consequence of the diabetic state.

Nerve Blood Flow in Diabetic Patients

The invasive nature of accurate measurement of nerve perfusion and its consequence, tissue oxygen tension, has meant that there are relatively few studies that have directly addressed this very important issue.

Measurement of sural nerve blood flow by fluorescein videoangiography [429] confirmed the presence of reduced perfusion in neuropathic subjects. Using

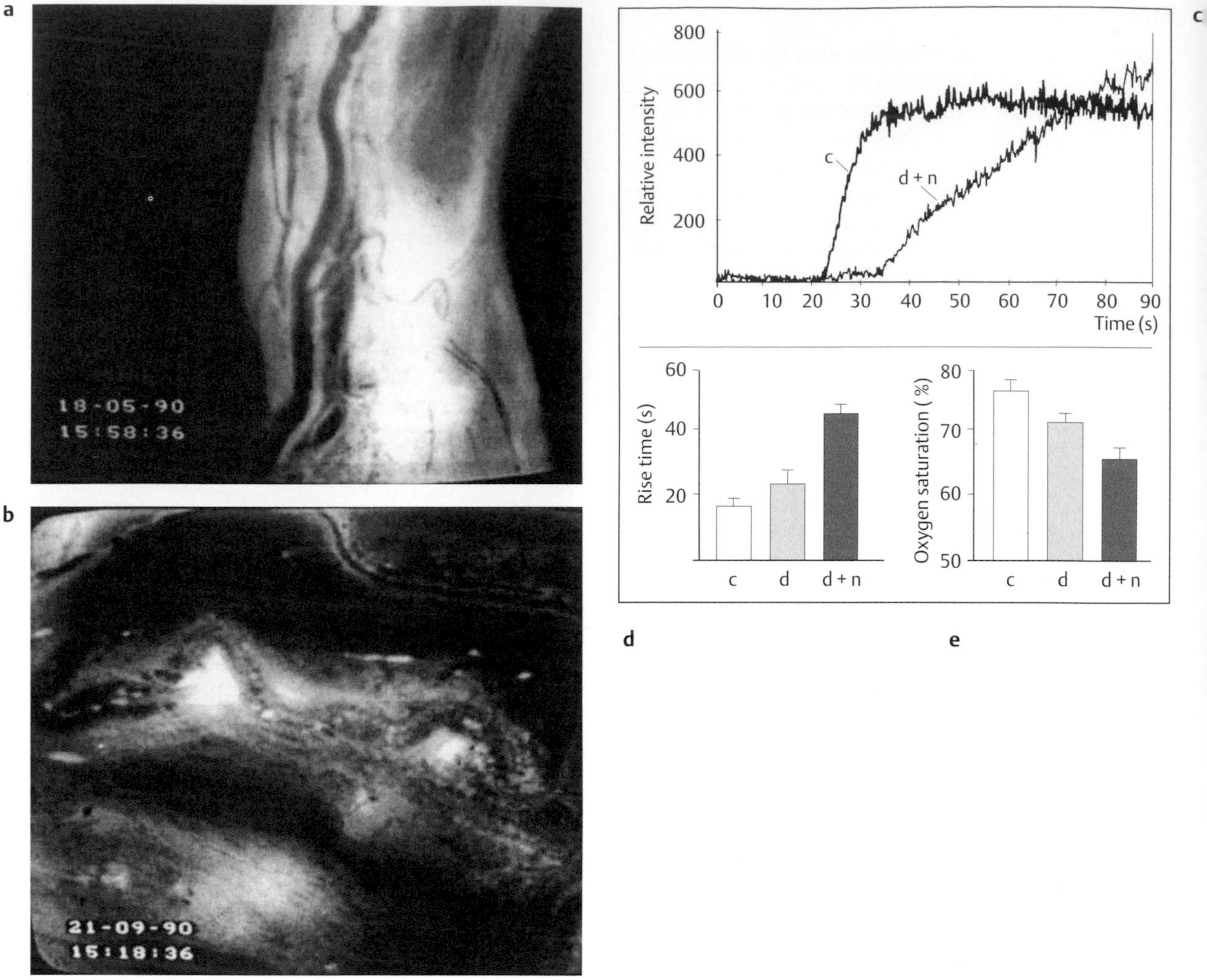

Fig. 4.**16** Fluorescein angiograms of the sural nerve from a nonneuropathic diabetic subject **a** showing normal intensity of fluorescence and a subject with chronic neuropathy **b** showing gross reduction in fluorescence due to impaired blood flow. The timecourse of the appearance of fluorescence **c** was markedly slowed in a neuropathic diabetic subject (d+n) compared with a nondiabetic control subject (c), indicating impaired nerve blood flow. This was reflected in the fluorescein rise time **d** for groups of nondiabetic control (c; $n = 9$), non-neuropathic diabetic (d; $n = 9$) and neuropathic diabetic (d+n; $n = 10$) subjects. The mean sural nerve intravascular oxygen saturation (e) was reduced in diabetic subjects with chronic neuropathy, strongly correlating with the elevation of fluorescein rise time. (From [562], with permission)

microelectrode polarography, Newrick and colleagues [430] demonstrated that the diabetic sural nerve was hypoxic. Furthermore, there was a strong correlation between peroneal motor nerve conduction velocity and leg transcutaneous oxygen tension measurements in type 1 and type 2 patients [431]. The development of combined lightguide spectrophotometry and microendoscopy [432] allows measurement of both intravascular oxygen saturation and blood flow. Comparison was made of sural nerves in a group of mildly to moderately neuropathic patients and in nonneuropathic and nondiabetic subjects. Data are shown in Figure 4.**16** and reveal a significant decrease in oxygen saturation and a near four-fold increase in fluorescein rise time in the neuropathic subjects compared with the nondiabetic control group, suggesting gross impairment of nerve blood flow. There was a doubling of rise time in the group of nonneuropathic patients, although this did not reach significance. Fluorescein rise time, nerve oxygen saturation, glycemic control, and sural nerve sensory nerve conduction velocity showed a strong correlation [432].

An exacerbating factor in the impoverished endoneurial microenvironment is the marked increase in arteriovenous shunting at the level of the epineurial vasculature, diverting blood away from the endoneurial circulation [429]. This, together with parallel changes in skin circulation, results in an endoneurial

PO_2 less than that of the veins [430,433]. Alterations in the distribution of flow between nutritive and shunt vessels may be an early phenomenon since early changes in autonomic innervation of the vascular supply to nerve trunks have been described [36,434,435].

Indirect Measures of Nerve Perfusion

In view of the difficulty of measuring nerve blood flow in humans, some indirect methods of studying perfusion have been utilized. Exercise normally causes a perfusion-dependent increase in nerve temperature, resulting in increased nerve conduction velocity. This response is absent in neuropathic patients [436]. Interestingly, the response to direct limb warming (immersion in 44 °C water) caused comparable increases in sural sensory nerve conduction velocity in diabetic subjects with and without neuropathy, as well as controls, indicating that the lack of an exercise effect in the neuropathic subjects was due to an impaired nerve blood flow response to the normal physiological stressor.

Contralateral cooling of the limbs produces a rapid decrease in blood flow in the ipsilateral limb. This neurovascular reflex arc is dependent on the integrity of small sensory and autonomic nerve fibers and the spinal cord, as well as a normal microcirculatory response. It is impaired in diabetic patients both with and without neuropathy [437].

Nerves in the limbs of diabetic patients are able to maintain electrical impulse conduction for a much longer time after blood supply has been occluded by the application of a sphygmomanometer cuff than those of nondiabetic subjects [438]. This phenomenon of increased resistance to ischemic conduction block is also observed in terms of vibration sensitivity [439,440,441]. Moreover, it is an early phenomenon and can be reversed by restitution of good glycemic control [442,443]. The apparently paradoxical finding of resistance to ischemic conduction block is best explained as an adaptation to chronic endoneurial hypoxia [444,445] by increasing the nerve's ability to utilize anaerobic metabolism. This also renders it better able than nondiabetic nerve to cope with an acute episode of hypoxia. The true impoverished endoneurial microenvironment is revealed when recovery of nerve function *after* ischemic block is studied [441]. Thus, while diabetic patients took twice as long as age-matched controls for their median nerve compound action potential amplitude (CNAP) to fall by 50% and nearly three times longer for their vibratory threshold to be doubled after cuff occlusion, once the cuff was released, in seven minutes restoration of CNAP was complete in nondiabetics but had only reached 75% in the diabetic group. Similarly, half-time for recovery of vibratory threshold was three times longer in the patients with diabetes. Reactive hyperemia, or postischemic hyperemia [446], is a response to hypoxia and the accumulation of vasodilator metabolites. Thus, as with the impaired response to exercise [436], the diabetic limb, including peripheral nerve, is demonstrated to be impaired in terms of its ability to respond appropriately to increased tissue demand for blood flow.

Evidence of Generalized Vascular Impairment

While these studies measured nerve function directly, reactive hyperemia is also used as a tool to study more general aspects of peripheral flow changes in diabetes. The underlying mechanism is flow-mediated vasodilation and is dependent on endothelium-derived NO. When blood flow at the ankle was occluded for four minutes [447], the subsequent hyperemia was reduced in both neuropathic and nonneuropathic diabetic patients. While the nondiabetic controls responded with a doubling of their ankle blood flow, nonneuropaths increased flow by only 33% and neuropaths by only 12%. This was despite the apparent increase in flow in the neuropathic foot at rest, the consequence of sympathetic neuropathy and therefore increased shunt flow. Measurement of brachial artery diameter changes in response to reactive hyperemia revealed reduced responses not only in type 1 [448] and type 2 [421,449] diabetic patients, but also in subjects with impaired glucose tolerance and in first-degree relatives [421]. There were interesting changes in markers of endothelial cell activation. Compared with control subjects, endothelin-1 was significantly higher in all three groups, von Willebrand factor was higher in the diabetic subjects, soluble intercellular adhesion molecule (sICAM) was higher in the impaired glucose tolerance and diabetic groups, and soluble vascular cell adhesion molecule (sVCAM) was elevated in the relatives and the diabetics. Thus, widespread evidence of disturbed endothelial function was seen, even in first-degree relatives [421]. Acute hyperglycemia caused by oral glucose loading was sufficient to cause impairment of endothelium-dependent vasodilation of brachial artery after reactive hyperemia, and this was paralleled by increased production of oxygen free radicals [450]. In patients with type 2 diabetes, a high-fat meal reduced the vasodilatory response by 81%. This gross impairment was associated with increased plasma levels of the endogenous NO synthase inhibitor asymmetric dimethylarginine (ADMA) [451]. ADMA is produced by endothelial cells, among others, and is increased in atherosclerosis [452]. When a subset of the diabetic patients were fed an isocaloric diet without fat, there was no significant effect on either vasodilatory response or ADMA [451].

Skin Blood Flow Changes

Another approach is to study skin microcirculation, especially in view of the association between neuropathy and the diabetic foot [453]. It seems reasonable to suggest that similar changes to those observed at the level of diabetic foot skin will also be present in the nerve. The initial studies used single pointer laser probes [454] and results may be difficult to interpret because of poor repeatability. The maximal hyperemic response to heat is unable to discriminate between endothelium-dependent and endothelium-independent vasodilation. The development of laser scanners that scan a relatively large skin area improved the reliability of skin blood flow measurements considerably. Furthermore, the iontophoresis of acetylcholine and sodium nitroprusside allowed the separate measurement of endothelium-dependent and endothelium-independent vasodilation in the microcirculation. Acetylcholine binds to endothelial receptors, which leads to an increase in endothelial cytosolic Ca^{2+}, activating constitutive endothelial nitric oxide synthase (eNOS) and thus stimulating the release of NO from the endothelial cells. The NO rapidly diffuses to the adjacent smooth muscle, activating guanylate cyclase and causing an increase in cGMP and smooth muscle relaxation. Nitric oxide donors such as sodium nitroprusside bring about vasodilation by a direct effect on the smooth muscle. The impairment of both endothelium-dependent and independent vasodilation is a constant finding in studies from various centers and indicates that diabetes can affect the endothelium and/or the vascular smooth muscle cell [421,455]. In diabetic neuropathic patients, the impairment in response to both acetylcholine and sodium nitroprusside is in contrast to patients with peripheral vascular disease, in whom the major deficit was in the smooth muscle responses [456].

Correspondence Between Pattern of Flow Changes and Risk of Complications

There are marked differences in vascular reactivity between skin areas at low and at high risk of diabetic complications. Measurements of capillary blood cell velocity (by videophotometric capillaroscopy) in the nailfolds of the great toe and the fourth finger in response to arterial occlusion in type 1 diabetics showed reduced capillary flow in the toes during reactive hyperemia. The ratio between capillary blood cell velocity and total skin microcirculation (laser Doppler flux) was reduced in the toes, indicating a maldistribution of blood away from the nutritive capillary supply [457]. Moreover, the deficit in nutritional supply was similar in patients without complications and in those who had complications [458], compatible with it having a causative role in their development. Subsequent studies have shown that even in healthy subjects, endothelium-dependent and endothelium-independent vasodilation are lower at foot level than in the forearm, and that the generalized impairment of the microcirculation in diabetic patients with neuropathy preserves this forearm-foot gradient [459]. The expression of eNOS in the forearm microcirculation is not affected by diabetes or the prediabetic state, despite pronounced functional impairment [460]. In contrast, eNOS expression at foot level was reduced in diabetic neuropathic patients with or without peripheral vascular disease [461]. The predisposition of the foot to vascular vulnerability, which is related to the effects of posture [462], is compounded by autonomic nerve fiber dysfunction, which affects both sympathetic vasoconstrictor tone [463,464] and sympathetic cholinergic function [465]. Moreover, the changes in autonomic function are early phenomena. Significant reduction of the sympathetic vasoconstrictor response to gravity was seen in type 2 patients with no evidence of peripheral neuropathy, progressing to extreme deficits in neuropathic patients with foot ulceration [465]. This loss of the normal postural response would lead to venous stasis and produce profound ischemic effects contributing to the etiology of diabetic neuropathy. In chronic venous insufficiency in nondiabetic subjects, reductions in nerve conduction velocity, reduced thresholds for warm and cold detection, and reduced vibration sensitivity were found [466]. The wide-ranging effects on Aα, Aβ, Aδ, and C fibers reproduce the spectrum of involvement of diabetic neuropathy. Evidence of venous tortuosities and engorgement has been shown in sural nerves of diabetic neuropathic patients [429] as well as in patients who developed insulin neuritis prior to the establishment of an appropriate insulin regime in newly diagnosed type 1 subjects [278].

Interpretation of Flow Changes

There is need for caution in interpreting measurements of blood flow in man. In a model of insulin neuritis, Low and colleagues showed in rat nerve that, while insulin increased total flow, it reduced endoneurial flow to such an extent that the nerve became hypoxic [467], thus providing an explanation for the sometimes devastating consequences of instigating rigorous glycemic control. The differential effects on shunt flow and nutritional flow, which can be monitored with the hydrogen clearance technique in animal models, is not available for measures of flow performed in human subjects. Thus, apparent increases in total flow have to be interpreted carefully, since if all the flow is going through shunts, as may occur in some end-stage neuropaths, the interpretation of the results may be misleading. The potential pitfalls of clinical evaluation of peripheral blood supply have been reviewed [468].

Nerve Axon Reflex

Diabetic neuropathy can also directly affect the microcirculation through the impairment of the nerve axon reflex. Normally, stimulation of the nociceptive C fiber results in both orthodromic conduction to the spinal cord and antidromic conduction to other axon branches, that is, the axon reflex. One function of this reflex is the secretion of several active peptides, such as substance P and calcitonin gene-related peptide, which cause vasodilation and increased permeability both directly and indirectly (through mast cell release of histamine). This neurogenic vasodilatory response accounts for approximately one-third of the total endothelium-dependent vasodilation at both forearm and foot level. Therefore, the presence of peripheral neuropathy further reduces the hyperemic response when it is most needed, that is, under conditions of injury and inflammation, and render the neuropathic foot functionally ischemic even in the absence of arterial occlusive disease [456,469,470].

Blood Vessel Morphology in Diabetic Nerves

A number of studies have shown thickening of the basement membrane in endoneurial capillaries in nerves from diabetic subjects due to reduplication of the basal lamina [24,27,471]. Such changes would increase the average diffusion distance for oxygen and nutrients to axons and Schwann cells. Endothelial cell hyperplasia [472] and swelling into the lumen sufficient to cause occlusion [30,33], as well as thrombosis [32], have all been demonstrated in nerve biopsies from diabetic subjects. In another interesting parallel with microvascular changes in the eye, a loss of pericytes was also found in vessels of diabetic nerve [471]. The severity of the microvascular changes was associated with the degree of diabetic peripheral neuropathy [24,27]. Crucially, the vascular changes preceded the development of peripheral neuropathy [471].

Structural changes to the blood vessels within the nerve reflect the final pathology; it is the epineurial and transperineurial arterioles that control endoneurial flow, so these are the most likely sites of the initial physiological insult mediating impaired perfusion that would be followed by structural changes. Moreover, they are well supplied by unmyelinated fibers with varicosities containing a number of distinct vesicles, suggestive of their role in neurogenic control of endoneurial flow [473]. Despite the obvious importance of these vessels, there have been few studies in human diabetic nerve. However, it has been demonstrated that the intimal area and the number of nuclei in epineurial arteries are increased in nerves from neuropathic diabetic subjects compared with control subjects [34]. Endothelial cell hyperplasia and hypertrophy, reducing lumen size, have also been reported [474]. In addition, innervation of epineurial and transperineurial arterioles was reduced [36,475], particularly for the smaller vessels most involved in determining vascular resistance. This denervation of vessels could contribute to both the reduced endoneurial blood flow and the increased epineurial arteriovenous shunting seen in diabetic neuropathic patients [429]. Similar structural changes are found in the blood vessels of nerves from patients with nondiabetic atherosclerotic peripheral vascular disease [476].

Superfusion of vasa nervorum with drug solutions in animal models primarily targets the epi-/perineurial resistance vessels. Reactivity to vasoconstrictors such as norepinephrine is markedly increased (30-fold greater) even after relatively short durations of diabetes. This is largely due to defective endothelium-derived vasodilation, particularly impaired NO production [477,478]. Acute effects of intra-arterial injection of norepinephrine in type 2 diabetic subjects revealed a marked reduction in nerve conduction in the diabetic subjects but no effect in control subjects, indicating greater sensitivity to its vasoconstrictor effects in type 2 diabetes [479].

Treatments to Test the Vascular Hypothesis in Peripheral Diabetic Neuropathy

If impaired endoneurial perfusion is central to the etiology of diabetic neuropathy, then vasodilators would be expected to have some beneficial effects in patients. In experimental diabetes, where invasive measurements of blood flow can be performed relatively easily, the reduction in endoneurial perfusion is a very early phenomenon, occurring within one week of chemical induction of the hyperglycemic state [480]. Vasodilators of every major class have been shown to be effective in preventing and reversing nerve perfusion and functional abnormalities, including nerve conduction velocity slowing, resistance to ischemic conduction block, and impaired nerve regeneration [481]. Drug treatments which manipulate the angiotensin system—ACE inhibitors [482] or angiotensin II AT_1 receptor antagonists [227,483]—are particularly effective in experimental diabetes. This may be related to up-regulation of the angiotensin system by hyperglycemia, since neither acute nor chronic use of ACE inhibitors or AT_1 receptor antagonists had any effect on vasa nervorum blood flow of nondiabetic rats, but both had considerable effects in animals that had been diabetic for several months [227,483]. This contrasts with other vasodilators such as α_1-adrenergic antagonists, β_2 agonists, or nitrodilators which increased flow in both nondiabetic and diabetic nerve [484,485]. Local vascular and circulating ACE levels are elevated in diabetic patients [226].

Small, short-term, open-label trials of ACE inhibitor effects on nerve function in diabetic subjects gave encouraging results [486,487]. Improvements in quantitative sensory tests and increased nerve conduction velocity were found. Increased parasympathetic activity was reported in patients with diabetic autonomic neuropathy given quinapril [488]. In a placebo-controlled study over 12 months, it was shown that trandalopril produced significant effects in halting progression of neuropathy [489]. None of the studies used high doses of the ACE inhibitors, near the bottom of the dose-response curve for reversal of nerve conduction deficits in diabetic rats [490]. This is illustrated for lisinopril in Figure 4.**17**. Improvements in endothelial function in type 1 [448,491], type 2 [449], and mixed groups of diabetic patients [492] have been reported

Presence of Nerve Ischemia in Diabetic Neuropathy

Experimental Diabetic Neuropathy

Ischemia results in the generation of hypoxanthine from ATP, NADPH (the cofactor), and conversion of the inactive enzyme to xanthine oxidase [604, 605]. The diabetic state and endoneurial ischemia increase lipolysis resulting in an increase in ω-6 fatty acids, such as linoleic acid or arachidonic acid [606], whose peroxidation results in 4-hydroxynonenal, an aldehydic product of membrane lipid peroxidation, and causes prominent cytotoxic effects in cultured endothelial cells, manifested by morphological changes, diminished cellular viability, and impaired endothelial barrier function [607]. 4-Hydroxynonenal has relatively long half-life within cells (minutes to hours), allowing multiple interactions with cellular components [608]. It impairs glutamate transport and mitochondrial function in neurons [609] and mediates oxidative stress-induced neuronal apoptosis [610].

Human Diabetic Neuropathy

Three pathologic alterations—increased intercapillary distance [24,611], thickening of capillary wall and basal lamina, and multifocal fiber loss [1]—suggest ischemic fiber degeneration. More direct evidence of endoneurial ischemia and hypoxia is also available. Oxygen tension is reduced in human diabetic neuropathy [430]. Nerve photography and fluorescein angiography demonstrated delayed fluorescein appearance time and intensity of fluorescence in human diabetic neuropathy [612]. These investigators demonstrated direct epineurial arteriovenous shunting in the majority of diabetic neuropathic patients they studied. A novel approach using microlightguide spectrophotometry to measure intravascular oxygen saturation and blood flow in human sural nerve after an intravenous injection of sodium fluorescein has confirmed impaired nerve blood flow and tissue deoxygenation. There was a correlation between rise time, nerve oxygen saturation, glycemic control, and sural nerve sensory conduction velocity [613].

Excessive Lipolysis and γ-Linolenic Acid Deficiency

The diabetic state and endoneurial ischemia increase lipolysis, resulting in an increase in ω-6 fatty acids, such as linoleic acid or arachidonic acid [606], whose peroxidation results in 4-hydroxynonenal [607] (discussed above). Malondialdehyde is also generated in the cyclooxygenase pathway. In the treatment of experimental diabetic neuropathy with GLA, correction of conduction deficit [614] occurred pari passu with correction of deficits in blood flow and oxygen tension [615]. Cameron and Cotter demonstrated synergism between threshold doses of GLA and ARI and between GLA and antioxidant [558] in reversing the neurovascular and conduction deficits in experimental diabetic neuropathy. They also reported synergism between GLA and ascorbate [504].

Auto-oxidative Lipid Peroxidation

Hyperglycemia, by a process of auto-oxidation, in the presence of decompartmentalized, redox-active trace transitional metals, can generate highly reactive oxidants and result in lipid peroxidation [616]. We have demonstrated, using an in vitro lipid peroxidation model (ascorbate-iron-EDTA preparation), that a high-glucose medium will result in lipid peroxidation in vitro of brain and sciatic nerve. The addition of 20-mM glucose to the incubation medium increased lipid peroxidation four-fold, confirming rapid and marked glucose-mediated auto-oxidative lipid peroxidation [617]. These studies confirm the observation in plasma of auto-oxidative glycation/oxidation [618,619]. Glucose auto-oxidation results in the production of protein-reactive ketoaldehydes, hydrogen peroxide, and other highly reactive oxidants, and the fragmentation of proteins (indicative of free radical mechanisms).

AGE-RAGE-NF-κB

Chronic hyperglycemia results in the generation of advanced glycosylation endproducts (AGE) [620]. Binding of AGE to its receptor (RAGE) results in the activation of NF-κB [621] and the generation of ROS and an inflammatory response [622]. There is induction of specific DNA binding activity for NF-κB in the VCAM-1 promoter region. The necessity for RAGE and the role of ROS was demonstrated by a block of this induction by anti-RAGE IgG or *N*-acetylcysteine (GSH donor). The application of this finding to humans is supported by the finding that peripheral blood mononuclear cells isolated from patients with diabetic nephropathy show increased activation of NF-κB [623]. There is a vicious cycle with AGE producing superoxide, superoxide accelerating AGE generation, and AGE quenching NO [624]. In experimental diabetic neuropathy studied over six months, lipoic acid normalized nerve conduction and nerve perfusion in a dose-dependent manner [219]. Cameron et al. [625] demonstrated that aminoguanidine improved nerve conduction without an effect on polyol pathway metabolites and surmised that its effect was vascular.

Polyol Pathway Overactivity Generates ROS

Polyol pathway overactivity generates ROS in a number of ways. Depletion in NADPH results in NO deficiency and an increase in leukocyte superoxide anion generation (see above). Since NADPH is also required for the regeneration of GSH, its depletion results in a reduction of GSH [626]. Sorbitol dehydrogenase, the second enzyme in the polyol pathway that converts sorbitol to fructose, also contributes to oxidative stress, most likely because depletion of its cofactor

NAD$^+$ leads to more glucose being channeled through the polyol pathway [626]. Polyol pathway overactivity results in reductions in *myo*-inositol and taurine. The latter is a potent antioxidant, and its depletion [367] further contributes to oxidative stress.

Endoneurial NO deficiency has a number of important consequences in microvasculature. It normally inhibits expression of P-selectin, ICAM-1, VCAM-1, and other adhesion molecules [600], a mechanism that is mediated through inhibition of protein kinase C and by preventing the activation of NF-κB [601]. NO also inhibits the cytoassembly of NADPH oxidase [602], thereby attenuating the release of superoxide by leukocytes [603]. Inhibition of NO, therefore, explains a number of changes seen in experimental diabetic neuropathy (expression of adhesion molecules, NF-κB activation, cytokine expression, and superoxide anion generation).

Protein Kinase C

While the activity of PKC in nerve is uncertain, it is known that inhibition of PKC-β will reduce oxidative stress [627] and will normalize the deficits in blood flow and nerve conduction [234]. In endothelial cell, high glucose causes NF-κB activation. Coincubation with a selective PKC inhibitor, calphostin C, produced a concentration-dependent inhibition of glucose-induced NF-κB activation, suggesting that PKC is important at the endothelial cell level in the activation of adhesion molecules and generation of ROS.

Growth Factor Deficit

Lipid peroxidation is aggravated by a reduction in nerve growth factor [253]. Nerve growth factor reduction will reduce, and its administration will restore, glutathione peroxidase and catalase [628,629].

Inflammatory Response

The main sources of ROS in mammals are the leukocyte and the mitochondrion. The quantitative role of the leukocyte, cytokines, and of catecholamine oxidation in diabetic nerve is uncertain. Leukocytic infiltration is not a feature in most cases of experimental diabetic neuropathy. In human diabetic neuropathy, there are some suggestions of an immune-mediated process, as suggested by the presence of iritis and inflammatory infiltrates in sympathetic ganglia [630]. Some forms of diabetic neuropathy, such as acute autonomic neuropathy and the subacute proximal neuropathies, might be associated with prominent round cell infiltration. A role of associated ROS and oxidative stress should be considered.

Changes in Pro-oxidant Status

Altered pro-oxidant status occurs in the diabetic state, with an increase in polyunsaturated fatty acids increasing arachidonic acid [606]. With ischemia, superoxide anion is converted to H_2O_2, but its further decomposition, which is mediated by glutathione peroxidase [631], may be compromised if the low content of this enzyme is further reduced. 4-Hydroxynonenal, an aldehydic product of membrane lipid peroxidation, is especially pertinent in that ischemia, by increasing arachidonic acid, provides substrate for 4-hydroxynonenal [608], which mediates neuronal apoptosis [610]. The occurrence of other alterations, especially increases in free iron and copper, has been proposed, but definitive evidence has not yet appeared.

Neural Targets of Oxidant Stress

The focus of investigations has been on nerve trunk. Recent emphasis has been based on the realization that human diabetic neuropathy is primarily a distal and sensory neuropathy, and emphasis has shifted to the sensory neuron and nerve terminals. In humans, skin biopsy studies of epidermal axons comprising unmyelinated sensory fibers have indeed demonstrated that these alterations precede and are more pronounced than changes seen in nerve trunk. Functional deficits of unmyelinated fibers also occur before deficits are demonstrable in nerve trunk [632].

Recent studies on spinal roots [633] and dorsal root ganglion have demonstrated the presence of prominent myelin alterations of dorsal and ventral roots after six months of diabetes. Changes in dorsal root ganglion are prominent [555], consisting of vacuolar degeneration. Pigmentary changes are present and are associated with both distal sensory loss [534] and conduction slowing of proximal nerves (including nerve roots). Another recent focus is the Schwann cell as a target in hyperglycemic ischemic nerves. The Schwann cell is suggested to be a target of oxidative stress and its apoptosis responsible for delayed ischemic demyelination [634,635].

The specificity of targets needs to be coupled with specificity of mechanisms. 4-Hydroxynonenal, a highly toxic product of lipid peroxidation, is a potent inhibitor of mitochondrial respiration [636]. 4-Hydroxy-2-nonenal mediates oxidative stress-induced apoptosis of neurons and terminals [610]. It disrupts neuronal calcium homeostasis and perturbs mitochondrial function, resulting in caspase activation. Activated caspases, in turn, induce activation of JNK (c-Jun *N*-terminal kinase), resulting in stimulation of AP-1 DNA-binding protein production [637]. This action of 4-hydroxynonenal can be blocked by GSH, which is reduced in diabetes [534]. More recently, apoptosis of dorsal root ganglion neurons, neuritis, and Schwann cells in vitro and in vivo has been reported in experimental diabetic neuropathy [638].

Synthesis of Pathogenetic Hypothesis

The above information has been synthesized into a pathogenetic model of diabetic neuropathy (Fig. 4.**19**).

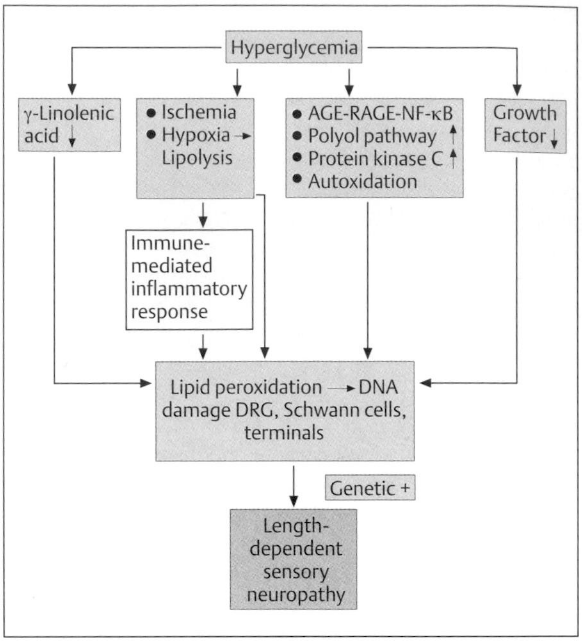

Fig. 4.**19** Role of oxidative stress in the pathogenesis of diabetic neuropathy

Hyperglycemia results in a reduction in nerve blood flow by altering vasoregulation (at the endothelial cell and arteriolar smooth muscle levels) of nerve microvessels and increasing blood viscosity.

Microvascular vasoconstrictor tone is increased (increased α-adrenergic and endothelin tone), and vasodilator tone is reduced (reduced endothelial activities of NO, calcitonin-gene-related peptide [CGRP], and substance P). NO deficiency, in addition to reducing microvascular flow, could enhance expression of adhesion molecules, impair blood-nerve barrier, generate superoxide radical, and activate PKC and NF-κB. Insulin administration could aggravate hypoxia (by increasing arteriovenous shunt flow and reducing nutritive flow). The ensuing endoneurial ischemia and hypoxia with resultant increased lipolysis, hyperglycemia-induced γ-linolenic acid deficiency, AGE generation (with binding to RAGE and NF-κB activation), polyol pathway and PKC overactivity, autooxidation, and growth factor deficiency result in a lipid peroxidation. The diabetic state exacerbates the inflammatory response to ischemia [639]. 4-Hydroxynonenal is particularly important in its ability to cause apoptosis of neurons, their appendages, and support cells. The pathways are simplified and depict all mechanisms as going through oxidative stress and lipid peroxidation. In fact, it is likely that a number of the mechanisms could cause neuropathy by other mechanisms. For instance, PKC increase and polyol pathway overactivity/*myo*-inositol deficiency could work in significant part via Na^+,K^+-ATPase deficiency. Growth factor deficiency could work independently of oxidative stress. The synergism of antioxidants with ARI and GLA suggest that there are significant interactions and synergism between mechanisms.

The targets of lipid peroxidation are probably multiple. Diabetic neuropathy is primarily a distal sensory neuropathy, so it is not surprising that dorsal root ganglion appears to be a key target. Dendrites, nerve terminals, Schwann cells, and microvessels could also be important. Dorsal root ganglion has an especially high concentration of mitochondria because of its high-energy metabolism. As in all tissues with vigorous oxidative metabolism, there is free radical generation and a susceptibility to oxidative damage. The mitochondrion is an important microtarget. Impairment in mitochondrial function is manifested as a reduction in membrane potential, opening of mitochondrial permeability transition pores, and vacuolar and pigmentary degeneration. Mitochondrial DNA is unusually susceptible to oxidative damage. There is normally about 1 % leakage of free radicals. Increased free radical leakage over time leads to increased mutations, as occurs with aging. These dysfunctional mitochondria have increased ROS leakage. A vicious cycle of oxidative damage to inner membrane proteins (of mitochondria) leading to imbalances in the electron transport chain, resulting in increased superoxide and hydrogen peroxide production, which in turn further damages membrane proteins, is suggested. Leakage of cytochrome *c* leads to activation of apoptotic cascade, and cells stain positively for activated caspase 3 and TUNEL. The process is slow, with only modest cell loss of large neurons (apoptosis lente). The physiologic alterations (distal sensory neuropathy, reduced sensory threshold, spontaneous firing) in experimental diabetic neuropathy could be due to the sensory neuropathy and radiculopathy described above.

Concluding Thoughts

In the past decade and a half, a number of pathogenetic advances have been made. First is the validation that glucose is indeed a neurotoxin and that tight glycemic control will prevent target complications. Second is the appreciation that pathogenetic mechanisms are probably interactive and interlinked. The simplistic view of the metabolic versus vascular hypothesis no longer obtains. The major candidate mechanisms are interlaced and may converge. Conversely, synergism appears to exist in methods to treat diabetic neuropathy, e. g., antioxidant with ARI, GLA with antioxidant. Third is the evolving improved understanding of targets of glucotoxicity. Evidence is still patchy, but a major target may be the dorsal root ganglion neurons, in addition to the Schwann cells and terminals. Fourth is a better understanding of molecular pathophysiologic mechanisms, especially in apoptosis.

Neurotrophic Factors

A. Vinik, G. Pittenger, K. Stansberry, T.S. Park, T. Erbas, and M. Skeen

Introduction

Diabetic neuropathy is not a single entity but rather, a number of different syndromes, each with a range of clinical and subclinical manifestations. According to the San Antonio Conference [639a], the main groups of neurological disturbance in diabetes mellitus are: (a) subclinical neuropathy determined by abnormalities in electrodiagnostic and quantitative sensory testing; (b) diffuse clinical neuropathy with distal symmetric sensorimotor and autonomic syndromes; and (c) focal syndromes. The spectrum of clinical neuropathic syndromes described in patients with diabetes mellitus includes dysfunction of almost every segment of the somatic peripheral and autonomic nervous system. Each syndrome can be distinguished by its pathophysiologic, therapeutic, and prognostic features. Diabetes may damage small fibers, large fibers, or both. Small-nerve fiber dysfunction usually (although not always) occurs early and is often present before objective signs or electrophysiologic evidence of large-fiber deficit. It is manifested first in the lower limbs, with pain and hyperalgesia, and is followed by loss of thermal sensitivity and reduced light touch and pin prick sensation. In diabetes, a reduction of protein gene product 9.5 (PGP 9.5), substance P, and CGRP in sensory neurons has been shown [640–644]. PGP 9.5 is a neuronal cytoplasmic protein and is found in all types of efferent and afferent nerve fibers. Studies have shown a loss of cutaneous nerve fibers that stain positive for the neuronal antigen PGP 9.5 in small-fiber neuropathy [645–647]. These neurons are dependent on NGF for their integrity and survival [648]. The effect of NGF depletion may be mediated through down-regulation of neurofilament gene expression or RNAs that encode the precursor molecule of substance P or CGRP, both of which are NGF-dependent and down-regulated in diabetes [648].

Large-fiber neuropathies may involve sensory and/or motor nerves. They are manifested by reduced sensitivity to vibration (often the first objective evidence of neuropathy) and position sense, weakness, muscle wasting, and depressed tendon reflexes. Most patients with distal symmetric polyneuropathy (DSPN) have a “mixed” variety with both large and small nerve fiber involvement. In the case of DSPN, a “glove and stocking” distribution of sensory loss is almost universal. Figure 4.**20** illustrates the cross-section of different nerve fibers, the modalities they subserve, and the sites targeted by various growth factors.

The characteristic histopathologic findings in diabetic neuropathy, which typify the disease, are axonal degeneration, demyelination, and atrophy. These are accompanied by futile attempts at axonal regeneration, remyelination, and synaptogenesis [649]. While a major focus of investigation has been upon those factors participating in nerve destruction, attention has recently been directed to the role of factors in diabetic neuropathy which may enhance nerve regeneration and protect nerves from programmed cell death and the noxious effects of apoptotic agents in the diabetic milieu. Since neuronal growth factors can promote the survival, maintenance, and regeneration of neurons subject to the noxious effects of diabetes, the success of diabetic patients in maintaining normal nerve morphology and function may ultimately depend on the expression and efficacy of these factors. Many of the neuronal changes characteristic of diabetic neuropathy are similar to those observed following either removal of target-derived growth factors by axotomy, or depletion of endogenous growth factors by experimental induction of growth factor autoimmunity as well as failure of their delivery and transport to the appropriate targets. Selective ablation of high- or low-affinity receptors using elegant molecular biologic techniques in transgenic animals has confirmed and refined our understanding of the role of receptors with differing affinities for certain of the growth factors, and a new awareness of the role of binding and basal lamina proteins has altered our perceptions of the actions of certain ligands. Current concepts of the knowledge of growth factors and their possible role in the pathogenesis of diabetic neuropathy are indicated in Figure 4.**21**.

Throughout life there is an intimate neuron-target interaction which affects the normal functioning, survival, and maintenance of both components. This interaction includes neuronal dependence upon retrograde transport of target-derived growth factors and nonneuronal supporting cells. In the cell body, these growth factors regulate neuronal gene expression and protein synthesis, and thereby play a role in cell

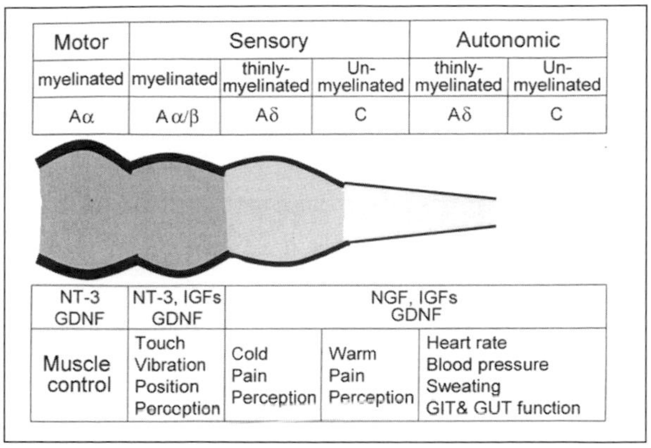

Fig. 4.**20** Peripheral nervous system, nerve fiber types, and the potential growth factors responsible for the integrity of the different fiber types

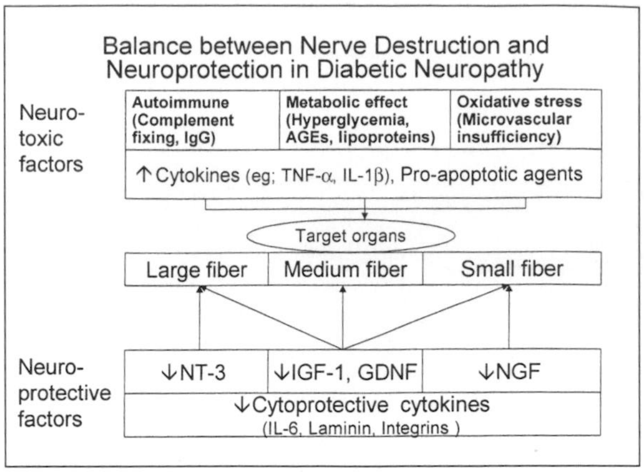

Fig. 4.**21** Pathways to nerve damage in diabetes, the types of nerve fiber involved, and the potential for neuroprotection by growth factors, integrins, and cytokines

survival, maintenance, and function. Moreover, during development or following axonal injury, a variety of growth factors enhance axonal growth. The major growth factors considered here are the neurotrophin family, which includes NGF, insulin, IGFs, basal laminar proteins such as laminin and the saposins, cytokines, and endogenous growth factor-releasing agents. The basic neurotrophic factor concept is defined by the hypothesis that trophic proteins are synthesized in target tissues and delivered via retrograde transport to the neuronal soma, where they exert a trophic and survival effect [650]. The growth factors and cytokines are a varied group of polypeptides produced by different cell types and show overlapping actions. Growth factors appear to be constitutively produced whereas cytokines are inducible.

The Family of Nerve Growth Factors

NGF, discovered nearly 50 years ago, is the most thoroughly studied of a growing list of growth promoting proteins. It has been known since the pioneering work of Levi-Montalcini [651] that neural crest-derived cells, sympathetic neurons, and dorsal root ganglion (DRG) neurons, are developmentally dependent on NGF. More recently, it has been shown that adult DRG and sympathetic neurons, both populations of neurons affected in diabetic neuropathy, are dependent on NGF for either their maintenance [649] or their survival [652].

Following sciatic nerve section in normal adult rats, a significant number of the axotomized neurons in the involved DRGs die [649,653,654]. This cell loss can be completely eliminated by the application of exogenous NGF to the cut proximal end of the nerve [652]. Moreover, those DRG neurons that do not die following sciatic nerve section [652] or in vivo NGF depletion [649] exhibit significant atrophy of their cell bodies and axons. This atrophy is at least partially reversed by the application of exogenous NGF [652].

NGF is also an important regulator of substance P synthesis in adult DRG neurons [655,656]. Substance P is found in the sympathetic nervous system as well as in a subpopulation of DRG neurons. It has been implicated in diverse and widespread activities including vasodilatation, gut motility, and nociception, all of which are perturbed in diabetic neuropathy. Lindsay and Harmar [656] have shown that NGF is involved in the regulation of mRNAs that encode the precursor molecules of substance P and CGRP. In vitro NGF deprivation caused cultured adult DRG neurons to down-regulate substance P and CGRP precursor molecule mRNA [656]. Moreover, when adult rats were immunized against mouse NGF—a procedure which caused an autoimmune depletion of NGF—substance P levels were reduced in the DRG, spinal cord, and skin by approximately 65% [655]. Calcutt and colleagues [657] concluded that in streptozotocin-induced diabetic rats a selective down-regulation of substance P precursor gene expression was due to a decline in retrogradely transported NGF reaching the ganglia, which in turn could explain the reduction in substance P synthesis and transport found in diabetic rats. It remains to be established, however, whether the reduction in substance P is pertinent to the symptom complex of neuropathy.

A number of functional disturbances are found in the dermal microvasculature of diabetic subjects. These include (1) decreased microvascular blood flow, (2) increased vascular resistance, (3) decreased tissue Po_2, and (4) altered vascular permeability characteristics, such as loss of the anionic charge barrier and decreased charge selectivity. Decreased microvascular blood flow and increased vascular resistance in diabetes could result from alterations in dermal neurovascular function, such as impaired dilator responses to substance P, CGRP, and reactivity to nociceptive stimulation. Diabetes also disrupts vasomotion, the rhythmic contraction exhibited by arterioles and small arteries [658,659]. Unmyelinated C fibers, which constitute the central reflex pathway, are assumed to be damaged in diabetic neuropathy, contributing to abnormalities in cutaneous blood flow [660]. These neurons are dependent on NGF for their integrity and survival [652,661]. The effect of NGF depletion may be mediated through down-regulation of neurofilament gene expression or RNAs that encode the precursor molecule of substance P or CGRP, both of which are NGF-dependent and down-regulated in diabetes [661] (Fig. 4.**22**).

Neurotrophin Receptors

It has recently been established that NGF belongs to a gene family encoding structurally and functionally related proteins called neurotrophins. The neurotrophin family includes NGF, brain-derived neurotrophic factor (BDNF), neurotrophin-3 (NT-3), NT-4, and NT-5 (Fig. 4.**23**).

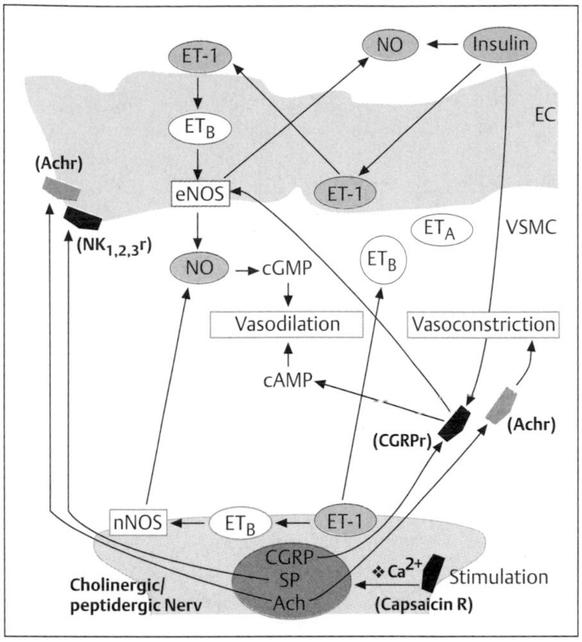

Fig. 4.22 The important role of neuropeptides regulating the microvascular system. Loss of the neurotrophic effects of NGF is accompanied by reduction in substance P (SP) and CGRP, vasodilators acting via the generation of nitric oxide (NO), leaving unopposed actions of the vasoconstrictors such as endothelin-1, (ET-1 acting through endothelin receptors, ET_A and ET_B), thereby compromising skin blood flow as well as contributing to nerve ischemia. In a normal blood vessel, endothelial cell agonists such as ADP and bradykinin (BK), acting via specific cell receptors, increase the release of NO, via the activation of endothelial cell NO synthase (eNOS). Mechanical forces, such as stretch and shear, acting through as yet not well-defined mechanoreceptors, produce a similar effect. Once formed, NO may pass into the vascular smooth muscle, where it promotes vasodilatation and decreases proliferation, or towards the vessel lumen, where it acts to decrease platelet and white blood cell adhesion and, possibly, aggregation. ET-1 may diffuse into the vascular smooth muscle, where it promotes vasoconstriction and cell proliferation. In a diseased vessel in diabetes, eNOS and endothelial production of NO may be compromised, thereby increasing the effectiveness of the vasoconstrictor ET-1 [717,718]. Also shown is the direct vasodilatory action of insulin and how insulinopenia and/or insulin resistance may contribute to the effects of loss of neurotrophism

These proteins have diverse actions on distinct populations of developing neurons [664–669]. Neurotrophins bind two classes of receptors: tyrosine receptor kinases, or trks (trkA, trkB, trkC), and a low-affinity receptor, p75 [670–673] . Functionally the trks contribute to high-affinity neurotrophin binding, subserve signal transduction, and largely mediate the biological actions of neurotrophins. In contrast, p75 (a 75-kDa glycoprotein) has been identified as a low-affinity receptor for NGF. It was initially thought only to participate in forming the functional NGF receptor and to alter the binding affinity of trkA for NGF [670–673]. It is, however, widely expressed by nonneuronal

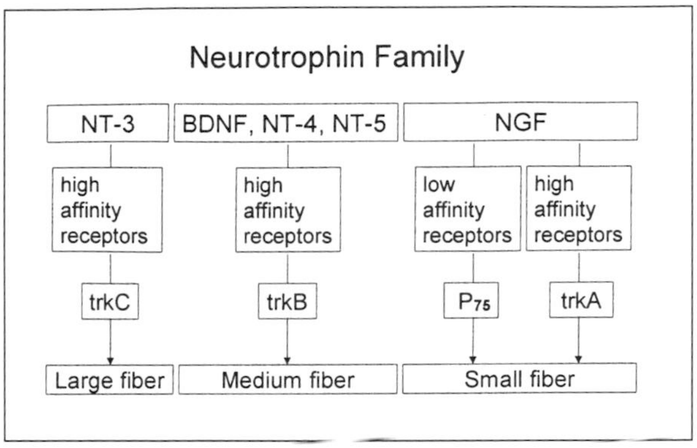

Fig. 4.23 The neurotrophin family of peptides, their receptors, and the nerve fibers targeted

peripheral tissues such as Schwann cells and increases following nerve injury.

In a study of the role of p75 in neuronal development, knockout of the p75 locus in mice was found to result in loss of small sensory ganglia, decreased pain sensitivity, and cutaneous innervation [674]. Sympathetic innervation of superior cervical ganglion targeting the iris and salivary glands was not affected [674]. Striking abnormalities in the pineal gland and the sweat glands were also found. A null mutation of p75 also caused a decrease in tyrosine hydroxylase in the pineal gland and the footpad, which was accompanied by a reduction in pain sensitivity and impaired sweating. Furthermore, the neuronal defect in p75 mutants was not due to a direct deleterious effect on the target organ, but rather was due to a failure of its development. It is not known how p75 receptor expression supports axonal growth, but it might guide developing axons or facilitate the actions of the neurotrophins at the target level. p75 interacts with the high-affinity trk receptors to enhance their sensitivity to neurotrophins. Whatever the case, it is apparent that the low-affinity neurotrophin receptor is essential to the integrity of small nerve fibers involved in pain, warm thermal perception, and sweating and as such constitutes an important target for corrective therapy in diabetic neuropathy.

Contrasting with the role of the low-affinity receptor for neurotrophins in sensory and autonomic function, it seems that the high-affinity trks may subserve motor and coordinating functions. Rüdiger Klein and colleagues [675] examined the role of the trkC gene, which is expressed throughout the mammalian nervous system and encodes a series of protein kinase isoforms that serve as receptors for NT-3 [673,676–681]. One of these isoforms, $gp145^{trkC}$/trkC K1, mediates the trophic properties of NT-3 in cultured cells. The homozygous trkC mutant mice appeared normal at birth, but they grew poorly and most of them died soon after birth. Those animals that survived demonstrated motor deficits and develop athetotic movements. The *trk*C mutants do, however, take nourishment and respond to painful stimuli in their whisker pads.

In contrast to mice that lack trkC, mice defective in trkB receptors [682] lose pain perception, as do mice that lack trkA. Smeyne and colleagues [683] studied the role of trks in vivo, by ablating the gene in embryonic stem cells by homologous recombination. Mice lacking trkC were found to have a severe sensory and sympathetic neuropathy and most died within one month of birth. They were found to have extensive neuronal loss in the trigeminal, sympathetic, and dorsal root ganglia, as well as a decrease in the cholinergic basal forebrain projections to the hippocampus and cortex. NGF induces neuron outgrowth and promotes survival of embryonic sensory and sympathetic neurons in culture, decreases the extent of naturally occurring cell death in developing sympathetic ganglia, and protects cholinergic neurons of the basal forebrain, putamen, and caudate [684–686]. Behaviorally, the animals show reduced sensitivity to vibration and painful stimuli and have myotic pupils and ptosis. Therefore, these findings were thought to demonstrate that trkA is the primary mediator of the trophic actions of NGF in vivo, at least for certain sensory pathways [684–686]. Hence, the signaling pathway for neurotrophins via their high-affinity receptors plays a crucial role in the development of both the peripheral and the central nervous system.

The transgenic mouse ablation experiments have provided a sophisticated model for the study of the importance of these growth factors and their receptors in various regions and the functioning of the nervous system. The diverse nature of the manifestations of the neurologic deficiencies in these transgenic animals is of great interest to any diabetologist familiar with the heterogeneity of diabetic polyneuropathy, and begins to shed light on the possible mechanisms whereby there is variable expression of the deficits in motor, sensory, and autonomic nerve function in different individuals. They further suggest that therapies will have to be tailored to the individual needs of patients with diabetic neuropathy.

Nerve Growth Factor in Diabetes

Data suggest that a decline in NGF synthesis in diabetes has a role in diabetic neuropathy. NGF levels in streptozotocin (STZ)-induced diabetic rats are dramatically reduced in the superior cervical ganglion, an NGF-dependent population of neurons [687]. Hellweg and colleagues [688] have shown retrograde transport of NGF in the sciatic nerve to be reduced in STZ-induced diabetic rats. Decreased retrograde NGF transport in axons of the STZ-induced diabetic rat ileal mesenteric nerves has also been reported [653], preceding the development of frank distal axonopathy. It seems reasonable to suspect that perturbations in NGF availability in some way contribute to the development of diabetic neuropathy. Perturbations of pain sensation are characteristic of diabetic neuropathy, and the levels of substance P, a nociceptive transmitter, are reduced in diabetic rats in parallel with increased tolerance to pain [689]. In addition, the amount of anterogradely transported substance P was reduced in STZ-induced diabetic rats [689,690]. Treatment with the ARI sorbinil, or its combination with gangliosides, increases the amount of substance P transported in sciatic nerves of diabetic rats and is accompanied by pain hypersensitivity [689,690]. This suggests that by increasing substance P production and transport, NGF may restore disordered pain perception towards normal in diabetic neuropathy.

In normal skin, NGF is produced by basal keratinocytes and acts via its high-affinity receptor (trk A) on nociceptor nerve fibers to increase their sensitivity, particularly in inflammation [691]. In vitro studies show that keratinocytes express both NGF and its high-affinity receptor, trkA, and that NGF may increase keratinocyte proliferation and its own expression via an autocrine loop [692]. A recent study suggests a correlation between NGF expression in skin and the early onset of small-fiber neuropathy. Diabetic subjects without symptomatic neuropathy were found to have an early dysfunction of small-fiber sensory and autonomic fibers as measured by temperature sensitivity and capsaicin-induced axon reflex vasodilation. NGF is reduced in epidermal keratinocytes in human diabetic skin, and this decrease has been related to dysfunction of cutaneous sensory fibers. These data can be interpreted to suggest that abnormal availability of target-derived NGF may be responsible in part for early small-fiber neuropathy [693] (Fig. 4.**24**).

Alterations in endogenous blood concentrations of NGF may be associated with hyperglycemia and/or diabetes and may be relevant to the development of neuropathy. Hellweg and colleagues [688] found that endogenous NGF concentrations were low in STZ-diabetic rats and could be restored by allogenic islet transplantation [694]. Similarly, NGF serum concentrations were diminished and tissue content was decreased in the submaxillary gland and sciatic nerve of mice made diabetic with STZ compared with matched controls [694,695]. Low levels of NGF could be due to both decreased production and decreased transport of NGF in diabetes. In addition, autoimmunity may play a role in the NGF deficiency in diabetes by mechanisms related to immune neutralization of available NGF. There are structural and biochemical similarities between NGF and the insulin family of peptides, and it has been suggested that antibodies to insulin may cross-react with NGF and contribute to an effective reduction in NGF available to nerves, thereby contributing to the development of neuropathy [696]. Since NGF selectively induces tyrosine hydroxylase, and dopamine β-hydroxylase is necessary for the survival of sympathetic nerve fibers [664] and is required for the expression of substance P and CGRP in adult

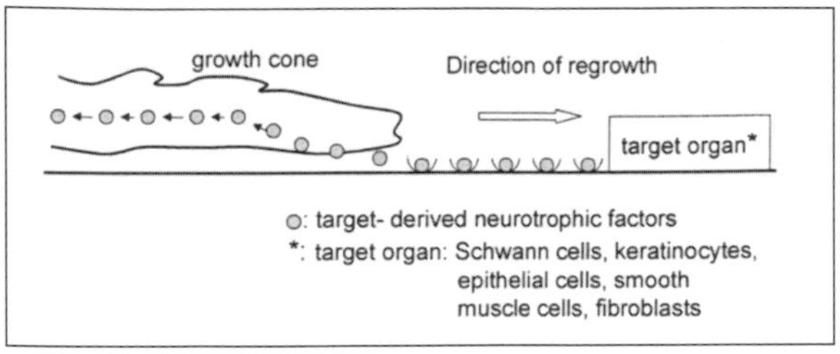

Fig. 4.24 Production of neurotrophic factors in the target cells and retrograde transport of the factor to maintain viability of the cell body

sensory neurons, it is apparent that immune neutralization of NGF could generate a clinical syndrome not unlike that found in diabetic neuropathy [697].

NGF in Treatment of Diabetic Neuropathy

It has now been shown that NGF treatment ameliorates diabetic sensory neuropathy in animals. Apfel and colleagues [698] administered NGF to rats at a dose of 3 µg/g or 5 µg/g three times weekly, starting one week after STZ administration. Reduction in pain sensation was prevented, as was the fall in CGRP in dorsal root ganglia in the untreated diabetic animals. NGF also prevented reduction in levels of another peptide, substance P, in sensory ganglia of diabetic animals. NGF did not, however, prevent the deficit in tibial motor conduction in diabetic rats, suggesting that NGF may be a useful adjunct for the treatment of diabetic sensory and autonomic but not motor neuropathy [699].

Diemel and colleagues [700] have also shown that rats with STZ-induced diabetes are depleted of both substance P and CGRP peptides in the sciatic nerve, as well as having depletion of CGRP and γ-preprotachykinin A mRNA in the fourth and fifth lumbar dorsal root ganglia. Treatment of rats with NGF prevented the deficits in the levels of CGRP and γ-preprotachykinin mRNA as well as normalizing the levels of CGRP and substance P peptides in lumbar DRGs. The effects in the diabetic animals were much more marked than those in the nondiabetic animals. There was no response to BDNF. The demonstration that in vivo administration of NGF can reverse the deficits in substance P and CGRP in peripheral sensory neurons of diabetic rats lends support to the notion that deficient expression or response to NGF may be important for development of diabetic neuropathy. The authors further suggest that systemic administration of NGF may be of value in treating the sensory forms of diabetic neuropathy.

Two randomized, placebo-controlled clinical trials of recombinant human NGF (rhNGF) administered to patients with polyneuropathy were initiated. In a phase II clinical trial of rhNGF in 250 patients with diabetic polyneuropathy, improvements in signs and symptoms were seen after treatment with either 0.1 or 0.3 µg/kg body weight rhNGF subcutaneously three times a week for six months. A second phase II trial in 270 patients with HIV-associated sensory neuropathy demonstrated significant improvements in neuropathic pain and sensitivity to pinprick, following 18 weeks of treatment with either 0.1 or 0.3 µg/kg rhNGF twice a week [260]. In addition, both studies suggested that administration of rhNGF was well tolerated, with the exception of self-limited injection site hyperalgesia and other pain-related syndromes. In the phase II trial on the efficacy of NGF in 250 patients with diabetic neuropathy, NGF improved a composite score that included measures of small-fiber function, warm thermal threshold, cooling detection threshold, and nerve impairment scores in the lower limb [701]. As a result of this success, a 48-week randomized, placebo-controlled phase III study of rhNGF in a dose of 0.1 µg/kg ($n = 504$) or placebo ($n = 515$) given subcutaneously three times a week was carried out. The primary outcome measure was change in baseline on the Neuropathy Impairment Score for the lower limbs. Secondary outcome measures included quantitative sensory test using the Case IV device, Neuropathy Symptom and Change score, and the patient benefit questionnaire. Nerve conduction studies were also performed and the incidence of foot ulcers was observed. Eighty-three percent of patients in the treatment arm completed the study, compared with 90% of the placebo group. rhNGF induced significant injection site hyperalgesia, which made true blinding difficult, and there was no significant difference in the primary outcome ($P = 0.25$). Furthermore, rhNGF did not induce significant improvement in the secondary endpoints. However, there were significant, albeit modest, improvements in the global assessment scores ($P < 0.03$) and 2 of 32 comparisons in improvement in global symptoms ($P = 0.05$ for leg pain; $P = 0.003$ for 6 months symptoms in the hands and feet). The reasons for these poor results compared with the phase II study are not entirely clear. We noted a surprising lack of progression in neuropathy in the placebo-treated group, suggesting that modern management of patients with diabetes has resulted in a change in the natural history of the condition, dictating a more robust endpoint and possibly longer duration studies. If the effect of rhNGF is not robust, and if all it can do is prevent the progression of neuropathy, it would not be possible to show an effect in a one-year trial. Among the possible other reasons for the conflicting data between the phase II [701] and this phase III study [702] were possible differences in the dose, concentration, and preparation of NGF, choice of endpoints, measurements of neuropathy (no direct estimation of small-fiber changes in the skin were made), and patient populations. With the recent developments of improved methods for identifying C fibers in skin by immunohistochemistry, quantification of nerve fiber density using the panneuronal marker

PGP-9.5 [703–760,644], and functional tests of C fiber integrity [660,705], it might be possible to overcome the endpoint limitations inherent in the study design and rescue NGF from a premature demise as a therapeutic agent in diabetic neuropathy.

Insulin and IGFs as Neurotrophic Factors

IGFs, which share structural homology with insulin, are widely distributed throughout the nervous system and exert profound effects on developing neurons. IGF-I and IGF-II are well-characterized growth factors that have been implicated in the growth and differentiation of neurons. Both IGF-I and IGF-II promote neurite outgrowth of neuroblastoma cells in vitro [706], and IGF-I has been implicated in the survival and differentiation of fetal rat brain neurons in culture [706]. The liver is the predominant source of serum IGF-I in rats [707,708], and hepatic IGF-I [709–711] and IGF-I mRNA [712,713] are greatly reduced in diabetes. This reduction apparently precedes the impairment of conduction velocity in spinal cord and peripheral nerves [714]. Plasma concentrations of IGF-II, unlike IGF-I, are not regulated by insulin. Fetal concentrations of IGF-II are high and correlate well with tissue differentiation and development including nervous system maturation, but serum concentrations fall before birth and remain fairly constant postnatally. Metabolic perturbations such as are caused by diabetes can reduce circulating levels of IGF-II further [715].

In contrast to IGF-I, the major sites of production and secretion of circulating IGF-II in the postnatal animal are the choroid plexus and leptomeninges [716,717]. mRNA for IGF-II also exists primarily in nervous tissue in the adult [718,719]. Using solution hybridization-ribonuclease protection assays, IGF-II mRNA has been found to be abundant in glia separated from neurons by culture techniques, whereas IGF-I mRNA has been found in both neurons and glia [720]. Other investigators have reported IGF-II mRNA and protein in neurons using in situ hybridization and immunohistochemical analysis.

The relative contribution of locally synthesized IGFs versus circulating IGFs in nervous system function has not been determined. It is probable that spinal cord ganglia and peripheral nerves may be dependent, not on circulating levels of IGFs, but rather on locally produced IGFs. Whether acting via paracrine, autocrine, or endocrine mechanisms, the rationale for implicating IGFs in diabetic neuropathy comes from several lines of research. To discuss all of these would be beyond the scope of this review. However, the following observations generally constitute the basis for the belief that IGFs play an integral part in normal nervous system function and a possible major role in the nerve impairments observed in diabetes: (1) IGFs in nervous tissue are regulated by insulin; (2) IGF receptors are present in the appropriate tissues (i. e., neurons, Schwann cells, ganglia) involved in diabetes-associated nerve disorders; (3) IGFs exert numerous effects on nervous tissue growth and function, including indirect effects such as those mediated through NGF; and (4) IGF-binding proteins (IGF-BPs) are present in the nervous system, are regulated by insulin and glycemic state, and have been shown to modulate IGF action in nervous tissue.

Insulin Regulation of IGFs

IGF-I mRNA in spinal cord is significantly reduced at one and two weeks after induction of diabetes in rats by STZ [721]. The reduction in IGF-I and IGF-II mRNAs in diabetic sciatic nerves can be prevented by insulin infusion [264]. Others report that insulin treatment can restore, in part, IGF-I mRNA levels in some, but not all tissues [722,723]. In contrast, serum IGF-II levels are not really altered in diabetes [724–726], and intensive insulin therapy does not seem to alter these levels [724]. However, insulin has been shown to regulate expression of IGF-II mRNA in nervous tissue [727], resulting in subsequent peptide concentration changes. In addition, both insulin and glucose utilization affected by insulin alters IGF-II protein levels in hypothalamic nuclei [728,729]. Thus, insulin status is an important determinant of both IGF-I and II concentrations at the tissue level where effects are exerted. Furthermore, it has now become apparent that resistance to insulin even in the prediabetic state may be a contributor to deficient neurotrophic factor support.

Dermal Neurovascular Dysfunction and Insulin Resistance

The study by Stansberry and colleagues [660] demonstrated significant inverse correlations between systolic blood pressure and the hyperemic response to ischemia and heated arm lowering. Significant correlations also existed between flow at 35 °C and levels of LDL-C, triglycerides, and C-peptide. It seems, therefore, that these defects in skin blood flow are part of the metabolic syndrome and may play a role in the pathogenesis of the condition as well as its complications. Jaap and colleagues [420] suggested that the failure of skin vasodilation occurs before the onset of type 2 diabetes and that this failure is related to insulin resistance. More recently, these researchers showed that failure of endothelial-dependent vasodilatation and direct vasodilation occurs in family members of patients with type 2 diabetes [730]. Caballero and colleagues [421] have shown that vascular reactivity in the skin microcirculation is impaired in individuals with impaired glucose tolerance and in normoglycemic subjects with a parental history of type 2 diabetes. They found a significant inverse correlation between microvascular reactivity and systolic blood pressure, fasting plasma glucose, HDL-C, fasting plasma insulin, and homeostasis model assessment (HOMA) values as an index of insulin resistance [421].

These data support the concept that an abnormality may precede the onset of hyperglycemia.

Stansberry and colleagues [660] showed that abnormalities exist in C-fiber-mediated nociceptive vasodilatation in the upper limb of people with diabetes in the absence of overt neuropathy. Once again this correlates with the metabolic markers of the insulin resistance syndrome. Knockout of capsaicin-sensitive sensory neurons result in impaired glucose tolerance and insulin sensitivity as well [731]. These findings suggest that defective neurogenic vasodilatation, in addition to its pathophysiologic role in causing complications, may be mechanistically responsible for as much as 25 % of impaired glucose utilization [732,733], although Avogaro and others question its significance [734].

IGF Receptors

In order for IGFs to elicit effects on growth and regeneration of nervous tissue, receptors must be present on the appropriate target cells. Just as receptors for insulin are found throughout the nervous system [735,736], type 1 IGF [737], and type 2 IGF receptors [738] have also been found in brain and other regions [739,740]. In particular, retina neurons [741] and glia [742] are enriched in IGF receptors. Two types of IGF receptors exist and these are generally referred to as the type 1 and type 2 receptors on the basis of their affinity for the respective IGF ligands. The type 1 IGF receptor is structurally similar to that of insulin, being a heterotetramer with a molecular weight of approximately 130 kDa and having innate tyrosine kinase activity. In contrast, the type 2 IGF receptor is a single polypeptide that does not have a tyrosine kinase domain. The type 2 receptor has been shown to be identical to the previously isolated mannose-6-phosphate receptor [743]. While the type 1 receptor binds IGF-II and insulin with lower affinity, the type 2 receptor does not bind insulin [744]. Also, like to the insulin receptor, the type 1 nervous tissue receptor differs from its peripheral counterpart [745]. Insulin has also been shown to modulate IGF-I effects indirectly, possibly by affecting postreceptor events that are shared by the two peptides [746]. The presence of IGF receptors is accompanied by facilitation of IGF-mediated effects in the nervous system. For example, a correlation between binding of the IGFs with neurite outgrowth has been shown by Recio-Pinto and Ishii [747]. At low ligand concentrations (< 1 nM], insulin acts through insulin receptors and IGFs through their own receptors. At supraphysiologic doses, cross-occupancy of the ligands occurs, which may be responsible for induction of neurite growth. IGF receptors are found on the cell bodies and all along the axon shafts, including the terminals [748], and insulin has been shown to bind to these axons [749]. As evidence that insulin and IGFs induce neurite outgrowth, both insulin and the IGFs [750,751] have been shown to increase both α- and β-tubulin mRNAs during neurite outgrowth. In addition, they stabilize α- and β-tubulin transcripts against degradation [751,268]. Insulin, IGF-I, and IGF-II also increase neurofilament (the other major structural protein of neurites) mRNAs during neurite growth [751]. In most systems examined, insulin needs to be present at much higher doses than IGFs to elicit the same response. This suggests that the predominant effect is that of IGFs, and under certain circumstances, such as in type 2 diabetes, insulin may act directly in vivo by cross-reaction. Most of insulin's effects are probably indirect by regulation of IGF peptides and receptor binding.

IGFs Effects on Nervous Tissue

In vitro, physiologic concentrations of insulin, IGF-I, and IGF-II can increase neurite outgrowth in cultured human neuroblastoma SH-SY5Y cells [706,651] as well as in embryonic sensory, sympathetic [753], spinal cord [754], and motor neurons [748]. All these populations of neurons are sensitive to insulin and the IGFs, suggesting that the ligands may indeed cooperate to regulate neural responses in some way. It has been shown that IGF-II gene expression in muscle correlates with the development of neuromuscular synapses. Regenerating axons use the distal nerve below a lesion as a conduit for growth back to denervated muscles [755]. The IGF-I and IGF-II mRNAs are significantly increased per nerve in regions distal to the site of crush [756,757], predominantly in Schwann cells, suggesting that during regeneration IGF mRNAs are up-regulated in denervated nerves.

There may of course be a factor within muscle that causes feedback inhibition and suppresses IGF-II expression, suggesting that maturation of synapses may suppress IGF-II expression, resulting in elimination of polyneuronal synapse formation [758]. It is postulated, therefore, that nerve crush concurrently leads to a loss of this feedback inhibition, causing up-regulation of IGF-II mRNAs in the adult rat muscle [756]. Furthermore, these transcripts are particularly enriched in regions of muscle fibers containing neuromuscular junctions and, as has been suggested by Pu and Ishii [759], this may be the explanation why regenerating axons tend to return to their original endplates. Direct application of IGFs to nondenervated muscle causes axonal sprouts to extend from motor nerve terminals [748], suggesting that IGF-II helps regulate the development and regeneration of mammalian synapses.

IGF-Binding Proteins

The IGFs (I and II) do not exist as free peptides, but are bound to one of several characterized binding proteins (Fig. 4.**23**). So far, six IGF-binding proteins (IGFBPs) have been cloned, sequenced, and characterized [760]. IGFBP-3 is the major form in plasma and is responsible for regulating the half-life of both IGF-I and IGF-II. This

IGFBP, however, exists primarily as a ternary complex, with the growth factor and an acid-labile subunit comprising the circulating unit. Formation of the complex involves the initial binding of IGFs to the IGFBP, and then this binary complex in turn has increased affinity for the acid labile unit forming the ternary complex. When in this state, IGF-I has reduced bioavailability and its half-life is increased. In the binary complex, when IGF-I is bound to any of the IGFBPs including IGFBP-3 without the acid labile subunit, IGF-I has a shorter turnover rate and its bioavailability increases. While it is known that IGF-I circulating concentrations decrease in diabetes [761], the contribution of the IGFBPs to this phenomenon has received little attention. Diabetes is also accompanied by a decreased synthesis and secretion of IGFBP-3 which could profoundly alter IGFBP-IGF interactions and thus IGF-I effects. Recently, it has been shown that there is increased proteolysis of IGFBP-3 in type 2 diabetic individuals compared to age-matched controls, which could account at least in part for the observed reduction in IGF-I [762]. The effects of this proteolytic cleavage on IGF-I action have yet to be determined.

IGFBP-1 and IGFBP-3 are regulated by insulin, and secretion of IGFBP-2 is altered profoundly by hypoglycemia, which increases IGFBP-2 levels, or hyperglycemia, which depresses secretion and synthesis. IGFBP-2 and IGFBP-6 are the major forms found in cerebrospinal fluid [763,764], but most IGFBPs are present in nervous tissue. IGFBP-2, IGFBP-5, and IGFBP-6 have a higher affinity for IGF-II than IGF-I. As with the ligands themselves, it is unknown whether circulating or local levels of IGFBPs are most important, but there appears to be an emerging general consensus that many binding-protein effects are exerted locally. Hence it is probable these IGFBPs may play a role in the activity of the IGFs in terms of nerve growth and regeneration. IGFBP-1, for example, is generally regarded as an inhibitor of IGF action, and levels are increased with diabetes [761]. Insulin therapy restores IGFBP-1 levels towards normal and consequently should restore IGF-mediated effects on nerve regeneration. However, in extreme insulin-resistant states, the positive effect of insulin on IGFBP synthesis may be impaired as the ability to stimulate insulin-mediated cellular events is compromised. This has been demonstrated recently in a study of patients with Mendenhall syndrome, in whom rhIGF-I was infused in order to overcome insulin resistance [765]. In subjects with this insulin resistance syndrome, rhIGF-I infusion was able to elevate IGFBP-3 concentrations, but failed to modulate IGFBP-1 levels. These data suggest that type 2 diabetic patients may have abnormal local production of IGFBP-1 and hence altered IGF effects that may contribute to neuropathy, but definitive data need to be collected.

In addition to the inhibitory effects of IGFBP-1, other IGFBPs may play an important role in the development of neuropathy. For example, IGFBP-4 and IGFBP-5 have also been shown to block IGF response in paralyzed skeletal muscle when infused locally. However, the levels of these IGFBPs in patients with neuropathy have not been reported. The above data, along with other data not presented here, suggest that IGFBP status of tissues and cells needs to be considered when examining IGF effects in diabetics. Further, the role of these proteins in the development of neurological disorders needs to be determined in order to fully evaluate the effectiveness potential of growth factor treatment in neuropathy. Such studies may indicate the use of IGF isoforms which have differential binding affinities for the various binding proteins.

Insulin and NGF: The Pleiotrophic Response

Aside from the direct effects insulin and the IGFs have on neurite outgrowth and regeneration, it is possible that IGFs exert a major action through modulation of other growth factors and their receptors. An example of this is the effect of IGF-II on NGF receptors. In serum-free medium, NGF receptor binding diminishes and NGF fails to have a physiological effect on the neuron as a result. Addition of IGF-II to this serum-free medium can induce NGF receptor binding and thus restore NGF function in neurons. While IGFs and NGF can work together to maintain normal nerve integrity, there appears to be a separate role for each of these neurotrophins in neurite outgrowth. Antisera to NGF, for example, do not block the effects of IGF on tubulin synthesis and differentiation.

It has been known for some time that insulin stimulates many anabolic processes in its target cells. Recently this has been stated in a more unified concept designated as the pleiotrophic response [661]. The processes that have been found to be under pleiotypic control are uridine uptake, RNA synthesis, polysome formation, protein synthesis, protein degradation, and glucose utilization [661]. The response to insulin closely parallels that of sensitive neurons to NGF in vitro. Sensory ganglia respond to NGF with an increase in uridine uptake, synthesis of all classes of RNA, protein synthesis, and glucose utilization. NGF also increases lipid synthesis, an aspect which might be related to a pleiotypic growth response [766]. The striking similarity between the structure of NGF and proinsulin suggests an evolution of NGF from an ancestral proinsulin. This may be an example of converging evolution, with formation of a new function from a preexisting protein, and may be compared with the evolution of α-lactalbumin from lysozyme and the development of several pancreatic serine proteases with varying specificity from a primitive precursor [767]. Thus, NGF might best be considered among the growth factors as occupying a position intermediate between protein hormones and inducers. Frazier and colleagues [767a] have developed a model in which they suggest that an ancestral proinsulin comprised of a B, C, and A chain finally gives rise to a fragment of 50 residues, which comprises the insulin A and B chain and undergoes contiguous reduplication, deletion, and modification, with final translation into an NGF with 118 residues comprised of a B, C, A, and B.

The stimulating pathways or pleiotropic actions of insulin and NGF may include two distinct but related pathways involving stimulation of both serine/threonine kinases and phosphatases [768,769]. The sequence of events following the initial interaction with NGF and insulin and the receptor bears remarkable similarities. The NGF receptors bear considerable structural homology with the insulin receptor. Within the tyrosine kinase domain, all of the trk proteins showed 40–50% sequence identity with the insulin receptor and over 80% sequence similarity. The similarities between NGF and insulin in structure, cellular actions, early signaling events, and receptor structure/function have led to renewed interest in the biology of newly discovered and previously recognized neurotrophic factors. It is indeed for this reason that we are interested in the overlap between the actions and mechanisms of insulin and neurotrophins and their involvement in the pathogenesis of diabetic polyneuropathy.

Insulin and IGFs in Diabetic Neuropathy

Recent advances in understanding the neurobiology of insulin and the IGFs have led to the suggestion that IGFs may be involved in the pathogenesis of diabetic neuropathy [714,770,770a,771]. Focus is being placed upon the relationship of these ligands to cell survival, synaptogenesis, neurite (axon and dendrite) outgrowth, and nerve regeneration affected by diabetes. In the model of the crushed sciatic nerve [772], IGF-II has been shown to increase the distance of motor axon regeneration. Locally infused IGF-I [757] and IGF-II [754] also significantly increases the distance of regeneration of sensory axons in lesioned sciatic nerves. Infused IGF-II increased the rate of regeneration [754], whereas insulin was only marginally effective [754, 772]. This suggests not only that the above effect is mediated through the IGF receptors, but also that it is the type 1 receptor rather than the type 2 which is responsible. Further support for the notion that IGF-I mediates the action of insulin in diabetes derives from the observation that sciatic nerve regeneration, which is impaired in diabetic rats [773–775], can be restored toward normal by infusion of insulin, which restores IGF levels. The assertion that IGF-I is the mediator of the regenerative response gains further support from studies showing inhibition of spontaneous nerve regeneration in the presence of anti-IGF antisera. Administration of anti-IGF antisera reduced the spontaneous regeneration distance of both motor [772] and sensory [757,776] axons. Administration of IGF-I to nerve repair sites via miniosmotic pumps significantly enhanced nerve regeneration [757,777] and regeneration was inhibited if the nerve was perfused with antibodies directed against native IGF-I. It appears therefore that endogenous IGF activity is required for nerve regeneration, and that the action of insulin requires the local presence of IGF-I for the regenerative response to be elicited.

To date, little research has been conducted associating reduced IGF protein levels, whether due to impaired transport or to impaired synthesis, with the occurrence of diabetic neuropathy. In one study, animals with decreased plasma concentrations of IGF-I due to experimentally induced diabetes show a marked impairment in peripheral nerve regeneration [755,778]. The molecular basis of this impairment is at present unknown. Unidentified soluble neuronal and Schwann cell-promoting factors are produced and released during normal conditions of peripheral nerve repair [779]. It is possible that the expression of these factors is compromised in a diabetic state, and that the absence of IGFs contributes to the impairment in nerve regeneration. There are however, no studies to support this notion.

Since one of the metabolic consequences of diabetes is a reduction in circulating IGF-I, it is reasonable to hypothesize that abnormal IGF-I or IGF-II metabolism plays a causative role in some aspect of diabetic neuropathy. Currently little is known regarding the effect of diabetes on local expression, synthesis, and transport of these growth factors in the nervous tissue. Complicating the interpretation of IGF-I changes reported in diabetes mellitus is the influence of nutritional status. Protein and carbohydrate intake and metabolism are primary regulators of IGF-I production by the tissues. Metabolic pathways for these nutrients may be disturbed in humans or animal models of diabetes, making the effects observed due to diabetes difficult to distinguish from those due to malnutrition. Factors such as the method of inducing diabetes, duration of symptoms, degrees of insulin treatment, or variability in glucose status often differ from laboratory to laboratory. In some cases, the IGF-I or IGF-II response observed may be more indicative of malnutrition than of diabetes, particularly when uncontrolled diabetic animals are used as the experimental model. IGF-I synthesis is altered in a tissue-specific manner by diabetes [780], whereas nutritional insufficiency represents a general decline in expression [781,782]. The decrease in IGF-I with protein malnutrition is thought to be due to induction of a growth-hormone-resistant state [782], which may or may not coexist with the appearance of diabetes. Another example of a nutritional versus diabetes-induced effect might be that of malnutrition on CNS, where protein restriction decreases IGF-II synthesis, but not that of IGF-I [783,784]. On the other hand, data generated in our laboratory suggest that IGF-II is up-regulated in dorsal root ganglia obtained from diabetic animals treated with insulin to partially correct the hyperglycemia [785]. IGFBP synthesis and secretion will also differ in diabetes and malnutrition [715,786]. In poorly controlled STZ-diabetic rats IGFBP-1, an inhibitor of IGF-I action in cartilage assays, is up-regulated as a function of both degree of hyperglycemia and duration of disease [787]. This suggests that more tightly controlled insulin and glucose levels would lead to smaller and perhaps insignificant differences in IGFBP-1 synthesis. IGFBP-2 is regulated differently in malnutrition versus diabetes, but exhibits a tissue-specific response in either case [783].

Role of Laminin in Nerve Growth and Development

Laminin is a large, heterotrimeric, cruciform glycoprotein composed of three subunits, a large A chain and two smaller B chains, B_1 and B_2 [788,789] (Fig. 4.**24**). In peripheral nervous tissue, the A chain is replaced by the A chain variant, the merosin, M chain [790]. It is a major component of basal lamina. In peripheral nerve, basal laminar components are synthesized by Schwann cells and form continuous basal laminar tubes within the endoneurium. Laminin has been shown to promote neurite extension by cultured neurons [779,791–794]. Moreover, studies of peripheral nerve injury have implicated Schwann cell basal laminae as the substrates along which axonal growth cones proceed [795,796].

Glycation may prevent binding of laminin to members of the integrin family and thus compromise its metabolic activity. Federoff and colleagues [213] found that nonenzymatic glycosylation of laminin and the laminin peptide IKVAV, which is a lysine-containing sequence within the laminin molecule, inhibits neuritic outgrowth by cultured neuroblastoma cells. The normal carbohydrate moieties of laminin appear to be essential for neurite outgrowth and cell migration [797]. Nonenzymatic glycosylation of laminin, however, results in the formation of cross-links, which alter the cruciform shape of the molecule [798]. Self-assembly of the molecule is also impaired [798]. These changes could inhibit laminin receptor binding as well as laminin interactions with heparin sulfate and type IV collagen within basal laminae. Moreover, impairment of laminin self-assembly may affect the normal turnover of Schwann cell basal laminae within the nerve.

Laminin in Diabetic Neuropathy

Advanced glycation of Schwann cell basal laminar components is likely to occur in the high-glucose environment of diabetic nerves. Examination of STZ-diabetic rat nerves indicates the presence of advanced glycosylation endproducts (AGEs) [346]. Whether Schwann cell basal laminae are specifically subjected to advanced glycation in diabetic nerves has not as yet been demonstrated. Moreover, while an inhibitor of advanced glycation, aminoguanidine, improved motor nerve conduction velocities and affected myelinated fiber size and axon diameter in STZ-diabetic rat peripheral nerves [346], a hypothesis of how advanced glycation might specifically affect those functional and morphological parameters has not been proposed. More importantly, since advanced glycation of laminin specifically inhibits neurite outgrowth in culture, it will be interesting to see whether such treatment improves axonal regeneration in diabetic rat nerves.

Our laboratory has been interested in laminin as a neurotrophic factor and specifically in neuronal laminin gene expression. We showed, using in situ hybridization, that all normal adult DRG neurons express the laminin B_2 chain gene [799]. Moreover, a subpopulation of small DRG neurons express the B_1 subunit gene [799]. This more restricted neuronal gene expression might have implications for the specificity of neuron-target interaction in the periphery as well as within the spinal cord. DRG neurons fail to express the A chain gene or the merosin M chain gene [799]. The merosin M chain gene is expressed by satellite and Schwann cells in the ganglia [799]. It does appear that glycation of laminin involves the A chain and thus is unlikely to be an explanation for our findings of impaired expression of laminin B_2 in STZ-diabetic animals (see below).

We have found that during sciatic nerve regeneration, laminin B_2 gene expression is up-regulated by nondiabetic axotomized DRG neurons [800,801]. This up-regulation of laminin B_2 in neurons during regeneration implicates neuronal B_2 laminin in the regenerative process. Laminin may act locally, within the DRG, in a paracrine and possibly autocrine fashion, or it may be anterogradely transported to the growth cone region, where it may influence local cellular events in the regenerating nerve.

Studies of laminin gene expression in STZ-diabetic rats suggest that neuronal laminin gene expression is decreased in diabetes. Both laminin B_1 and B_2 chain neuronal gene expression is reduced in diabetic DRGs [802]. Moreover, diabetic DRG neurons, unlike nondiabetic DRG neurons, fail to up-regulate laminin B_2 gene expression during sciatic nerve regeneration [802,803]. Reduced B_2 neuronal gene expression in uninjured diabetic DRG neurons may be another example of reduced neurotrophic factor support in diabetes. Future experiments will address the cause of decreased DRG B_2 laminin gene expression in diabetes. A number of possible explanations can be explored. For example, if laminin B_2 is normally anterogradely transported down the axon, perturbations in axonal transport, which occur in diabetes, might cause an accumulation of B_2 protein within the neuronal cell body that inhibits transcription of B_2 message. Alternatively, the B_2 message might be less stable in diabetic neurons than in nondiabetic neurons. A third possibility might be that laminin B_2 gene expression in neurons is regulated by another neurotrophic factor which is reduced in diabetes. Regardless of the cause of reduced DRG neuronal laminin B_2 gene expression in diabetes, failure of up-regulation of B_2 message in diabetic DRG neurons may contribute to the slowed axonal-regeneration observed in diabetic rats [799]. It will be important to determine how neuronal laminin gene expression is regulated and whether therapeutic treatment of diabetic rats with insulin or other neurotrophic factors affects laminin gene expression and restores the regenerative response of DRG neurons. Alternatively, it may be relevant to explore the effects of local perfusion of injured nerves with the B_2 subunit of laminin to determine efficacy in induction of nerve regeneration, and if this proves to be positive, it might lay the foundations for exploring a therapeutic potential.

Prosaposins as Neurotrophic Factors

Prosaptide TX14(A) is a 14-amino-acid peptide derived from prosaposin, a cytokine and a naturally occurring protein found in human milk and cerebrospinal fluid [804,805]. Prosaptide peptides induce differentiation and prevent cell death in a variety of neuronal cells [806–809]. Prosaptide TX14(A) has been shown to relieve neuropathic pain and attenuate and/or reverse the effects of peripheral neuropathy in several animal models [806,807,809,810].

Prosaptide has been shown to promote the survival and differentiation of both neuronal and nonneuronal cell types in vitro. Prosaptide induces neurite outgrowth in NS20Y neuroblastoma cells, CHAT activity in SK-N-MC neuroblastoma cells [804,805], and sulfatide synthesis in both primary Schwann cells and CG4 oligodendrocytes [809], and promotes cell survival in the face of apoptotic stimuli [808,811,812] without inducing cell proliferation [811]. Cellular responses to prosaptide are initiated by ligand binding to a G-protein-coupled receptor (GPCR) [810] with subsequent downstream activation of signaling pathways, e. g., MAP kinase [813] and Akt kinase [811] pathways. Such activation has demonstrated an apparent bimodal effect with high prosaptide or prosaposin concentrations attenuating or decreasing receptor responses [810]. This apparent bimodal response is not without precedent for other GPCRs. For the prosaposin GPCR, Hiraiwa and colleagues [810] showed that prosaptide-induced [^{35}S]-GTPγS binding to SHSY5Y neuroblastoma cell membranes was concentration-dependent and reduced at prosaptide concentrations exceeding 2 nM.

Animal model studies have provided evidence of efficacy of prosaptide in the treatment of diabetic peripheral neuropathy. Prosaptide prevented and reversed both thermal hypoalgesia and nerve conduction velocity deficits (both motor and sensory) in STZ-induced diabetic rats [808]. The compound does not act as an ARI, nor is there any evidence that it has any effect on the vascular perfusion of the nerve. Additionally, in a rat chemotherapeutic model prosaptide was shown to mitigate the sensory loss associated with paclitaxel treatment [808].

In vivo studies supporting prosaptide's therapeutic effect on neuropathic pain have been derived from several animal models including the STZ-diabetic rat and the Seltzer rat. In the STZ-diabetic rat prosaptide was able to reduce both tactile allodynia and formalin-induced hyperalgesia. In the Seltzer model of neuropathic pain induced by physical nerve trauma, prosaptide TX14(A) was able to relieve the thermal hyperalgesia associated with that rat model [814]. In a chemical trauma nerve injury model, prosaptide TX14(A) was able to prevent the thermal hyperalgesia associated with the application of TNFα directly to rat sciatic nerve [807]. In keeping with the aforementioned bimodal nature of the prosaposin GPCR response, Otero and colleagues [814] were unable to obtain additional analgesic benefit using prosaptide in a dose exceeding 50–100 µg/kg in the Seltzer rat hyperalgesia pain model.

In a recently completed phase II clinical trial for relief of diabetic pain, efficacy of prosaptide compared with placebo was evaluated using five different pain scales, all of which showed statistically significant or near-significant pain score reduction compared with placebo. The analgesic effect was demonstrable throughout the study period in all five pain scales. Patients in all four arms of the study had a substantial decrease in McGill visual analogue scale scores during placebo lead-in prior to randomization. Exploratory analysis applied the minimum pain score study entry requirement to patients at the end of placebo lead-in. In addition, patient pain scores were normalized to their individual prerandomization baseline scores. The population that responded to prosaptide experienced mean pain relief of approximately 45–80% over the course of the study. Once this agent is approved for use in painful diabetic neuropathy we can anticipate further prying into its neurotrophic or anti-apoptotic potential.

Interleukins

The cytokine interleukin-6 (IL-6) has multiple functions in the immune and hemopoietic systems. IL-6 is structurally related to ciliary neurotrophic factor (CNTF), a trophic factor for motoneurons, sensory DRG neurons, and other neuronal subpopulations. Both act via related receptor complexes, consisting of one ligand-specific α-subunit (IL-6R and CNTF-R) respectively and two signal-transducing components. Accumulating evidence suggests that IL-6 has a pivotal role in nerve lesion and repair [815]. IL-6 and IL-6R are upregulated in Schwann cells and neurons after nerve injury [816,817], indicating a role in the promotion of axonal growth. In experimental models of neuron destruction, addition of exogenous IL-6 alone or in combination with its soluble receptor (sIL-6R) produced marked neuroprotection of neurons from either the central or peripheral nervous system [818,819]. IL-6 synthesis in the peripheral nervous system occurs mainly in neurons, Schwann cells, and glia [820]. In intact and injured nerves, macrophages, lymphocytes, mastocytes, and fibroblasts can be major contributors to IL-6 production [817,821]. Furthermore, sympathetic neurons produce IL-6 in vitro, and their survival is enhanced by IL-6 and sIL-6R in the absence of nerve growth factor [822].

Elevated serum IL-6 is associated with several neurodegenerative disorders including Alzheimer's disease [823], Guillain-Barré syndrome, chronic inflammatory demyelinating polyneuropathy, and the POEMS syndrome [823–826], and elevated IL-6 levels are also reported in autoimmune neuronal diseases such as multiple sclerosis and diabetes [825,827].

Our laboratory has used murine N1E-115 neuroblastoma cells as a model for in vitro detection of serum neurotoxicity in diabetic patients with neuropathy [828–830]. The toxic effects appear to be at least partially mediated by immune effectors [829]. We have shown that toxicity correlates with increased neuropathy symptom scores, decreased vibration perception, and with HbA_{1c}. In a previous study, we demonstrated that N1E-115 cells express IL-6, but not the IL-6 receptor [831]. Furthermore, IL-6 in combination with sIL-6R was able to abrogate serum-induced apoptosis. We postulated that serum neurotoxicity in patients with diabetic neuropathy might be mediated by disruption of the IL-6/IL-6R axis. We have also shown [831] that IL-6 alone or IL-6 plus sIL-6R is neuroprotective. These results suggested an autocrine role for IL-6 on certain neurons. Since, however, many neuronal cells do not express the receptor, it has been suggested that a designer cytokine linking IL-6 and the α-receptor component may prove an effective therapy for certain neuropathies [832]. This has not been realized yet as far as we are aware.

Neuroimmunophilins

It has recently been found that both cyclosporin A and neuroimmunophilin ligands (e. g., FK506), both used in the immunosuppression during transplantation, exhibit significant neuroprotective and neuroregenerative capacities. This discovery by serendipity raised the question of their mode of action as well as whether their immunosuppressive properties could be obviated and their neuroprotective effects enhanced. It now appears that an analogue of FK506 which lacks the calcineurin-binding properties of the native compound (calcineurin binding is essential for immunosuppression) has been identified which in preliminary studies may fulfill this potential. The neuroimmunophilin ligands are a class of compounds which, in contrast to the neuropeptide neurotrophins, readily cross the blood-brain and blood-nerve barrier and have been shown to be orally active in a variety of ischemic and traumatic nerve injury as well as human neurodegenerative disorders. These compounds do not appear to bind to the traditional neurotrophic receptors such as the trks, but may enhance the release of a variety of neurotrophic agents such as NGF, NT-3, and BDNF, amongst others. A number of binding proteins for the FK506 compound have been identified and shown to mediate the immunosuppressive action (FKBP-12) and neuroprotection (FKBP-52), the latter being a part of the nuclear receptor complex. In animal studies, reduction in NF-κB correlates with the ability to induce the production of BDNF and improved motoneuron function. Thus, steroid receptor chaperone proteins may represent novel targets for the future drug development of novel classes of compounds for the treatment of a variety of neurologic disorders including diabetic neuropathy [833]. The great advantage of this approach over that of using individual neurotrophic agents is the apparent increase in a multitude of neurotrophic peptides, e. g., BDNF, NGF, and NT-3, thereby targeting the multifaceted aspects of diabetic neuropathy with a single agent. It is further possible that these agents will survive the gastrointestinal tract and reach concentration gradients in nerves that are considerably greater than those found in plasma, obviating the necessity for local delivery. An immunophilin ligand analogue, VX-853 (Vertex), is undergoing a phase II clinical study for diabetic neuropathy. Another analogue, Tak-428 (Takeda), is an advancing competitor in this field and shows considerable promise based upon several animal models of diabetic neuropathy. With the harsh lessons we have learned on translation of animal data to man in the recent past, however, the need for hypothesis-testing phase II studies in humans is mandatory.

Programmed Cell Death and Neuropathy

Homeostasis of multicellular organisms is controlled not only by the proliferation and differentiation of cells, but also by cell death. In addition to the many growth factors, there are a number of other circulating factors that regulate cell survival, differentiation, and death. It is beyond the scope of this section to enter into great detail on the importance of apoptosis in the development of neuropathy. Nor is it feasible to engage in the argument on the differences between necrosis, programmed cell death, and apoptosis. However, it is pertinent in any discussion of neurotrophism to mention that apoptosis (in the generic sense) may be a mechanism whereby diabetes induces nerve damage and wherein diabetes opposes the antiapoptotic mechanisms that normally protect nerves. It is of interest that NGF and IGFs can rescue neuronal cells from apoptosis [834,835], and that certain cytokines can activate the apoptotic mechanisms. We have reported on the presence of complement-mediated induction of apoptosis of the murine N1E-115 neuroblastoma cell line cultured in the presence of sera from type 1 diabetic patients [829,836], and others have made similar observations indicating that complement may not be necessary for this to occur in type 2 diabetic patients [837]. Our previous studies indicate that the effect occurs through the action of an autoantibody [829], resulting in apoptosis of the adrenergic neuron cell line. Therefore, it is important to identify the antigen recognized by the autoantibody and its relationship to induction of apoptosis.

Apoptosis is regulated by many extrinsic and intrinsic cellular signals, and the threshold of apoptotic cell death is also dynamically regulated by multiple inducers and inhibitors of gene products [838]. Several apoptosis-related oncogene products are also expressed and regulated in neurons. Bcl-2, a cell-death suppressor, is found in the mitochondrial membrane, the nucleus, and the endoplasmic reticulum. A high level of expression of bcl-2 in sympathetic neurons prevents cell death induced by deprivation of NGF [839]. However, we were unable to detect bcl-2 in neuroblastoma cells by immunofluorescence. The apparent lack of bcl-2 in the neuroblastoma cell line might simply reflect the lack of bcl-2 in neuroblasts, or it may result from gene loss during tumorigenesis. Furthermore, the lack of bcl-2 may be associated with an increased propensity for apoptosis in this cell line. Because we were unable to show the presence of bcl-2 in resting N1E-115 cells, it was unlikely that bcl-2 participated in the regulation of the apoptotic response studied here. Hence, we sought an alternative antigen.

Fas (APO-1, CD95) is a type I cell-surface receptor with a molecular weight of 35–40 kDa, depending on the source species, belonging to the TNF/NGF receptor superfamily. Fas is expressed in many cell lines, but the largest body of research shows that Fas mediates apoptosis in susceptible T-lymphocyte target cells [840]. Fas-mediated apoptosis may be antibody-dependent. When Fas ligand or anti-Fas antibodies bind to the Fas receptor, the target cell undergoes apoptosis. The apoptotic signal through Fas requires the cross-linking and trimerization of Fas receptors [841]. The trimerized Fas complex can then be activated by antibody action, resulting in the transduction of the signal for induction of apoptosis. Polymerization of Fas can be accomplished either with Fas ligand or with antibodies to Fas recognizing specific epitopes [842]. Consistent with this hypothesis, immunofluorescence revealed a clustering of Fas on the neuroblastoma cell surface in response to type 1 diabetic serum (data not shown), in contrast to its normal diffuse distribution on the cell membrane. This clustering appears to be a consequence of molecular cross-linking of Fas by a factor in type 1 diabetic serum. According to our previous study, the cytotoxic factor is likely to be an autoantibody [829]. Our finding that type 1 diabetic serum blocks the Fas cell-surface immunofluorescence using a Fas-specific antiserum suggests competition of the IgG in type 1 diabetic serum and the rabbit anti-Fas antibody, indicating that Fas might be one of the membrane antigens recognized by autoantibodies in type 1 diabetic serum. Further supporting this hypothesis is the observation that treatment with anti-Fas monoclonal antibody caused neuroblastoma cell death in a dose-dependent fashion, just as did the type 1 diabetic immunoglobulin in serum. Cytotoxicity of type 1 diabetic serum might be enhanced by the expression of Fas or an increase in circulating Fas ligand. It remains to be determined whether Fas expression in neuroblastoma cells is altered by exposure to type 1 diabetic serum, and whether circulating Fas ligand is increased in type 1 diabetic serum. Furthermore, there is no evidence in the literature for or against the presence of Fas or Fas ligand on cells in peripheral nerves.

Thus, autoimmune-induced apoptotic neuronal death could be involved in the pathogenesis of diabetic neuropathy. Fas, as we have just seen, may be a key mediator of pathogenetic neuronal apoptosis. However, we cannot exclude the possibility that other unknown antigens or death factors, such as glycolipids, the low-affinity NGF receptor (p75), the TNFα receptor, or other as yet unknown regulators of apoptosis, may also play a part. The roles of these regulators in apoptotic neuronal death and whether they might contribute to the development of diabetic neuropathy remain to be elucidated. These findings support the possibility that alternate treatments for diabetic neuropathy may include antiapoptotic maneuvers. Indeed, there is now a suggestion that blockade of the pathway that leads to the formation of excitatory neurotransmitters may be just such a mechanism.

Glutamate Neurotoxicity and Its Prevention

Glutamate is a major excitatory neurotransmitter in the nervous system and plays an important role in neuronal plasticity and neurotoxicity [843]. Under physiologic conditions glutamate is released into the synapse and activates postsynaptic receptors, e. g., NMDA, AMPA, kainate or metabotropic glutamate receptor subtypes. In pathophysiologic states such as ischemia and certain neurodegenerative disorders, there is a large release of glutamate which activates postsynaptic receptors, culminating in cell toxicity and neurodegeneration. Compounds developed so far in the attempt to antagonize these receptors, e. g., MK-801 and CGS197555, have been too toxic. An alternative strategy has evolved that inhibits the hydrolysis of the neuropeptide *N*-acetylaspartylglutamate (NAAG) to NAA and glutamate by the carboxypeptidase, NAALADase (*N*-acetylated-alpha linked-acidic dipeptidase). NAAG is a major membrane component in nervous tissues, present in millimolar amounts [843]. NAAG is released from neurons after depolarization and is both an agonist at group II metabotropic glutamate receptors [844] and a mixed agonist/antagonist at the NMDA receptor [845]. It has been suggested that the enzyme functions to terminate the neurotransmitter activity of NAAG and liberate glutamate from NAAG, which subsequently acts on various glutamate receptor subtypes [843,846,847]. Inhibition of the enzyme could thus provide neuroprotection by increasing NAAG and decreasing glutamate [848–852]. The enzyme exists in very high concentration in Schwann cells and has been postulated to be involved in the signaling between axons and Schwann cells and in myelination [853]. Scientists at Guilford Pharmaceuticals (Baltimore, Md.) have implanted a silicone implant into a sciatic nerve crush and shown a 1.5-fold increase in the number of myelinated axons and a 20% increase in myelin thickness.

NAAGS in Diabetic Neuropathy

Male Sprague-Dawley rats (200–225 g) were made diabetic with STZ (70 mg/kg) and treated once a day with vehicle or GPI 5232 or 5421. Drug or vehicle treatment began 45 days after STZ administration and there was no attempt to control the diabetes. Diabetic rats displayed heat hyperalgesia tested with infrared thermal nociception starting at 45 days after STZ and progressing thereafter. The hyperalgesic response was reversed in the drug-treated animals. Motor and sensory nerve conductions were impaired in the STZ-diabetic animals, and treatment with drug daily for 4, 8, and 12 weeks prevented the decline in both motor and sensory conduction velocities [854]. These studies are being extended to nerve morphometry, skin biopsies, and other diabetic animals, Zucker, BB/W and BB/Z diabetic rats, and Trembler mice. The unique potential of these compounds to relieve pain, protect against neurodegeneration, and remyelinate damaged nerve fibers holds great promise for patients with diabetic neuropathies.

Therapeutic Potential for Growth Factors

As we understand the role of growth factors in the control of growth initiation, proliferation of neurons, and the apoptotic process, it becomes possible to consider the use of neurotrophic factors in the treatment of diabetic neuropathy. Aided by the availability of large quantities of recombinant neurotrophic factors, it is feasible to consider their possible place in the management of diabetic neuropathy. The choice of the optimal neurotrophic factor is dependent upon an awareness of the neuronal population involved in the disease process and an understanding of the specificity of each factor for a specific neuronal population affected by the disease process. This emphasizes the need for more specific delineation of the neuronal population involved in the disease process as well as the specific syndrome present in a particular patient.

Sympathetic and dorsal root ganglia express receptors for the neurotrophins NGF and basic fibroblast growth factor (bFGF). These agents may thus prove efficacious for the treatment of the small-fiber sensory and autonomic neuropathies. The motor neuropathies are candidates for treatment with a variety of growth factors including CNTF, IGF-1, and bFGF, and certain other muscle-derived growth factors [855,856]. NT-3 administration prevented a reduction in nerve conduction velocity in sensory nerves but not motor nerves [857]. Local application of exogenous NT-3 not only prevents the progressive decline in nerve conduction velocities of the sensory and motor neurons [858], but also promotes peripheral nerve regeneration [859].

The optimum approach to mixed sensory neuropathies may be the use of factors with less specificity for motor or sensory neurons. Some factors such as CNTF exert trophic actions on both sensory and motor neurons [860] and will be worthy of trial in mixed neuropathies. Alternatively, the use of combinations of growth factors each with actions on a component of the neuropathic process may prove to be the appropriate approach. Glial-derived neurotrophic factor (GDNF) was purified as a new member of neurotrophic family in 1993 [861]. Approximately a third of primary sensory neurons do not express trk receptors, and can be identified by the binding of the lectin IB4. These neurons have been found to express Ret mRNA, the signal transduction component of the receptor for GDNF, a member of the transforming growth factor-β superfamily [861]. Ret is a common receptor for GDNF and neurturin, and it interacts with either of two other receptor subunits, GFRα1 and GFRα2. Ret receptors have been identified in small-diameter primary sensory neurons, and colocalize with GFRα-1 and GFRα-2 subunits [862]. Initially, GDNF was thought to support survival of only dopaminergic neurons, but recent reports have shown it to be a potent neurotrophic factor for many other neuronal populations. GDNF prevents the slowing of conduction velocity that normally occurs after axotomy in a population of small-diameter dorsal root ganglion cells and the A-fiber sprouting into lamina II of the dorsal horn [862]. GDNF has a trophic effect on motoneurons and autonomic neurons [862] as well as Schwann cells that implicate its diverse role in promoting peripheral nerve regeneration.

By stimulating nerve growth and regeneration as well as remodeling, administration of growth factors that target neurons may decrease the vulnerability to damage by the diabetic disease process. NGF has been considered for the treatment of Alzheimer's disease because of the loss of cholinergic neurons in this disease and the pronounced and selective trophic action of NGF upon cholinergic neurons [863]. Recombinant NGF has been shown to reverse experimental cholinergic injury in animals [864]. bFGF and BDNF also protect cholinergic cell bodies, although less well than NGF [865, 866]. The major brunt of diabetic neuropathy is initially borne by the long parasympathetic, cholinergic nerves and their neurons, suggesting that NGF, alone or in combination with BDNF or bFGF, may have a place in the treatment of parasympathetic neuropathy.

There is also evidence that dopaminergic neurons may be responsive to treatment with the growth factors. BDNF, bFGF, IGF-1, and epidermal growth factor (EGF) promote developmental differentiation of the dopaminergic neurons affected in Parkinson's disease [867,868]. It is not clear, however, that these fibers are affected in diabetes, and confirmation of a place for this particular combination of growth factors must await the documentation of a dopaminergic deficit in diabetes.

There is reason to consider other prospects for growth factor therapy in diabetes. Even motoneurons may be protected from cell death. CNTF rescues motoneurons from naturally occurring cell death during chick embryo development and may retard motoneuron degeneration in the adult [856]. Among a variety of approaches being used to enhance peripheral nerve regeneration is the manipulation of Schwann cells and the use of neurotrophic factors. Such factors include NGF and the members of the neurotrophin family, namely, BDNF, NT-3, NT-4/5, the neurokines, CNTF, and leukemia inhibitory factor (LIF), and also the transforming growth factors (TGFs)-β and their distant relative, glial cell line-derived neurotrophic factor (GDNF) [869].

Early results of treatment of toxic neuropathies with growth factors are encouraging. The small-fiber sensory neuropathy induced by paclitaxel can be prevented by the administration of NGF [870]. The large-fiber neuropathy induced by the antitumor agent cisplatin, with prominent proprioceptive deficits, can be prevented in rodents treated with NGF [810], which has also been shown to prevent or delay the development of sensory neuropathy in STZ-induced diabetes. CNTF supports the survival of cultured neurons and promotes motoneuron survival after axotomy [856], and thus shows special promise for the treatment of the pure motor neuropathies in diabetes.

The question as to how the growth factors will gain access to neurons may not be as difficult as once believed. Implantable pumps, now used extensively in the treatment of diabetes, may permit delivery of adequate concentration of growth factors to peripheral nerves, where they may act locally. The future is also promising for the implanting of genetically engineered cells [871]. It is also within the realm of possibility that pharmacological agents will be able to selectively modify the activity of neurotrophic agonists, as has been shown for certain alkaloid-like compounds [872,873] and the immunophilins [833].

In summary, although the mechanism of action is as yet unknown, the current knowledge of growth factors and their relationship to diabetic neuropathy suggests a pathophysiological role for reduced levels of NGF and laminin, and possibly the IGFs available to neuronal cell bodies. In this regard it is now conceivable that neuronal function may be compromised, and atrophy of nerves and possibly even cell death may be a consequence of growth factor reduction in diabetic neuropathy. Whether the growth factor deficiency is due to decreased synthesis, an inability of the factor to bind to its receptor, disturbances in retrograde axonal transport, or intraneuronal processing also remains to be established. Further studies aimed at understanding the disturbances in expression of the genes and the proteins potentially involved in diabetic neuropathy, as well as their receptor binding and subsequent transport from sites of synthesis to sites of action, should shed considerable light on the relationship between growth factor expression and diabetic neuropathy.

Caveats on the Use of Neurotrophic Factors in the Clinic

The first disease to be targeted for neurotrophic factor treatment in a major clinical trial was amyotrophic lateral sclerosis (ALS). Motoneurons, accessible to protein drugs introduced into the bloodstream, should be very amenable to growth factor treatment because the affected neurons lie outside the blood-brain barrier, the physiological wall that keeps large molecules like proteins from entering the brain. Three growth factors became early candidates for treating ALS: BDNF and IGF-1, both made by muscles, and CNTF, made by Schwann cells that form an insulating sheath around the neurons. Regeneron Pharmaceuticals and Synergen began clinical trials with CNTF and a third company, Cephalon, began trials with IGF-1. Regeneron, in collaboration with Amgen, was also developing BDNF and NT-3.

Following a small trial, Regeneron announced that 12 patients with ALS who had received CNTF injections showed less of a decline in muscle strength than did 14 patients receiving placebo. The results were not statistically significant, but in 2001 Regeneron began a full-scale trial including 720 patients at 36 clinical sites. However, in a preliminary safety trial of CNTF by Synergen, patients suffered side effects, including coughing, fever, weight loss, and activation of herpesvirus, which can hide in latent form in some neurons. In Regeneron's large-scale trial, researchers announced that they had unblinded the data on 550 patients who had completed six months of the trial and found that they had fared worse on measures of muscle strength than did patients receiving placebos!

The question remains whether anything more than modest effects can be expected of CNTF. It is thought that the best that can be expected is a modest slowing of the deterioration rate, with the question of whether these modest effects would improve a patient's life enough to justify the use of the drug. It has recently been found that CNTF has a half-life of only three minutes. It has been suggested that a better result might be obtained if CNTF were delivered directly to the cerebrospinal fluid, which bathes the spinal roots of the motoneurons. Practical issues may thus limit its application to people with diabetic neuropathy.

Researchers hope that IGF-1 will have fewer drawbacks as an ALS therapy. It has been used in large-scale drug trials for diabetes, dwarfism, and osteoporosis without showing serious side effects. The Cephalon trial aims to answer the question of whether IGF-1 will have efficacy in ALS.

The successful phase II clinical trial on NGF by Genentech for diabetic sensory neuropathy raised hopes and then immediately dashed them with the larger phase III study. The reasons for this failure are not clear, but hopefully NGF will not be shelved because of a failed clinical trial. Trials may fail even with active compounds, and absence of evidence is not evidence of absence of an effect. Those of us who had many patients in both studies were very encouraged with the earlier study and very depressed by the later one. The mystery continues.

There is a further caveat regarding the possible value of the IGFs in the therapy of diabetic neuropathy. While the data regarding the potential of IGF-I and/or IGF-II for therapy are encouraging, there are many possible problems with their use as therapeutic agents administered systemically. For example, in transgenic mice that overexpress IGF, numerous tissue abnormalities have been reported [874]. These include red blood cell hematopoeisis in spleen, aberrant collagen bundle formation in skin, and enlarged glomeruli. IGF-I also has been reported to counteract the beneficial effect of bFGF on neuronal survival [875]. In humans, IGF-I administration increases glomerular filtration and renal plasma flow acutely, and has been associated with a number of undesirable side effects, including the development of entrapment neuropathies when it is administered for longer periods of time [876,877]. This is particularly disconcerting when considered in light of the increased predisposition of diabetic subjects to entrapment syndromes. It remains to be shown whether IGF-II shares this side effect with IGF-I.

There is significant potential for neurotrophic factors, cytokines, integrins, immunophilin ligands, and basement membrane proteins to provide neuroprotection, nerve regeneration, and remyelination. In addition, the potential for release of endogenous neurotrophins is enough to fuel several generations of clinical trials. This is an exciting era for those involved in diabetic neuropathy research. Not too long ago it was said: "There is nothing we can do for the person with diabetes and their neuropathy except listen and commiserate," and today we are in the midst of a plethora of possibilities. It no longer seems unreasonable to anticipate that neurotrophic factor therapy for diabetic neuropathy is around the corner.

■ Autoimmunity

P.J. Watkins and G. Sundkvist

Introduction

History

Severe symptomatic autonomic neuropathy in diabetes (DAN) is an awful and debilitating disorder [878]. Yet it occurs relatively rarely amongst the many people with diabetes known to have peripheral neuropathy accompanied by defective autonomic function and thus appears to be a specific and distinctive disorder of uncertain pathogenesis.

The observation at autopsy of a cellular infiltration in sympathetic ganglia and autonomic nerve bundles in five patients with severe DAN led Duchen et al. [55] to postulate the possible role of autoimmunity. Soon afterwards Bennett [696] speculated that antibodies to insulin might cross-react with NGF and cause immunologically mediated damage to peripheral nerves. The description in 1984 of iritis as a feature of DAN further enhanced the concept of potential immunological mechanisms [879]. Indeed, most patients with severe symptomatic DAN are females with type 1 diabetes and thus prone to autoimmune disorders. Furthermore, both islets and the nervous system have some antigenic components in common, including gangliosides, sulfatides, and glutamic acid decarboxylase [880]. There seemed a case to answer.

Nature of Autonomic Neuropathy

Small myelinated and unmyelinated nerve fibers support autonomic transmission and thermal (and pain) sensory perception. A proportion of patients with severe symptomatic DAN have a highly selective neuropathy affecting predominantly these small nerve fibers, leaving sensory modalities transmitted by large nerve fibers (notably light touch and vibration perception) almost intact [7,881] (Fig. 4.**25**). The highly selective neuropathy that characterizes some of these cases again suggests that they form a specific subset of the neuropathies with a distinctive pathogenesis. Since NGF may specifically sustain the smaller nerve fibers, its depletion [882] may play a role in the selective neurological damage seen in these cases. This is discussed below.

Autoimmunity and the Nervous System

Diverse diseases of the nervous system have an established autoimmune basis. Various forms of peripheral neuropathy occur in patients with polyarteritis and Wegener syndrome, systemic lupus erythematosus, and rheumatoid arthritis, and Guillain-Barré syndrome represents a response to cell-mediated hypersensitivity. Neuropathies occur too in patients with paraproteinemias. Multiple sclerosis, stiff man syndrome, and chronic inflammatory demyelinating polyradiculopathy also have an immune basis [880]. There are therefore several precedents for the existence of neuropathies with an autoimmune basis.

Iritis

Iritis is an immune-mediated inflammatory condition associated with circulating immune complexes. Whittington and Lawrence [883] had described its

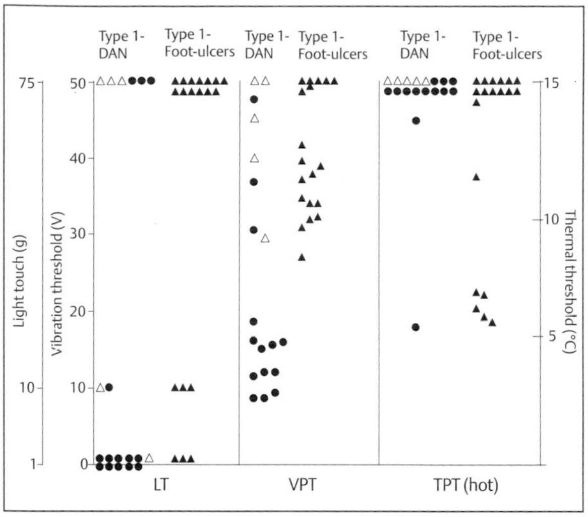

Fig. 4.25 Light touch (LT), vibration perception (VPT), and thermal thresholds (TPT hot) of type 1 diabetic patients with severely symptomatic autonomic neuropathy without (solid circles) and with (open triangle) foot ulcers, compared to those of type 1 neuropathic diabetic patients, selected for the presence of neuropathic foot ulcers (solid triangles). All patients in both groups had severely abnormal autonomic function tests. This demonstrates the distinctive relative preservation of large-fiber sensory modalities (light touch and vibration perception) in some patients with symptomatic diabetic autonomic neuropathy. (From [912], with permission)

occurrence in diabetes, and as early as 1868 Noyes had suggested that diabetes might cause iritis [884].

One of us described its occurrence in nearly one-third of a group of 47 young (21–40 years old) type 1 diabetic patients with DAN [879]. In every case the iritis had been treated by an ophthalmologist with topical steroids, and in most with mydriatic eye drops as well. It preceded the first appearance of autonomic symptoms by two to 60 months in 12 of the 14 patients, and no other cause of the iritis was ever discovered. In most but not all of the patients it has not recurred, and has not left serious residual deformities. Subsequently, some corroboration of these observations came from a Dutch center describing an association between uveitis and diabetes [885]. Furthermore, syphilis and leprosy are conditions that may cause iritis and neuropathies and they have several characteristics similar to diabetic autonomic neuropathy.

Role of Nerve Growth Factor

Why should an immune-mediated iritis be associated with DAN? Presumably antibodies might attack common antigens in both iris and peripheral nerve. NGF is a potential candidate. NGF is known to stimulate and maintain growth and differentiation of sensory and sympathetic neurons and ganglion cells during early development, and in adults it is required for their survival [882]. In fact, NGF is required for gene expression of some neuropeptides including substance P and calcitonin-gene-related peptide (CGRP) in sensory fibers. In in vitro experiments, ganglion cells from animals at early developmental stages cannot survive more than 48 hours without NGF in the medium.

Experimental immunosympathectomy [886] can be induced by NGF antiserum, which causes degeneration of sympathetic ganglion cells and other postganglionic fibers. Presynaptic nerve fibers in sympathetic ganglia and adrenal medulla are also damaged by injection of monoclonal antibodies to neural acetylcholinesterase. Administration of anti-NGF serum to newborn animals results in almost complete destruction of autonomic ganglia. Peripheral nerves in diabetes have been shown to be NGF-depleted, and serum levels may be low.

The iris contains large amounts of NGF, which increase substantially when it is denervated [887]. In theory, at least, antibodies to NGF might therefore cause both damage to the autonomic nervous system and iritis. NGF is also known to act as a cytokine and induce inflammation. It has been suggested that insulin antibodies might cross-react with NGF with which insulin has some structural similarities [696]. Specific antibodies to NGF have not, however, been detected [888].

Cellular Mechanisms In Autonomic And Proximal Diabetic Neuropathies

Lymphocytic cellular infiltrations are well established in a range of autoimmune endocrine disorders including type 1 diabetes. They have been described in pancreatic islets, the thyroid gland, adrenal medulla, pituitary gland, and ovary. The extensive cellular infiltration of sympathetic ganglia (Fig. 4.**26**) and autonomic bundles in five cases of severe DAN which included lymphocytes, macrophages and some plasma cells was strongly suggestive of an immune mechanism [55]. Minor infiltration of lymphocytes and macrophages in the superior cervical ganglion, and of lymphocytes in dorsal root ganglia and trigeminal ganglion, were more recently described in a long-term type 1 diabetic patient suffering both severe DAN and autoimmune polyendocrine disease [889]. Focal collections of inflammatory cells in relation to the autonomic innervation of the esophagus in neuropathic diabetics have also been described [890]. The concept of a cell-mediated immunity has been further enhanced by the observation of increased activated T cells in severe DAN cases [891].

Epineurial vasculitis and nonvasculitic epineurial inflammatory infiltrates have also been described in diabetic patients with proximal diabetic neuropathy (also known as diabetic amyotrophy or femoral neuropathy) [52,53]. These patients have asymmetric proximal pain and weakness associated in some with radicular sensory involvement. The inflammatory

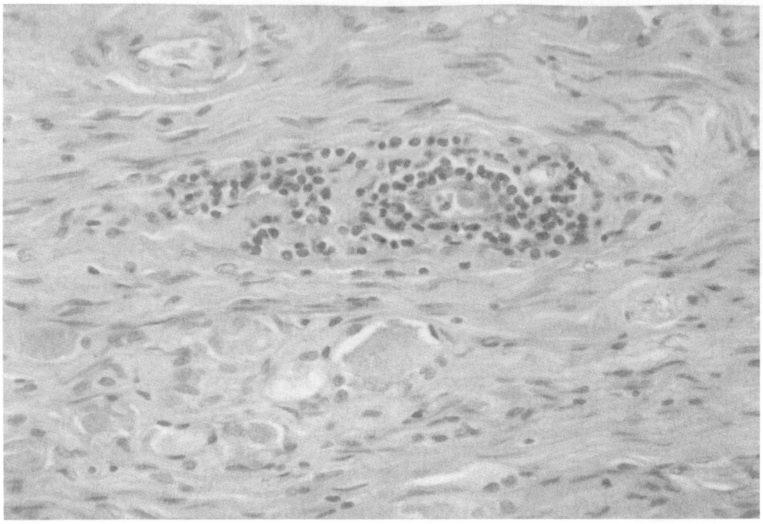

Fig. 4.26 Autopsy section of superior cervical ganglion from a patient with severe symptomatic autonomic neuropathy, showing an extensive infiltration of lymphocytes, macrophages, and plasma cells

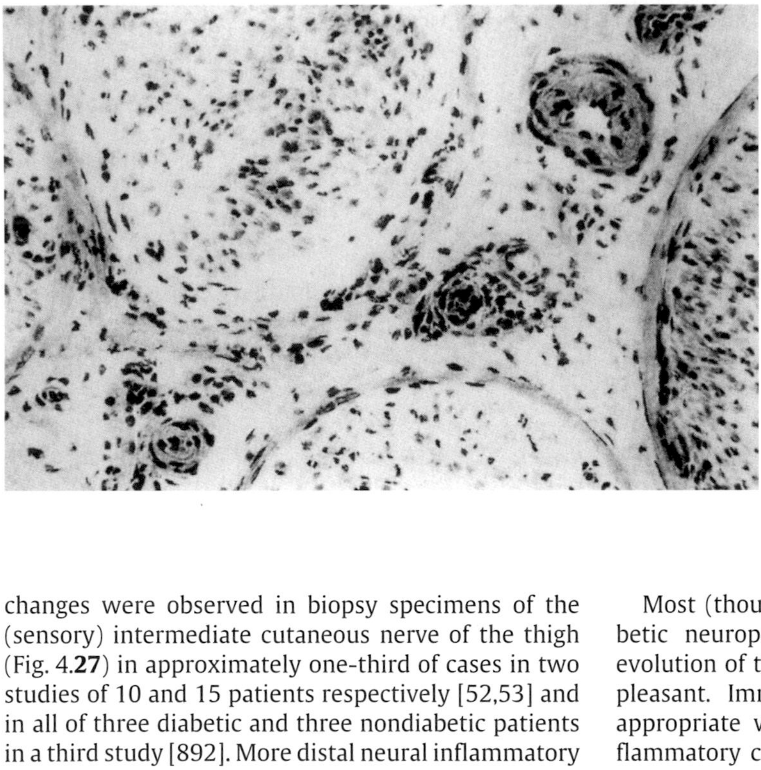

Fig. 4.27 Biopsy of intermediate cutaneous nerve of the thigh from a patient with proximal diabetic neuropathy; cryostat section showing an inflammatory infiltrate related to epineurial microvessels with invasion of the wall of the centrally located vessel [12]

changes were observed in biopsy specimens of the (sensory) intermediate cutaneous nerve of the thigh (Fig. 4.27) in approximately one-third of cases in two studies of 10 and 15 patients respectively [52,53] and in all of three diabetic and three nondiabetic patients in a third study [892]. More distal neural inflammatory changes have been described in the sural nerve in a small number of cases described by P.J. Dyck (personal communication). In contrast, inflammatory changes have not been seen in sural nerve biopsies of patients with symmetrical distal sensory neuropathy.

Vasculitic or other inflammatory processes thus occur in some patients with proximal diabetic neuropathy and in some with autonomic neuropathy. There may be an autoimmune basis for these changes: Said et al. [52] have suggested that diabetes may render the nerves more susceptible to an intercurrent inflammatory process. Indeed, the occurrence of chronic inflammatory demyelinating polyneuropathy appears to be increased in diabetic patients.

Most (though not all) patients with proximal diabetic neuropathy recover completely, though the evolution of the disease is lengthy and its course unpleasant. Immunosuppressive treatment might be appropriate where nerve biopsy has confirmed inflammatory changes, and indeed one such trial is in progress (P.J. Dyck, personal communication).

Antibody-Mediated Immunity

Autoantibodies to neural tissues have been described in a disparate range of neurological disorders. These include stiff man syndrome, Guillain-Barré syndrome, and Behçet disease, as well as some cases of diabetic peripheral neuropathy [880]. Anti-GAD antibodies, though often present in type 1 diabetes, are not, as first thought [893], associated with neuropathy [894–896]. Rabinowe first described the presence of complement fixing autoantibodies to sympathetic ganglion [897] and vagus nerve [898] and their association with

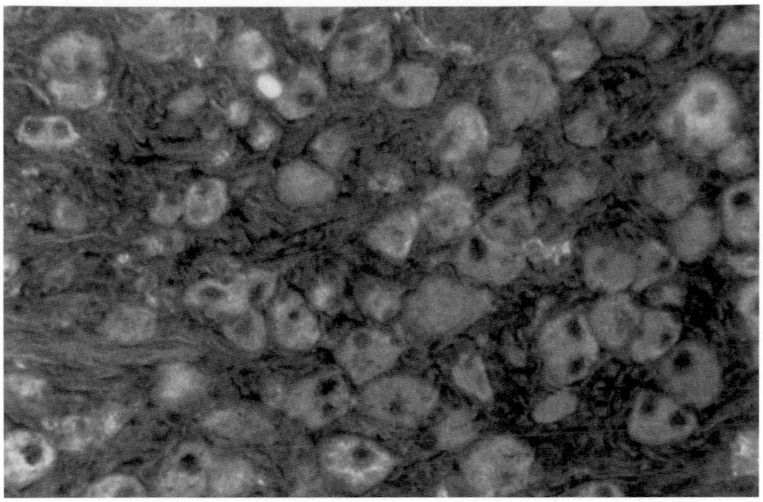

Fig. 4.**28** Immunofluorescence studies (complement fixing) using sera from patients with diabetic autonomic neuropathy staining sympathetic ganglion [907]

diabetic autonomic neuropathy. Adrenal medullary antibodies have a long-established relationship with type 1 diabetes; however, it is unlikely that these antibodies are involved in the pathogenesis of diabetic autonomic neuropathy [899].

The presence of autoantibodies to sympathetic ganglion (Fig. 4.**28**) and vagus nerve in type 1 diabetes, albeit in low titers, has now been well established by groups in Boston [880], Munich [900,901], Malmö [902], and London [903]. The findings are consistent and reproducible, and, once present, a longitudinal study has shown that they persist at least over a 2.5-year period [904]. They are found in approximately one-fifth to one-third of all type 1 diabetic patients (Table 4.**9**). They are demonstrable at any diabetes duration from one to 72 years, with views differing as to whether they increase or decrease over time [905]. They have also been described in some nondiabetic first-degree relatives of type 1 diabetic patients [880]. In contrast, they occur in only 3.1–4.4% of nondiabetic subjects, and they may [902] or may not [904] be found in some patients with type 2 diabetes. In this context, it might be mentioned that cytotoxic sera against neuroblastoma cells have been associated with peripheral sensorimotor neuropathy but not with autonomic neuropathy [906].

The putative autoantigen generating neural antibody responses is not known. Negative findings for targets relating to catecholamine synthesis have been described, and autoantibodies to GAD and IA-2 do not correlate with the presence of neuropathy, indicating that antineural antibodies exist independently [907]. Furthermore, Zanone et al. [908] showed no relationship between the subcellular distribution of GAD and that of cervical ganglion or vagal nerve antibodies, suggesting selective targeting of peripheral nervous system antigens.

Neural Autoantibodies and Autonomic Function

Early work by Rabinowe et al. described an association between the presence of neural autoantibodies with postural hypotension: sympathetic ganglion antibodies were associated with a defective catecholamine response to standing [897], and there was also an association between vagal nerve antibodies and heart rate changes on tilting [898]. Earlier observations also demonstrated that neural autoantibodies were more frequently seen in patients with severe symptomatic autonomic neuropathy than in those without [903]. New and sophisticated methods of demonstrating cardiac sympathetic denervation have recently been described, and such denervation may correlate weakly with the presence of sympathetic ganglion antibodies [900,901]. Determination of neural autoantibodies in a large group of type 1 diabetic patients ($n = 394$) [905] demonstrated their presence at all durations of the disease. Although autonomic function was not determined in this group of patients, there was no relation with vibration perception, making a correlation with autonomic dysfunction unlikely. In agreement with this, no correlation between the presence of sympathetic ganglion antibodies and disturbed autonomic function was shown in another

Table 4.**9** Presence of neural autoantibodies in type 1 diabetes

Symptomatic tissue neuropathy	Type 1 diabetic patients			Nondiabetic controls	
	Boston [903]	London [905]	Munich [900]	London [905]	Munich [900]
Vagus nerve	37%	22%	–	3.1%	–
Cervical ganglion	30%	31%	25%	4.4%	4%

group of type 1diabetic patients; in type 2 diabetic patients, however, there was a correlation between the presence of vagal nerve antibodies and parasympathetic neuropathy [902]. Whether the presence of neural autoantibodies predicts a later development of autonomic dysfunction is not known. A recently found association between autonomic neuropathy versus antibodies against sympathetic ganglion and vagal nerve at the diagnosis of type 1 diabetes implies, however, that these antibodies may be involved in the pathogenesis of autonomic neuropathy [909].

Conclusions

Type 1 diabetes is an autoimmune disorder associated with an increased prevalence of a wide range of organ-specific autoantibodies that include islet cell, anti-GAD, anti IA-2, antigastric, antithyroid, adrenal cortical, and antisteroidal cell antibodies. Recently, anti-transglutaminase antibodies have also been found in about 8% of these patients [910], indicating the presence of clinical celiac disease in the majority. Several studies during the last decade have demonstrated that neural autoantibodies occur in a substantial proportion of type 1 diabetic patients. Their clinical significance is unclear. It has not yet been determined whether they predict autonomic damage, and the association with disturbed autonomic nerve function has to be established.

There remains, however, some powerful evidence that autoimmune mechanisms play some role in the development of severe symptomatic autonomic neuropathy in a small subgroup of diabetic patients. They usually have type 1 diabetes, are likely to be female, have sometimes developed associated iritis, and autonomic tissues show a striking cellular infiltration. These are tantalizing observations that still leave the field in uncertainty and require further elucidation.

References

[1] Sugimura K, Dyck PJ. Multifocal fiber loss in proximal sciatic nerve in symmetric distal diabetic neuropathy. J Neurol Sci 1982; 53: 501–9.

[2] Behse F, Buchthal F, Carlsen F. Nerve biopsy and conduction studies in diabetic neuropathy. J Neurol Neurosurg Psychiatry 1977; 40: 1072–82.

[3] Ohnishi A, Harada M, Tateishi J, Ogata J, Kawanami S. Segmental demyelination and remyelination in lumbar spinal roots of patients dying with diabetes mellitus. Ann Neurol 1983; 13: 541–8.

[4] Sima AAF, Nathaniel V, Bril V, McEwen TA, Greene DA. Histopathological heterogeneity of neuropathy in insulin-dependent and non-insulin-dependent diabetes, and demonstration of axo-glial dysjunction in human diabetic neuropathy. J Clin Invest 1988; 81: 349–64.

[5] Yagihashi S, Matsunaga M. Ultrastructural pathology of peripheral nerves in patients with diabetic neuropathy. Tohoku J Exp Med 1979; 129: 357–66.

[6] Bischoff A. Morphology of diabetic neuropathy. Horm Metab Res Suppl 1980; 9: 18–28.

[7] Said G, Slama G, Selva J. Progressive centripetal degeneration of axons in small fiber type diabetic polyneuropathy. A clinical and pathological study. Brain 1983; 106: 791–807.

[8] King RHM, Llewelyn JG, Thomas PK, Gilbey SG, Watkins PJ. Diabetic neuropathy: abnormalities of Schwann cell and perineurial basal laminae. Implications for diabetic vasculopathy. Neuropathol Appl Neurobiol 1989; 15: 339–55.

[9] Thomas PK, Lascelles RG. The pathology of diabetic neuropathy. Q J Med 1966; 140: 489–509.

[10] Sima AAF, Prashar A, Nathaniel V, Bril V, Werb MR, Greene DA. Overt diabetic neuropathy: repair of axo-glial dysjunction and axonal atrophy by aldose reductase inhibition and its correlation to improvement in nerve conduction velocity. Diabet Med 1993; 10: 115–21.

[11] Britland ST, Young RJ, Sharma AK, Clarke BF. Association of painful and painless diabetic neuropathy with different patterns of nerve fiber degeneration and regeneration. Diabetes 1990; 39: 898–908.

[12] Llewelyn JG, Gilbey SG, Thomas PK, et al. Sural nerve morphometry in diabetic autonomic and painful sensory neuropathy. Brain 1991; 114: 867–92.

[13] Sugimura K, Dyck PJ. Sural nerve myelin thickness and axis cylinder caliber in human diabetes. Neurology 1981; 31: 1087–91.

[14] Engelstad JK, Davies JL, Giannini C, O'Brien PC, Dyck PJ. No evidence for axonal atrophy in human diabetic polyneuropathy. J Neuropathol Exp Neurol 1997; 56: 255–62.

[15] Thomas PK, Lascelles RG. Schwann-cell abnormalities in diabetic neuropathy. Lancet 1965; 62: 1355–7.

[16] Chopra JS, Hurwitz LJ, Montgomery DAD. The pathogenesis of sural nerve changes in diabetes mellitus. Brain 1969; 92: 391–418.

[17] Lamontagne A, Buchthal F. Electrophysiological studies in diabetes mellitus. J Neurol Neurosurg Psychiatry 1970; 33: 442–50.

[18] Kalichman MW, Powell HC, Mizisin AP. Reactive, degenerative and proliferative Schwann cell responses in experimental galactose and human diabetic neuropathy. Acta Neuropathol (Berl) 1998; 95: 47–56.

[19] Veves A, Malik RA, Lye RH, et al. The relationship between sural nerve morphometric findings and measures of peripheral nerve function in mild diabetic neuropathy. Diabet Med 1991; 8: 917–21.

[20] Ballin RHM, Thomas PK. Hypertrophic changes in diabetic neuropathy. Acta Neuropathol (Berl) 1968; 11: 93–102.

[21] Thomas PK, Beamish NG, Small JR, et al. Paranodal structure in diabetic sensory polyneuropathy. Acta Neuropathol (Berl) 1996; 92: 614–20.

[22] Behse F, Buchthal F, Carlsen F, Knappheis GG. Unmyelinated fibers and Schwann cells of sural nerve in neuropathy. Brain 1975; 98: 493–510.

[23] Fagerberg SE. Diabetic neuropathy. A clinical and histological study on the significance of vascular affections. Acta Med Scand 1959; 86: 345.

[24] Malik RA, Newrick PG, Sharma AK, et al. Microangiopathy in human diabetic neuropathy: relationship between capillary abnormalities and the severity of neuropathy. Diabetologia 1989; 32: 92–102.

[25] Malik RA, Tesfaye S, Thompson SD, et al. Endoneurial localization of microvascular damage in human diabetic neuropathy. Diabetologia 1993; 36: 454–9.

[26] Powell HC, Rosoff J, Myers RR. Microangiopathy in human diabetic neuropathy. Acta Neuropathol (Berl) 1985; 68: 295–305.

[27] Yasuda H, Dyck PJ. Abnormalities of endoneurial microvessels and sural nerve pathology in diabetic neuropathy. Neurology 1987; 37: 20–8.

[28] Bradley J, Thomas PK, King RHM, Llewelyn JG, Muddle JR, Watkins PJ. Morphometry of endoneurial capillaries in diabetic sensory and autonomic neuropathy. Diabetologia 1990; 33: 611–8.

[29] Sima AAF, Nathaniel V, Prashar A, Bril V, Greene DA. Endoneurial microvessels in human diabetic neuropathy. Endothelial cell dysjunction and lack of treatment effect by aldose reductase inhibitor. Diabetes 1991; 40: 1090–9.
[30] Williams E, Timperley WR, Ward JD, Duckworth T. Electron microscopical studies of vessels in diabetic peripheral neuropathy. J Clin Pathol 1980; 33: 462–70.
[31] Giannini C, Dyck PJ. Ultrastructural morphometric abnormalities of sural nerve microvessels in diabetes mellitus. Ann Neurol 1994; 36: 408–15.
[32] Timperley WR, Ward JD, Preston FE, Duckworth T, O'Malley BC. Clinical and histological studies in diabetic neuropathy. A reassessment of vascular factors in relation to intravascular coagulation. Diabetologia 1976; 12: 237–43.
[33] Dyck PJ, Hansen S, Karnes J, et al. Capillary number and percentage closed in human diabetic sural nerve. Proc Natl Acad Sci USA 1985; 82: 2513–17.
[34] Korthals JK, Gieron MA, Dyck PJ. Intima of epineurial arterioles is increased in diabetic neuropathy. Neurology 1988; 38: 1582–6.
[35] Malik RA, Tesfaye S, Thompson SD, et al. Transperineurial abnormalities in the sural nerve of patients with diabetic neuropathy. Microvasc Res 1994; 48: 236–45.
[36] Beggs J, Johnson PC, Olafsen A, Watkins CJ. Innervation of the vasa nervorum: changes in human diabetics. J Neuropathol Exp Neurol 1992; 51: 612–29.
[37] Bradley JL, King RHM, Muddle JR, Thomas PK. The extracellular matrix of peripheral nerve in diabetic polyneuropathy. Acta Neuropathol (Berl) 2000; 99: 539–46.
[38] Johnson PC, Doll SC, Cromey DW. Pathogenesis of diabetic neuropathy. Ann Neurol 1986; 19: 450–7.
[39] Griffey RH, Eaton RP, Sibbitt RR, Sibbitt WI, Bicknell JM. Diabetic neuropathy. Structural analysis of nerve hydration by magnetic resonance spectroscopy. JAMA 1988; 260: 2872–8.
[40] Eaton RP, Qualls C, Sibbitt WL, King MK, Griffey RH. Structure-function relationships within peripheral nerves in diabetic neuropathy: the hydration hypothesis. Diabetologia 1996; 39: 439–46.
[41] Johnson PC, Brendel K, Meezan E. Human diabetic perineurial cell basement membrane thickening. Lab Invest 1981; 44: 265–70.
[42] Johnson PC, Doll SC. Dermal nerves in human diabetic subjects. Diabetes 1984; 33: 244–50.
[43] Bradley JL, Thomas PK, King RHM, Watkins PJ. A comparison of perineurial and vascular basal lamina changes in diabetic neuropathy. Acta Neuropathol (Berl) 1994; 88: 426–32.
[44] King RHM, Llewelyn JG, Thomas PK, Gilbey SG, Watkins PJ. Perineurial calcification. Neuropathol Appl Neurobiol 1988; 14: 105–23.
[45] Dyck PJ, Sherman WR, Hallcher LM, et al. Human diabetic endoneurial sorbitol, fructose, and myo-inositol related to sural nerve morphometry. Ann Neurol 1980; 8: 590–6.
[46] Vital C, Vallat JM, Le Blanc M, Martin F, Coquet M. Les neuropathies périphériques du diabète sucre. Etude ultrastructurale de 12-cas biopsies. J Neurol Sci 1973; 18: 381–98.
[47] Bradley JL, Thomas PK, King RHM, et al. Myelinated nerve fiber regeneration in diabetic sensor neuropathy: correlation with type of diabetes. Acta Neuropathol (Berl) 1995; 90: 403–10.
[48] Britland ST, Young RJ, Sharma AK, Clarke BF. Acute and remitting painful diabetic polyneuropathy: a comparison of peripheral nerve fiber pathology. Pain 1992; 48: 361–70.
[49] Dreyfus PM, Hakim S, Adams RD. Diabetic ophthalmoplegia. AMA Arch Neurol Pysch 1957; 77: 337–49.
[50] Asbury AK, Aldredge H, Hershberg R, Fisher CM. Oculomotor palsy in diabetes mellitus: a clinico-pathologic study. Brain 1970; 93: 555–66.
[51] Smith BE, Dyck PJ. Subclinical histopathological changes in the oculomotor nerve in diabetes mellitus. Ann Neurol 1992; 32: 376–85.
[52] Said G, Goulon-Goeau C, Lacroix C, Moulonguet A. Biopsy findings in different patterns of proximal diabetic neuropathy. Ann Neurol 1994; 35: 559–69.
[53] Llewelyn JG, Thomas PK, King RHM. Epineurial microvasculitis in proximal diabetic neuropathy. J Neurol 1998; 245: 159–65.
[54] Dyck PJB, Norell JE, Dyck PJ. Microvasculitis and ischemia in diabetic lumbosacral radiculoplexus neuropathy. Neurology 1999; 53: 2113–21.
[55] Duchen LW, Anjorin A, Watkins PJ, MacKay JD. Pathology of autonomic neuropathy in diabetes. Ann Intern Med 1980; 92: 301–5.
[56] Appenzeller O, Richardson EP Jr. The sympathetic chain in patients with diabetic and alcoholic polyneuropathy. Neurology 1966; 16: 1205–9.
[57] Olsson Y, Sourander P. Changes in the sympathetic nervous system in diabetes mellitus. J Neuro-Visceral Relations 1968; 31: 86–95.
[58] Schmidt RE, Plurad SB, Parvin CA, Roth KA. The effect of diabetes and aging on human sympathetic autonomic ganglia. Am J Pathol 1993; 143: 143–53.
[59] Schmidt RE. The neuropathology of human sympathetic autonomic ganglia. Microsc Res Tech 1996; 35: 107–21.
[60] Rabinowe SL. Immune mechanisms in diabetic autonomic and related neuropathies. In: Low PA, editors. Clinical autonomic disorders. Philadelphia, Pa.: Lippincott-Raven; 1997: 509–24.
[61] Stroud CR, Heller SR, Ward JD, Hardisty CA, Weetman AP. Analysis of antibodies against components of the autonomic nervous system in diabetes mellitus. Q J Med 1997; 90: 577–85.
[62] Sejnowski TJ. Peptidergic synaptic transmission in sympathetic ganglia. Fed Proc 1982; 441: 2923–8.
[63] Schmidt RE, Beaudet LN, Plurad SB, Dorsey DA. Axonal cytoskeletal pathology in aged and diabetic human sympathetic autonomic ganglia. Brain Res 1997; 769: 375–83.
[64] Appenzeller O, Ogin G. Myelinated fibers in human paravertebral sympathetic chain: white rami communicantes in alcoholic and diabetic patients. J Neurol Neurosurg Psychiatry 1974; 37: 1155–61.
[65] Low PA, Walsh JC, Huang CY, McLeod JG. The sympathetic nervous system in diabetic neuropathy—a clinical and pathological study. Brain 1975; 98: 341–56.
[66] Said G, Goulon-Goeau C, Tchbroutsky G. Severe early-onset polyneuropathy in insulin dependent diabetes mellitus: a clinical and pathological study. N Engl J Med 1992, 326: 1257–63.
[67] Beggs J, Johnson PC, Olafsen A, Watkins CJ. Innervation of the vasa nervorum: changes in human diabetics. J Neuropathol Exp Neurol 1993; 51: 612–29.
[68] Kristensson K, Nordborg C, Olsson Y, Sourander P. Changes in the vagus nerve in diabetes mellitus. Acta Pathol Microbiol Scand 1971; 79A: 684–5.
[69] Guo Y-P, McLeod JG, Baverstock J. Pathologic changes in the vagus nerve in diabetes and chronic alcoholism. J Neurol Neurosurg Psychiatry 1987; 50: 1449–53.
[70] Guy RJC, Dawson JL, Barrett JR, Laws JW, Thomas PK, Sharma AK, et al. Diabetic gastroparesis from autonomic neuropathy: surgical considerations and changes in vagus nerve morphology. J Neurol Neurosurg Psychiatry 1984; 47: 686–91.
[71] Yoshida MM, Schuffler MD, Sumi SM. There are no morphological abnormalities of the gastric wall or abdominal vagus in patients with diabetic gastroparesis. Gastroenterology 1988; 94: 907–14.
[72] Gu J, Polak JM, Lazarides M, Morgan R, Pryor JP, Marangos PJ, et al. Decrease of vasoactive intestinal polypeptide (VIP) in the penises from impotent men. Lancet 1984; 2: 315–7.
[73] Crowe R, Lincoln J, Blacklay PF, Pryor JP, Lumnley JSP, Burnstock G. Vasoactive intestinal polypeptide-like immunoreactive nerves in diabetic penis. A comparison between streptozotocin-treated rats and man. Diabetes 1983; 32: 1075–7.
[74] Lysy J, Karmeli F, Goldin E. Substance P levels in the rectal mucosa of diabetic patients with normal bowel function and constipation. Scand J Gastroenterol 1993; 28: 49–52.
[75] Faerman I, Glocer L, Celener D, Jadzinsky M, Fox D, Maler M, et al. Autonomic nervous system and diabetes: histological and histochemical study of the autonomic nerve fibers of the urinary bladder in diabetic patients. Diabetes 1973; 22: 225–37.
[76] Faerman I, Glocer L, Fox D, Jadzinsky MN, Rapaport M. Impotence and diabetes: histological studies of the autonomic nervous fibers of the corpora cavernosa in impotent diabetic males. Diabetes 1974; 23: 971–6.
[77] Drewes VM, Olsen S. Histological changes in the small bowel in diabetes mellitus—a study of peroral biopsy specimens. Acta Pathol Microbiol Scand 1965; 63: 478–80.

[78] Schmidt H, Riemann JF, Schmid A, Sailer D. Ultrastruktur der diabetischen autonomen Neuropathie des Gastrointestinaltraktes. Klin Wochenschr 1984; 62: 399–405.
[79] Stevens MJ, Raffel DM, Allman KC, Dayanikli F, Ficaro E, Sandford T, et al. Cardiac sympathetic dysinnervation in diabetes—implications for enhanced cardiovascular risk. Circulation 1998; 98: 961–8.
[80] Schmidt RE, Plurad SB. Ultrastructural and biochemical characterization of autonomic neuropathy in rats with chronic streptozotocin diabetes. J Neuropathol Exp Neurol 1986; 45: 525–44.
[81] Yagihashi S, Sima AAF. The distribution of structural changes in sympathetic nerves of the BB rat. Am J Pathol 1985; 121: 138–47.
[82] Schmidt RE, Plurad DA, Plurad SB, Cogswell BE, Diani AR, Roth KA. Ultrastructural and immunohistochemical characterization of autonomic neuropathy in genetically diabetic Chinese hamsters. Lab Invest 1989; 61: 77–92.
[83] Schmidt RE, Dorsey DA, Beaudet LN, Plurad SB, Parvin CA, Miller MS. Insulin-like growth factor I reverses experimental diabetic autonomic neuropathy. Am J Pathol 1999; 155: 1651–60.
[84] Ishii DN. Insulin and related neurotrophic factors in diabetic neuropathy. Diabet med 1993; 10 (Suppl 2): 14S–5.
[85] Loesch A, Belai A, Lincoln J, Burnstock G. Enteric nerves in diabetic rats: electron microscopic evidence for neuropathy of vasoactive intestinal polypeptide-containing fibres. Acta Neuropathol 1986; 70: 161–8.
[86] Belai A, Burnstock G. Selective damage of intrinsic calcitonin gene-related peptide-like immunoreactive enteric nerve fibers in streptozotocin-induced diabetic rats. Gastroenterology 1987; 92: 730–4.
[87] Ballman M, Conlon JM. Changes in the somatostatin, substance P and vasoactive intestinal polypeptide content of the gastrointestinal tract following streptozotocin induced diabetes in the rat. Diabetologia 1985; 28: 355–8.
[88] Belai A, Lincoln J, Milner P, Burnstock G. Differential effect of streptozotocin-induced diabetes on the innervation of the ileum and distal colon. Gastroenterology 1991; 100: 1024–32.
[89] Belai A, Lincoln J, Burnstock G. Lack of release of vasoactive intestinal peptide and calcitonin gene-related peptide during electrical stimulation of enteric nerves in streptozotocin-diabetic rats. Gastroenterology1987; 93: 1034–40.
[90] Scott LD, Ellis TM. Small intestinal transit and myoelectric activity in diabetic rats. In: Christensen J, editors. Gastrointestinal motility. New York, N.Y.: Raven Press; 1980: 395–9.
[91] Diani AR, Grogan DM, Yates ME, Risinger DL, Gerritsen GC. Radiologic abnormalities and autonomic neuropathology in the digestive tract of the ketonuric diabetic Chinese hamster. Diabetologia 1979; 17: 33–40.
[92] Nowak TV, Harrington B, Kalbfleisch JA, Anatruda JM. Evidence for abnormal cholinergic transmission in diabetic rat small intestine. Gastroenterology 1986; 91: 124–32.
[93] Lucas PD, Sardar AM. Effects of diabetes on cholinergic transmission in two rat gut preparations. Gastroenterology 1991; 100: 123–8.
[94] Chang EM, Fedorak RN, Field M. Experimental diabetic diarrhea in rats. Intestinal mucosal denervation hypersensitivity and treatment with clonidine. Gastroenterology 1986; 91: 364–9.
[95] Turpeinen AK, Vanninen E, Kuikka JT, Uusitupa MIJ. Demonstration of regional sympathetic denervation of the heart in diabetes. Comparison between patients with NIDDM and IDDM. Diabetes Care 1996; 19: 1083–90.
[96] Pinna C, Bolego C, Puglisi L. Effect of substance P and capsaicin on urinary bladder of diabetic rats and the role of the epithelium. Eur J Pharmacol 1994; 271: 151–8.
[97] Luiten PGM, Horst GJ ter, Buijs RM, Steffens AB. Autonomic innervation of the pancreas in diabetic and non-diabetic rats. A new view on intraneural sympathetic structural organization. J Auton Nerv Syst 1986; 15: 33–44.
[98] Felten DL, Felten SY, Melman A. Noradrenergic innervation of the penis in control and streptozotocin-diabetic rats: evidence of autonomic neuropathy. Anat Rec 1983; 206: 49–59.
[99] Li H, Grimes P. Adrenergic innervation of the choroid and iris in diabetic rats. Curr Eye Res 1993; 12: 89–94.
[100] Zhang W-X, Chakrabarti S, Greene DA, Sima AAF. Diabetic autonomic neuropathy in BB-rats: the effect of ARI-treatment on heart-rate variability and vagus nerve structure. Diabetes 1990; 39: 613–8.
[101] Yagihashi S, Sima AAF. Diabetic autonomic neuropathy. Ultrastructural and morphometric changes in parasympathetic nerves. Diabetes 1986; 35: 733–43.
[102] Paro M, Prosdocimi M, Zhang W-X, Sutherland G, Sima AAF. Autonomic neuropathy in the BB-rat. Alterations in bladder function. Diabetes 1989; 38: 1023–30.
[103] Cellek S, Rodrigo J, Lobos E, Fernandez P, Serrano J, Moncada S. Selective nitrergic neurodegeneration in diabetes mellitus - a nitric oxide-dependent phenomenon. Br J Pharmacol 1999; 128: 1804–12.
[104] Purves D. Functional and structural changes of mammalian sympathetic neurons following interruption of their axons. J Physiol 1975; 252: 429–63.
[105] Schmidt RE. Synaptic dysplasia in sympathetic autonomic ganglia. J Neurocytol 1996; 25: 777–91.
[106] Marchal Calvi J de. Recherches sur les accidents diabétiques. Paris: Asselin, 1864.
[107] Santiago JV. Lessons from the Diabetes Control and Complications Trial. Diabetes 1993; 42: 1549–54.
[108] Lasker RD. The Diabetes Control and Complications Trial. Implications for policy and practice. N Engl J Med 1993; 329: 1035–6.
[109] The Diabetes Control and Complications Trial Research Group. The effect of intensive treatment of diabetes on the development and progression of long-term complications in insulin-dependent diabetes mellitus. N Engl J Med 1993; 329: 977–86.
[110] Prospective Diabetes Study UK (UKPDS) Group. Intensive blood-glucose control with sulphonylureas or insulin compared with conventional treatment and risk of complications in patients with type 2 diabetes (UKPDS 33). Lancet 1998; 352: 837–53.
[111] Prospective Diabetes Study UK (UKPDS) Group. Effect of intensive blood-glucose control with metformin on complications in overweight patients with type 2 diabetes (UKPDS 34). Lancet 1998; 352: 854–65.
[112] Nathan DM. Some answers, more controversy, from UKPDS. Lancet 1998; 352: 832–3.
[113] McCormack J, Greenhalgh T. Seeing what you want to see in randomised controlled trials: versions and perversions of UKPDS data. Br Med J 2000; 320: 1720–3.
[114] Hreidarsson AB. Acute, reversible autonomic nervous system abnormalities in juvenile insulin-dependent diabetes. Diabetologia 1981; 20: 457–81.
[115] Davenport A, Ahmad R. Hyperosmolar nonketotic hyperglycemia manifested as ascending polyneuropathy. South Med J 1990; 2: 250–2.
[116] Gregersen G. Variations in motor conduction velocity produced by acute changes of the metabolic state in diabetic patients. Diabetologia 1968; 4: 273–7.
[117] Fraser DM, Campbell IW, Ewing DJ, Murray A, Neilson JMM, Clarke BF. Peripheral and autonomic nerve function in newly diagnosed diabetes mellitus. Diabetes 1977; 6: 546–50.
[118] Terkildsen AB, Christensen NJ. Reversible nervous abnormalities in juvenile diabetics with recently diagnosed diabetes. Diabetologia 1971; 7: 113–7.
[119] Frost-Larsen K, Sandahl-Christiansen J, Parving H-H. The effect of strict short-term metabolic control on retinal nervous system abnormalities in newly diagnosed type-1 (insulin-dependent) diabetic patients. Diabetologia 1983; 24: 207–9.
[120] Troni W, Carta Q, Cantelle R, Caselle MT, Rainero I. Peripheral nerve function and metabolic control in diabetes mellitus. Ann Neurol 1984; 16: 178–83.
[121] Gallai V, Agostini L, Rossi A, Massi-Benedetti M, Calabrese G, Puxeddu A, Brunetti P. Evaluation of the motor and sensory conduction velocity (MCV, SCV) in diabetic patients before and after a three days treatment with the artificial beta cell (biostator). In: Canal N, Pozza G, editors. Peripheral neuropathies. Amsterdam: North Holland Press;1978: 287–9.
[122] Campbell IW, Ewing DJ, Harrower ABD, Neilson JMM, Fraser DM, Baldwa VS, Murray A, Clarke BF. Peripheral and autonomic nerve function in diabetic ketoacidosis. Lancet 1976; 24: 167–9.
[123] Holman RR, Mayon-White V, Orde-Peckar C, Steemson J, Smith B, McPherson K, Rizza C, Knight AH, Dornan TL, Howard-Williams J, Jenkins L, Rolfe R, Barbour D, Poon P,

Mann JI, Bron AJ, Turner RC. Prevention of deterioration of renal and sensory-nerve function by more intensive management of insulin-dependent diabetic patients. Lancet 1983; 1: 204–8.
[124] Dahl-Jörgensen K, Brinchmann-Hansen O, Hanssen KF, Ganes T, Kierulf P, Smeland E, Sandivik L, Aagenaes O. Effect of near normoglycaemia for two years on progression of early diabetic retinopathy, nephropathy, and neuropathy: the Oslo study. Br Med J 1986; 293: 1195–9.
[125] Jakobsen J, Christiansen JS, Kristoffersen I, Christensen CK, Hermansen K, Schmitz A, Mogensen CE. Autonomic and somatosensory nerve function after 2 years of continuous subcutaneous insulin infusion in Type 1 diabetes. Diabetes 1988; 37: 452–5.
[126] Service FJ, Daube JR, O'Brien PC, Zimmerman BR, Swanson CJ, Brennan MD, Dyck PJ. Effect of blood glucose control on peripheral nerve function in diabetic patients. Mayo Clin Proc 1983; 58: 283–9.
[127] Lauritzen T, Frost-Larsen K, Larsen H-W, Deckert T, and the Steno Study Group. Two-year experience with continuous subcutanous insulin infusion in relation to retinopathy and neuropathy. Diabetes 1985; 34: 74–9.
[128] Schneider U, Jund R, Nees S, Grafe P. Differences in sensitivity to hyperglycemic hypoxia of isolated rat sensory and motor nerve fibers. Neurology 1992; 31: 605–10.
[129] Llewelyn JG, Thomas PK, Fonseca V, King RHM, Dandona P. Acute painful diabetic neuropathy precipitated by strict glycaemic control. Acta Neuropathol 1986; 72: 157–63.
[130] Caravati CM. Insulin neuritis: a case report. Va Med Mon 1933; 59: 745–6.
[131] Ward JD, Barnes CG, Fisher DJ, Jessop JD, Baker RWR. Improvement in nerve conduction following treatment in newly diagnosed diabetics. Lancet 1971; 1: 428–31.
[132] Boulton AJM, Drury J, Clarke B, Ward JD. Continuous subcutaneous insulin infusion in the management of painful diabetic neuropathy. Diabetes Care 1982; 5: 386–90.
[133] Gambardella S, Napoli A, Spallone V, Verrastro AM, Lazzari R, Geraldini C, Sideri G, Menzinger G. Influence of glucoregulation with continuous subcutaneous insulin infusion on nerve conduction velocity and beat to beat variation in diabetics. J Endocrinol Invest 1983; 6: 363–7.
[134] Krönert K, Hülser J, Luft D, Stetter T, Eggstein M. Effects of continuous subcutaneous insulin infusion and intensified conventional therapy on peripheral and autonomic nerve dysfunction. J Clin Endocrinol Metab 1986; 64: 1219–23.
[135] Dyck PJ. Detection, characterization, and staging of polyneuropathy: assessed in diabetics. Muscle Nerve 1988; 11: 21–32.
[136] Dyck PJ, O'Brien PC. Meaningful degrees of prevention or improvement of nerve conduction in controlled clinical trials of diabetic neuropathy. Diabetes Care 1989; 9: 649–52.
[137] Ziegler D, Dannehl K, Wiefels K, Gries FA. Differential effects of near-normoglycaemia for 4 years on somatic nerve dysfunction and heart rate variation in type 1 diabetic patients. Diabet med 1992; 9: 622–9.
[138] Reichard P, Pihl M, Rosenqvist U, Sule J. Complications in IDDM are caused by elevated blood glucose level: The Stockholm Diabetes Intervention Study (SDIS) at 10-year follow-up. Diabetologia 1996; 39: 1483–8.
[139] Amthor K-F, Dahl-Jörgensen K, Berg TJ, Skard Heier M, Sandvik L, Aagenaes A, Hanssen KF. The effect of 8 years of strict glycaemic control on peripheral nerve function in IDDM patients: the Oslo Study. Diabetologia 1994; 37: 579–84.
[140] Diabetes Control and Complications Trial Research Group. The effect of intensive diabetes treatment on nerve conduction in the Diabetes Control and Complications Trial (DCCT). Ann Neurol 1995; 38: 869–80.
[141] The Diabetes Control and Complications Trial Research Group. The effect of intensive diabetes therapy on measures of autonomic nervous system function in the Diabetes Control and Complications Trial (DCCT). Diabetologia 1998; 41: 416–23.
[142] The Diabetes Control and Complications Trial/Epidemiology of Diabetes Interventions and Complications Research Group. Retinopathy and nephropathy in patients with type 1 diabetes four years after a trial of intensive therapy. N Engl J Med 2000; 342: 381–9.
[143] Ohkubo Y, Kishikawa H, Araki E, Miyata T, Isami S, Motoyoshi S, Kojima Y, Furuyoshi N, Shichiri M. Intensive insulin therapy prevents the progression of diabetic microvascular complications in Japanese patients with non-insulin-dependent diabetes mellitus: a randomized prospective 6-year study. Diabetes Res Clin Pract 1995; 28: 103–17.
[144] Wake N, Hisashige A, Katayama T, Kishikawa H, Ohkubo Y, Sakai M, Araki E, Shichiri M. Cost-effectiveness of intensive insulin therapy for type 2 diabetes: a 10-year follow-up of the Kumamoto study. Diabetes Res Clin Pract 2000; 48: 201–10.
[145] Gæde P, Vedel P, Parving H-H, Pederson O. Intensified multifactorial intervention in patients with type 2 diabetes mellitus and microalbuminuria: the Steno type 2 randomised study. Lancet 1999; 353: 617–22.
[146] Azad N, Emanuele NV, Abraira C, Henderson WG, Colwell J, Levin SR, Nuttall FQ, Comstock JP, Sawin CT, Silbert C, Rubino FA, the VA CSDM Group. The effects of intensive glycemic control on neuropathy in the VA Cooperative Study on Type II diabetes mellitus. J Diabetes Complications 2000; 13: 307–13.
[147] Tattersall R. Is pancreas transplantation for insulin-dependent diabetics worthwhile? N Engl J Med 1989; 2: 112–4.
[148] Kennedy WR, Navarro X, Goetz FC, Sutherland DER, Najarian JS. Effects of pancreatic transplantation on diabetic neuropathy. N Engl J Med 1990; 15: 1031–7.
[149] Solders G, Tyden G, Persson A, Groth C-G. Improvement of nerve conduction in diabetic neuropathy. A follow-up study 4 years after combined pancreatic and renal transplantation. Diabetes 1992; 41: 946–51.
[150] Müller-Felber W, Landgraf R, Scheuer R, Wagner S, Reimers CD, Nusser J, Abendroth D, Illner W-D, Land W. Diabetic neuropathy 3 years after successful pancreas and kidney transplantation. Diabetes 1993; 42: 1482–6.
[151] Navarro X, Sutherland DER, Kennedy WR. Long-term effects of pancreatic transplantation on diabetic neuropathy. Ann Neurol 1997; 42: 727–36.
[152] Allen RDM, Al-Habri IS, Morris JGL, Clouston PD, O'Connell PJ, Chapman JR, Nankivell BJ. Diabetic neuropathy after pancreas transplantation: determinants of recovery. Transplantation 1997; 63: 830–8.
[153] Martinenghi S, Comi G, Galardi G, Di Carlo V, Pozza G, Secchi A. Amelioration of nerve conduction velocity following simultaneous kidney/pancreas transplantation is due to the glycaemic control provided by the pancreas. Diabetologia 1997; 40: 1110–2.
[154] Krolewski AS, Laffel LMB, Krolewski M, Quinn M, Warram JH. Glycosylated hemoglobin and the risk of microalbuminuria in patients with insulin-dependent diabetes mellitus. N Engl J Med 1995; 332: 1251–5.
[155] Warram JH, Manson JE, Krolewski AS. Glycosylated hemoglobin and the risk of retinopathy in insulin-dependent diabetes mellitus. N Engl J Med 1995; 332: 1305–6.
[156] Haffner SM. Is there a glycemic threshold? Arch Intern Med 1997; 157: 1791.
[157] The Diabetes Control and Complications Trial Research Group. The relationship of glycemic exposure (HbA1c) to the risk of development and progression of retinopathy in the Diabetes Control and Complications Trial. Diabetes 1995; 44: 968–83.
[158] The Diabetes Control and Complications Trial Research Group. The absence of a glycemic threshold for the development of long-term complications: the perspective of the Diabetes Control and Complications Trial. Diabetes 1996; 45: 1289–98.
[159] Orchard TJ, Forrest KY-Z, Ellis D, Becker DJ. Cumulative glycemic exposure and microvascular complications in insulin-dependent diabetes mellitus. The glycemic threshold revisited. Arch Intern Med 1997; 157: 1851–6.
[160] Pirart J. Diabetes mellitus and its degenerative complications: a prospective study of 4400 patients observed. Diabetes Care 1978; 1: 168–88.
[161] Heesom AE, Hibberd ML, Millward A, Demaine AG. Polymorphism in the 5′-end of the aldose reductase gene is strongly associated with the development of diabetic nephropathy in type I diabetes. Diabetes 1997; 46: 287–91.
[162] Ko BC, Lam KS, Wat NM, Chung SS. An (A-C)n dinucleotide repeat polymorphic marker at the 5′-end of the aldose reductase gene is associated with early onset diabetic retinopathy in NIDDM patients. Diabetes 1995; 46: 727–32.
[163] Dyck PJ, Kratz KM, Karnes JL, Litchy WJ, Klein R, Pach JM, et al. The prevalence by staged severity of various types of diabetic neuropathy, retinopathy, and nephropathy in a pop-

ulation based cohort: the Rochester Diabetic Neuropathy Study. Neurology 1993; 43: 817–24.
[164] Ido Y, Vindigni A, Chang K, et al. Prevention of vascular and neural dysfunction in diabetic rats by C-peptide. London: Science; 1996.
[165] Johansson B-L, Borg K, Fernquist-Forbes E, Odergren T, Remahl S, Wahren J. C-peptide improves autonomic nerve function in patients with type-1 diabetes. Diabetologia 1996; 39: 687–95.
[166] Sima AAF, Zhang W, Xu G, Sugimoto K, Guberski D, Yorek MA. A comparison of diabetic polyneuropathy in type II diabetic BBZDR/Wor rats and in type I diabetic BB/Wor rats. Diabetologia 2000; 43: 786–93.
[167] Sima AAF, Zhang W, Sugimoto K, Henry D, Li Z, Wahren J, Grunberger G. C-peptide prevents and improves chronic type I diabetic neuropathy in the BB/Wor-rat. Diabetologia 2001; 44: 889–97.
[168] Yagihashi S. Pathology and pathogenetic mechanisms of diabetic neuropathy. Diab Metab Rev 1995; 11: 193–225.
[169] Sima AAF, Ristic H, Merry A, Kamijo M, Lattimer SA, Stevens MJ, Greene DA. The primary preventional and secondary interventative effects of acetyl-L-carnitine on diabetic neuropathy in the BB/W-rat. J Clin Invest 1996; 97: 1900–7.
[170] Greene DA, Sima AAF, Feldman E, Stevens MJ. Diabetic neuropathy. In: Porte D, Sherwin R, editors. Ellenberg and Rifkin's Diabetes Mellitus. Stamford, Conn.: Appleton and Lange; 1997.
[171] Dyck PJ, Zimmerman BR, Vilen TH, Minnerath SR, Karnes JL, Yao JK, et al. Nerve glucose, fructose, sorbitol, myo-inositol and fiber degeneration and regeneration in diabetic neuropathy. N Engl J Med 1988; 319: 542–8.
[172] Ishii DN. Implications of insulin-like growth factors in the pathogenesis of diabetic neuropathy. Brain Res Rev 1995a; 20: 47–67.
[173] Greene DA, Sima AAF, Stevens MJ, et al. Aldose reductase inhibitors: as approach to the treatment of diabetic nerve damage. Diabetes Metab Rev 1993; 9: 189–217.
[174] Chakrabarti S, Sima AAF, Nakajima T, Yaghihashi S, Greene DA. Aldose reductase in the BB rat: isolation, immunological identification and localization in the retina and peripheral nerve. Diabetologia 1987; 30: 244–51.
[175] Powell HC, Rosoff J, Myers RR. Microangiopathy in human diabetic neuropathy. Acta Neuropathol (Berl) 1991; 81: 529–39.
[176] Stevens MJ, Lattimer SA, Kamijo M, Huysen C Van, Sima AAF, Greene DA. Osmotically induced nerve taurine depletion and the compatible osmolyte hypothesis in experimental diabetic neuropathy in the rat. Diabetologia 1993; 36: 608–14.
[177] Aruoma O, Halliwell B, Hoey BM, Butler J. The antioxidant action of taurine, hypotaurine and their metabolic precursors. Biochem J 1988; 256: 251–5.
[178] El Idrissi A, Trenkner E. Growth factors and taurine protect against excitotoxicity by stabilizing calcium homeostasis and energy metabolism. J Neurosci 1999; 19: 9459–68.
[179] Greene DA, Chakrabarti S, Lattimer SA, Sima AAF. Role of sorbitol accumulation and myoinositol depletion in paranodal swelling of large myelinated nerve fibers in the insulin-deficient spontaneously diabetic biobreeding rat. J Clin Invest 1987; 79: 1479–85.
[180] Mayer JH, Tomlinson DR. Prevention of defects of axonal transport and nerve conduction velocity by oral administration of myo-inositol or an ARI in streptozotocin diabetic rats. Diabetologia 1983; 25: 433–8.
[181] Brismar T, Sima AAF. Changes in nodal function in nerve fibers of the spontaneously diabetic BB-Wistar rat. Potential clamp analysis. Acta Physiol Scand 1981; 113: 499–506.
[182] Williamson JR, Chang K, Frangos M, et al. Hyperglycemic pseudohypoxia and diabetic complications. Diabetes 1993; 42: 801–13.
[183] Sonobe M, Yasuda H, Hisanaga T, et al. Amelioration of nerve Na^+K^+-ATPase activity independently of myo-inositol level by PGE1 analogue OP-1206 α-CD in streptozocin-induced diabetic rats. Diabetes 1991; 40: 726–30.
[184] Yasuda H, Sonobe M, Hatanaka I, et al. A new prostaglandin E1 analogue (TFC-612) prevents a decrease in motor nerve conduction velocity in streptozocin-diabetic rats. Biochem Biophys Res Commun 1988; 150: 225–30.
[185] Cameron NE, Cotter MA, Archibald V, Dines KC, Maxfield EK. Anti-oxidant and pro-oxidant effects on nerve conduction velocity, endoneurial blood flow and oxygen tension in non-diabetic and streptozocin-diabetic rats. Diabetologia 1994; 37: 449–59.
[186] Stevens MJ, Lattimer SA, Feldman EL, et al. Acetyl-L-carnitine deficiency as a cause of altered nerve myo-inositol content, Na^+K^+-ATPase activity and motor conduction velocity in the streptozocin diabetic rat. Metabolism 1996; 45: 865–72.
[187] Hotta N, Koh N, Sakakibata F, et al. Effect of proprionyl-L-carnitine on motor nerve conduction, autonomic cardiac function and nerve blood flow in rats with streptozocin-induced diabetes. J Pharmacol Exp Ther 1996; 276: 49–55.
[188] Cotter MA, Cameron NE, Keegan A, Dines KC. Effect of acetyl- and propionyl-L-carnitine on peripheral nerve function and vascular supply in experimental diabetes. Metabolism 1995; 44: 1209–14.
[189] Wahren J, Ekberg K, Johansson J, Henriksson M, Pramanika A, Johansson B-L, et al. Role of C-peptide in human physiology. Am J Physiol Endocrinol Metab 2000; 278: E759–768.
[190] Hohman TC, Banas D. Basso M, Cotter MA, Cameron NE. Increased oxidative stress in experimental diabetic neuropathy. Diabetologia 1997; 40: A549.
[191] Tilton RG, Chang K, Nyengaard JR, Eden M Van Den, Kilo C, Williamson JR. Inhibition of sorbitol dehydrogenase. Effects on vascular and neural dysfunction in streptozocin-induced diabetic rats. Diabetes 1995; 44: 234–42.
[192] Cameron NE, Cotter MA, Basso M, Hohman TC. Comparison of the effects of inhibitors and aldose reductase and sorbitol dehydrogenase on neurovascular function, nerve conduction and tissue polyol-pathway metabolites in streptozocin-diabetic rats. Diabetologia 1997; 40: 271–81.
[193] Schmidt RE, Dorsey DA, Beaudet LN, Plurad SB, Williamson JR, Ido Y. Effect of sorbitol dehydrogenase inhibition on experimental diabetic autonomic neuropathy. J Neuropathol Exp Neurol 1998; 57: 1175–89.
[194] Sima AAF, Brismar T. Reversible diabetic nerve dysfunction. Structural correlates to electrophysiological abnormalities. Ann Neurol 1985; 18: 21–9.
[195] Yagihashi S, Yamagishi SI, Wada R, et al. Galactosemic neuropathy in transgenic mice for human aldose reductase. Diabetes 1996; 45: 56–9.
[196] Robertson DM, Sima AAF. Diabetic neuropathy in the mutant mouse [C57/BL/KS(db/db)]. A morphometric study. Diabetes 1980; 29: 60–7.
[197] Vlassara H, Brownlee M, Cermi A. Excessive non-enzymatic glycosylation of peripheral and central nervous system components in diabetic rats. Diabetes 1983; 32: 670–4.
[198] Vlassara H, Brownlee M, Cermi A. Recognition and uptake of human diabetic peripheral nerve myelin by macrophages. Diabetes 1985; 34: 553–7.
[199] Vlassara H. Recent progress on the biologic and clinical significance of advanced glycation end products. J Lab Clin Med 1994; 124: 19–30.
[200] Wells-Knecht KJ, Lyons TJ, McCance DR, Thorpe SR, Feather MS, Baynes JW. 3-Deoxyfructose concentrations are increased in human plasma and urine in diabetes. Diabetes 1994; 43: 1152–6.
[201] Glomb M, Monnier VM. Mechanism of protein modification by glyoxal and glycoaldehyde, reactive intermediates in the Maillard reaction. J Biol Chem 1995; 270: 10017–26.
[202] Requena JR, Baynes JW. Studies in animal models on the role of glycation end products (AGEs) in the pathogenesis of diabetic complications: pitfalls and limitations. In: Sima AAF, editor. Frontiers in animal diabetes research. Chronic complications in diabetes. Amsterdam: Harwood Academic; 2000: 43–69.
[203] Takagi Y, Kashiwagi A, Tanaka Y, Asahina T, Kikkawa R, Shigeta Y. Significance of fructose-induced protein oxidation and formation of advanced glycation end product. J Diabetes Complications 1995; 9: 87–91.
[204] Baynes JW, Thorpe SR. Role of oxidative stress in diabetic complications. A new perspective on an old paradigm. Diabetes 1999; 48: 1–9.
[205] Hoshi A, Takahashi M, Fujii J, et al. Glycation and inactivation of sorbitol dehydrogenase in normal and diabetic rats. Biochem J 1999; 318: 119–23.

[206] Soulis-Liparota T, Cooper ME, Dunlop M, Jerums G. The relative roles of advanced glycation, oxidation and aldose reductase inhibition in the development of experimental diabetic nephropathy in the Sprague-Dawley rat. Diabetologia 1995; 38: 387–94.

[207] Weimbs T, Stoffel W. Topology of CNS myelin proteolipid protein: evidence for the nonezymatic glycosylation of extracytoplasmic domains in normal and diabetic animals. Biochemistry 1994; 33: 10408–15.

[208] Schmidt AM, Vianna M, Gerlach M, et al. Isolation and characterization of two binding proteins for advanced glycation end products from bovine lung which are present on the endothelial cell surface. J Biol Chem 1992; 267: 14987–97.

[209] Neeper M, Schmidt AM, Brett J, et al. Cloning and expression of a cell surface receptor for advanced glycosylation end products of proteins. J Biol Chem 1992; 267: 14998–5004.

[210] Yan SD, Schmidt AM, Anderson GM, Zhang J, Brett J, Zou YS, et al. Enhanced cellular oxidative stress by the interaction of advanced glycation end products with their receptor/binding proteins. J Biol Chem 1994; 269: 9889–97.

[211] Wautier JL, Wautier MP, Schmidt AM, Anderson GM, Hori O, Zoukourian C, et al. Advanced glycation end products (AGEs) on the surface of diabetic erythrocytes bind to the vessel wall via a specific receptor inducing oxidant stress in the vasculature: a link between surface-associated AGEs and diabetic complications. Proc Natl Acad Sci USA 1994; 91: 7742–6.

[212] Vlassara H, Brownlee M, Cerami A. Nonenzymatic glycosylation of peripheral nerve protein in diabetes mellitus. Proc Natl Acad Sci USA 1981; 78: 5190–92.

[213] Federoff JH, Lawrence D, Brownlee M. Nonenzymatic glycation glycosylation of laminin and the laminin peptide CIKVAVS inhibits neurite outgrowth. Diabetes 1993; 42: 509–13.

[214] Baynes JW. Role of oxidative stress in the development of complications of diabetes. Diabetes 1991; 40: 405–12.

[215] Sugimoto K, Nishizawa Y, Horiuchi S, Yagihashi S. Localization in human diabetic peripheral nerve of N^{ε}-carboxymethyllysine protein adducts, one of the advanced glycation end products. Diabetologia 1997; 40: 1380–7.

[216] Arai K, Maguchi S, Fujii S, Ishibashi H, Oikawa K, Taniguchi N. Glycation and inactivation of human Cu-Zn-superoxide dismutase. Identification of the in vitro glycated sites. J Biol Chem 1987; 262: 16969-72.

[217] Bierhaus A, Chevion S, Chevion M, et al. Advanced glycation end product-induced activation of NF-κB is suppressed by α-lipoic acid in cultured endothelial cells. Diabetes 1997; 46: 1481–90.

[218] Yagihashi S, Kamijo M, Baba M, Yagihashi N, Hagai K. Effect of aminoguanidine of functional and structural abnormalities in peripheral nerve of STZ-induced diabetic rats. Diabetes 1992; 41: 47–52.

[219] Kihara M, Schmelzer JD, Podulso JF, Curran FF, Nickander KK, Low PA. Aminoguanidine effect on nerve blood flow, vascular permeability, electrophysiology and oxygen free radicals. Proc Natl Acad Sci USA 1991; 88: 6107–11.

[220] Wada R, Sugo M, Nakano M, Yagihashi S. Only limited effects of aminoguanidine treatment on peripheral nerve function, (Na^+,K^+)-ATPase activity and thrombomodulin expression in streptozocin-induced diabetic rats. Diabetologia 1999; 42: 743–7.

[221] Sugimoto K, Yagihashi S. Effects of aminoguanidine on structural alterations of microvessels in peripheral nerve of streptozocin diabetic rats. Microvasc Res 1997; 53: 105–12.

[222] 222. Cameron NE, Cotter MA. The relationship of vascular changes to metabolic factors in diabetes mellitus and their role in the development of peripheral nerve complications. Diabetes Metab Rev 1994; 10: 189–224.

[223] Van Dam PS, Van Asbeck BS, Erkeleus DW, Marx JM, Gispen W-H, Bravenboer B. The role of oxidative stress in neuropathy and other diabetic complications. Diabetes Metab Rev 1995; 11: 181–92.

[224] Wolff SP. Diabetes mellitus and free radicals. Free radicals, transition metals and oxidative stress in the aetiology of diabetes mellitus and complications. Br Med Bull 1993; 49: 642–52.

[225] Cameron NE, Cotter MA. Oxidative stress and abnormal lipid metabolism in diabetic complications. In: Sima AAF, editor. Frontiers in animal diabetes research. Chronic complications in diabetes. Amsterdam: Harwood Academic; 2000: 97–130.

[226] Hallab M, Bled F, Ebrau JM, et al. Elevated serum angiotensin I converting enzyme in type I, insulin dependent diabetic subjects with persistent microalbuminuria. Acta Diabetol 1992; 29: 82–5.

[227] Maxfield EK, Cameron NE, Cotter MA, Dines KC. Angiotensin II receptor blockade improves nerve function, modulates nerve blood flow and stimulates endoneurial angiogenesis. Diabetologia 1993; 36: 1230–7.

[228] Quehenberger P, Bierhaus A, Fasching P, Muellner C, Klevesath M, Hong M, et al. Endothelin 1 transcription is controlled by nuclear factor-κB in AGE stimulated cultured endothelial cells. Diabetes 2000; 49: 1561–70.

[229] Cameron NE, Cotter MA. Effects of a non-peptide endothelin 1 ET_A antagonist on neurovascular function in diabetic rats: interaction with the renin-angiotensin system. J Pharmacol Exp Ther 1996; 278: 1262–8.

[230] Stevens EJ, Tomlinson DR. Effects of endothelin receptor antagonism with bosentan on peripheral nerve function in experimental diabetes. Br J Pharmacol 1995; 115: 373–79.

[231] Gryglewski RJ, Palmer RMJ, Moncado S. Super-oxide anion is involved in the breakdown of endothelium-derived relaxing factor. Nature 1986; 320: 454–6.

[232] Ceriello A. Coagulation activation in diabetes mellitus: the role of hyperglycemia and theraputic prospects. Diabetologia 1993; 36: 1119–25.

[233] Faruqi D, Motte C de la, DiCorleto PE. α-Tocopherol inhibits agonist-induced monocytic cell adhesion to cultured human endothelial cells. J Clin Invest 1994; 94: 592–600.

[234] Cameron NE, Cotter MA, Jack AM, Basso MD, Hohman TC. Protein kinase C effects on nerve function, perfusion, Na(+) K(+)-ATPase activity and glutathione content in diabetic rats. Diabetologia 1999; 42: 1120–30.

[235] Nakamura J, Kato K, Hamada Y, et al. A protein kinase C beta-selective inhibitor ameliorates neural dysfunction in streptozocin-induced diabetic rats. Diabetes 1999; 48: 2090–95.

[236] Kishi Y, Schmelzer JD, Yao JK, et al. Alpha-lipoic acid: effect on glucose uptake, sorbitol pathway, and energy metabolism in experimental diabetic neuropathy. Diabetes 1999; 48: 2045–51.

[237] Hotta N, Kakura H, Fukasawa H, et al. Effect of niceritrol on streptozocin-induced diabetic neuropathy in rats. Diabetes 1992; 41: 587–91.

[238] Tesfamariam B, Cohen RA. Free radicals mediate endothelial cell dysfunction caused by elevated glucose. Am J Physiol 1992; 263: H231–326.

[239] Taylor PD, Poston L. The effect of hyperglycemia on function of rat isolated mesenteric resistance artery. Br J Pharmacol 1994; 113: 801–8.

[240] Keegan A, Cotter MA, Cameron NE. Autonomic neuropathy, corpus cavernosum innervation and endothelial responses: diabetic defects prevented by alpha-lipoic acid in rats. J Peripher Nerv Syst 1997; 2: 277.

[241] Love A, Cotter MA, Cameron NE. Effects of the sulphydryl donor N-acetyl-L-cysteine on nerve conduction, perfusion, maturation and regeneration following freeze damage in diabetic rats. Eur J Clin Invest 1996; 26: 698–706.

[242] Love A, Cotter MA, Cameron NE. Effects of alpha tocopherol on nerve conduction velocity and regeneration following freeze lesion in immature diabetic rats. Naunyn Schmiedebergs Arch Pharmacol 1997; 355: 126–30.

[243] Zochodne DW, Verge MK, Hoke A, Jolley C, Thomsen K, et al. Nitric oxide synthase activity and expression in experimental diabetic neuropathy. J Neuropathol Exp Neurol 2000; 59: 798–807.

[244] Johansson B-L, Pernow J, Wahren J. Muscle vasodilation by C-peptide is NO-mediated. Diabetologia 1999a; 42: A324.

[245] Horrobin DF, Carmichael H. Essential fatty acids in relation to diabetes. In: Horrobin DF, editor. Treatment of diabetic neuropathy, a new approach. Edinburgh, UK: Churchill Livingstone; 1992: 21–39.

[246] Ward KK, Low PA, Schmelzer JD, Zochodne DW. Prostacyclin and noradrenaline in peripheral nerve of chronic experimental diabetes in rats. Brain 1989; 112: 197–208.

[247] Karasu D, Dewhurst M, Stevens EJ, Tomlinson DR. Effects of antioxidant treatment on sciatic nerve dysfunction in streptozocin-diabetic rats; comparison with essential fatty acids. Diabetologia 1995; 38: 129–34.

[248] Cameron NE, Cotter MA, Robertson S. Essential fatty acid supplementation: effects on peripheral nerve and skeletal muscle function and capillarization in streptozocin-induced diabetic rats. Diabetes 1991; 40: 532–9.
[249] Ido Y, McHowat J, Chang KC, et al. Neural dysfunction and metabolic imbalances in diabetic rats: prevention by acetyl-L-carnitine. Diabetes 1994; 43: 1469–77.
[250] Tomlinson DR, Fernyhough P. Neurotrophism in diabetic neuropathy. In: Sima AAF, editor. Frontiers in animal diabetes research. Chronic complications in diabetes. Amsterdam: Harwood Academic; 2000: 167–82.
[251] DiStefano PS,. Freidman B, Radziejewski C, Alexander C. The neurotrophins BDNF, NT-3 and NGF display distinct patterns of retrograde axonal transport in peripheral and central axons. Neuron 1992; 8: 983–93.
[252] Schmidt RE, Graban GG, Yip HK. Retrograde axonal transport of [^{125}I]-nerve growth factor in ileal mesenteric nerves in vitro: effect of streptozocin diabetes. Brain Res 1986; 378: 325–36.
[253] Hellweg R, Hartung H-D. Endogenous levels of nerve growth factor (NGF) are altered in experimental diabetes mellitus: a possible role for NGF in the pathogenesis of diabetic neuropathy. J Neurosci Res 1990; 26: 258–67.
[254] Fernyhough P, Brewster NJ, Diemel LT, Tomlinson DR. Nerve growth factor mRNA in diabetic rat sciatic nerve; effects of neurotrophic factor treatment. Br J Pharmacol 1993; 110: 173P.
[255] 255. Sima AAF, Merry AC, Levitan I. Increased regeneration in ARI-treated diabetic nerve is associated with up-regulation of IGF-1 and NGF receptors. Exp Clin Endocrinol Diabetes 1997; 105: 60–2.
[256] Gold BG, Mobley WC, Matheson SF. Regulation of axonal caliber, neurofilament content, and nuclear localization in mature sensory neurons by nerve growth factor. J Neurosci 1991; 11: 943–55.
[257] Verge VNK, Tetzlaff W, Bisby MA, Richardson PM. Influence of nerve growth factor on neurofilament gene expression in mature primary sensory neurons. J Neurosci 1990; 10: 2018–25.
[258] Wang C, Li Y, Wible B, Angelides KJ, Ishii DN. Effects of insulin and insulin-like growth factors on neurofilament mRNA and tubulin mRNA content in human neuroblastoma cell SH-SY5Y cells. Brain Res Mol Brain Res 1992; 13: 289–300.
[259] Yagihashi S, Kamijo M, Watanabe K. Reduced myelinated fiber size correlates with loss of axonal neurofilaments in peripheral nerve of chronically streptozocin diabetic rats. Am J Pathol 1990; 136: 5–1373.
[260] Apfel SC, Kessler JA, Adornato BT, Litchy WJ, Sanders C, Rask CA. Recombinant human nerve growth factor in the treatment of diabetic polyneuropathy. NGF Study Group. Neurology 1998; 51: 695–702.
[261] Dyck PJ, Peroutka S, Rask C, et al. Intradermal recombinant human nerve growth factor induces pressure allodynia and lowered heat-pain threshold in humans. Neurology 1997; 48: 501–5.
[262] Heumann R, Hengerer B, Brown M, Perry H. Molecular mechanisms leading to lesion-induced increases in nerve growth factor synthesis. Ann NY Acad Sci 1991; 633: 581–2.
[263] Whitworth IH, Terenghi G, Green CJ, Brown RA, Stevens E, Tomlinson DR. Targeted delivery of nerve growth factor via fibronectin conduits assists nerve regeneration in control and diabetic rats. Eur J Neurosci 1995; 7: 2220–5.
[264] Ishii DN, Lupien SB. Insulin-like growth factors protect against diabetic neuropathy: effects on sensory nerve regeneration in rats. J Neurosci Res 1995; 40: 138–44.
[265] Sugimoto K, Murakawa Y, Zhang W, Xu G, Sima AAF. Insulin receptor in rat peripheral nerve: its localization and alternatively spliced isoforms. Diabetes Metab Res Rev 2000; 16: 354–63.
[266] Rigler R, Pramanik A, Jonasson P, Kratz G, Jansson T, Nygren P-A, et al. Specific binding of proinsulin C-peptide to human cell membranes. Proc Natl Acad Sci USA 1999; 96: 13318–23.
[267] Grunberger G, Quiang X, Li Z-G, Mathews S, Sbriessa D, Shisheva A, et al. Molecular basis for the insulinomimetic effects of C-peptide. Diabetologia 2001; 44: 247–57.
[268] Fernyhough P, Mill JF, Roberts JL, Ishii DN. Stabilization of tubulin mRNAs by insulin and insulin-like growth factor 1 during neurite formation. Mol Brain Res 1989; 6: 109–20.
[269] Feldman EL, Sullivan KA, Kim B, Russell JW. Insulin-like growth factors upregulate neuronal differentiation and survival. Neurobiol Dis 1997; 4: 201–14.
[270] Rosner L, Elsted R. The neuropathy of hypoglycemia. Neurology 1964; 14: 1–6.
[271] Danta G. Hypoglycemic peripheral neuropathy. Arch Neurol 1969; 21: 121–32.
[272] Jaspan JB, Wollman RL, Bernstein L, Rubenstein AH. Hypoglycemic peripheral neuropathy in association with insulinoma: implication of glucopenia rather than hyperinsulinism. Case report and review of the literature. Medicine (Baltimore) 1982; 61: 33–44.
[273] Dyer KR, Messing A. Peripheral neuropathy associated with functional islet cell adenomas in SV40 transgenic mice. J Neuropathol Exp Neurol 1989; 48: 388–412.
[274] Sugimoto K, Yagihashi S. Peripheral nerve pathology in rats with streptozotocin-induced insulinoma. Acta Neuropathol (Berl) 1996; 91: 616–23.
[275] Tom MI, Richardson JC. Hypoglycemia from islet cell tumor of pancreas with amyotrophy and cerebrospinal nerve cell changes. J Neuropathol Exp Neurol 1951; 10: 57–66.
[276] Mohseni S, Lillesaar C, Theodorsson E, Hildebrand C. Hypoglycemic neuropathy: occurrence of axon terminals in plantar skin and plantar muscle of diabetic BB/Wor rats treated with insulin implants. Acta Neuropathol (Berl) 2000; 99: 257–62.
[277] Mohseni S. Hypoglycemic neuropathy in diabetic BB/Wor rats treated with insulin implants affects ventral root axons. Acta Neuropathol (Berl) 2000; 100: 415–20.
[277a]Murakawa Y, Zhang W, Brismar T, Efendic S, Östenson C-G, Sima AAF. Mild neuropathy in glucose intolerant GK-rats is associated with impaired neuotrophism. Diabetes 2002; 51 (Suppl 2): A192.
[278] Tesfaye S, Malik R, Harris N, et al. Arterio-venous shunting and proliferating new vessels in acute painful neuropathy of rapid glycemic control (insulin neuritis). Diabetologia 1996; 39: 329–35.
[279] Sugimoto K, Baba M, Yagihashi S. Characterization of peripheral neuropathy in rats with insulinoma induced by streptozotocin and nicotinamide. Diabetes 1998; 47: A538.
[280] Sima AAF, Sugimoto K. Experimental diabetic neuropathy: an update. Diabetologia 1999; 42: 773–88.
[281] Sugimoto K, Murakawa Y, Sima AAF. Diabetic neuropathy—a continuing enigma. Diabetes Metab Res Rev 2000; 16: 408–33.
[282] Ohtomo Y, Aperia A, Sahlgren B, Johansson B-L, Wahren J. C-peptide stimulates rat renal tubular Na^+K^+-ATPase activity in synergism with neuropeptide Y. Diabetologia 1996; 39: 199–205.
[283] Forst T, DeLa Tour DD, Kunt T, Pfutzner A, Goitman K, Pohlmann T, et al. Effects of proinsulin C-peptide on nitric oxide, microvascular blood-flow and erythrocyte Na^+K^+-ATPase activity in diabetes mellitus type 1. Clin Sci 2000; 98: 283–90.
[284] Kunt T, Forst T, Closs E, Wallerath U, Forstermann R, Lehman R, et al. Activation of endothelial nitric oxide synthase (eNOS) by C-peptide. Diabetologia 1998; 41: A176.
[285] Jensen ME, Messina EJ. C-peptide induces a concentration dependent dilatation of skeletal muscle arterioles only in the presence of insulin. Am J Physiol 1999; 276: H1223–1228.
[286] Johansson B-L, Sjoberg S, Wahren J. The influence of human C-peptide on renal function and glucose utilization in type I (insulin-dependent) diabetic patients. Diabetologia 1999; 35: 121–8.
[287] Johansson B-L, Linde B, Wahren J. Effects of C-peptide on blood-flow, capillary diffusion capacity and glucose utilization in the exercising forearm of type I (insulin-dependent) diabetic patients. Diabetologia 1992; 35: 1151–8.
[288] Zierath J, Handberg A, Tally H, Wallberg-Henriksson H. C-peptide stimulates glucose transport in isolated human skeletal muscle independent of insulin receptor and tyrosine kinase activation. Diabetologia 1996; 39: 306–13.
[289] Johansson B-L, Kernell A, Sjoberg S, Wahren J. Influence of combined C-peptide and insulin administration on renal function and metabolic control in diabetes type I. J Clin Endocrin Metab 1993; 77: 976–81.

[290] Johansson B-L, Borg K, Fernquist-Forbes E, Kernall A, Odergren T, Wahren J. Beneficial effects of C-peptide on incipient nephropathy and neuropathy in patients with type I diabetes—a three month study. Diabet Med 2000; 17: 181–9.

[291] Li Z-G, Zhang W, Grunberger G, Sima AAF. C-peptide corrects IGF's and prevents apoptosis in type I BB/Wor-rat hippocampus. Diabetes 2000; 49 (Suppl 1): A168.

[292] Sima AAF, Zhang W-X, Tai J, Tze WJ, Nathaniel V. Diabetic neuropathy in STZ-induced diabetic rat and effect of allogenic islet cell transplantation. Morphometric analysis. Diabetes 1988; 37: 1129–36.

[293] Bischoff A. Ultrastructural pathology of the nervous system in early diabetes. In: Camerini-Davalos RA, Cole HS, editors. Vascular and neurological changes in early diabetes. New York, N.Y.: Academic Press; 1973: 441–9.

[294] Sharma AK, Richard PA. Diabetic neuropathy in various animal models. In: Sima AAF, editor. Frontiers in animal diabetes research. Chronic complications in diabetes. Amsterdam: Harwood Academic; 2000: 131–65.

[295] Sharma AK, Thomas PK. Animal models: pathology and pathophysiology. In: Dyck PJ, Thomas PK, Ashbury AK, Winegrad AL, Porte D Jr, editors. Diabetic neuropathy. Philadelphia, Pa.: Saunders; 1987: 237–52.

[296] Yagihashi S, Kamijo M, Ido Y, Mirrless D. Effects of long-term aldose reductase inhibition on development of experimental diabetic neuropathy: ultrastructural and morphometric studies of sural nerve in streptozotocin-induced diabetic rats. Diabetes 1990; 39: 690–6.

[297] Sima AAF, Lattimer SA, Yagihashi S, Greene DA. Axo-glial dysjunction. J Clin Invest 1986; 77: 474–84.

[298] Medori R, Antilio-Gambetti L, Jenich H, Gambetti P. Changes in axon size and slow axonal transport are related in experimental diabetic neuropathy. Neurology 1988; 38: 597–601.

[299] Schmidt RE, Scharp DW. Axonal dystrophy in experimental diabetic neuropathy. Diabetes 1982; 32: 761–70.

[300] Sugimura K, Windebank AJ, Natarajan V, Lambert EH, Schmidt HH, Dyck PJ. Interstitial hyperosmolality may cause axis cylinder shrinkage in streptozotocin-induced diabetic nerve. J Neuropathol Exp Neurol 1980; 39: 710–21.

[301] Sharma AK, Bajada S, Thomas PK. Influence of streptozotocin-induced diabetes on myelinated nerve fiber maturation and on body growth in the rat. Acta Neuropathol (Berl) 1981; 53: 257–65.

[302] Felton DL. Spinal cord alterations in streptozotocin-induced diabetes. Anat Rec 1979; 193: 741.

[303] Sidenius P, Jakobsen J. Reduced perikaryal volume of lower motor and primary sensory neurons in early experimental diabetes. Diabetes 1980; 29: 182–6.

[304] Russel JW, Windebank AJ, Schenone A, Feldman EL. Insulin-like growth factor-1 prevents apoptosis in neurons after growth factor withdrawal. J Neurobiol 1998; 36: 455–67.

[305] Marliss EB, Nakhooda AF, Poussier P, Sima AAF. The diabetic syndrome of the BB-Wistar rat. Possible relevance to type-1 (insulin dependent) diabetes in man. Diabetologia 1982; 22: 225–32.

[306] Sima AAF. Can the BB-rat help to unravel diabetic neuropathy? Neuropathol Appl Neurobiol 1985; 11: 253–64.

[307] Sima AAF, Prashar A, Zhang W-X, Chakrabarti S, Greene DA. Preventive effect of long term aldose reductase inhibition (Ponalrestat) on nerve conduction and sural nerve structure in the spontaneously diabetic BB-rat. J Clin Invest 1990; 85: 1410–20.

[308] Cherian PV, Kamijo M, Angelides KJ, Sima AAF. Nodal Na^+-channel displacement is associated with nerve conduction slowing in the chronically diabetic BB/W-rat. Prevention by an aldose reductase inhibitor. J Diabetes Complications 1996; 10: 192–200.

[309] Magnani P, Cherian PV, Gould GW, Greene DA, Sima AAF, Brosius FC. III. Glucose transporters in rat peripheral nerve: paranodal expression of GLUT1 and GLUT3. Metabolism 1996; 45: 153–60.

[310] Merry AC, Yamamoto K, Sima AAF. Imbalances in N-CAM, SAM and polysialic acid may underlie he paranodal ion channel barrier defect in diabetic neuropathy. Diabetes Res Clin Pract 1998; 40: 153–60.

[311] Einheber S, Zanazzi G, Cing W, Scherer S, Milner TA, Peles E, et al. The axonal membrane protein Caspr, a homologue of Neurexin IV, is a component of the septate-like paranodal junctions that assemble during myelination. J Cell Biol 1997; 139: 1495–506.

[312] Menegoz M, Gaspar P, LeBert M. Galvez, Bugaya F, Palfrey C, et al. Paranodin, a glycoprotein of neuronal paranodal membranes. Neuron 1997; 19: 319–31.

[313] Baumgartner S, Littleon JT, Broadie K, Bhat MA, Harbecke R, Lengyel JA, et al. A Drosophila neurexin is required for septate junction and blood nerve barrier formation and function. Cell 1996; 87: 1059–68.

[314] Peles E, Nativ M, Lustig M, Grumet A, Schilling J, Martinez R, et al. Identification of a novel contactin-associated transmembrane receptor with multiple domains implicated in protein-protein interactions. EMBO J 1997; 16: 978–88.

[315] Singhal A, Cheng C, Hong S, Zochodne DW. Near nerve local insulin prevents conduction slowing in experimental diabetes. Brain Res 1997; 763: 209–14.

[316] Kordeli E, Lambert S, Bennett V. Ankyrin$_G$, a new ankyrin gene with neural-specific isoforms localized at the axon initial segment and node of Ranvier. J Biol Chem 1995; 270: 232–9.

[317] Davis JQ, Bennett V. Ankyrin binding activity shared by the neurofascin/L1/NrCAM family of nervous system cell adhesion molecules. J Biol Chem 1994; 269: 27163-6.

[318] Lambert S, Bennett V. Axonal ankyrins and ankyrin binding proteins: potential participants in lateral membrane domains and transcellular connections at the node of Ranvier. Curr Top Membranes 1996; 43: 129–45.

[319] Sima AAF, Lorusso AC, Thibert P. Distal symmetric polyneuropathy in the spontaneously diabetic BB-Wistar rat: an ultrastructural and teased fiber study. Acta Neuropathol (Berl) 1982; 58: 39–47.

[320] Kamijo M, Mer AC, Akdas G, Cherian PV, Sima AAF. Nerve fiber regeneration following axotomy in the diabetic biobreeding Worchester rat: the effect of ARI treatment. J Diabetes Complications 1996; 10: 183–91.

[321] Srinivasan S, Stevens M, Wiley JW. Diabetic peripheral neuropathy evidence for apoptosis and associated mitochondrial dysfunction. Diabetes 2000; 49: 1932–8.

[322] Mathew CE, Berdanier CD. Noninsulin-dependent diabetes mellitus as a mitochodrial genomic genomic disease. Proc Soc Exper Biol Med 1998; 219: 97–108.

[323] Malik RA, Williason S, Abbot C, et al. Effect of angiotensin-converting enzyme (ACE) inhibitor trandolapril on human diabetic neuropathy: randomized double-blind controlled trial. Lancet 1998; 352: 1978–81.

[324] Yagihashi S, Yamagishi S-I, Nihimura C. Utility of the transgenic mouse in diabetes research. In: Sima AAF, editor. Frontiers in animal diabetes research. Chronic complications in diabetes. Amsterdam: Harwood Academic; 2000: 71–96.

[325] Thorpe SR, Baynes JW. Role of the Maillard reaction in diabetes mellitus and diseases of aging. Drugs Aging 1996; 9: 69–77.

[326] Baynes JW, Thorpe SR. Glycation and advanced glycation reactions. In: Turtle JR, Kaneko T, Osato S, editors. Diabetes in the new millennium. Sydney: Endocrinology and Diabetes Research Foundation; 1999: 337–50.

[327] Monnier VM, Bautista O, Kenny D, Sell DR, Fogarty J, Dahms W, Cleary PA, Lachin J. Genuth S, and the DCCT Skin Collagen Ancillary Study Group. Skin collagen glycation, glycoxidation, and crosslinking are lower in subjects with long-term intensive versus conventional therapy of type 1 diabetes. Diabetes 1999; 48: 870–80.

[328] Thorpe SR, Lyons TJ, Baynes JW. Glycation and glycoxidation in diabetic vascular disease. In: Keaney JF, editor. Oxidative stress and vascular disease. Norwell, Mass.: Kluwer; 1999: 259–83.

[329] Qian M, Eaton JW. Glycochelates and the etiology of diabetic peripheral neuropathy. Free Radic Biol Med 2000; 28: 652–6.

[330] Yan SD, Schmidt AM, Anderson GM, Zhang J, Brett J, Zou YS, Pinsky D, Stern D. Enhanced cellular oxidant stress by the interaction of advanced glycation end products with their receptors/binding proteins. J Biol Chem 1994; 269: 9889–97.

[331] Thornalley PJ. Advanced glycation and the development of diabetic complications. Unifying the involvement of glucose, methylglyoxal and oxidative stress. Endocrinol Metab 1996; 3: 149–66.

[332] Brownlee M, Vlassara H, Cerami A. Trapped immunoglobulins on peripheral nerve myelin from patients with diabetes mellitus. Diabetes 1986; 35: 999–1003.
[333] Brownlee M, Pongor S, Cerami A. Covalent attachment of soluble proteins by nonenzymatically glycosylated collagen: role in the in situ formation of immune complexes. J Exp Med 1983; 158: 1739–44.
[334] Vlassara H, Brownlee M, Cerami A. Recognition and uptake of human diabetic peripheral nerve myelin by macrophages. Diabetes 1985; 34: 553–7.
[335] Sugimoto K, Nishizawa Y, Horiuchi S, Yagihashi S. Localization in human diabetic peripheral nerve of N^{ϵ}-carboxymethllysine-protein adducts, an advanced glycation endproduct. Diabetologia 1997; 40: 1380–7.
[336] Sensi M, Morano S, Morelli S, Castaldo P, Sagratella E, Grazia Rossi M De, Andreani M, Caltabiano V, Vetri M, Purrello F, DiMario U. Reduction of advanced glycation end-product (AGE) levels in nervous tissue proteins of diabetic Lewis rats following islet transplants is related to different durations of poor metabolic control. Eur J Neurosci 1998; 10: 2768–75.
[337] Morano S, Sensi M, Di Gregorio S, Pozzessere G, Petrucci AF, Valle E, Pugliese G, Caltabiano V, Vetri M, Di Mario U, Purrello F. Peripheral, but not central, nervous system abnormalities are reversed by pancreatic islet transplantation in diabetic Lewis rats. Eur J Neurosci 1996; 8: 1117–23.
[338] Sensi M, Morano S, Valle E, Petrucci AF, Pozzessere G, Caltabiano V, Vetri M, Purrello F, Andreani D, Di Mario U. Effect of islet transplantation on neuroelectrophysiological abnormalities in diabetic inbred Lewis rats: comparison of primary vs. secondary intervention. Transplantation 1999; 68: 1453–9.
[339] Nilsson BO. Biological effects of aminoguanidine: an update. Inflamm Res 1999; 48: 509–15.
[340] Khalifah RG, Baynes JW, Hudson BG. Amadorins: novel post-Amadori inhibitors of advanced glycation reactions. Biochem Biophys Res Commun 1999; 257: 251–8.
[341] Nakamura S, Makita Z, Ishikawa S, Yasumura K, Fujii W, Yanagisawa K, Kawata T, Koike T. Progression of nephropathy in spontaneous diabetic rats is prevented by OPB-9195, a novel inhibitor of advanced glycation. Diabetes 1997; 46: 895–9.
[342] Miyata T, Ueda Y, Asahi K, Izuhara Y, Inagi R, Saito A, Ypersele Strihou C De, Kurokawa K. Mechanism of the inhibitory effect of OPB-9195 [(+/-)-2-isopropylidenehydrazono-4-oxo-thiazolidin-5-ylacetanilide] on advanced glycation end product and advanced lipoxidation end product formation. J Am Soc Nephrol 2000; 11: 1719–25.
[343] Philis-Tsimikas A, Parthasarathy S, Picard S, Palinski W, Witztum JL. Aminoguanidine has both pro-oxidant and antioxidant activity toward LDL. Arterioscler Thromb Vasc Biol 1995; 15: 367–76.
[344] Onorato JM, Jenkins AJ, Thorpe SR, Baynes JW. Pyridoxamine, an inhibitor of advanced glycation reactions, also inhibits advanced lipoxidation reactions. Mechanism of action of pyridoxamine. J Biol Chem 2000; 275: 21177–84.
[345] Cameron NE, Cotter MA, Dines K, Love A. Effects of aminoguanidine on peripheral nerve function and polyol pathway metabolites in streptozotocin-diabetic rats. Diabetologia 1992; 35: 946–50.
[346] Yagihashi S, Kamijo M, Baba M, Yagihashi N, Nagai K. Effect of aminoguanidine on functional and structural abnormalities in peripheral nerve of STZ-induced diabetic rats. Diabetes 1992; 41: 47–52.
[347] Sugimoto K, Yagihashi S. Effects of aminoguanidine on structural alterations of microvessels in peripheral nerve of streptozotocin diabetic rats. Microvasc Res 1997; 53: 105–12.
[348] Ino-ue M, Ohgiya N, Yamamoto M. Effect of aminoguanidine on optic nerve involvement in experimental diabetic rats. Brain Res 1998; 800: 319–22.
[349] Miyauchi Y, Shikama H, Takasu T, Okamiya H, Umeda M, Hirasaki E, Ohhata I, Nakayama H, Nakagawa S. Slowing of peripheral motor nerve conduction was ameliorated by aminoguanidine in streptozocin-induced diabetic rats. Eur J Endocrinol 1996; 134: 467–73.
[350] Way KJ, Reid JJ. Effect of aminoguanidine on the impaired nitric oxide-mediated neurotransmission in anococcygeus muscle from diabetic rats. Neuropharmacology 1994; 33: 1315–22.
[351] Schmidt RE, Dorsey DA, Beaudet LN, Reiser KM, Williamson JR, Tilton RG. Effect of aminoguanidine on the frequency of neuroaxonal dystrophy in the superior mesenteric sympathetic autonomic ganglia of rats with streptozocin-induced diabetes. Diabetes 1996; 45: 284–90.
[352] Birrell AM, Heffernan SJ, Ansselin AD, McLennan S, Church DK, Gillin AG, Yue DK. Functional and structural abnormalities in the nerves of type 1 diabetic baboons: aminoguanidine treatment does not improve nerve function. Diabetologia 2000; 43: 110–6.
[353] Ruggiero-Lopez D, Lemomte M, Moinet G, Patereau G, Lagarde M, Wiernsperger N. Reaction of metformin with dicarbonyl compounds. Possible implication for inhibition of advanced glycation end product formation. Biochem Pharmacol 1999; 58: 1765–73.
[354] Tanaka Y, Iwamoto H, Onuma T, Kawamori R. Inhibitory effect of metformin on formation of advanced glycation end products. Curr Ther Res 1997; 58: 693–7.
[355] Beisswenger P, Howell S, Touchette A, Lal S, Szwergold B. Metformin reduces systemic methylglyoxal levels in type 2 diabetes. Diabetes 1999; 48: 198–202.
[356] Tanaka Y, Uchino H, Shimizu T, Yoshii H, Niwa M, Ohmura C, Mitsuhashi N, Onuma T, Kawamori R. Effect of metformin on advanced glycation endproduct formation and peripheral nerve function in streptozotocin-induced diabetic rats. Eur J Pharmacol 1999; 376: 17–22.
[357] Cameron NE, Cotter MA. Rapid reversal by aminoguanidine of the neurovascular effects of diabetes in rats: modulation by nitric oxide synthase inhibition. Metabolism 1996; 45: 1147–52.
[358] Roufail E, Soulis T, Boel E, Cooper ME, Rees S. Depletion of nitric oxide synthase-containing neurons in the diabetic retina: reversal by aminoguanidine. Diabetologia 1998; 41: 1419–25.
[358a]Degenhardt TP, Alderson NL, Arrington DD, et al. Pyridoxamine inhibits early renal disease and dyslipidemia in the streptotocin-diabetic rat. Kidney Internat 2002; 61: 939–50.
[359] Windebank AJ, Feldman EL. Diabetes and the nervous system. In: Aminoff MJ, editors. Neurology and General Medicine, 3rd edition. Edinburgh, UK: Churchill Livingstone; 2001: 341–64.
[360] Young MJ, Boulton AJM, Macleod AF, Williams DRR, Sonksen PH. A multicentre study of the prevalence of diabetic peripheral neuropathy in the United Kingdom hospital clinic population. Diabetologia 1993; 36: 150–4.
[361] DCCT Research Group. The effect of intensive treatment of diabetes on the development and progression of long-term complications in insulin-dependent diabetes mellitus. N Engl J Med 1993; 329: 977–86.
[362] The DCCT Research Group. The effect of intensive diabetes therapy on the development and progression of neuropathy. Ann Intern Med 1995; 122: 561–8.
[363] Intensive blood-glucose control with sulphonylureas or insulin compared with conventional treatment and risk of complications in patients with type 2 diabetes (UKPDS 33). UK Prospective Diabetes Study (UKPDS) Group. Lancet 1998; 352: 837–53.
[364] Stevens MJ, Feldman EL, Thomas TP, Greene DA. The pathogenesis of diabetic neuropathy. In: Veves A, Conn PMC, editors. Clinical management of diabetic neuropathy. Totowa, N.J.: Humana Press; 1997: 13–47.
[365] Dvornik D. Hyperglycemia in the pathogenesis of diabetic complications. In: Porte D, editors. Aldose reductase inhibition. An approach to the prevention of diabetic complications. New York: Biomedical Information Corporation; 1987: 69–151.
[366] Tuck RR, Schmelzer JD, Low PA. Endoneurial blood flow and oxygen tension in the sciatic nerves of rats with experimental diabetic neuropathy. Brain 1984; 107: 935–50.
[367] Stevens MJ, Lattimer SA, Kamijo M, VanHuysen C, Sima AAF, Greene DA. Osmotically induced nerve taurine depletion and the compatible osmolyte hypothesis in experimental diabetic neuropathy in the rat. Diabetologia 1993; 36: 608–14.
[368] Greene DA, Stevens MJ. The sorbitol-osmotic and sorbitol-redox hypotheses. In: LeRoith D, Olefsky JM, Taylor S, editors. Diabetes mellitus: a fundamental and clinical text. Philadelphia, Pa.: Lippincott-Raven, 1996: 801–9.
[369] Nakamura J, Monte DA Del, Shewach D, Lattimer SA, Greene DA. Inhibition of phosphatidylinositol synthase by glucose

in human retinal pigment epithelial cells. Am J Physiol 1992; 262: E417–426.

[370] Keogh RJ, Dunlop ME, Larkins RG. Effects of inhibition of aldose reductase on glucose flux, diacylglycerol formation, protein kinase C, and phospholipase A2 activation. Metabolism 1997; 46: 41–7.

[371] Ishii H, Tada H, Isogai S. An aldose reductase inhibitor prevents glucose-induced increase in transforming growth factor-beta and protein kinase C activity in cultured mesangial cells. Diabetologia 1998; 41: 362–4.

[372] Suarez G, Rajaram R, Bhuyan KC, Oronsky AL, Gold JA. Administration of an aldose reductase inhibitor induces a decrease of collagen fluorescence in diabetic rats. J Clin Invest 1988; 82: 624–7.

[373] Cameron NE, Cotter MA, Dines KC, Maxfield EK, Carey F, Mirrlees DJ. Aldose reductase inhibition, nerve perfusion, oxygenation and function in streptozotocin-diabetic rats: dose-response considerations and independence from a myo-inositol mechanism. Diabetologia 1994; 37: 651–63.

[374] Mizisin AP, Calcutt NA, DiStefano PS, Acheson A, Longo FM. Aldose reductase inhibition increases CNTF-like bioactivity and protein in sciatic nerves from galactose-fed and normal rats. Diabetes 1997; 46: 647–52.

[375] Ohi T, Saita K, Furukawa S, Ohta M, Hayashi K, Matsukura S. Therapeutic effects of aldose reductase inhibitor on experimental neuropathy through synthesis/secretion of nerve growth factor. Exp Neurol 1998; 151: 215–20.

[376] Dyck PJ, Karnes JL, O'Brien P, Okazaki H, Lois A, Engelstad J. The spatial distribution of fiber loss in diabetic polyneuropathy suggests ischemia. Ann Neurol 1986; 19: 440.

[377] Tomlinson DR, Sidenius P, Larsen JR. Slow component-a of axonal transport, nerve myo-inositol and aldose reductase inhibition in streptozotocin-diabetic rats. Diabetes 1986; 34: 398–402.

[378] Mayer JH, Tomlinson DR. The influence of aldose reductase inhibition and nerve myoinositol on axonal transport and nerve conduction velocity in rats with experimental diabetes. J Physiol (London) 1983; 340: 25P–26P.

[379] Williamson JR, Ostrow E, Eades D, Chang K, Allison W, Kilo C, Sherman WR. Glucose-induced microvascular functional changes in nondiabetic rats are stereospecific and are prevented by an aldose reductase inhibitor. J Clin Invest 1990; 85: 1167–72.

[380] Greene DA, Lattimer SA. Action of sorbinil in diabetic peripheral nerve. Relationship of polyol (sorbitol) pathway inhibition to a myo-inositol-mediated defect in sodium-potassium ATPase activity. Diabetes 1984; 33: 712–6.

[381] Yasuda H, Masanobu S, Yamashita M, Teradam M, Hatanaka I, Huitian Z, Shigeta Y. Effect of prostaglandin E, analogue TFC612 on diabetic neuropathy in streptozotocin-induced diabetic rats; comparison with aldose reductase inhibitor ONO2235. Diabetes 1989; 38: 832–8.

[382] Dent MT, Tebbs SE, Gonzales AM, Ward JD, Wilson RM. Neutrophil aldose reductase activity and its association with established diabetic microvascular complications. Diabet Med 1991; 8: 439–42.

[383] Vinores SA, Campochiaro PA, Williams EH, May EE, Green R, Sorenson RL. Aldose reductase expression in human diabetic retina and retinal pigment epithelium. Diabetes 1988; 37: 1658–64.

[384] Takahashi Y, Tachikawa T, Ito T, Takayama S, Omori Y, Iwamoto Y. Erythrocyte aldose reductase protein: a clue to elucidate risk factors for diabetic neuropathies independent of glycemic control. Diabetes Res Clin Pract 1998; 42: 101–7.

[385] Hamada Y, Kitoh R, Raskin P. Increased activity of erythrocyte aldose reductase in insulin dependent diabetes with severe diabetic complications. Diabetes 1991; 40 (Suppl 1): 35.

[386] Shah VO, Dorin RI, Sun Y, Braun M, Zager PG. Aldose reductase gene expression is increased in diabetic nephropathy. J Clin Endocrinol Metab 1997; 82: 2294–8.

[387] Maeda S, Haneda M, Yasuda H, Tachikawa T, Isshiki K. Koya D, terada M, Hidaka H, Kashiwagi A, Kikkawa R. Diabetic nephropathy is not associated with the dinucleotide repeat polymorphism upstream of the aldose reductase (ALR2) gene but with erythrocyte aldose reductase content in Japanese subjects with type 2 diabetes. Diabetes 1999; 48: 420–2.

[388] Burg MB. Molecular basis of osmotic regulation. Am J Physiol 1995; 268: F983–996.

[389] Rim JS, Atta MG, Dahl SC, Berry GT, Handler JS, Kwon HM. Transcription of the sodium/myo-inositol cotransporter gene is regulated by multiple tonicity-responsive enhancers spread over 50 kilobasepairs in the 5′-flanking region. J Biol Chem 1998; 273: 20615–20621.

[390] Henry DN, Monte M Del, Greene DA, Killen PD. Aldose reductase gene regulation in cultured human retinal pigment epithelial cells. J Clin Invest 1993; 92: 617–23.

[391] Stevens MJ, Henry DN, Thomas TP, Killen PD, Greene DA. Aldose reductase gene expression and osmotic dysregulation in cultured human retinal pigment epithelial cells. Am J Physiol 1993; 265: E428–438.

[392] Stevens MJ, Hosaka Y, Masterson JA, Jones SM, Thomas TP, Larkin DD. Downregulation of the human taurine transporter by glucose in cultured retinal pigment epithelial cells. Am J Physiol 1999; 277: E760–771.

[393] Stevens MJ, Larkin DR, Hosaka Y, Porcellati F, Thomas TP, Masterson JM, Killen PD, Greene DA. Suppression of endogenous osmoregulatory genes in human retinal pigment epithelial cells transfected to overexpress aldose reductase. Diabetologia 1997; 40 (Suppl 1): A491.

[394] Kao YL, Donaghue K, Chan A, Knight J, Silink M. A novel polymorphism in the aldose reductase gene promoter region is strongly associated with diabetic retinopathy in adolescents with type 1 diabetes. Diabetes 1999; 48: 1338–40.

[395] Fujisawa T, Ikegami H, Kawaguchi Y, Yamato E, Nakagawa Y, Shen G-Q, Fukuda M, Ogihara T. Length rather than a specific allele of dinucleotide repeat in the 5′ upstream region of the aldose reductase gene is associated with diabetic retinopathy. Diabet Med 1999; 16: 1044–7.

[396] Ichikawa F. Yamada K, ishiyama-Shigemoto S, Yuan X, Nonaka K. Association of an (A-C)n dinucleotide repeat polymorphic marker at the 5′-region of the aldose reductase gene with retinopathy but not with nephropathy or neuropathy in Japanese patients with type 2 diabetes mellitus. Diabet Med 1999; 16: 744–8.

[397] Heesom AE, Millward A, Demaine AG. Susceptibility to diabetic neuropathy in patients with insulin dependent diabetes mellitus is associated with a polymorphism at the 5′ end of the aldose reductase gene. J Neurol Neurosurg Psychi\try 1998; 64: 213–6.

[398] Moczulski DK, Burak W, Doria A, et al. The role of aldose reductase gene in the susceptibility to diabetic nephropathy in type II (non-insulin dependent) diabetes mellitus. Diabetologia 1999; 42: 94–7.

[399] Vallabh OS, Marina S, Jovanka N, Yijuan S. Z-2 microsatellite allele is linked to increased expression of the aldose reductase gene in diabetic nephropathy. J Clin Endocrinol Metab 1998; 83: 2886–91.

[400] Dyer PH, Chowdhury TA, Dronsfield MJ, Dunger D, Barnett AH, Bain SC. The 5′-end polymorphism of the aldose reductase gene is not associated with diabetic nephropathy in Caucasian type 1 diabetic patients. Diabetologia 1999; 42: 1030–1.

[401] Isermann B, Schmidt S, Bierhaus A, Schiekofer S, Borcea V, Ziegler R, Nawroth P, Ritz E. (CA)n dinucleotide repeat polymorphism at the 5′-end of the aldose reductase gene is not associated with microangiopathy in Caucasians with long-term diabetes mellitus 1. Nephrol Dial Transplant 2000; 15: 918–20.

[402] Pfeifer MA, Schumer MP, Gelber DA. Aldose reductase inhibitors: the end of an era or the need for different trial designs? Diabetes 1997; 2: S82–89.

[403] Hotta N, Sakamoto N, Shigeta Y, Kikkawa R, Goto Y. Clinical investigation of epalrestat, an aldose reductase inhibitor, on diabetic neuropathy in Japan: multicenter study. Diabetic Neuropathy Study Group in Japan. J Diabetes Complications 1996; 10: 168–72.

[404] Goto Y, Hotta N, Shigeta Y, Sakamoto N, Kikkawa R. Effects of an aldose reductase inhibitor, epalrestat, on diabetic neuropathy. Clinical benefit and indication for the drug assessed from the results of a placebo-controlled double-blind study. Biomed Pharmacother 1995; 49: 269–77.

[405] Greene DA, Arezzo JC, Brown MB. Effect of aldose reductase inhibition on nerve conduction and morphometry in diabetic neuropathy. Zenarestat Study Group. Neurology 1999; 53: 580–9.

[406] Stevens MJ, Dayanikli F, Raffel DM, Allman KC, Sandford T, Feldman EL, Wieland DM, Corbett J, Schwaiger M. Scinti-

graphic assessment of regionalized defects in myocardial sympathetic innervation and blood flow regulation in diabetic patients with autonomic neuropathy. J Am Coll Cardiol 1998; 31: 1575–84.
[407] Mantysaari M, Kuikka J, Mustonen J, et al. Noninvasive detection of cardiac sympathetic nervous dysfunction in diabetic patients using [^{123}I] metaiodobenzylguanidine. Diabetes 1992; 41: 1069–75.
[408] Ziegler D, Weise F, Langen K-J, Piolot R, Boy C, Hubinger A, Muller-Gartner H-W, Gries FA. Effect of glycemic control on myocardial sympathetic innervation assessed by [123]metaiodobenzylguanidine scintigraphy: a 4-year prospective study in IDDM patients. Diabetologia 1998; 41: 443–51.
[409] Stevens MJ, Raffel DM, Allman KC, Schwaiger M, Wieland DM. Regression and progression of cardiac sympathetic dysinnervation in diabetic patients with autonomic neuropathy. Metabolism 1999; 48: 92–101.
[410] Utsunomiya K, Narabayashi I, Nakatani Y, Tamura K, Onishi S. I-123 MIBG cardiac imaging in diabetic neuropathy before and after epalrestat therapy. Clin Nucl Med 1999; 24: 418–20.
[411] The UK Prospective Diabetes Study (UKPDS) Group. Intensive blood-glucose control with sulphonylureas or insulin compared with conventional treatment and risk of complications in patients with type 2 diabetes (UKPDS 33). Lancet 1998; 352: 837–53.
[412] Gabir MM, Hanson RL, Dabelea D, Imperatore G, Roumain J, Bennett P, Knowler WC. Plasma glucose and prediction of microvascular disease and mortality. Diabetes Care 2000; 23: 1113–8.
[413] Maser RE, Steenkiste AR, Dorman JS, et al. Epidemiological correlates of diabetic neuropathy. Report from the Pittsburgh Epidemiology of Diabetes Complications Study. Diabetes 1989; 38: 1456–61.
[414] Tesfaye S, Stevens L, Stephenson J, et al. The prevalence of diabetic peripheral neuropathy and its relation to glycaemic control and potential risk factors: The EURODIAB IDDM complications study. Diabetologia 1996; 39: 1377–84.
[415] Forrest K, Maser R, Pambianco G, Becker D, Orchard T. Hypertension as a risk factor for diabetic neuropathy: a prospective study. Diabetes 1997; 46: 665–70.
[416] Dyck PJ, Davies JL, Wilson DM, Service FJ, Melton LJ, O'Brien PC. Risk factors for diabetic polyneuropathy— intensive longitudinal assessment of the Rochester Diabetic Neuropathy Study cohort. Diabetes Care 1999; 22: 1479–86.
[417] Karamanos B, Porta M, Songini M, Metelko Z, Kerenyi Z, Tamas G, Rottiers R, Stevens LK, Fuller JH. Different risk factors of microangiopathy in patients with type I diabetes mellitus of short versus long duration. The EURODIAB IDDM complications study. Diabetologia 2000; 43: 348–55.
[418] Zander E, Herfurth S, Bohl B, Heinke P, Herrman U, Kohnert K-D, Kerner W. Maculopathy in patients with diabetes mellitus type 1 and type 2: associations with risk factors. Br J Ophthalmol 2000; 84: 871–6.
[419] Fuller JH, Chaturvedi N. Abnormalities of nerve conduction velocity are related to other microvascular complications in type I diabetic subjects without clinically detectable diabetic neuropathy. Diabetes 2000; 49 (Suppl 1): 673.
[420] Jaap AJ, Hammersley MS, Shore AC, Tooke JE. Reduced microvascular hyperaemia in subjects at risk of developing type 2 (non-insulin-dependent) diabetes mellitus. Diabetologia 1994; 37: 214–6.
[421] Caballero AE, Arora S, Saouaf R, Lim SC, Smakowski P, Park JY, King GL, LoGerfo FW, Horton ES, Veves A. Microvascular and macrovascular reactivity is reduced in subjects at risk for type 2 diabetes. Diabetes 1999; 48: 1856–62.
[422] Stehouwer CDA, Fischer HRA, Kuijk AWR Van, Polak BCP, Donker AJM. Endothelial dysfunction precedes development of microalbuminuria in IDDM. Diabetes 1995; 44: 561–4.
[423] Plater ME, Ford I, Dent MT, Preston FE, Ward JD. Elevated von Willebrand factor antigen predicts deterioration in diabetic peripheral nerve function. Diabetologia 1996; 39: 336–43.
[424] Feng DL, Bursell S-E, Clermont AC, Lipinska I, Aiello LP, Laffel L, King GL, Tofler GH. Von Willebrand factor and retinal circulation in early-stage retinopathy of type I diabetes. Diabetes Care 2000; 23: 1694–8.
[425] Standl E, Balletshofer B, Dahl B, Weichenhain B, Stiegler H, Hormann A, Holle R. Predictors of 10-year macrovascular and overall mortality in patients with NIDDM: The Munich general practitioner project. Diabetologia 1996; 39: 1540–5.
[426] Young MJ, Veves A, Smith JV, Walker MG, Boulton AJM. Restoring lower limb blood flow improves conduction velocity in diabetic patients. Diabetologia 1995; 38: 1051–4.
[427] Akbari CM, Gibbons GW, Habershaw GM, LoGerfo FW, Veves A. The effect of arterial reconstruction on the natural history of diabetic neuropathy. Arch Surg 1997; 132: 148–52.
[428] Malik R, Masson EA, Sharma AK, et al. Hypoxic neuropathy: relevance to human diabetic neuropathy. Diabetologia 1990; 33: 311–8.
[429] Tesfaye S, Harris N, Jakubowski JJ, Mody C, Wilson RM, Rennie IG, Ward JD. Impaired blood flow and arterio-venous shunting in human diabetic neuropathy: a novel technique of nerve photography and fluorescein angiography. Diabetologia 1993; 36: 1266–74.
[430] Newrick PG, Wilson AJ, Jakubowski J, Boulton AJM, Ward JD. Sural nerve oxygen tension in diabetes. BMJ 1986; 293: 1053–4.
[431] Young MJ, Veves A, Walker MG, Boulton AJM. Correlation between nerve function and tissue oxygenation in diabetic patients: further clues to the aetiology of diabetic neuropathy? Diabetologia 1992; 35: 1146–50.
[432] Ibrahim S, Harris ND, Radatz M, Selmi F, Rajbhandari S, Brady L, Jakubowski J, Ward JD. A new minimally invasive technique to show nerve ischaemia in diabetic neuropathy. Diabetologia 1999; 42: 737–42.
[433] Boulton AJM, Scarpello JHB, Ward JD. Venous oxygenation in the diabetic neuropathic foot: evidence of arterio-venous shunting? Diabetologia 1982; 22: 6–8.
[434] Koistinaho J, Wadhwani KC, Rapoport SI. Adrenergic innervation in the tibial and vagus nerves of rats with streptozotocin-induced diabetes. Brain Res 1990; 513: 106–12.
[435] Milner P, Apenzeller O, Qualls C, Burnstock G. Differential vulnerability of neuropeptides in nerves of the vasa nervosum to streptozotocin-induced diabetes. Brain Res 1992; 574: 56–62.
[436] Tesfaye S, Harris N, Wilson RM, Ward JD. Exercise induced conduction velocity increment: a marker of impaired nerve blood flow in diabetic neuropathy. Diabetologia 1992; 35: 155–9.
[437] Haak E, Haak T, Grozinger P, Krebs G, Usadel KH, Kusterer K. The impact of contralateral cooling on skin capillary blood cell velocity in patients with diabetes mellitus. J Vasc Res 1998; 35: 245–9.
[438] Gregersen G. A study of the peripheral nerves in diabetic subjects during ischaemia. J Neurol Neurosurg Psychiatry 1968; 31: 175–81.
[439] Steiness I. Vibratory perception in diabetics during arrested blood flow to the limb. Acta Med Scand 1959; 163: 195–205.
[440] Gregersen G. Vibratory perception threshold and motor conduction velocity in diabetics and non-diabetics. Acta Med Scand 1968; 183: 61–5.
[441] Lindstrom P, Lindblom U, Brismar T. Delayed recovery of nerve conduction and vibratory sensibility after ischaemic block in patients with diabetes mellitus. J Neurol Neurosurg Psychiatry 1997; 63: 346–50.
[442] Steiness I. Influence of diabetic status on vibratory perception during ischaemia. Acta Med Scand 1961; 170: 319–38.
[443] Kuriya N, Mori M, Miyake S, Takamori M, Nagataki S. Effect of ischaemia on peripheral nerve function in diabetes mellitus. Diab Res Clin Pract 1986; 2: 277–82.
[444] Low PA, Ward K, Schmelzer JD, Brimijoin S. Ischemic conduction failure and energy metabolism in experimental diabetic neuropathy. Am J Physiol 1985; 248: E457–462.
[445] Low PA, Yao JK, Kishi Y, Tritschler H-J, Schmelzer JD, Zollman PJ, Nickander KK. Peripheral nerve energy metabolism in experimental diabetic neuropathy. Neurosci Res Commun 1997; 21: 49–56.
[446] Levick R. Control of blood vessels. In: Levick IR, editor. An in introduction to cardiovascular physiology. Oxford: Butterworth-Heinemann; 1995: 201–230.
[447] Vigilance JE, Reid HL, Richards GP, Mills J. Impaired vasodilatory reserve in diabetics with and without neuropathy. Med Sci Res 1997; 25: 561–4.
[448] O'Driscoll G, Green D, Rankin J, Stanton K, Taylor R. Improvement in endothelial function by angiotensin convert-

ing enzyme inhibition in insulin-dependent diabetes mellitus. J Clin Invest 1997; 100: 678–84.
[449] O'Driscoll G, Green D, Maiorana A, Stanton K, Colreavy F, Taylor R. Improvement in endothelial function by angiotensin-converting enzyme inhibition in non-insulin-dependent diabetes mellitus. J Am Coll Cardiol 1999; 33: 1506–11.
[450] Kawano H, Motoyama T, Hirashima O, Hirai N, Miyao Y, Sakamoto T, et al. Hyperglycaemia rapidly suppresses flow-mediated endothelium dependent vasodilation of brachial artery. J Am Coll Cardiol 1999; 34: 146–54.
[451] Fard A, Tuck CH, Donis JA, Sciacca R, Di Tullio MR, Wu HD, et al. Acute elevations of plasma asymmetric dimethylarginine and impaired endothelial function in response to a high-fat meal in patients with type 2 diabetes. Arterioscler Thromb Vasc Biol 2000; 20: 2039–49.
[452] Vallance P, Leone A, Calver A, Collier J, Moncado S. Endogenous dimethylarginine as an inhibitor of nitric oxide synthesis. J Cardiovasc Pharmacol 1992; 20 (Suppl 12): S60–62.
[453] Boulton AJM. Late sequelae of diabetic neuropathy. In: Boulton AJM, editor. Diabetic neuropathy. Carnforth: Marius Press; 1997: 63–75.
[454] Rayman G, Williams SA, Spencer PD, Smaje LH, Wise PH, Tooke JE. Impaired microvascular hyperemic response to minor skin trauma in type-I diabetes. London: BMJ Publishing; 1986.
[455] Morris SJ, Shore AC, Tooke JE. Responses of the skin microcirculation to acetylcholine and sodium nitroprusside in patients with NIDDM. Diabetologia 1995; 38: 1337–44.
[456] Veves A, Akbari CM, Primavera J, Donaghue VM. Zacharoulis D, Chrzan JS et al. Endothelial dysfunction and the expression of endothelial nitric oxide synthetase in diabetic neuropathy, vascular disease and foot ulceration. Diabetes 1998; 47: 457–63.
[457] Jorneskog G, Fagrell B. Discrepancy in skin capillary circulation between fingers and toes in patients with type I diabetes. Int J Microcirc Clin Exp 1996; 16: 313–9.
[458] Jorneskog G, Brismar K, Fagrell B. Skin capillary circulation severely impaired in toes of patients with IDDM, with and without late diabetic complications. Diabetologia 1995; 38: 474–80.
[459] Arora S, Smakowski P, Frykberg RG, Freeman R, LoGerfo FW, Veves A. Differences in foot and forearm skin microcirculation in diabetic patients with and without neuropathy. Diabetes Care 1998; 21: 1339–44.
[460] Veves A, Quist WC, Caballero AE, LoGerfo FW, Horton ES. Expression of endothelial nitric oxide synthase (eNOS) in the skin microvasculature. Diabetes 2000; 49 (Suppl)(1): A150.
[461] Jude EB, Boulton AJM, Ferguson MW, Appleton I. The role of nitric oxide synthase isoforms and arginase in the pathogenesis of diabetic foot ulcers: possible modulatory effects by transforming growth factor beta 1. Diabetologia 1999; 42: 748–57.
[462] Rayman G, Hassan A, Tooke JE. Blood flow in the skin of the foot related to posture in diabetes-mellitus. London: BMJ Publishing; 1986.
[463] Ward JD. The diabetic leg. Diabetologia 1982; 22: 141–7.
[464] Watkins PJ, Edmonds ME. Sympathetic nerve failure in diabetes. Diabetologia 1988; 25: 73–7.
[465] Cacciatori V, Dellera A, Bellavere F, Bongiovanni LG, Teatini F, Gemma ML, Muggeo M. Comparative assessment of peripheral sympathetic function by postural vasoconstriction arteriolar reflex and sympathetic skin response in NIDDM patients. Am J Med 1997; 102: 365–70.
[466] Reinhardt F, Wetzel T, Vetten S, Radespiel-Troger M, Hilz MJ, Heuss D, Neundorfer B. Peripheral neuropathy in chronic venous insufficiency. Muscle Nerve 2000; 23: 883–7.
[467] Kihara M, Zollman PJ, Smithson IL, Lagerlund TD, Low PA. Hypoxic effect of exogenous insulin on normal and diabetic peripheral nerve. Am J Physiol 1994; 266: E980–985.
[468] Fagrell B Advances in microcirculation network evaluation. an update. Int J Microcirc Clin Exp 1995; 15: 34–40.
[469] Parkhouse N, LeQueen PM. Impaired neurogenic vascular response in patients with diabetes and neuropathic foot lesions. N Engl J Med 1988; 318: 1306–9.
[470] Hamdy O, Abou-Elenin K, LoGerfo FW, Horton ES, Veves A. Contribution of nerve-axon reflex-related vasodilation to the total skin vasodilation in diabetic patients with and without neuropathy. Diabetes Care 2001; 24: 344–9.
[471] Giannini C, Dyck PJ. Ultrastructural morphometric features in human sural nerve microvessels. J Neuropathol Exp Neurol 1993; 52: 361–9.
[472] Timperley WR, Boulton AJM, Davies Jones GAB, Jarrat JA, Ward JD. Small vessel disease in progressive diabetic neuropathy associated with good metabolic control. J Clin Pathol 1985; 38: 1030–8.
[473] Beggs J, Johnson PC, Olafsen A, Watkins CJ, Cleary C. Transperineurial arterioles in human sural nerve. J Neuropathol Exp Neurol 1991; 50: 704–18.
[474] Tesfaye S, Malik R, Ward JD. Vascular factors in diabetic neuropathy. Diabetologia 1994; 37: 847–54.
[475] Grover-Johnson NM, Baumann FG, Imparato AM, Kim GE, Thomas PK. Abnormal innervation of lower limb epineurial arterioles in human diabetics. Diabetologia 1981; 20: 31–8.
[476] McKenzie D, Nukuda H, Rij AM van, McMorran PD. Endoneurial microvasculature abnormalities of sural nerve in non-diabetic chronic atherosclerotic occlusive disease. J Neurol Sci 1999; 162: 84–8.
[477] Kihara M, Low PA. Impaired vasoreactivity to nitric oxide in experimental diabetic neuropathy. Exp Neurol 1995; 132: 180–5.
[478] Maxfield EK, Cameron NE, Cotter MA. Effect of diabetes on reactivity of sciatic vasa nervorum in rats. J Diabetes Complications 1997; 11: 47–55.
[479] Hogikyan RV, Wald JJ, Feldman EL, Greene DA, Halter JB, Supiano MA. Acute effects of adrenergic-mediated ischemia on nerve conduction in subjects with type 2 diabetes. Metab Clin Exp 1999; 48: 495–500.
[480] Cameron NE, Cotter MA, Low PA. Nerve blood flow in early experimental diabetes in rats: relation to conduction deficits. Am J Physiol 1991; 261: E1–8.
[481] Cameron NE, Cotter MA. Metabolic and vascular factors in the pathogenesis of diabetic neuropathy. Diabetes 1997; 46 (Suppl 2): S31–37.
[482] Cameron NE, Cotter MA, Robertson S. Angiotensin converting enzyme inhibition prevents the development of muscle and nerve dysfunction and stimulates angiogenesis in streptozotocin-diabetic rats. Diabetologia 1992; 35: 12–18.
[483] Maxfield EK, Love A, Cotter MA, Cameron NE. Nerve function and regeneration in diabetic rats: effects of ZD-7155, an AT_1 receptor antagonist. Am J Physiol 1995; 269: E530–537.
[484] Cameron NE, Cotter MA. Effects of chronic treatment with a nitric oxide donor on nerve conduction abnormalities and endoneurial blood flow in streptozotocin-diabetic rats. Eur J Clin Invest 1995; 25: 19–24.
[485] Cotter MA, Cameron NE. Correction of neurovascular deficits in diabetic rats by β_2 agonist and α_1 adrenoceptor antagonist treatment: interactions with the nitric oxide system. Eur J Pharmacol 1998; 343: 217–23.
[486] Reja A, Tesfaye S, Harris ND, Ward JD. Is ACE inhibition with lisinopril helpful in diabetic neuropathy? Diabet Med 1995; 12: 307–9.
[487] Al-Memar A, Wimalaratana HSK, Millward BA. Lisinopril improves nerve function in insulin-dependent diabetic patients with neuropathy: a preferential effect on small fibres (abstract). Diabet Med 1996; 13 (Suppl 1): 91.
[488] Kontopoulos AG, Athyros VG, Didangelos TP, Papageorigiou AA, Avramidis MJ, Mayroudi MC, et al. Effect of chronic quinapril administration on heart rate variability in patients with diabetic autonomic neuropathy. Diabetes Care 1997; 20: 355–61.
[489] Malik R, Williamson S, Abbott C, Carrington AL, Iqbal J, Boulton AJM. Effect of the angiotensin converting enzyme inhibitor trandalopril on human diabetic neuropathy: a randomised controlled trial. Lancet 1998; 352: 1978–81.
[490] Cotter MA, Mirrlees DJ, Cameron NE. Neurovascular interactions between aldose reductase and angiotensin converting enzyme inhibition in diabetic rats. Eur J Pharmacol 2001; 417: 223–30.
[491] Arcaro G, Zenere BM, Saggiani F, Zenti MG, Monauni T, Lechi A, et al. ACE inhibitors improve endothelial function in type I diabetic patients with normal arterial pressure and microalbuminuria. Diabetes Care 1999; 22: 1536–42.
[492] Haak E, Haak T, Kusterer K, Reschke B, Faust H, Usadel KH. Microcirculation in hyperglycaemic patients without diabetic complications—effect of low-dose angiotensin converting enzyme inhibition. Exp Clin Endocrinol Diabetes 1998; 106: 45–50.

[746] Heaton JH, Krett NL, Alvarez JM, Gelehrter TD, Romanus JA, Rechler MM. Insulin regulation of insulin-like growth gactor action in rat hepatoma cells. J Biol Chem 1984; 259: 2396–402.

[747] Recio-Pinto E, Ishii DN. Insulin and related growth factors: effects on the nervous system and mechanism for neurite growth and regeneration. Neurochem Inter 1988; 12: 397–414.

[748] Caroni P, Grandes P. Nerve sprouting in innervated adult skeletal muscle induced by exposure to elevated levels of insulin-like growth factor I receptor. J Cell Biol 1990; 110: 1307–17.

[749] Houten M Van, Posner BI, Kopriwa BM, Brawer JR. Insulin binding sites localized to nerve terminals in rat median eminence and arcuate nucleus. Science 1979; 207: 1081–3.

[750] Mill JF, Chao MV, Ishii DN. Insulin, insulin-like growth factor II, and nerve growth factor effects on tubulin mRNA levels and neurite formation. Proc Natl Acad Sci USA 1985; 82: 7126–30.

[751] Wang C, Li Y, Wible B, Angelides KJ, Ishii DN. Effects of insulin and insulin-like growth factors on neurofilament mRNA and tubulin mRNA content in human neuroblastoma SH-SY5Y cells. Mol Brain Res 1992; 13: 289–300.

[752] Ishii DN, Recio-Pinto E. Role of insulin, insulin-like growth factors, and nerve growth factor in neurite formation. In: Raizada MK, Phillips MI, LeRoith D, editors. Insulin-like growth factors, and their receptors in the central nervous system. New York, N.Y.: Plenum Press; 1987: 315–48.

[753] Recio-Pinto E, Rechler MM, Ishii DN. Effects of insulin, insulin-like growth factor II, and nerve growth factor on neurite formation and survival in cultured sympathetic and sensory neurons. J Neurosci 1986; 6: 1211–9.

[754] Glazner GW, Ishii DN. Insulin, insulin-like growth factor-I and nerve growth factor stimulate neurite formation in rat spinal cord cultures. Soc Neurosci Abstr 1988; 14: 1040.

[755] Liuzzi FJ, Tedeschi B. Peripheral Nerve Regeneration. In: Burchiel KR, editors. Neurosurg.Clin.North Am. 3 no. 1. Philadelphia, Pa.: W. B.Saunders, 1991: 31–42.

[756] Glazner GW, Wright WG, Ishii DN. Kinetics of insulin-like growth factor (IGF) mRNA changes in rat nerve and muscle during IGF-dependent nerve regeneration (abstract). Soc Neurosci Abstr 1993; 19: 253.

[757] Kanje M, Skottner A, Sjoberg J, Lundborg G. Insulin-like growth factor I (IGF-I) stimulates regeneration of the rat sciatic nerve. Brain Res 1989; 486: 396–8.

[758] Ishii DN. Relationship of insulin-like growth factor II gene expression in muscle to synaptogenesis. Proc Natl Acad Sci U S A 1989; 86: 2898–902.

[759] Pu SF, Ishii DN. Distribution of insulin-like growth factor mRNAs in rat nerve and muscle during nerve regeneration by in situ hybridization (abstract). Soc Neurosci Abstr 1993; 19: 253.

[760] Shimasaki S, Shimonaka M, Zhang H-P, Ling N. Identification of five different insulin-like growth factor binding proteins (IGFBPs) from adult rat serum and molecular cloning of a novel IGFBP-5 in rat and humans. J Biol Chem 1991; 266: 10646–53.

[761] Tan K, Baxter RC. Serum insulin-like growth factor I levels in adult diabetic patients: the effect of age. J Clin Endocrinol Metab 1986; 63: 651–5.

[762] Bang P, Brismar K, Rosenfeld RG. Increased proteolysis of insulin-like growth factors-binding protein-3 (IGFBP-3) in non-insulin dependent diabetes mellitus serum, with elevation of a 29-kilodalton (kDa) glycosylated IGFBP-3 fragment contained in the approximately 130-to150 kDa ternary complex. J Clin Endocrinol Metab 1994; 78: 1119–27.

[763] Tseng LY-H, Brown AL, Yang YW-H, Romanus JA, Orlowski CC, Taylor T, Rechler MM. The fetal rat binding protein for insulin-like growth factors is expressed in the choroid plexus and cerebrospinal fluid of adult rats. Mol Endocrinol 1989; 3: 1559–68.

[764] Roghani M, Hossenlopp P, Lepage P, Balland A, Binoux M. Isolation from human cerebrospinal fluid of a new insulin-like growth factor-binding protein with a selective affinity for IGF-II. FEBS Lett 1989; 255: 253–8.

[765] Quin JD, Checkley A, Gallagher A, Jones J, MacCuish AC, Miell JP. Response of insulin-like growth factor (IGF)-binding protein-1 and IGFBP-3 to IGF-1 treatment in severe insulin resistance. J Endocrinol 1994; 141: 177–82.

[766] Watkins AD. Perceptions, emotions and immunity: an integrated homoeostatic network. Q J Med 1995; 88: 283–94.

[767] Hill RL, Brew K, Vanaman TC, Trayer IP, Mattock P. Function, and evolution of alpha-lactalbumin. Brookhaven Symp Biol 1968; 21: 139–54.

[767a] Bradshaw RA, Hogue-Angeletti RA, Frazier WA. Nerve growth factor and insulin: evidence of similarities in structure, function, and mechanism of action. Recent Prog Horm Res 1974; 30: 575–96.

[768] Saltiel AR, Cuatrecasas P. In search of a second messenger for insulin. Am J Physiol 1988; 255: C1–C11.

[769] Saltiel AR. Signal transduction in insulin. J Nutr Biochem 1990; 1: 180–8.

[770] Ishii DN. Neurobiology of insulin and insulin-like growth factors. In: Loughlin SE, Fallow JH, editors. Neurotrophic factors. New York, N.Y.: Academic Press; 1993: 415–42.

[770a] Ishii DN. Insulin and related neurotrophic factors in diabetic neuropathy. Diabetic Med 1993; 10 (Suppl 2): 14S–15S.

[771] Recio-Pinto E, Ishii DN. Insulin and insulin-like growth factor receptors regulating neurite formation in cultured human neuroblastoma cells. J Neurosci Res 1988; 19: 312–20.

[772] Near SL, Whalen LR, Miller JA, Ishii DN. Insulin-like growth factor-II stimulates motor nerve regeneration. Proc Natl Acad Sci USA 1992; 89: 11716–20.

[773] Bisby MA. Axonal transport of labeled protein and regeneration rate in nerves of streptozocin-diabetic rats. Exp Neurol 1980; 69: 74–84.

[774] Ekstrom AR, Kanje M, Skottner A. Nerve regeneration and serum levels of insulin-like growth factor-I in rats with streptozotocin-induced insulin deficiency. Brain Res 1989; 496: 141–7.

[775] Ekstrom AR, Tomlinson DR. Impaired nerve regeneration in streptozotocin-diabetic rats. Effects of treatment with an aldose reductase inhibitor. J Neurol Sci 1989; 93: 231–7.

[776] Glazner GW, Lupien S, Miller JA, Ishii DN. Insulin-like growth factor-II increases the rate of sciatic nerve regeneration in rats. Neuroscience 1993; 54: 791–7.

[777] Sjoberg J, Kanje M. Insulin-like growth factor (IGF-I) as a stimulator of regeneration in the freeze-injured rat sciatic nerve. Brain Res 1989; 485: 102–8.

[778] Mosier CI. On the reliability of a weighted composite. Psychometrika 1943; 8: 341–8.

[779] Longo FM, Hayman EG, Davis GE, Ruoslahti E, Engvall E, Manthorpe MA, Varon S. Neurite-promoting factors and extracellular matrix components accumulating in vivo within nerve regeneration chambers. Brain Res 1984; 309: 105–17.

[780] Catanese VM, Sciavolino PJ, Lango MN. Discordant, organ-specific regulation of insulin-like growth factor-I messenger ribonucleic acid in insulin-deficient diabetes in rats. Endocrinology 1993; 132: 496–503.

[781] Bornfeldt KE, Arnqvist BE, Mathews LS, Norstedt G. Regulation of insulin-like growth factor-I and growth hormone receptor gene expression by diabetes and nutritional state in rat tissues. J Endocrinol 1989; 122: 651–6.

[782] Maes M, Kateslegers JM, Underwood LE. Low circulating somatomedin-C/insulin-like growth factor I in insulin-dependent diabetes and malnutrition: growth hormone receptor and post-receptor defects. Acta Endocrinol (Copenh) 1987; 112: 86–92.

[783] Straus DS. Nutritional regulation of hormones and growth factors that control mammalian growth. FASEB J 1994; 8: 6–12.

[784] Straus DS, Takemoto CD. Effect of dietary protein deprivation on insulin-like growth factor (IGF)-I and -II, IGF binding protein-2, and serum albumin gene expression in rat. Endocrinology 1990; 127: 1849–60.

[785] Liuzzi FJ, Depto AS. Increased insulin-like growth factor II gene expression in diabetic rat dorsal root ganglia (abstract). Diabetes 1994; 43: 335.

[786] Taylor AM, Dunger DB, Preece MA, Holly JMP, Smith CP, Wass JAH, Patel S, Tate VE. The growth hormone independent insulin-like growth factor-I binding protein BP-28 is associated with serum insulin-like growth factor-I inhibitory bioactivity in adoloscent insulin-dependent diabetics. Clin Endocrinol (Oxf) 1990; 32: 229–39.

[787] Luo J, Murphy LJ. Differential expression of insulin-like growth factor-I and insulin-like growth factor binding protein-1 in the diabetic rat. Mol Cell Biochem 1991; 103: 41–40.

[788] Timple R, Rhode H, Gehron Robey P, Rennard SI, Foidart JMa, Martin GR. Laminin: a glycoprotein from basement membranes. J Biol Chem 1979; 254: 9933–7.
[789] Timple R. Structure and biological activity of basement membrane proteins. Eur J Biochem 1989; 180: 487–502.
[790] Ehrig K, Leivo I, Argraves WS, Ruoslahti EA, Engvall E. Merosin, a tissue-specific basement membrane protein, is a laminin-like protein. Proc Natl Acad Sci USA 1990; 87: 3264–8.
[791] Baron-Van Evercooren A, Kleiman HK, Ohno S, Marangos P, Schwarz JP, Dubois-Dalq ME. Nerve growth factor, laminin and fibronectin promote neurite growth from human fetal sensory ganglion cultures. J Neurosci Res 1982; 8: 179–94.
[792] Lander AD, Fujii D, Reichardt LF. Laminin is associated with the "neurite outgrowth-promoting factors" found in conditioned media. Proc Natl Acad Sci USA 1985; 82: 2183–7.
[793] Manthrorpe M, Engvall E, Ruoslahti E, Longo FM, Davis GE, Varon S. Laminin promotes neuritic regeneration from cultured peripheral and central neurons. J Cell Biol 1983; 97: 1882–90.
[794] Rivas RJ, Burneister DW, Goldberg DJ. Rapid effects of laminin on the growth cone. Neuron 1992; 8: 107–15.
[795] Ide C. Nerve regeneration and Schwann cell basal lamina: observations of the long-term regeneration. Arch Histol Jpn 1983; 46: 243–57.
[796] Ide C, Tohyama K, Yokata R, Nitatori TA, Onocera S. Schwann cell basal lamina and nerve regeneration. Brain Res 1990; 288: 61–75.
[797] Dean JWI, Chandrasekaran S, Tanzer ML. A biological role for carbohydrate moieties of laminin. J Biol Chem 1990; 265: 12553–62.
[798] Charonis AS, Reger LA, Dege JE, Kouzi-Koliakos K, Furcht LT, Wohlhueter RM, Tsilibary EC. Laminin alterations after in vitro nonenzymatic glycosylation. Diabetes 1990; 39: 807–14.
[799] Le Beau JM, Liuzzi FJ, Depto AJ, Vinik AI. Up-regulation of laminin B2 gene expression in dorsal root ganglion neurons and non-neuronal cells during sciatic nerve regeneration. Exp Neurol 1995; 134: 150–5.
[800] Wassermann A, Neisser A, Bruck C. Eine serodiagnostische Reaktion bei Syphilis. Dtsch Med Wochenschr 1906; 32: 745–6.
[801] Le Beau JM, Liuzzi FJ. Laminin B2 mRNA is up-regulated in sensory neurons and Schwann cells during peripheral nerve regeneration (abstract). Soc Neurosci Abstr 1991; 17: 1500.
[802] Depto AS, Le Beau JM, Liuzzi FJ, Suwanwalaikorn S, Mamplata N, Newlon PG, Vinik AI. Laminin gene expression in diabetic rat dorsal root ganglia (abstract). Soc Neurosci Abstr 1993; 19: 835.
[803] Le Beau JM, Liuzzi FJ, Vinik AI. Differential expression of laminin genes in dorsal root ganglia during sciatic nerve regeneration (abstract). Soc Neurosci Abstr 1993; 19: 679.
[804] O'Brien J, Carson G, Seo H, Hiraiwa M, Kishimoto Y. Identification of prosaposin as a neurotrophic factor. Proc Natl Acad Sci USA 1994; 91: 9593–6.
[805] O'Brien J, Carson G, Seo H, Hiraiwa M, Weiler S, Tomich J, Barranger J, Kahan M, Azuma N, Kishimoto Y. Identification of the neurotrophic factor sequence of prosaposin. FASEB J 1995; 9: 681–5.
[806] Calcutt NA, Capana W, Eskeland N, Mohiuddin L, Dines K, Mizisin A, O'Brien J. Prosaposin gene expression and the efficacy of a prosaposin-derived peptide in preventing structural and functional disorders of peripheral nerve in diabetic rats. J Neuropathol Exp Neurol 1999; 58: 628–36.
[807] Wagner R, Myers R, O'Brien J. Prosaptide prevents hyperalgesia and reduces peripheral TNFR1 expression following TNF-α nerve injection. Neuroreport 1998; 9: 2827–31.
[808] Campana W, Eskeland N, Calcutt NA, Misasi R, Myers R, O'Brien J. Prosaptide prevents paclitaxel neurotoxicity. Neurotoxicology 1998; 19: 237–44.
[809] Hiraiwa M, Taylor M, Campana W, Darin S, O'Brien J. Cell death prevention, mitogen-activated protein kinase stimulation, and increased sulfatide concentrations in Schwann cells and oligodendrocytes by prosaposin and prosaptides. Proc Natl Acad Sci USA 1997; 94: 4778–81.
[810] Hiraiwa M, Martin B, Kishimoto Y, Conner G, Tsuji S, O'Brien J. Lysosomal proteolysis of prosaposin, the precursor of saposins (sphingolipid activator proteins): its mechanism and inhibition by ganglioside. Arch Biochem Biophys 1997; 341: 17–24.
[811] Campana W, Darin S, O'Brien J. Phosphatidylinositol 3-kinase and Akt protein kinase mediate IGF-I- and prosaptide-induced survival in Schwann Cells. J Neurosci Res 1999; 57: 332–41.
[812] Tsuboi K, Hiraiwa M, O'Brien JS. Prosaposin prevents programmed cell death of rat cerebellar granule neurons in culture. Brain Res Dev Brain Res 1998; 110: 249–55.
[813] Campana W, Hiraiwa M, O'Brien J. Prosaptide activates the MAPK pathway by a G-protein-dependent mechanism essential for enhanced sulfatide synthesis by Schwann cells. FASEB J 1998; 12: 307–14.
[814] Otero D, Conrad B, O'Brien J. Reversal of the thermal hyperalgesia in a rat partial sciatic nerve ligation model by prosaptide TX14(A). Neurosci Lett 1999; 270: 29–32.
[815] Gadient R, Otten U. Postnatal expression of interleukin-6 (IL-6) receptor (IL-6R) mRNAs in rat sympathetic and sensory ganglia. Brain Res 1996; 724: 41–6.
[816] Hirota H, Kiyama H, Kishimoto T, Taga T. Accelerated nerve regeneration in mice by upregulated expression of interleukin(IL)6 and IL-6 receptor after trauma. J Exp Med 1996; 183: 2627–34.
[817] Creange A, Barlovatz-Meimon G, Gherardi RK. Cytokines and peripheral nerve disorders. Eur Cytokine Netw 1997; 8: 145–51.
[818] Loddick SA, Takao T, Hashimoto K, Souza EB De. Interleukin-1 receptors: cloning studies and role in central nervous system disorders. Brain Res Brain Res Rev 1998; 26: 306–19.
[819] Ikeda SR. Voltage-dependent modulation of N-type calcium channels by G-protein $\beta\gamma$ subunits. Nature 1996; 380: 255–8.
[820] Murwani R, Hodgkinson S, Armati P. Tumor necrosis factor alpha and interleukin-6 mRNA expression in neonatal Lewis rat Schwann cells and a neonatal rat Schwann cell line following interferon gamma stimulation. J Neuroimmunol 1996; 71: 65–71.
[821] Reichert F, Levitzky R, Rotshenker S. Interleukin 6 in intact and injured mouse peripheral nerves.Eur J Neurosci 1996; 8: 530–5.
[822] Marz P, Cheng JG, Gadient RA, Patterson PH, Stoyan T, Otten U, Rose-John S. Sympathetic neurons can produce and respond to interleukin 6. Proc Natl Acad Sci USA 1998; 95: 3251–6.
[823] Hull M, Fiebich BL, Lieb K, Strauss S, Berger SS, Volk B, Bauer J. Interleukin-6-associated inflammatory processes in Alzheimer's disease: new therapeutic options. Neurobiol Aging 1996; 17: 795–800.
[824] Hamdy O, Abouelenin K, Logefo F, Horton E, Veves A. The contribution of nerve axon reflex-related vasodilation (NARRV) to the total endothelium-dependent vasodilation in the skin of diabetic patients with and without neuropathy. Diabetes 2000; 49: A164.
[825] Shimada K, Koh CS, Yanagisawa N. Detection of interleukin-6 in serum and cerebrospinal fluid of patients with neuroimmunological diseases. Arerugi 1993; 42: 934–40.
[826] Rose C, Zandecki M, Copin MC, Gosset P, Labalette M, Hatron PY, Jauberteau MO, Devulder B, Bauters F, Facon T. POEMS syndrome: report on six patients with unusual clinical signs, elevated levels of cytokines, macrophage involvement and chromosomal aberrations of bone marrow plasma cells. Leukemia 1997; 11: 1318–23.
[827] Pittenger G, Erbas T, Burcus N, Vinik A. Serum from patients with diabetic neuropathy impairs laminin neuroprotection by altering laminin receptor integrin expression. Diabetes 2000; 49: A34.
[828] Pittenger GL, Liu D, Vinik AI. The toxic effects of serum from patients with type I diabetes mellitus on mouse neuroblastoma cells: a new mechanism for development of autonomic neuropathy. Diabet Med 1993; 10: 925–32.
[829] Pittenger GL, Liu D, Vinik AI. The neuronal toxic factor in serum of type 1 diabetic patients is a complement-fixing autoantibody. Diabet Med 1995; 12: 380–6.
[830] Pittenger GL, Liu D, Vinik AI. The apoptotic death of neuroblastoma cells caused by serum from patients with insulin-dependent diabetes and neuropathy may be Fas-mediated. J Neuroimmunol 1997; 76: 153–60.
[831] Knezevic-Cuca J, Stansberry KB, Johnston G, Zhang J, Keller ET, Vinik AI, Pittenger GL. Neurotrophic role of interleukin-6

and soluble interleukin-6 receptors in NIE-115 neuroblastoma cells. J Neuroimmunol 2000; 102: 8–16.
[832] Thier M, Marz P, Otten U, Weis J, Rose-John S. Interleukin-6 (IL-6) and its soluble receptor support survival of sensory neurons. J Neurosci Res 1999; 55: 411–22.
[833] Gold BG. Neuroimmunophilin ligands: evaluation of their therapeutic potential for the treatment of neurological disorders. Expert Opin Investig Drug 2000; 9: 2331–42.
[834] Rabizadeh S, Oh J, Zhong LT, Yang J, Bitler CM, Butcher LL, Bredesen DE. Induction of apoptosis by the low-affinity NGF receptor. Science 1993; 261: 345–8.
[835] Jensen LM, Zhang Y, Shooter EM. Steady-state polypeptide modulations associated with nerve growth factor (NGF)-induced terminal differentiation and NGF deprivation-induced apoptosis in human neuroblastoma cells. J Biol Chem 1992; 267: 19325.
[836] Pittenger GL, Milicevic Z, Vinik AI. Autoimmune mechanisms of diabetic neuropathy. In: LeRoith D, Olefsky JM, Taylor S, editors. Diabetes mellitus: a fundamental and clinical text D. Philadelphia, Pa.: Lippincott-Raven; 1996: 751–8.
[837] Srinivasan S, Stevens MJ, Sheng H, Hall KE, Wiley JW. Serum from patients with type 2 diabetes with neuropathy induces complement-independent, calcium-dependent apoptosis in cultured neuronal cells. J Clin Invest 1998; 102: 1454–62.
[838] Steller H. Mechanism and genes of cellular suicide. Science 1995; 267: 1445–9.
[839] Garcia I, Martinou I, Tsujimoto Y, Martinou JC. Prevention of programmed cell death of sympathetic neurons by the bcl-2 proto-oncogene. Science 1992; 258: 302–4.
[840] Weller M, Frei K, Groscurth P, Krammer PH, Yonekawa Y, Fontana A. Anti-Fas/APO-1 antibody-mediated apoptosis of cultured human glioma cells. Induction and modulation of sensitivity by cytokines. J Clin Invest 1994; 94: 954–64.
[841] Peitsch MC, Tschopp J. Comparative molecular modelling of the Fas-ligand and other members of the TNF family. Mol Immunol 1995; 32: 761–72.
[842] Nagata S, Golstein P. The Fas death factor. Science 1995; 267: 1449–56.
[843] Coyle JT. The nagging question of the function of N-acetylaspartylglutamate. Neurobiol Dis 1997; 4: 231–8.
[844] Wrobleska B, Wrobleska JT, Pshenichkin S, Surin A, Sullivan SE, Neale JH. NAAG selectively activates mGluR3 receptors in transfected cells. J Neurochem 1997; 69: 174–81.
[845] Puttfarcken PS, Handen JS, Montgomery DT, Coyle JT, Werling LL. N-Acetyl-aspartylglutamate modulation of N-methyl-D-aspartate-stimulated [3H]norepinephrine release from rat hippocampal slices. J Pharmacol Exp Ther 1993; 266: 796–803.
[846] Fuhrman S, Palkovits M, Cassidy M, Neal JH. the regional distribution of N-acetylaspartylglutamate (NAAG) and peptidase activity against NAAG in the rat nervous system. J Neurochem 1994; 62: 275–81.
[847] Meyerhoff C, Bischof F, Sternberg F, Zier H, Pfeiffer EF. On line continuous monitoring of subcutaneous tissue glucose in men by combining portable glucosensor with microdialysis. Diabetologia 1992; 35: 1087–92.
[848] Pernis A, Gupta S, Gollob KJ, Garfein E, Coffman RL, Schindler C, Rothman P. Lack of interferon γ receptor β chain and the prevention of interferon γ signaling in T_H1 Cells. Science 1995; 269: 245–7.
[849] Choi DW, Rothman SM. The role of glutamate neurotoxicity in hypoxic ischemic neuronal death. Annu Rev Neurosci 1990; 13: 171–82.
[850] Meldrum BS. Protection against ischaemic neuronal damage by drugs acting on excitatory neurotransmission. Cerebrovasc Brain Metab Rev 1990; 2: 27–57.
[851] Wahlgren NG. A review of earlier clinical studies on neuroprotective agents and current approaches. Int Rev Neurobiol 1997; 40: 337–63.
[852] Bruno V, Battaglia G, Copani A, Giffard RG, Raciti G, Raffaele R, Shinozaki H, Nicoletti F. Activation of class II or III metabotrophic glutamate receptors protects cultured cortical neurons against excitotoxic degeneration. Eur J Neurosci 1995; 7: 1906–13.
[853] Berger UV, Schwab ME. N-acetylated alpha-linked acidic dipeptidase may be involved in axon-Schwann cell signalling. J Neurocytology 1996; 25: 499–512.
[854] Vornov JJ. NMDA-receptor activation occurs during recovery in a tissue culture model of ischemia. J Neurochem 1995; 65: 1681–91.
[855] Arakawa Y, Sendtner M, Thoenen H. Survival effect of ciliary neurotrophic factor (CNTF) on chick embryonic motoneuron in culture: comparison with other neurotrophic factors and cytokines. J Neurosci 1990; 10: 3507–15.
[856] Sendtner M, Kreutzberg GW, Thoenen H. Ciliary neurotrophic factor prevents the degeneration of motor neurons after axotomy. Nature 1990; 345: 440–1.
[857] Tomlinson DR, Fernyhough P, Diemel LT. Role of neurotrophins in diabetic neuropathy and treatment with nerve growth factors. Diabetes 1997; 46 (Suppl 2): S43–49.
[858] Munson JB, Shelton DL, McMahon SB. Adult mammalian sensory and motor neurons: roles of endogenous neurotrophins and rescue by exogenous neurotrophins after axotomy. J Neurosci 1997; 17: 470–6.
[859] Sterne GD, Brown RA, Green CJ, Terenghi G. Neurotrophin-3 delivered locally via fibronectin mats enhances peripheral nerve regeneration. Eur J Neurosci 1997; 9: 1388–96.
[860] Barbin G, Manthorpe M, Varon S. Purification of the chick eye ciliary neuronotrophic factor. J Neurochem 1984; 43: 1468–78.
[861] Lin LF, Doherty DH, Lile JD, Bektesh S, Collins F. GDNF: a glial cell line-derived neurotrophic factor for midbrain dopaminergic neurons. Science 1993; 260: 1130–2.
[862] Bennett DL, Michael GJ, Ramachandran N, Munson JB, Averill S, Yan Q, Mcmahon SB, Priestley JV. A distinct subgroup of small DRG cells express GDNF receptor components and GDNF is protective for these neurons after nerve injury. J Neurosci 1998; 18: 3059–72.
[863] Hefti F, Schneider LS. Rationale for the planned clinical trials with nerve growth factor in Alzheimer's disease. Psychiatr Dev 1989; 7: 297–315.
[864] Goodman JI, Baumoel S, Frankel L. et al. The diabetic neuropathies. Springfield, Ill.: Charles C. Thomas; 1953.
[865] Anderson KJ, Dam D, Lee S, Cotman CW. Basic fibroblast growth factor prevents death of lesioned cholinergic neurons in vivo. Nature 1988; 332: 360–1.
[866] Schwaber JS, Due BR, Rogers WT, Junard EO, Hefti F. Use of a digital brain atlas to compare the distribution of NGF- and bFGF-protected cholinergic neurons. J Comp Neurol 1991; 309: 27–39.
[867] Ferrari G, Toffano G, Skaper SD. Epidermal growth factor exerts neuronotrophic effects on dopaminergic and GABAergic CNS neurons: comparison with basic fibroblast growth factor. J Neurosci Res 1991; 30: 493–7.
[868] Hyman C, Hofer M, Barde YA, Juhasz M, Yancopoulos GD, Squinto SP, Lindsay RM. BDNF is a neurotrophic factor for dopaminergic neurons of the substantia nigra. Nature 1991; 350: 230–2.
[869] Frostick SP, Yin Q, Kemp GJ. Schwann cells, neurotrophic factors, and peripheral nerve regeneration. Microsurgery 1998; 18: 397–405.
[870] Hayakawa K, Sobue G, Itoh T, Mitsuma T. Nerve growth factor prevents neurotoxic effects of cisplatin, vincristine and taxol, on adult rat sympathetic ganglion explants in vitro. Life Sci 1994; 55: 519–25.
[871] Whittemore SR, Holets VR, Keane RW, Levy DJ, McKay RD. Transplantation of a temperature-sensititve, nerve growth factor-secreting, neuroblastoma cell line into adult rats with fimbria-fornix lesions rescues cholinergic septal neurons. J Neurosci Res 1992; 267: 13–6.
[872] Berg MM, Sternberg DW, Parada LF, Chao MV. K-252a inhibits nerve growth factor-induced trk proto-oncogene tyrosine phosphorylation and kinase activity. J Biol Chem 1992; 267: 13–6.
[873] Knusel B, Hefti F. K-252b is a selective and nontoxic inhibitor of nerve growth factor action on cultured brain neurons. J Neurochem 1991; 57: 955–62.
[874] Quaife CJ, Mathews LS, Pinlert CA, Hammer RE, Brinster RL, Palmiter RD. Histopathology associated with elevated levels of growth hormone and insulin-like growth factor I in transgenic mice. Endocrinology 1989; 124: 40–8.
[875] Blottner D, Baumgarten HG. Insulin-like growth factor-I counteracts bFGF-induced survival of nitric oxide synthase (NOS)- positive spinal cord neurons after target-lesion in vivo. J Neurosci Res 1992; 32: 471–80.

[876] Guler HP, Eckardt KU, Zapf J, Bauer C, Froesch R. Insulin-like growth factor I increases glomerular filtration rate and renal plasma flow in man. Acta Endocrinol (Copenh) 1989; 121: 101-6.
[877] Bondy CA, Underwood LE, Clemmons DR, Guler HP, Bach MA, Skarulis M. Clinical uses of insulin-like growth factor I. Ann Intern Med 1994; 120: 593-601.
[878] Watkins PJ, Edmonds ME. Diabetic autonomic failure. In: Mathias CJ, Bannister R, editors. Autonomic failure. Oxford: Oxford University Press; 1999: 378-86.
[879] Guy RJC, Richards F, Edmonds ME, Watkins PJ. Diabetic autonomic neuropathy and iritis: an association suggesting an immunological cause. Br Med J 1984; 289: 343-5.
[880] Rabinowe SL. Immune mechanisms in diabetic autonomic and related neuropathies. In: Low PA, editors. Clinical autonomic disorders. Boston: Little, Brown; 1993: 445-61.
[881] Stevens MJ, Edmonds MD, Foster AVM, Watkins PJ. Selective neuropathy and preserved vascular response in the diabetic Charcot foot. Diabetologia 1992; 35: 148-54.
[882] Anand P. Nerve growth factors and the autonomic nervous system. In: Mathias CJ, Bannister R, editors. Autonomic failure. Oxford: Oxford University Press; 1999: 28-32.
[883] Whittington TD, Lawrence RD. Metabolic disorders. Diabetes mellitus. In: Sorsby A, editor. Systemic opthalmology. London: Butterworth; 1951: 334-48.
[884] Noyes HD. Retinitis in glycaemia. Trans Am Ophthalmol Soc 1868: 71-5.
[885] Rothova A, Meenken C, Michels RP, Kijlstra A. Uveitis and diabetes mellitus. Am J Ophthalmol 1988; 106: 17-20.
[886] McLeod JG. Autonomic dysfunction in peripheral nerve disease. In: Mathias J, Bannister R, editors. Autonomic failure. Oxford: Oxford University Press; 1999: 367-77.
[887] Edendal T, Olson L, Seiger A, Hedlund KO. Nerve growth factor in the rat iris. Nature 1980; 286: 25-8.
[888] Zanone MM, Banga JP, Peakman M, Edmonds ME, Watkins PJ. An investigation of antibodies to nerve growth factor in diabetic autonomic neuropathy. Diabet Med 1993; 11: 378-83.
[889] Watkins PJ, Gayle C, Alsanjari N, Scaravilli F, Zanone MM, Thomas PK. Severe sensory-autonomic neuropathy and endocrinopathy in insulin dependent diabetes. Q J Med 1995; 88: 795-804.
[890] Smith B. Neuropathology of the oesophagus in diabetes mellitus. J Neurol Neurosurg Psychiatry 1974; 37: 1151-4.
[891] Gilbey SG, Hussain MJ, Watkins PJ, Vergani D. Cell-mediated immunity and diabetic symptomatic autonomic neuropathy. Diabet Med 1988; 5: 845-8.
[892] Bradley WG, Chad D, Verghese JP, Liu HC, Good P, Gabbair AA, Adelman LS. Painful lumbosacral plexopathy with elevated erythrocyte sedimentation rate: a treatable inflammatory syndrome. Ann Neurol 1984; 15: 457-64.
[893] Kaufman DL, Erlander MG, Clare-Salzler M, Atkinson MA, Maclaren NK, Tobin AJ. Autoimmunity to two forms of glutamic decarboxylase in insulin-dependent diabetes mellitus. J Clin Invest 1992; 89: 283-92.
[894] Watkins PJ, Dyrberg T, Vergani D. High prevalence of autoantibodies to glutamic acid decarboxylase in long standing IDDM is not a marker of symptomatic autonomic neuropathy. Diabetes 1994; 43: 1146-51.
[895] Sundkvist G, Velloso LA, Kämpe O, Rabinowe SJ, Ivarsson SA, Lilja B, Karlsson FA. Glutamic acid decarboxylase antibodies, autonomic nerve antibodies and autonomic neuropathy in diabetic patients. Diabetologia 1994; 37: 293-9.
[896] Roll U, Nuber A, Schröder A, Gerlach E, Janka H-U, Ziegler A-G. No association of antibodies to glutamic acid decarboxylase and diabetic complications in patients with IDDM. Diabetes Care 1995; 18: 210-5.
[897] Brown FM, Brink SJ, Freeman R, Rabinowe S. Anti-sympathetic nervous system autoantibodies. Diminished catecholamines with orthostasis. Diabetes 1989; 38: 938-41.
[898] Rabinowe S, Brown FM, Watts M, Smith AM. Complement-fixing antibodies to sympathetic and parasympathetic tissues in IDDM. Autonomic brake index and heart rate variation. Diabetes Care 1990; 13: 1084-8.
[899] Husebye ES, Winqvist O, Sundkvist G, Kämpe O, Karlsson FA. Autoantibodies against adrenal medulla in type 1 and type 2 diabetes mellitus: no evidence for an association with autonomic neuropathy. J Intern Med 1996; 239: 139-46.
[900] Muhr D, Haslbeck M, Mollenhouer U, Standl E, Ziegler AG, Schnell O. Autoantibodies to sympathetic ganglia, GAD, or tyrosine phosphatase in long term IDDM with and without ECG based cardiac autonomic neuropathy. Diabetes Care 1997; 1: 1-4.
[901] Schnell O, Muhr D, Dresel S, Tatsch K, Ziegler AG, Haslbeck M, Standl E. Autoantibodies against sympathetic ganglia and evidence of cardiac sympathetic dysinnervation in newly diagnosed and long term IDDM patients. Diabetologia 1996; 39: 970-5.
[902] Sundkvist G, Lind P, Bergstrom B, Lilja B, Rabinowe S. Autonomic nerve antibodies and autonomic nerve function in type 1 and type 2 diabetic patients. J Intern Med 1991; 229: 505-10.
[903] Zanone MM, Peakman M, Purewal T, Watkins PJ, Vergani D. Autoantibodies to nervous tissue structures are associated with autonomic neuropathy in type 1 (insulin dependent) diabetes mellitus. Diabetologia 1993; 36: 564-9.
[904] Cachia MJ, Peakman M, Zanone MM, Watkins PJ, Vergani D. Reproducibility and persistence of neural and adrenal autoantibodies in diabetic autonomic neuropathy. Diabet Med 1997; 14: 461-5.
[905] Ejskjaer N, Arif S, Dodds W, Zanone MM, Vergani D, Watkins PJ, Peakman M. Prevalence of autoantibodies to autonomic nervous tissue structures in type 1 diabetes mellitus. Diab Med 1999; 16: 544-9.
[906] Pittenger GL, Malik RA, Burcus N, Boulton AJ, Vinik AL. Specific fiber deficits in sensorimotor diabetic polyneuropathy correspond to cytotoxicity against neuroblastoma cells of sera from patients with diabetes. Diabetes Care 1999; 22: 1839-44.
[907] Ejskjaer N, Zanone MM, Peakman M. Autoimmunity in diabetic autonomic neuropathy. Does the immune system get on your nerves ? Diabet Med 1998; 15: 723-9.
[908] Zanone MM, Petersen JS, Vergani D, Peakman M. Expression of glutamic acid decarboxylase in nervous tissue structures targeted by autoantibodies in patients with diabetic autonomic neuropathy. J Neuroimmunol 1997; 78: 1-7.
[909] Muhr-Becker D, Ziegler AG, Druschky A, Wolfram G, Haslbeck M, Neundörfer B, Standl E, Schnell O. Evidence for specific autoimmunity against sympathetic and parasympathetic nervous tissues in type 1 diabetes mellitus and the relation to cardiac autonomic dysfunction. Diabet Med 1998; 15: 467-72.
[910] Lampasona V, Bonfanti R, Bazzigaluppi E, Venerando A, Chiumello G, Bosi F, Bonifacio E. Antibodies to tissue transglutaminase C in type 1 diabetes. Diabetologia 1999; 42: 1195-8.
[911] Feldman EL, Stevens MJ, Greene DA. Pathogenesis of diabetic neuropathy. Clin Neurosci 1997; 4: 365-70.
[912] Winkler AS, Ejskjaer N, Edmonds M, Watkins PJ. Dissociated sensory loss in diabetic autonomic nuropathy. Diabet Med 2000; 17:457-62.

5 Clinical Features and Treatment of Diabetic Neuropathy

Severity and Staging of Diabetic Polyneuropathy

P.J. Dyck

Why Quantitate the Severity of Diabetic Polyneuropathy?

Patients and physicians need to know not only whether disease is present in a given patient but also its severity. This is especially true for diabetic polyneuropathy, which begins so insidiously that its presence and severity are not apparent without careful evaluation. Knowledge of whether diabetic polyneuropathy is present and how severe it is is needed for cohort and epidemiologic studies and for conduct of therapeutic trials. It is also needed for purposes of following the course of the neuropathy in clinical practice, and in order to decide when to initiate preventative or ameliorating treatments, assuming that such treatments are available.

To this date the health burden of diabetic polyneuropathy has been largely expressed in the form of the number or percentage of diabetic patients who have it. The percentage of diabetic patients who have diabetic polyneuropathy at a given date (the prevalence), or the number or percentage who develop it over a given period of time (the incidence), is not very meaningful unless one also knows the severity of the neuropathy or the health outcomes which it causes. For example, if most or all of the patients with diabetes mellitus have only asymptomatic neuropathy which does not give them health problems at this time or in the foreseeable future, then diabetic polyneuropathy is not a serious health problem. If, on the other hand, many or most of the patients develop symptoms, impairments, or adverse health outcomes as a result of diabetic polyneuropathy, then diabetic polyneuropathy is a major health problem. To date the health burden of diabetic polyneuropathy has not been adequately assessed. It will not be possible to do this until physicians adopt approaches to assessing its severity. In the following sections, we outline how we judge overall severity and stage it.

How Is Severity of Diabetic Polyneuropathy to Be Judged?

It is possible to judge the severity of symptoms, impairments, attributes of nerve conduction (NC), quantitative sensation tests (QST), quantitative autonomic tests (QAT), morphometry of biopsied nerves, counts of nerve endings in skin biopsies, and adverse health outcomes. We have suggested that no single measure is sufficiently representative that it can be used as the only measure of diabetic polyneuropathy. I advocate that severity of a patient's diabetic polyneuropathy be assessed by quantitating neuropathic symptoms, impairments (including clinical, NC, QST, and QAT), staged severity, and health outcomes [1,2].

Minimum Criteria for the Diagnosis of Diabetic Neuropathy

Many minimum criteria for the diagnosis of diabetic polyneuropathy have been proposed. Before considering specific criteria, I must emphasize that to begin with a correct judgment must be made that the patient has diabetic polyneuropathy and not another neuropathy or another variety of diabetic neuropathy. Other neurologic diseases or neuropathies occur in perhaps 10% of patients who have diabetes mellitus [3]. One diagnostic criterion is a physician's judgment that the patient has diabetic polyneuropathy. Without specifying what examinations should be done, what criteria for abnormality should be used, and minimum criteria for diabetic polyneuropathy, great inaccuracies would ensue from the use of this criterion alone. Decreased or absent ankle reflexes and decreased vibratory detection threshold of the foot as detected using a tuning fork is a widely used criterion [4,5]. This criterion has great appeal because it is simple and uses generally available expertise and tools, but it has major flaws. First, other tests are more sensitive and perhaps more reliable. Second, it is unclear that without special training or experience physicians can sensitively or accurately judge abnormality considering the influence of such anthropometric factors as age, sex, height, and weight. A third criterion is the presence of at least two abnormalities (from among symptoms, clinical deficits, NC, QST, or QAT) with one of the two being an abnormality of NC or quantitative autonomic examination [1]. Abnormality of NC was an abnormality ($\geq$99th or $\leq$1st percentile, whichever applied) of

Table 5.1 Calculating the NIS(LL)+7 tests score (items 17–24, 28–29, and 34–37 of NIS) (points)

1. Sum individual scores of the NIS for the lower limbs, NIS(LL).
2. Summate transformed points for percentile abnormality[a] of the five attributes of NC of lower limb (peroneal nerve [CMAP, MNCV, and MNDL], tibial nerve [MNDL], and sural [SNAP]), of VDT and of HBDB divided by the number of attributes with obtainable values,[b] multiply by 7 (the number of attributes), and add this number to the global score.

[a] < 95th = 0; ≥ 95th–99th = 1; ≥ 99th–99.9th = 2; ≥ 99.9th = 3 (or ≥ 5th = 0 to ≤ 0.1th = 3, whichever end of the distribution is abnormal)
[b] MNCV and MNDL cannot be estimated when CMAP is 0

Abbreviations:

CMAP = compound muscle action potential
SNAP = sensory nerve action potential
MNDL = motor nerve distal latency
VDT = vibration detection threshold
HBDB = heart beat deep breathing

Table 5.2 Calculating the NIS(LL)+7 tests (items 17–24, 28–29, and 34–37 of NIS) (normal deviate [nd])

1. Sum individual scores of the NIS for the lower limbs, NIS(LL).
2. Summate normal deviate[a] for percentile abnormality[b] of the five attributes of NC of lower limb (peroneal nerve [CMAP, MNCV, and MNDL], tibial nerve [MNDL], and sural [SNAP]), of VDT and of HBDB divided by the number of attributes with obtainable values,[c] multiply by 7 (the number of attributes), and add this number to the global score.

[a] Express all percentile values so that abnormality appears in the upper end of the distribution
[b] For tests or NC attributes which are abnormal at low percentile values (e. g., HBDB, NC conduction velocities and amplitudes), express their values as occurring at the high end of the distribution (e. g., 25th becomes 75th, 60th becomes 40th, and 4th becomes 96th). Estimate the normal deviate (nd) for each percentile value instead of point values as outlined in Table 5.1
[c] MNCV and MNDL cannot be estimated when CMAP is 0

attributes of NC in at least two separate nerves. Perhaps a better criterion (the fourth one) is to use a composite score such as NIS(LL)+7 tests [2]. The seven tests were: peroneal motor nerve conduction velocity, peroneal compound muscle action potential, peroneal motor distal latency, sural sensory nerve action potential and tibial motor distal latency, heart-pulse decrease with breathing, and vibratory detection threshold using CASE IV. In Tables 5.**1** and 5.**2**, we provide the algorithm of how to calculate the NIS(LL)+7 test. The NIS(LL) could be combined with varying numbers of tests (e. g., NIS(LL)+2, +3…+ *n*).

Can Neuropathic Abnormalities Be Demonstrated in Patients Who Do not Fulfill Minimum Criteria for Diabetic Polyneuropathy?

We studied this question in the Rochester Diabetic Neuropathy Study cohort. We characterized the QST results for the foot of each patient as hyperesthetic (≤ 2.5th percentile), low normal (> 2.5th to 50th), high normal (50th to < 97.5th), or hypoesthetic (≥ 97.5th). In Figure 5.**1**, we show the distribution of severity of diabetic polyneuropathy using NIS(LL)+4 tests in four cohorts studied. In Figure 5.**2**, we show the distribution of the percentile response categories for the four cohorts. In the normative population, we set values so that 50 % of vibratory detection thresholds were above and 50 % below the 50th percentile. In the Rochester Diabetic Neuropathy Study cohort, we found that there were more patients in the 50th–97.5th percentile range than were in the 2.5th–50th percentile range. Similar observations were made for attributes of nerve conduction and also for heart-pulse variation with deep breathing. These data clearly imply that there is a subtle shift of values from the below-50th percentile group to the above-50th percentile group prior to their fulfilling minimum criteria for diabetic polyneuropathy. This provides unequivocal evidence that subtle functional abnormalities precede defined minimum criteria for diabetic polyneuropathy.

Severity of Neuropathic Symptoms

Diabetic neuropathic symptoms can be characterized as negative (decreased function) and as positive (hyperfunction). The former symptoms relate to decreased feeling of tactile, mechanoreceptor, thermal, and painful stimuli; the latter are such spontaneous symptoms as feelings of asleep-numbness, tightness, swelling (without being swollen), prickling, and pain. Various approaches have been used to quantitate these symptoms. In the total symptom score (TSS) [6], the symptoms of asleep-numbness, prickling, pain, and burning are quantitated by intensity ("not present," "mild," "moderate," or "severe") and by frequency ("occasional," "often," or "continuous"). In the neuropathy symptom score, we tally the number of symptoms (from a list of 17 symptoms) encountered in neuropathy [7]. In the Neuropathy Symptoms and Change (NSC) score, we assess for number, severity, and change of symptoms [8].

Although this has not been studied adequately, symptoms relate poorly to severity or change of neuropathic impairment [2]. It may be that symptoms tend to be worse with the onset of neuropathy or with rapid progression of neuropathy, and to lessen as greater impairment occurs.

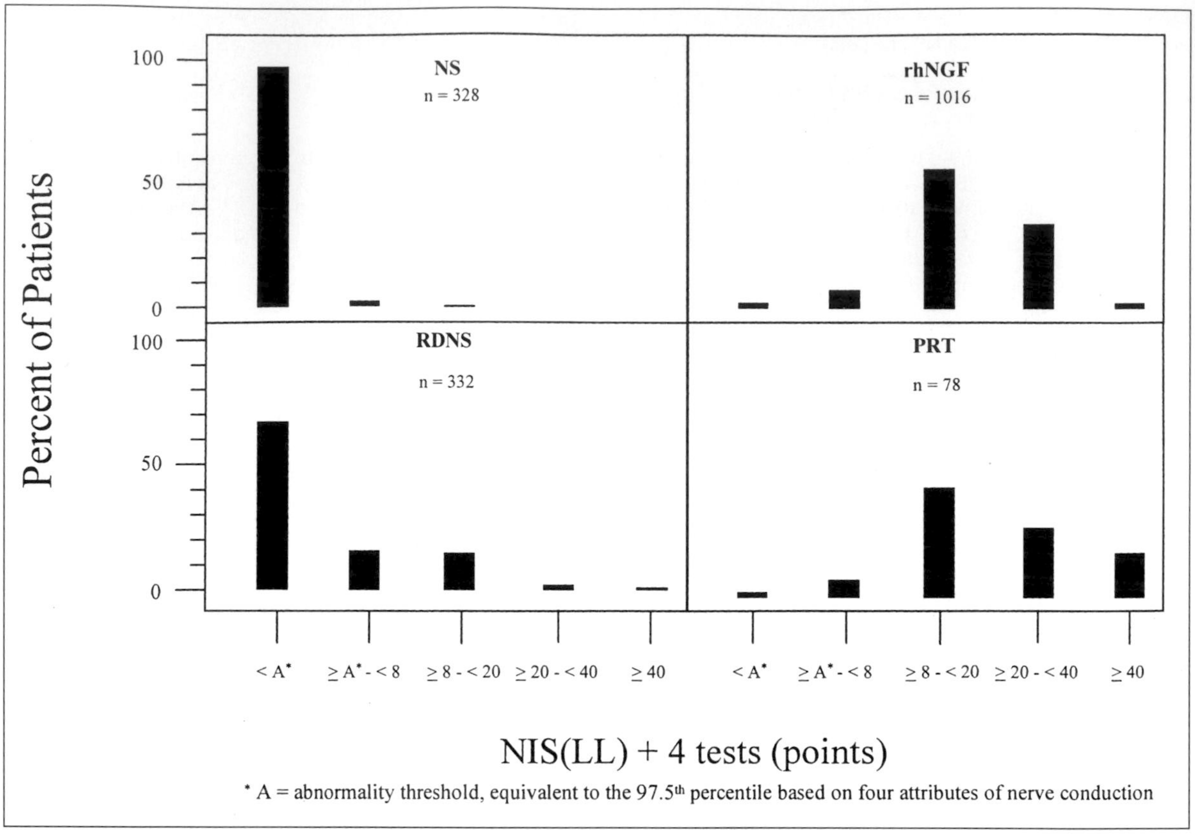

Fig. 5.1 Quantitative test abnormalities were estimated for the foot using CASE IV in four cohorts: healthy subjects (NS), the Rochester Diabetic Neuropathy Study (RDNS), the nerve growth factor therapeutic trial (rhNGF), and a pancreas renal transplant cohort (PRT). The NIS(LL)+4 tests score were used to estimate overall severity of diabetic polyneuropathy. Observe that the greatest severity of neuropathies was found in the rhNGF and PRT cohorts, while an intermediate severity was found in the RDNS cohort

Continuous Measures of Neuropathic Impairment

Several measures have been developed to encompass the weakness, reflex change, and sensory loss in diabetic polyneuropathy. We have developed the Neuropathy Impairment Score (NIS), which is a standard evaluation of muscle weakness, reflex decrease or loss, and sensation decrease or loss [7]. The various abnormalities are to be scored for the patient's age, gender, physical fitness, and anthropometric features. For each item a continuous measure of abnormality is allowed. In a second approach, a nurse does a screening evaluation; and if certain conditions are exceeded, a physician completes the examination to score severity of neuropathy [9].

Composite Scores for Diabetic Polyneuropathy Severity

We have developed two approaches to estimate NIS(LL)+n tests (where n is the chosen number of tests [e. g., n = 4, 7, or other]). For either approach, we add to the NIS of lower limbs (NIS[LL]) points for test abnormality. In order to be able to do this, it is necessary to have test abnormalities expressed as a percentile. We have provided details of how to estimate percentiles [10] and such normative results from a healthy subject cohort from Rochester, Minnesota [11].

In the first approach, we transform only values which are beyond a certain level of abnormality (e. g., ≥ 95th or ≤ 5th) and use whole number transformations (e. g., ≥ 95th to < 99th = 1 point, ≥ 99th to < 99.9th = 2, and ≥ 99.9th = 3). If abnormalities are at the lower end of the normal distribution, they are similarly transformed: ≤ 5th to > 1st = 1 point and so on. If a test was done but a value cannot be estimated (e. g., motor nerve conduction velocity [MNCV]) when the compound muscle action potential was zero, its effect on the score is included by dividing the summed values of attributes which can be measured by their number and multiplying this value by the total number of attributes assessed. The approach is outlined in Table 5.1. Note that in this approach, values falling below the 95th or above the 5th percentile (whichever applies) do not contribute to the score, and

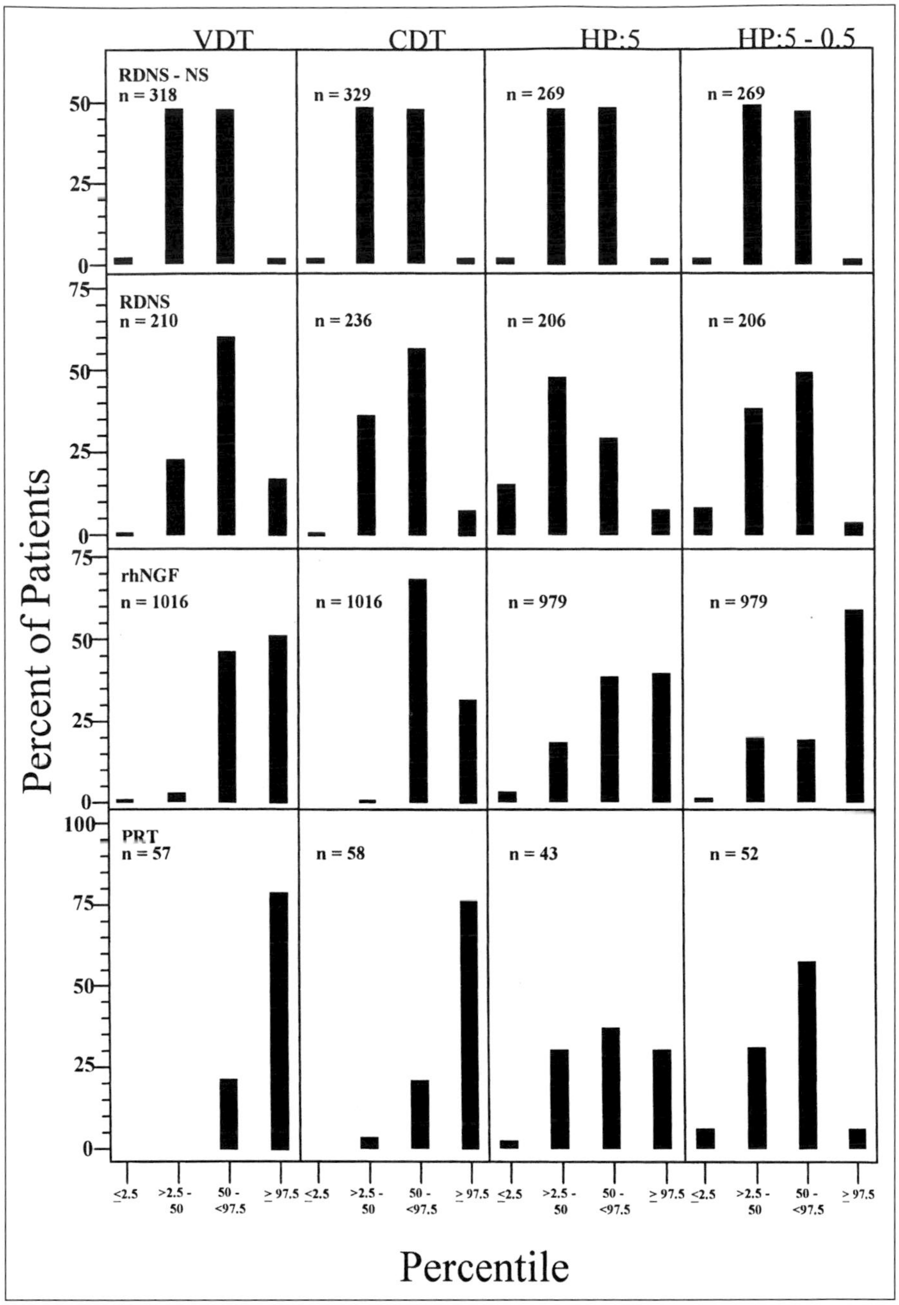

Fig. 5.2 Distribution of quantitative sensory abnormalities in the four cohorts described in the legend to Figure 5.1. For all modalities of sensation studied, there was a higher percentage of abnormalities between the 50th and 97.5th percentiles than between the 2.5th and 50th percentiles, reflecting a subclinical shift in abnormality as discussed in the text

there is no interpolation of transformed points within the range of percentile abnormality. We therefore call this the NIS(LL)+*n* tests (points).

In the second approach (NIS[LL]+*n* tests) (normal deviate [nd]), set out in Table 5.2, we interpolate normal deviate values for percentile values of test results. For each of the *n* test results employed, we estimate a percentile and normal deviate value. Before the normal deviate values are added to NIS(LL), percentile values which are in the lower end of the distribution are expressed as if they fell in the upper distribution (e. g., 1st becomes 99th, 95th becomes 5th, 49th becomes 51st, and so on). A normal deviate value relates each percentile value to a normal distribution. For example, for the 50th percentile the corresponding normal deviate is 0 since 50 % of values in a normal distribution fall below 0. The normal deviate corresponding to the 95th percentile is 1.96 since 95 % of values in a normal distribution fall below 1.96. Therefore, in this approach, we summate normal deviate values whether they fall within or fall outside of the normal range, but do not use normal deviate values corresponding to values higher than the 99.9th.

The second is the preferable of the two approaches because normal deviate values are calculated for each percentile value, and values within the normal range are also included.

Staging Severity of Diabetic Polyneuropathy

Composite scores such as NIS(LL)+*n* tests (points or normal deviate) are useful continuous measures of overall severity of neuropathy impairment. They are especially useful in epidemiologic or controlled clinical trials requiring continuous quantitative data. However, there is also a need for an approach that includes symptoms, as well as neurologic impairments and test abnormalities, and is directed at categorization of the health problem represented by the neuropathy. In the approach we developed, we divide diabetic polyneuropathy into four stages: N0 = no diabetic polyneuropathy; N1 = asymptomatic polyneuropathy; N2 = symptomatic polyneuropathy; and N3 = disabling polyneuropathy. In the recent reports and in our revision of *Diabetic Neuropathy*, we modify the staging approach [12].

The approach that we have developed is in some respects similar to the staging approach used in diabetic retinopathy. Taking some liberties with the staging of diabetic retinopathy, it may be staged as R0 = no retino-pathy; R1 = mild background retinopathy; R2 = severe background retinopathy; and R3 = proliferative retinopathy.

Patients without diabetic polyneuropathy are staged as N0. This includes diabetic patients who do not fulfill the minimal criteria for diabetic polyneuropathy discussed in a previous section. These patients have a lesser abnormality than N1a.

Patients with diabetes mellitus and neuropathic test abnormalities (NC, QST, or QAT abnormalities) due to diabetic polyneuropathy, but who do not have neuropathic symptoms or findings (NIS < 2 points) are staged as N1a.

Patients with neuropathic test abnormalities (findings of N1a), neuropathy impairment (NIS ≥ 2 points), both due to diabetic polyneuropathy, and no neuropathic symptoms are staged N1b.

Patients with stage N2a have neuropathic test abnormalities and neuropathic impairment ≥ 2 points, and symptoms of diabetic polyneuropathy but of a lesser degree than N2b.

Symptoms of diabetic polyneuropathy may consist of positive or negative symptoms. The positive symptoms are usually assumed to be due to hyperfunction and negative symptoms to hypofunction. Hypersensitivity symptoms include altered sensory experiences that may be likened to asleep-numbness (as if a hand had gone to sleep); prickling; a crusted or tight feeling; enlargement feeling; and so on. Other positive symptoms include burning pain, lancinating pain, deep throbs, and deep aching. Negative sensory symptoms include not being able to feel, tactile, mechanoreceptor, thermal or painful stimuli.

Patients staged as 2b fulfill minimum criteria for diabetic polyneuropathy and have positive or sensory symptoms of diabetic polyneuropathy resulting in ankle dorsiflexor weakness due to diabetic polyneuropathy of ≥ 50%. They have less involvement than those at stage 3.

Occurrence of any of the following ten conditions, when judged to be due to diabetic polyneuropathy, results in the diagnosis of the neuropathy as stage 3 (disabling neuropathy) [3].

Motor:

1. Symptoms of muscle weakness, confirmed by examination, of sufficient severity that the patient is unable to walk independently.

Sensory:

1. Symptoms of sensory loss of sufficient severity, confirmed by examination, that the patient could not walk independently because of sensory ataxia.
2. Absence of feeling in hands so that the patient is disabled.
3. Symptoms of pain, having the characteristics of neuropathic pain, that is disabling. Criteria a, b, and c have to be fulfilled:
   a. The patient has previously attended physicians for pain relief.
   b. Work and recreational activities have been curtailed by at least 25% because of pain.
   c. Medication for pain relief has been taken on a continuing basis (≥ 50% of days) for at least six weeks.

Autonomic:

1. Gastric atony as demonstrated by gastric retention tests and by exclusion of other gastric or psychiatric causes of emesis, causing emesis of retained (≥18 hours) food at least once weekly for at least six weeks.
2. Urinary retention as demonstrated by manometer evidence of detrusor hypoactivity and not due to psychiatric disturbance or urinary bladder disease, necessitating continuous use of a catheter for six weeks or longer.
3. Urinary incontinence due to loss of sphincter function, necessitating continuous (≥ 50% of time) use of diapers or leg urinal for at least six weeks and not due to psychiatric or bladder disease.
4. Rectal incontinence due to loss of anal sphincter function of at least six weeks' duration and not due to psychiatric or rectal disease.
5. Diarrhea to the degree that it causes weight loss (≥ 5 kg) and steatorrhea (≥ 10 mg/24 hours) and not due to psychiatric disturbance, laxative abuse, or other bowel disease.
6. Symptomatic light-headedness or fainting due to orthostatic hypotension (≥ 30 mmHg systolic) with concomitant blood pressure drop, present

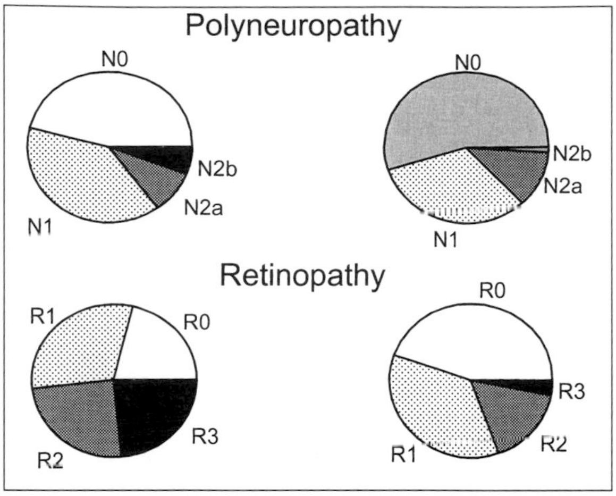

Fig. 5.3 Distribution of staged severity of diabetic polyneuropathy in a population-based study of diabetic patients in Rochester, Minnesota. Whereas approximately 50 % of both type 1 and type 2 diabetic patients have diabetic polyneuropathy, the spectrum of the staged severity is more severe in type 1 diabetes. N0, no diabetic polyneuropathy; N1, asymptomatic polyneuropathy as described in text; N2a, symptomatic diabetic polyneuropathy but with a degree of dorsiflexor muscle weakness at the ankle that is less than 50 %; N2b, symptomatic diabetic polyneuropathy with greater dorsiflexor muscle weakness than 50 %

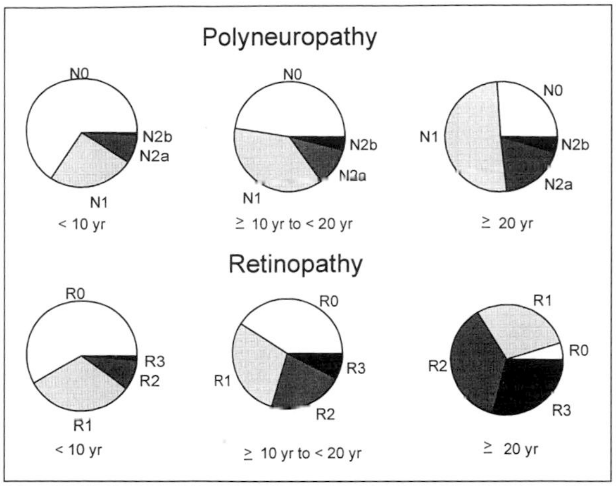

Fig. 5.4 Prevalence of staged severity of diabetic polyneuropathy by duration of diabetes mellitus. Note that the spectrum of staged severity is worse with greater duration of diabetes

continuously (light-headedness or fainting weekly) for at least six weeks.

In Figure 5.**3**, we show the frequency distribution of staged diabetic polyneuropathy as obtained in a prevalence study of diabetic patients in Rochester, Minnesota [3]. It was of note that patients with type 1 diabetes mellitus had more severe stages of diabetic polyneuropathy than did those with type 2. In Figure 5.**4**, we show that duration of diabetes also influences the staged severity of diabetic polyneuropathy.

Classification of the Diabetic Neuropathies

P.K. Thomas

A wide variety of syndromes affecting the peripheral nervous system may be encountered in patients with diabetes mellitus. This is probably a reflection of a range of underlying disease mechanisms. These syndromes may develop in isolation or in combination.

Neuropathy is an important complication both of type I and type 2 diabetes (see Chapter 3), but there are some significant differences between the two forms. Symptomatic autonomic neuropathy is almost always seen in type I patients. Reversible mononeuropathies, by contrast, are more common in older men with type 2 diabetes. The classification advocated here is based on the one originally proposed by Thomas [13] and is listed in Table 5.**3**.

Table 5.**3** Classification of the diabetic neuropathies

Hyperglycemic neuropathy
Generalized neuropathies
Sensorimotor polyneuropathy
Acute painful sensory neuropathy
Autonomic neuropathy
Acute motor neuropathy
Focal and multifocal neuropathies
Cranial neuropathies
Thoracolumbar radiculoneuropathy
Proximal diabetic neuropathy
Focal limb neuropathies (including entrapment and compression neuropathies)
Superimposed chronic inflammatory demyelinating polyneuropathy
Hypoglycemic neuropathy

Hyperglycemic Neuropathy

The older literature [14] described the occurrence of uncomfortable sensory symptoms experienced distally in the limbs in poorly controlled or newly diagnosed diabetics, or following an episode of diabetic ketosis (see pages 309–312). These consist of tingling paresthesias, pain, or hyperesthesia. They rapidly subside following establishment of euglycemia. More recently such symptoms have been referred to as hyperglycemic neuropathy [15]. Their explanation has not been established. Diabetic nerve has been found to be hypoxic [16]. From experimental observations in rats, hyperglycemic but not normoglycemic hypoxia has been shown to produce alterations in fast K^+ conductance and afterpotentials, related to axoplasmic acidification [17]. This could lead to the generation of ectopic impulses and the occurrence of positive sensory symptoms.

It is also known that nerve conduction velocity is reduced in poorly controlled diabetic patients. This improves rapidly on correction of the hyperglycemia [18,19]. A further feature of hyperglycemic neuropathy is an abnormal resistance to ischemic conduction failure [20]. This may be noticed by patients who find that they have a reduced tendency to develop ischemic paresthesias on nerve compression. This may be related to a switch by diabetic nerve to anaerobic glycolysis [21].

Diabetic Distal Sensory or Sensorimotor Polyneuropathy

This is the most frequent form of diabetic neuropathy and is discussed on pages 199–202. It is usually insidious in onset and may be the presenting feature in patients with type 2 diabetes. It may be asymptomatic and discovered incidentally on examination or when patients present with a neuropathic complication. When symptomatic, it gives rise to sensory manifestations that are most evident distally in the lower limbs, consisting of numbness, tingling, and pain. It is often accompanied by autonomic neuropathy, which is usually mild in patients with type 2 diabetes. A mild distal motor neuropathy may also coexist.

The most important consequences of diabetic sensory polyneuropathy are chronic ulceration and, to a lesser extent, neuropathic osteoarthropathy, as a result of loss of pain sense in the feet together with the effects of autonomic dysfunction (see pages 296–297).

Acute Painful Diabetic Neuropathy

Acute painful diabetic neuropathy is a separate entity from distal symmetric diabetic sensory polyneuropathy. Its onset is acute or subacute, with burning pain experienced mainly in the lower limbs but sometimes in the upper limbs or on the trunk. There is usually distressing contact hyperesthesia of the skin. Motor signs, tendon reflex depression, and autonomic dysfunction are not prominent, but impotence may develop in males. The syndrome can be precipitated by the initiation of treatment (see pages 308–309) or be associated with precipitous weight loss (see page 208). Recovery occurs with continued glycemic control over a matter of months. Recurrence is unlikely.

Autonomic Neuropathy

Autonomic neuropathy normally is an accompaniment of diabetic sensory polyneuropathy. A very wide range of manifestations may occur [15] (see pages 225–294). In patients with newly diagnosed diabetes [22,23], minor reversible disturbances of autonomic function can be detected that recover with establishment of euglycemia.

Symptomatic autonomic neuropathy, as already stated, is almost always encountered in type 1 diabetic patients who have reached middle age and have had diabetes for several years. Once established, it is largely irreversible [24].

Acute Motor Neuropathy

Patients have been described who have developed an acute primarily motor neuropathy accompanied by bilateral facial weakness following an episode of diabetic ketosis [25] associated with an elevated cerebrospinal fluid protein content. Recovery occurred over the course of a few weeks. Such cases have to be distinguished from examples of the Guillain-Barré syndrome and critical illness neuropathy [26].

Focal and Multifocal Neuropathies

The second broad category of diabetic neuropathies (see Table 5.**3**) consists of the occurrence of isolated peripheral nerve lesions or of multiple isolated lesions. These are best separated into focal cranial nerve lesions, truncal or thoracolumbar radiculoneuropathy, proximal diabetic neuropathy, and focal lesions of limb nerves. They are considered in more detail on pages 202–204.

Cranial Neuropathies

Amongst the cranial nerves, focal lesions most commonly affect the nerves to the external ocular muscles, particularly the third nerve. This usually has an acute onset with pain, and pupillary function is characteristically spared. Of the other cranial nerves, the seventh is most often implicated, but as the frequency of these lesions is low it is difficult to be certain of a clear association with diabetes.

Thoracolumbar Radiculoneuropathy

This manifestation of diabetic neuropathy consists of the occurrence of focal sensory symptoms either unilaterally or bilaterally on the trunk, with pain, cutaneous hyperesthesia, and sensory loss in a radicular distribution or in the territory of intercostal nerves. Focal weakness of the anterior abdominal wall may occur. The onset of symptoms is often acute or subacute, and recovery generally occurs over the course of some months.

Proximal Diabetic Neuropathy

Otherwise known as diabetic amyotrophy or lumbosacral plexus radiculoneuropathy, this syndrome is encountered most often in older males with type 2 diabetes. The onset can be subacute or insidious and is commonly accompanied by pain. It can be unilateral or bilateral and, if bilateral, asymmetric or symmetric. Radicular sensory loss may be present. At times distal lower limb muscles and occasionally those of the upper limbs may also be affected.

Focal Limb Nerve Lesions

These are probably more frequent in patients with diabetes than in the general population, but epidemiological data are scarce (see Chapter 3). Often they are at common sites of entrapment or external compression, indicating an increased susceptibility of diabetic nerve to compression injury, but they also occur at other locations.

Superimposed Chronic Inflammatory Demyelinating Polyneuropathy

Although a case control study has not been undertaken it seems likely that chronic inflammatory demyelinating polyneuropathy CIDP occurs more commonly in individuals with diabetes than in the general population [27,28]. Prominent motor involvement or a reduction of conduction velocity into the demyelinating range, particularly if conduction block at sites not subject to entrapment is demonstrated, would suggest this possibility. Confirmation of the diagnosis could be obtained by finding oligoclonal IgG bands on examination of the cerebrospinal fluid or by nerve biopsy. The important diagnostic findings on nerve biopsy are the presence of inflammatory infiltrates and stripping of myelin off axons by macrophages. These examples of CIDP probably represent a secondary immunologic response to nerve damage by diabetic neuropathy, as is thought to occur at times in hereditary motor and sensory neuropathy [29].

Hypoglycemic Neuropathy

Repeated or single episodes of severe hypoglycemia have been documented to give rise to a predominantly motor neuropathy or neuronopathy [30,31]. Severe hypoglycemic episodes are usually either the result of an insulinoma or insulin overdose. Whether recurrent hypoglycemic episodes that occur during the course of treatment of insulin-dependent diabetes can also cause hypoglycemic neuropathy is conceivable but not established. Animal studies suggest that this is possible [32].

Diabetic Sensorimotor Neuropathy: Methods of Assessment

Electrophysiologic Testing

V. Bril

Introduction to Electrophysiology

Electrophysiology comprises investigation of the electrical response characteristics of nerve and muscle. The synonymous term "nerve conduction studies" (NCS) encompasses properties of transmission of electrical current along nerve and muscle fiber membranes. Motor and sensory nerve fibers have different properties. Their responsiveness to electrical stimulation is measured in end organs (motor or sensory), or in nerve trunks, and these responses are recorded, measured, and quantified.

Electrophysiology can be thought of in the simplest terms as an extension of the clinical neurologic examination. The testing provides numerical values for peripheral nerve and muscle function. The measures are objective, independent of patient input, and unbiased. These are the most reliable measures of the peripheral neuromuscular system available currently [33–39].

The utility of NCS for evaluation of patients with neuromuscular disorders has been demonstrated in countless reports and texts [34,40–44]. This method of investigation is well established and widely available. Other diagnostic measures have not replaced nerve conduction studies or electromyography for the objective documentation of peripheral neuromuscular function.

The use of NCS has extended to ancillary evaluation of centrally mediated neurologic disorders such as multiple sclerosis, strokes, and movement disorders [45–47].

Nerve Conduction Studies in Neuropathies: An Overview

NCS document the presence, nature, distribution, and severity of peripheral nerve impairment. Subjects presenting with symptoms of numbness, tingling, and weakness may have a peripheral, central, or nonorganic cause of these complaints. The NCS can substantiate a peripheral neuromuscular basis for the symptoms. The absence of NCS abnormalities raises doubts as to the presence of neuromuscular dysfunction. The NCS provide information on whether the peripheral nerve process is primarily axonal or demyelinating, with implications for investigation and management. NCS can distinguish the presence of mononeuropathy (abnormalities falling within the territory of a single peripheral nerve), multiple mononeuropathy (multiple single nerves), or polyneuropathy (diffuse peripheral nerve disease). Finally, the severity of NCS abnormality reflects the severity of the underlying neuromuscular disorder and can help direct management. For example, early surgical decompression may be advised in those with severe NCS findings of carpal tunnel syndrome.

An important finding of NCS in polyneuropathy is whether the process is primarily axonal or demyelinating. This distinction aids in the diagnosis, directing therapeutic decisions and prognostication. Primary demyelinating disorders suggest etiologies such as hereditary polyneuropathy, monoclonal gammopathy of unknown significance with polyneuropathy, or chronic inflammatory demyelinating polyneuropathy (CIDP). All of these neuropathies can be found in association with diabetic sensorimotor polyneuropathy (DSP). In demyelinating disorders, NCS are helpful in diagnosis and in following the response to therapy, particularly for CIDP [48–54]. In the case of Guillain-Barré syndrome, large changes in motor conduction velocity can be expected during the course of the disorder, reflecting the underlying processes of demyelination and remyelination. The amplitude of the distal compound muscle action potential helps determine prognosis in that a low-amplitude compound muscle action potential at initial NCS testing indicates more severe involvement, a less benign course, and a less favorable prognosis [55–57]. In Guillain-Barré syndrome, large clinical changes occur relatively rapidly in a period of months to years, allowing accurate clinical determination of responses to therapy with corresponding changes in NCS [58]. In CIDP, improvements in NCS as well as clinical improvements help validate various therapeutic interventions [49,52,54,59].

The role of NCS in following responses to therapy in axonal neuropathies is more difficult to evaluate as few axonal neuropathies have effective therapeutic interventions. Changes in NCS parameters in axonal neuropathies are more difficult to ascertain. Only small changes in conduction velocities and amplitudes are expected [60–63]; the methodology must be rigorous and standardized [33,64]; and large numbers of patients are needed for demonstration of efficacy [64]. These considerations have led to the development of expert core laboratories [64] to standardize the methodology and provide quality control for clinical trials.

Core labs have optimized NCS in clinical trials (Table 5.**4**) [64]. Axonal neuropathies such as DSP [63], or toxic polyneuropathies can respond to therapeutic intervention [63,65,66], but the responses observed may be simply the prevention of more rapid disease progression such as that which typifies DSP, for example, rather than regression of NCS abnormalities.

In addition, in the case of toxic neuropathies, withdrawal of the offending toxin allows NCS to recover towards baseline values, but there are no active interventions which produce nerve regeneration. Future developments may lead to more positive therapy producing nerve regeneration and improved function, rather than simply the prevention of rapid disease progression. In that case, effective regeneration would be mirrored in the NCS by findings of increasing motor and sensory nerve potential amplitudes, and increasing nerve conduction velocities towards normal values.

Axonal Neuropathies: Diabetic Neuropathy as the Prototype

The prototype of axonal neuropathies is DSP. Polyneuropathy associated with diabetes is characterized by the progressive loss of nerve fibers, both large and small [67–73]. Recent attention has focused on those with isolated small-fiber neuropathy, but these cases are rare [74,75]. Progressive loss of all axons is the pathologic hallmark of DSP [68]. Other changes observed, such as axonal atrophy, secondary loss of myelin, and numerous vascular changes, contribute to DSP [68,76], but loss of axons is the essential process. This loss is reflected in NCS by the progressive loss of the amplitudes of the evoked motor and sensory potentials [34]. This loss is further illustrated in Figure 5.**5**, which shows the sural nerve mean myelinated fiber density in patients with differing clinical severity of DSP as defined by a clinical scoring system developed in Toronto [77]. The clinical scoring system (CSS), a clinician-relevant and uncomplicated instrument, was developed using expert logic to ensure that subjects with a broad spectrum of DSP entered a trial of simple screening tests for DSP in the clinic [77]. The CSS successfully stratified subjects with diabetes into four categories of DSP: none, mild, moderate, and severe [77]. The relationship between progressive nerve fiber loss and the NCS findings is further illustrated in Figure 5.**6**,

Table 5.4 Variability of repeat NCS testing

Parameter	Control subjects	Patients	
		Baseline	Completion
	(*n* = 253)	(*n* = 1345)	(*n* = 1144)
Median motor DL	4	4	4
Median motor amp wrist	7	10	9
Median motor amp elbow	8	11	10
Median motor CV	3	3	3
Median sensory DL	4	4	4
Median sensory amp wrist	8	11	11
Median sensory distal CV	3	4	4
Median sensory amp elbow	13	17	17
Median sensory proximal CV	3	4	3
Peroneal motor DL	5	6	6
Peroneal motor amp ankle	9	13	12
Peroneal motor amp knee	10	15	13
Peroneal motor CV	3	3	3
Right sural DL	5	6	6
Right sural amp	10	16	15
Right sural CV	3	5	4
Left sural DL	4	6	5
Left sural amp	10	16	15
Left sural CV	3	5	4

DL, distal latency (ms); amp, amplitude (motor: mV; sensory; μV); CV, conduction velocity (m/s); n, number
Values expressed as percentages. Data from a multicenter study containing 60 sites in Europe and North America [40]

which shows that sural nerve potential amplitudes decrease with nerve fiber loss in the sural nerves in patients with DSP. As the amplitudes decline, a secondary mild slowing of conduction velocity is observed. Greater degrees of conduction velocity slowing cast doubt on the diagnosis of DSP and raise the possibility of coexistent disease, such as CIDP [78,79]. Such unexpected NCS findings lead to a more detailed review of the patient, and perhaps, different therapeutic interventions. In DSP, the distal motor and F wave latencies are mildly increased, particularly along the median nerve, and not solely due to the presence of carpal tunnel syndrome, but rather as part of diffuse DSP [80,81]. The most distal nerve segments are affected first in this length-

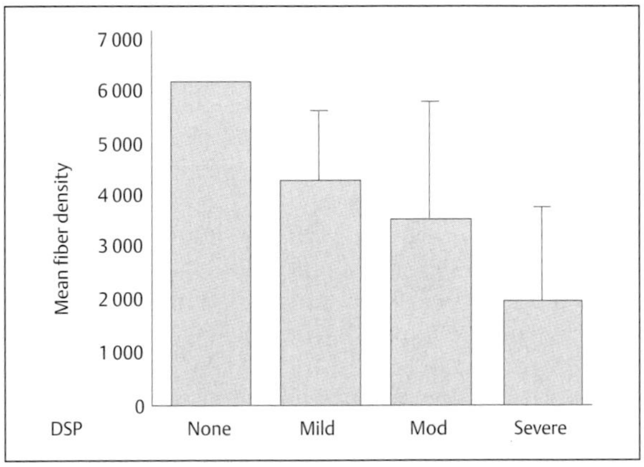

Fig. 5.5 Mean fiber density in the sural nerves of patients with diabetic sensorimotor polyneuropathy (DSP) of varying severity as defined by a clinical scoring system introduced in Toronto [77]. The scoring system allots points for different neuropathic findings distally in the lower limbs in the following manner: symptoms, six points; reflexes, eight points; and sensory deficits five points. Error bars show ± 1SD

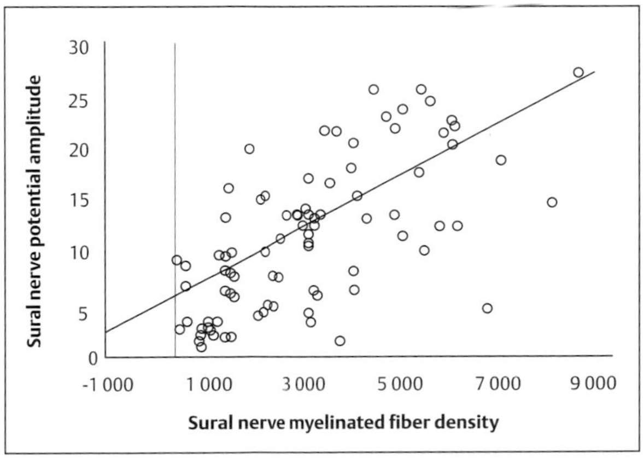

Fig. 5.6 Correlation of sural nerve myelinated fiber density with summed sural nerve potential amplitudes (linear regression). This highly significant correlation had a Pearson's correlation coefficient of 0.681 ($P < 0.0001$)

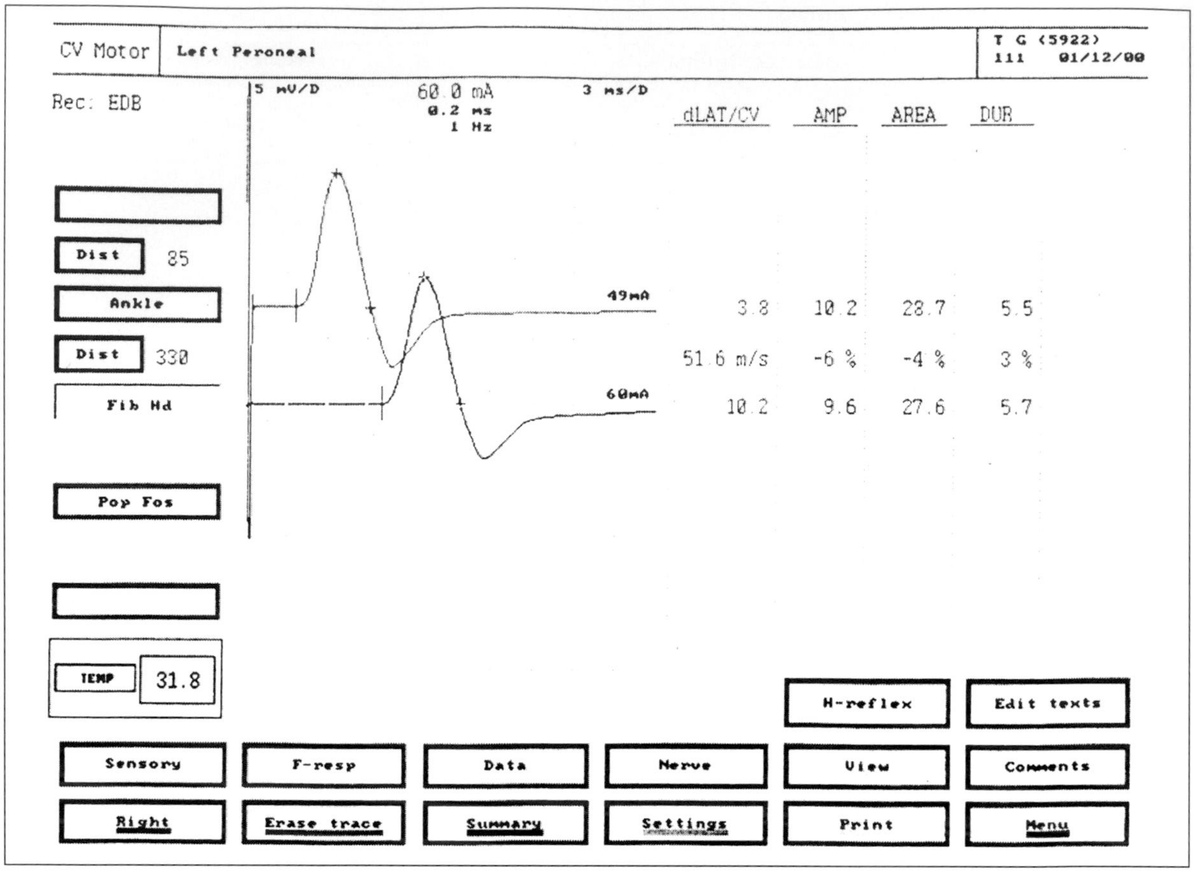

Fig. 5.7 Peroneal motor nerve conduction study (NCS) in a healthy volunteer: EMG equipment (Medtronic, Mississauga, Canada) printout. The evoked compound muscle action potentials are obtained after stimulation at the ankle (top tracing) and at the knee (bottom tracing). The amplitudes of the evoked compound muscle action potentials are normal at 10.2 mV with distal stimulation and 9.6 mV with proximal stimulation. The motor conduction velocity of 51.6 m/s is normal

dependent "dying-back" neuropathy characterized by centripetal degeneration of axons starting at the distal terminals and progressing centrally [80,82,83]. Thus, early changes are observed distally in the lower limbs. NCS reflect this pattern of nerve impairment and loss. For example, in younger patients, the plantar sensory nerves are affected before the sural nerve responses [84] as the nerve fibers to the plantar sensory nerves are longer than those to the sural nerves, and are affected earlier in any length-dependent dying-back neuropathy. Early abnormalities in F wave parameters can be observed in DSP as these responses are determined by conduction along the whole length of the nerve [85–88].

In NCS, parameters reported include the latency of the onset of the evoked motor or sensory response, the amplitude of that response, the conduction velocity, either motor or sensory, for the nerve being studied, and F wave latencies (Figs. 5.**7**, 5.**8**). These values are influenced by age, height, and anthropometric characteristics, and change in specific directions in disease states. The normative values are technique-dependent and must be established for each laboratory. Alternatively, published normative ranges can be used if the same techniques for NCS are employed.

Electromyography, which is the needle electrode examination of muscles, supplements the nerve conduction studies and has a limited role in DSP. Although the abnormal finding of fibrillation potentials in the intrinsic foot muscles may predate NCS parameter findings in the abnormal range [89], these changes are nonspecific. Typically, an electromyographic examination (EMG) would be performed to investigate the possibility of additional diagnoses to DSP, such as radiculopathy, inflammatory myopathy, or motor neuronopathy. In DSP, the EMG shows increased insertional activity in distal muscles, abnormal spontaneous activity, and some degree of chronic neurogenic change in motor unit potentials related to reinnervation following denervation, mainly in advanced neuropathy. These are nonspecific changes of an axonal process with involvement of motor fibers and may be observed in different polyneuropathies as well as radiculopathies.

The goals of doing NCS in subjects with suspected DSP are to document the presence and severity of DSP by abnormal findings, document the extent of the disorder, and identify any changes which would suggest an alternative diagnosis. Examples of such changes are: unexpected degrees of slowing of nerve

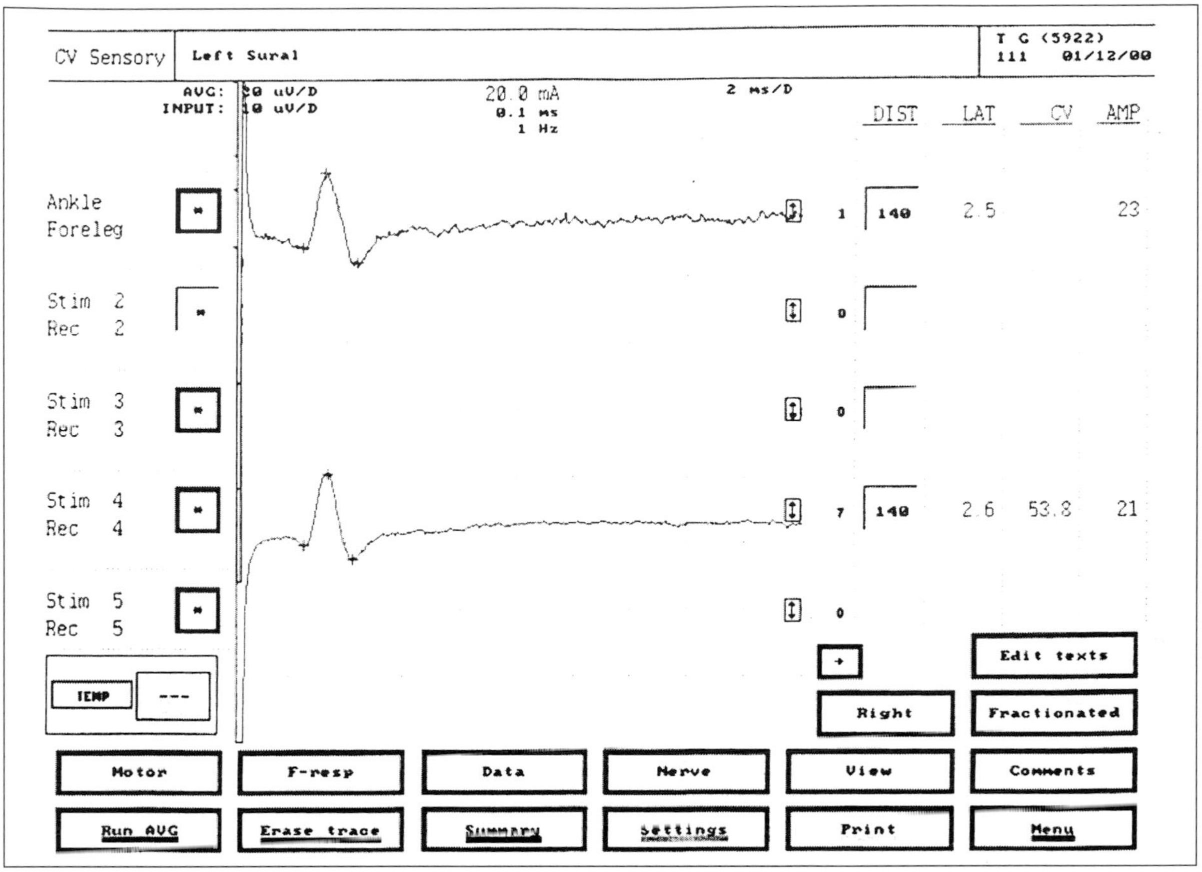

Fig. 5.**8** Sural sensory NCS in a healthy volunteer. The upper tracing is a recording of a single response. The + marks indicate sites at which latency and amplitude are measured. The lower tracing is obtained after averaging seven responses. The latency of 2.6 ms, amplitude of 21 μV, and conduction velocity of 53.8 m/s are all normal values

conduction velocities with preservation of evoked motor and sensory potential amplitudes, indicating a primary demyelinating process; normal sensory NCS findings with prominently abnormal motor NCS findings, indicating a primary motor neuropathy; normal NCS findings with absent deep tendon reflexes and elevated vibration perception thresholds, suggesting a polyradicular disease; or normal NCS findings with preserved deep tendon reflexes and elevated vibration perception thresholds, suggesting central neurologic disease in the spinal cord, or higher.

The presence of disease is reflected by abnormal NCS parameters, i. e., prolonged distal motor and sensory latencies, reduction in the evoked motor and sensory potential amplitudes, and secondary slowing of conduction velocity (Figs. 5.**9**, 5.**10**). These changes are less definite in mildly affected patients as the overlap between reference subjects and those with DSP is considerable even when adjusting for confounding anthropometric features. NCS can be insensitive to those rare patients with isolated small fiber disease. The severity of disease can be suspected by the degree of abnormality of the parameters in the study; in the most severe cases, the motor and sensory responses are lost distally in the lower limb, and diffuse upper limb changes are observed. The extent of disease can be demonstrated by the number and distribution of nerves affected. If the changes are within the territory of a single nerve, then a mononeuropathy is present. When diffuse changes in NCS are observed, then the presence of DSP is confirmed.

Methodology

Nerves Tested

The nerves tested for DSP include lower and upper limb peripheral nerves. Both motor and sensory nerves are studied. Unilateral NCS are acceptable as the process is symmetric [90]. Typically, the sural nerve response is measured. In subjects less than 40 years of age, the plantar sensory nerves can be assessed [84,91]. For motor nerve function in the lower limb, peroneal nerve testing is favored for technical reliability, but this procedure can be supplemented by posterior tibial nerve conduction studies. In the upper limb, median motor and sensory nerve function tests are utilized. Ulnar nerve conduction studies are also commonly tested. Some laboratories include radial nerve sensory conduction studies in the routine evaluation for DSP [92,93].

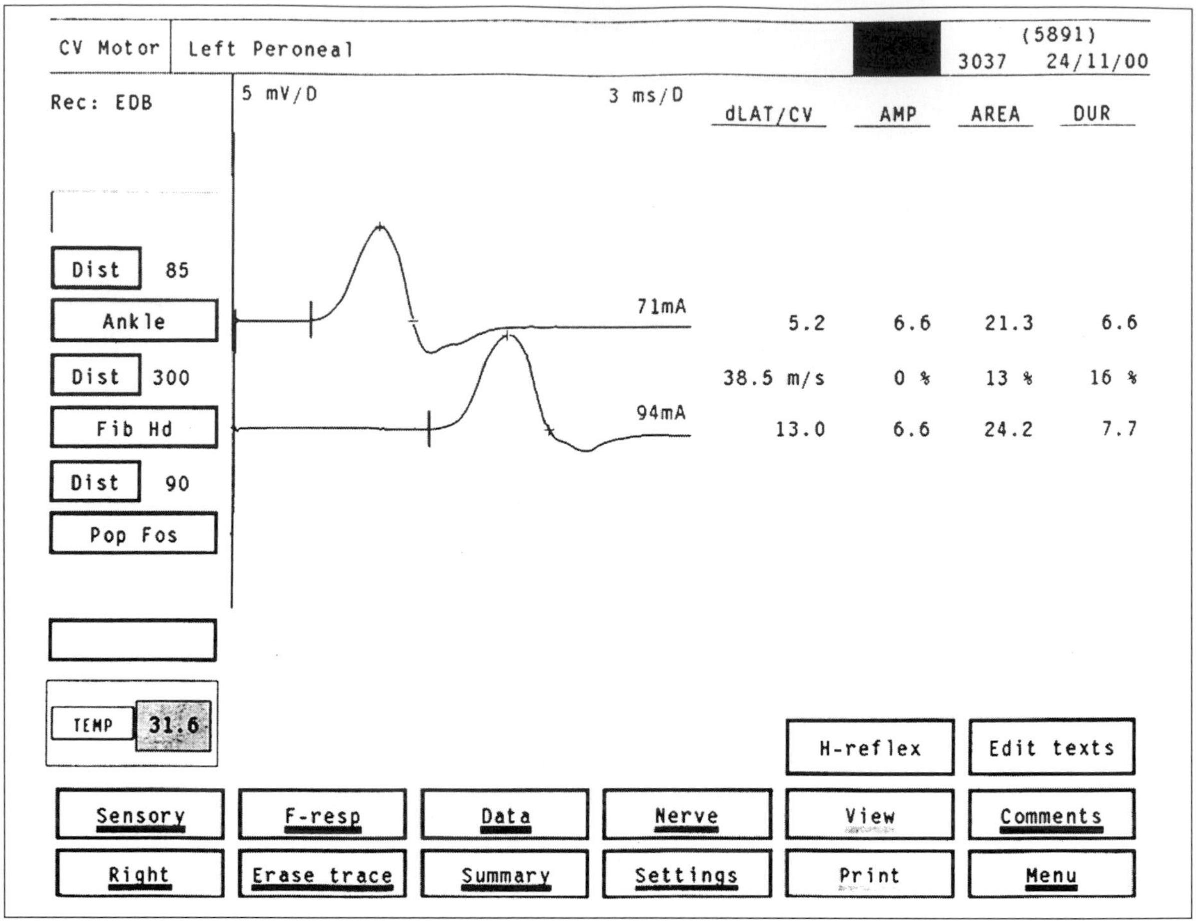

Fig. 5.9 Peroneal motor NCS in a patient with DSP: motor nerve responses after stimulation of the peroneal nerve at the ankle (upper tracing) and at the knee (lower tracing) in a patient with DSP. The conduction velocity of 38.5 m/s is mildly slowed. The amplitude of 6.6 mV is normal

Some laboratories use ratios of different nerve parameters, such as sural/radial sensory nerve potential amplitudes, in order to improve diagnostic accuracy in DSP [92,93]. A confounding factor in NCS for DSP can be abnormality of peripheral nerve function at sites of bony compression, producing NCS findings of mononeuropathy. This type of finding may be integral to DSP and not indicative of simple mononeuropathy [81,94–97].

Electromyography

Electromyographic examination in subjects with DSP is supplementary and exploratory to the routine NCS. This procedure has value if other diagnoses such as radiculopathy, motor neuronopathy, and inflammatory myopathy are under serious consideration in the differential diagnosis for an individual subject. Percutaneous needle insertion into muscles is required, a procedure most patients find uncomfortable. Consequently, electromyography is not well tolerated in serial studies and clinical trials. When electromyography is done in DSP, abnormal results are observed in the more distal muscles in moderately to severely advanced disease. Reportedly, fibrillation potential activity can be observed earlier than abnormal NCS findings in DSP [89], but the specificity of such results is in doubt. Increased insertional activity, abnormal spontaneous activity (fibrillation potentials), and loss of recruitment, i. e., loss of the normal amount of motor unit potential activity, are observed in any process affecting motor axons sufficiently. Remodeling of motor unit potentials due to denervation with subsequent reinnervation is indicated by the presence of motor unit potentials with increased durations, increased amplitudes, and polyphasic form. More specialized techniques such as single-fiber electromyography are useful mainly in a research capacity rather than in the routine diagnostic evaluation of DSP. These more sophisticated techniques may yield more information on motor unit remodeling in reinnervation [98], but are of limited value for routine evaluation of patients with DSP.

Results Expected

Typical tracings of motor and sensory NCS in patients with DSP are shown in Figures 5.**9** and 5.**10**. These

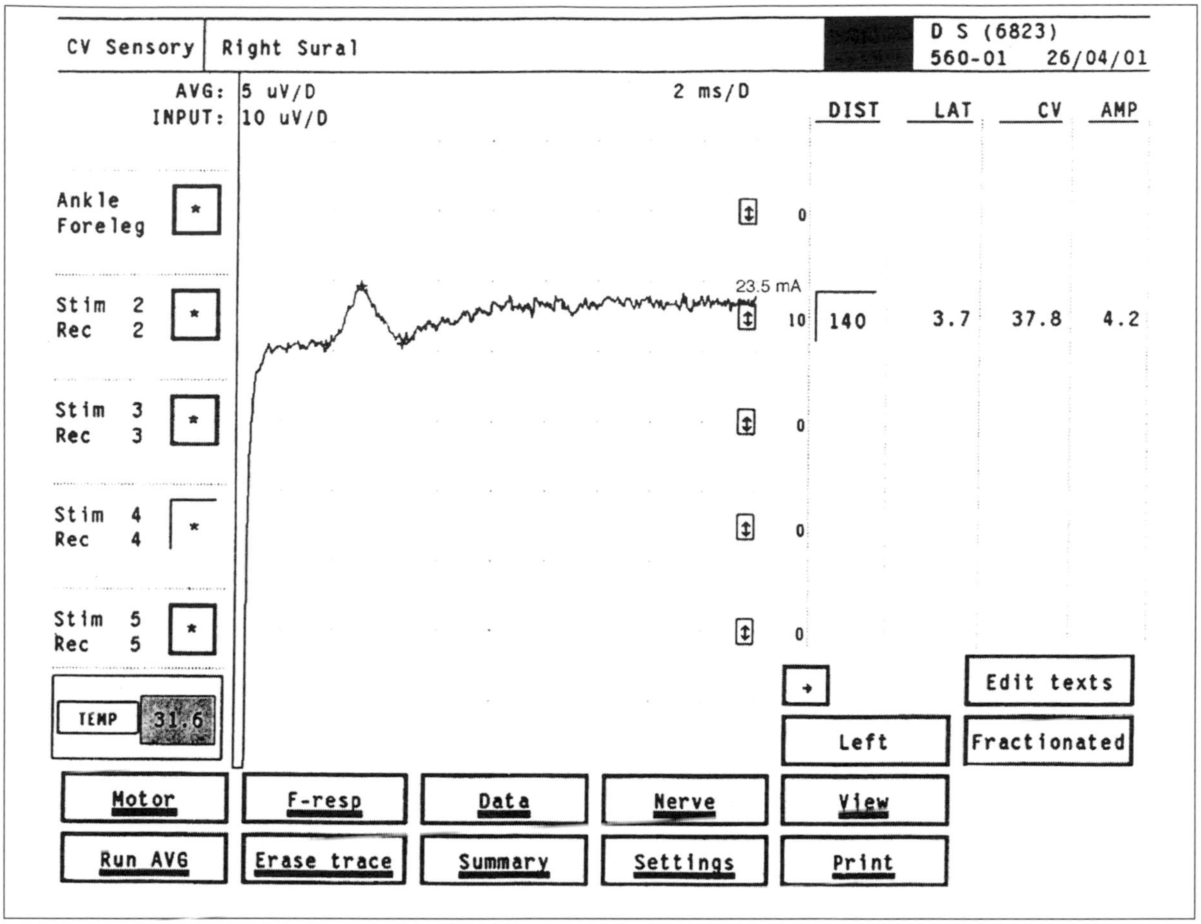

Fig. 5.**10** Sural sensory NCS in a patient with DSP. The amplitude of 4.2 μV is below normal, and the conduction velocity of 37.8 m/s is reduced

figures illustrate printouts from an electromyograph (Medtronic, Mississauga, Canada). The parameters reported most commonly are: distal latencies, amplitudes, conduction velocities, and F wave latencies. In mild and early neuropathy, all results may be within normal limits. In part, normal NCS findings may indicate that the disease process is mild and has not had discernible effects on the peripheral nerves in spite of the presence of symptoms and deficits of DSP on clinical testing. A more likely explanation is that the values in an individual patient are abnormal for that subject, but overlap with normative ranges for the particular laboratory. In other patients, marked changes in NCS are observed with minimal or no clinical symptoms. The first NCS abnormalities are observed in distal lower limb sensory responses, with a reduction in sensory potential amplitudes. As more large fibers are lost, the distal sensory latency increases and the conduction velocity decreases. As the disease progresses, similar changes in motor nerve conduction studies are observed. Early changes in the distal motor and sensory nerve conduction parameters of the median nerve are observed commonly [80,81,94,97]. With disease progression, more severe NCS changes are observed. Finally, the distal motor and sensory responses are lost completely.

The amount of information from NCS can be daunting. In order to comprehend the results clearly and to analyze the data, clinically relevant summary scores have been utilized. Rank sum scores for conduction velocity and amplitude [60], summed amplitude and conduction velocity scores [99], and a single index of polyneuropathy, IPN [100], are different ways to assimilate a large amount of confusing data.

Relationships to Clinical Measures and Pathologic Changes

The NCS are valuable as they provide reliable, quantitative information on nerve function. Coefficients of variation on repeat testing are lower than other testing methods such as quantitative sensory testing or clinical examination, as demonstrated in Table 5.**4** [33,64]. The NCS findings correlate both with morphologic severity of DSP [101] and with clinical severity of disease [77]. NCS reflect both the acute and the chronic stages of glycemic control [99]. Changes in conduction velocity mirror acute changes in metabolic control [102–105], but can also reflect long-term changes in glycemic levels [63,99]. Thus, NCS are a meaningful, reliable, and standardized way of measuring nerve function accurately in DSP. They carry implications as to underlying nerve structure (degree of nerve fiber loss), the clinical findings, and glycemic control. For these reasons, they continue to be of great value in the evaluation of DSP in clinical trials. Routine NCS testing of all subjects with diabetes may not be feasible for practical considerations, but NCS remain mandatory for patients in the clinic when there is any doubt about the diagnosis of DSP, or an alternative diagnosis is being considered in the differential diagnosis of an individual subject. Changes in NCS occur slowly in most DSP patients, with little to no change in parameters observed in 12 months. More rapid decline should raise concerns about the adequacy of glycemic control, or the presence of comorbid disease such as CIDP.

Limitations

Large-Fiber Activity Measure

One of the major criticisms of NCS in DSP is that large-fiber activity is measured, but that small-fiber function is not assessed. In rebuttal, it should be remembered that most subjects with DSP have diffuse nerve fiber impairments affecting all fiber sizes. The hallmark of the disorder is progressive loss of all fibers, both large and small. Thus, NCS remain a valid and important measure of nerve function in DSP.

Accuracy

The normative ranges for NCS parameters overlap with abnormal values in DSP, thus limiting the sensitivity and accuracy of testing. Nevertheless, NCS are the most sensitive measure of DSP; other testing modalities do not have the same degree of sensitivity [35,106]. As a result, NCS remain the best measure of DSP.

Small-Fiber Measures

Increasingly, tests of small-fiber function have been investigated for utility in the evaluation of subjects with DSP [107]. The sympathetic skin response (SSR) is one such method. In response to different stimuli, a long-latency response can be recorded from the palmar and plantar surfaces of the extremities. These responses are thought to represent activity of sympathetic peripheral nerve fibers. Unfortunately, the responses can be absent in healthy subjects. Changes in latency and amplitude parameters are not evident in a year, and the parameters do not correlate with small-fiber symptoms [108]. The simple absence or presence of the SSR does correlate with DSP duration and duration of diabetes mellitus; but no more refined information is obtained with this type of investigation [108,109].

Methods of testing of the autonomic system are diffuse, with many different methods, testing paradigms, and results [110–113]. Reproducibility has been a problem. Recently, a system was developed which showed lower test variability with a central reading group [114]. Such standardized approaches may improve the reliability of these investigations and lead to their more routine use in the future. Presently, these test methods are utilized mainly for clinical research trials and not in most clinics.

None of the small-fiber investigational methods is standardized, widespread, and practical. Newer methods including skin punch biopsy with evaluation of intradermal fibers are promising, but none is yet a standard way to evaluate DSP, even in clinical trials.

Summary

NCS are the most reliable and accurate measure of peripheral nerve function in DSP. Close relationships with morphologic and clinical measures of neuropathy confirm the validity of this type of testing. NCS are mandatory when alternative diagnoses in addition to DSP are being considered, and remain an essential element of clinical trials in DSP. If a therapeutic intervention for DSP does not produce an improvement in NCS, it is unlikely to be an effective therapy for this indication.

■ Quantitative Sensory Testing

J.C. Arezzo

Introduction

The progressive loss of distal cutaneous sensation is the hallmark of the most common form of neuropathy associated with diabetes, symmetric distal polyneuropathy. While individuals are usually acutely aware of abnormalities resulting in "positive symptoms," such as pain and paresthesias, changes in sensory function resulting in "negative symptoms," such as numbness, are often insidious and can remain undetected by both patient and physician. Accurate and reliable detection of the loss of sensation associated with diabetic neuropathy has gained increasing importance as new putative therapies emerge and as the link between diminished sensation, ulcerations, and ultimately amputations is solidified. For many, the sensory portion of the neurologic examination has remained unchanged for the past 100 years, relying almost exclusively on a tuning fork, pin, cotton wisp, and perhaps the "cold" end of a reflex hammer. Alternatively, the limits of sensation can be determined by combining quantitative methods for the accurate delivery of stimuli with established psychophysical procedures to assess signal detection. The term "quantitative sensory testing" (QST) is appropriately applied to procedures where the intensity and characteristics of the stimuli are well controlled (i. e., same on Tuesday as on Friday; same in Boston as in Düsseldorf) and where the detection threshold is determined in parametric units that can be compared to established "normal" values.

Standard instruments and highly accepted procedures have been adopted for quantitative evaluation of frequency specific auditory deficits, as well as changes in contrast sensitivity and visual acuity. However, the quantitative evaluation of distal cutaneous function, which is key for diabetic neuropathy, has proven a more formidable task. There are several reasons for the added difficulty of QST of somatosensory function:

1. Cutaneous sensation involves a wide variety of submodalities (vibration, light touch, cold, pain) which are often associated with specialized distal receptors and distinct spinal pathways, and are carried by peripheral axons of differing cross-sectional diameter and myelination patterns.
2. Due to the extreme length of the cutaneous sensory pathways, accurate assessment of change in sensation requires the measurement of sensory function at several points along a distal-to-proximal gradient.
3. Distal cutaneous sensory function is strongly influenced by the local modulation of receptor sensitivities. For instance, the threshold of nociceptors can be lowered by more than 100-fold by the triggered release of neuropeptides in the vicinity of stimulation, and adaptation can dramatically and rapidly alter the sensitivity of mechanoreceptors.

In spite of these difficulties, the past two decades have witnessed the development of a number of commercially available instruments for QST of cutaneous functions including touch, vibration, warmth, cold, and pain. Devices have ranged from complex computer-aided instruments (e. g., CASE IV, pioneered by Peter Dyck and colleagues [115,116]) to simple "handheld" tools with no moving parts (e. g., monofilaments) [117]. In the diabetic population, QST procedures have been used to document the presence of subclinical neuropathy [e. g., 118], to follow the progression of neuropathy in a large cohort of subjects [e. g., 119], as part of a comprehensive battery of neurologic measures [e. g., 120], to predict patients "at risk" for foot ulcerations [e. g., 121], and as primary efficacy endpoints in a series of multicenter clinical trials evaluating the prevention or treatment of diabetic polyneuropathy [e. g., 122]. There have been several reviews of QST procedures [123–131], and several "consensus expert panels" have considered the strengths and limitations of QST as a method of assessing sensory neuropathy [132–134]. This section is not intended as a comprehensive review of QST methodology. Rather, we will examine how diabetes may alter sensory thresholds, and will explore the impact of some recent developments on the use of QST for the assessment of diabetic neuropathy.

Pathophysiology Underlying the Elevation of Sensory Thresholds

Multiple mechanisms have been proposed to account for the pathogenesis of diabetic neuropathy, including microvascular disease [135], modification of proteins critical to neural function by glycation and glycosylation [136], altered metabolism of fatty acids [137], increased activity in the polyol pathway causing a reduction in Na^+/K^+ adenosine triphosphatase activity [138], basement membrane replication and pericyte degeneration [139], a reduction in the expression or binding of neurotrophic factors [149], and superoxide overproduction [141]. It is likely that several or all of these factors interact to cause diabetic neuropathy and that their relative contribution may differ across patients, reflecting both genetics and diet. Although the mechanisms of neuropathy are still controversial, it is generally agreed that in its most common manifestation, diabetic symmetric polyneuropathy is a type of "length-dependent distal axonopathy" [142]. In this condition, the neuronal soma remains relatively unaffected at a time when the distal peripheral axon begins to undergo pathologic alterations. Change in distal sensory function, specifically hypoesthesia, is the result of a series of structural alterations in the distal axon that underlie both acute and long-term deficits.

Transduction

The first critical step in sensory processing, termed transduction, is the conversion of energy as it occurs in the real world (e. g., mechanical, thermal) into "neural energy" in the form of depolarizing or hyperpolarizing transmembrane signals within neurons. Mechanoreceptors, such as those sensitive to vibration or discriminative touch, generally utilize a nonneural element to amplify energy or to aid in adaptation. However, in the somatosensory system, all sensory transduction occurs directly in myelinated or unmyelinated distal axons. At the distal extreme, the surface area of some afferent axons is expanded through a series of filopod extensions, which greatly facilitates transduction (Fig. 5.**11**). In a series of studies, Schaumburg and colleagues documented that the loss of the filopod extensions, and the consequent loss of axon surface area, was the initial pathologic alteration associated with an experimental distal axonopathy similar to that seen in many diabetic subjects [143,144]. These changes undoubtedly result in the loss or redistribution of transmembrane channels tuned to cutaneous energy (e. g., ion channels that change conformation due to

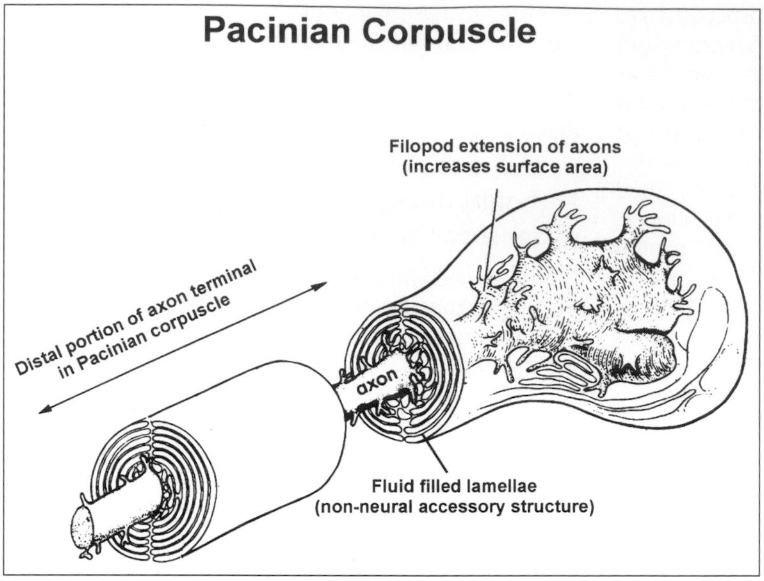

Fig. 5.11 Distal extreme of a "normal" axon innervating a Pacinian corpuscle. Note the filopod processes that characterize the axon terminal and thereby expand the surface area. These processes contain dense arrays of transmembrane channels, which change conformation as a function of mechanical energy (e. g., sensory transduction). In the early stages of a distal axonopathy, such as that associated with diabetic neuropathy, these filopod extensions are lost and the sensitivity of the receptor is diminished

mechanical stretch). Thus, the initial stages of a distal axonopathy can alter transduction, resulting in elevated sensory thresholds before axonal loss or altered conduction within sensory pathways has taken place.

Receptors may also increase their sensitivity to stimulation in the early stages of diabetic neuropathy, resulting in hyperesthesia [118]. These changes may in part reflect abnormalities in distal peptide neurotransmitter levels, which can be modified in peripheral nerve fibers of diabetic patients prior to axon loss [145].

Conduction

At threshold, the patient is required to detect a specific sensory signal against a background of transmitted neural events. As well documented in signal detection theory [146], the process can be modeled as a statistical signal-to-noise task on the sensory side, with a superimposed "decision criteria" on the output side. The integrity of the sensory signal is determined by the quality of receptor activation (i. e., transduction) and by the fidelity of the signal transmission along the remarkable length of the neuraxis from peripheral receptor to higher brain centers. The speed and synchrony of conduction is therefore a key component to the detection of low threshold stimulation. Several aspects of distal axonopathy interfere with optimal nerve conduction and consequently elevate sensory thresholds. These include changes in nodal environment, alterations in axonal cross-sectional diameter, and alterations in axo-glial junctions. In diabetic neuropathy, these early pathologic changes combine to reduce maximum conduction velocity and response synchrony (see [147] for a recent review). Deficits in conduction may be especially important in the loss of sensation critically dependent on the accurate transmission of temporal information, such as discriminating between vibration and pressure or determining the pattern of movement across a receptor surface.

Fiber Loss

In its later stages, distal axonopathy associated with diabetic neuropathy results in the frank loss of axons due to a dying-back process [148]. At these time points, Wallerian degeneration is evident, there is a reduction in fiber density, and there may be an alteration in the axon diameter histogram [149]. Sensory loss is usually extensive due to a combination of altered transduction and conduction in surviving axons and a reduction in the number of available sensory fibers.

Methodology

The sensitivity and reliability of QST procedures are determined by a combination of the equipment selected, the testing algorithm utilized, the site evaluated, and the population examined.

Equipment

Minimally, QST equipment should provide for: (1) accurate control of stimulus intensity in meaningful units (e. g., micrometers of vertical displacement for vibration), (2) control over stimulus characteristics (e. g., vibration waveform; thermal rate of change), (3) sufficient dynamic range of intensity to allow evaluation of multiple degrees of neuropathy, (4) calibration procedures to ensure consistency, (5) the ability to utilize multiple psychophysical procedures (e. g., forced choice; method of limits), and (6) the ability to measure sensation at multiple anatomical sites. There is no ideal QST device for all types of assessment of diabetic neuropathy. The instrument appropriate for the rapid screening of a large diabetic population for the magnitude of sensory loss that may indicate "risk" for foot ulceration is different from the device ideal for the detection of subclinical changes in asymptomatic diabetic subjects. The speed and ability to assess multiple points along a distal-to-proximal gradient afforded by a simple handheld device, such as the biothesiometer, may offset the greater control over stimulus characteristics and the precise adherence to a specified testing algorithm provided by a computer-assisted device.

Comparison of QST findings across instruments must be done with caution. In spite of the strong recommendations of several "consensus panels" [132–134], the units of measurement reported are often highly specific to the instrument utilized and difficult to relate to true physical intensity (e. g., volts for the biothesiometer). Although clumsy and inaccurate, comparisons of QST findings across some instruments can be approximated by considering the degree of deviance in the test scores from values in an appropriate norm population.

Algorithm

A number of different psychophysical QST procedures are available (see [150,151] for review), each with its strengths and limitations. For instance, a true multistep, forced-choice algorithm is very accurate, but time-consuming. The use of this procedure may result in fatigue and changes in attention level during testing and may not be appropriate for an evaluation requiring the assessment of multiple sites and/or multiple modalities in the same subject. In most subjects, the use of an alternative four-, two-, and one-stepping algorithm adds speed without significant loss of accuracy [152]. If ramp stimulation is utilized, as is often the case in assessing thermal sensitivity, the rate of the change in intensity and the use of both ascending and descending ramps are important considerations [153,154]. If the ramp is linear, the start point predictable, and the rate of change rapid, a critical temporal clue may be provided to the subject which could confound the accurate assessment of threshold values. There are substantial arguments in the QST literature regarding the optimal testing algorithm, and it is clear that the absolute value of thresholds may be under- or overestimated by the use of specific procedures. However, it is also clear that QST data obtained with a wide range of psychophysical procedures can provide a sensitive index of diabetic neuropathy if the data are compared to those of a normal population examined with the same testing method.

Anatomical Site

The distribution and density of cutaneous receptors differ substantially across the body surface, with different gradients evident for each modality. Thus, the density of Meissner corpuscles sensitive to light touch is more than an order of magnitude higher in the distal fingertips than the forearm, while thermoreceptors are more evenly distributed along a distal-to-proximal gradient. In selecting an anatomical site to evaluate, there is often a tradeoff between repeat test reliability and sensitivity to change in the induced neuropathy. For instance, thermal thresholds are more reliable if they are measured at a site on the wrist, which allows the positioning of a large stimulus probe. However, these sites may be relatively insensitive to the earliest change in transduction at the distal extreme of the longest sensory axons of the fingers. The threshold for detection of vibration is often lowest over a bony prominence, but the use of these sites may allow the transmission of the vibrating stimulus to more proximal receptors. Further, limiting QST measurement to a single site, by the use of a fixed stimulus probe, may miss deterioration or improvement in sensory function at a different point on the distal-to-proximal gradient. As is the case for instruments and algorithms, there is no one ideal site for QST evaluation; however, evaluation of regions of high receptor density and low sensory thresholds maximize sensitivity to alterations in transduction and conduction.

Population

The clinical or experimental population evaluated is usually fixed by the needs of the assessment, but it is critical that QST data in these subjects be compared to an appropriate normal population. Various QST measures are affected by anthropometric variables such as age [155,156], gender [157], body mass [157,158], and history of smoking and alcohol consumption [158]. These factors must always be considered in determining the "normal range" against which to evaluate deficits in diabetic subjects. The correlation of QST findings with other measures of neuropathy (e. g., maximum conduction velocity) and the repeat measure reliability of the QST data are also influenced by the severity of neuropathy in the population examined [118].

Vibration Perception Threshold

The relationship between elevated vibration perception threshold and diabetic neuropathy has been documented for almost 100 years [159]. The sensitive perception of vibration in the 50–300 Hz range principally reflects the activation of mechanoreceptors (i. e., Pacinian and Meissner corpuscles), conduction in large-diameter myelinated peripheral axons, and transmission through the dorsal column spinal pathways. The very nature of the temporal component of the vibrating stimuli, as opposed to simple mechanical pressure, requires high-fidelity afferent conduction and is thus sensitive to multiple aspects of a distal axonopathy.

There have been multiple studies and multiple instruments utilized to document the correlation between loss of vibration and a variety of indicators of progression of diabetic neuropathy [e.g., 115,125, 160–64]. Dyck and colleagues [118] used computer-assisted QST to compare vibration thresholds with signs and symptoms of neuropathy in three large cohorts: the Rochester Diabetic Neuropathy Study, the recombinant human growth factor study, and the pancreas-renal transplant cohort. In these patient groups, there was a "strong and consistent correlation" between sensory loss and other markers of diabetic neuropathy. Further, the data confirmed that vibration thresholds are especially sensitive to mild or subclinical neuropathy. Davis et al. [165] also demonstrated that vibratory thresholds can detect subclinical neuropathy in children and adolescents with type 1 diabetes. Nerve conduction velocity studies subsequently confirmed the neuropathy detected by QST in these young patients. At the other end of the severity spectrum, Boulton and colleagues [161] documented that vibration thresholds provided a strong indication of "risk" for future ulceration across a wide range of ages and durations of diabetes. In a four-year prospective study [166], patients with baseline threshold elevated above a fixed value (i. e., 25 V with the biothesiometer) were seven times more likely to develop foot ulcers. This trend was confirmed in a longer study in which patients with initial vibration thresholds above the same value had a much higher prevalence of foot ulcers over the course of a 10- to 13-year follow-up period [167]. A recent evaluation of 1035 patients with insulin-dependent or non-insulin-dependent diabetes reported that each one-unit increase in vibration threshold (voltage scale) at baseline increased the hazard of foot ulceration by 5.6% over a one-year study period [119].

Thermal Perception Threshold

Most mechanoreceptors and free nerve endings are responsive to thermal energy, but true cutaneous thermoreceptors are orders of magnitude more sensitive, responding to shifts in temperature of less than 1 °C. Separate cold and warm thermoreceptors have been identified, generally characterized by small receptor fields (usually less than 1 mm^2) and relatively slow conduction velocities. In primates, some cold receptors are innervated by thinly myelinated Aδ fibers with conduction between 3 and 20 m/s [168]. The sensation of "pain" is also elicited by the high-intensity stimulation of thermoreceptors, especially those sensitive to warming, leading to the identification of "heat pain" thresholds.

As is the case with vibration, elevated thermal thresholds have been well documented in patients with diabetic neuropathy defined by other criteria [116,118,123,125,160,169,170] and their alteration has been demonstrated to predict foot ulcerations [171]. Elevated thermal thresholds have been reported in up to 75% of subjects with moderate to severe diabetic neuropathy [172]. Generally, there is a high correlation between elevated thermal and vibration thresholds, but these measures can be dissociated, suggesting a predominant small- or large-fiber neuropathy in individual patients [164]. Lowered "heat pain" thresholds have also been reported in patients with diabetic neuropathy, and this condition may be an important indication of hypersensitivity associated with early changes in distal nerve segments [118]. The correlation of structure and function in distal small-diameter axons may now be possible by combining thermal thresholds with punch biopsy procedures [173–175].

As there is no reasonable zero energy level, the assessment of thermal thresholds has proven technically more challenging than the measurement of vibration thresholds. The testing procedures are generally longer and the obtained results more variable. Computer-assisted procedures may be especially valuable in examining thermal thresholds. Dyck and associates [176] recently reported that the reproducibility of thermal sensory testing with the CASE IV in normal subjects falls within ±1 stimulus step 88% of the time. However, they also noted that variables such as high or low baseline skin temperature can affect some measurements such as heat pain responses and must be carefully controlled.

Simple Devices

A recent trend is the introduction of simple, handheld QST devices, which are inexpensive and easy to operate. These devices are generally less sensitive and accurate than the more elaborate instruments and they usually assign thresholds to progressive categories (e. g. 10 g vs 5 g) rather than continuous variables. However, they can play a strong role in the rapid screening of a large "at risk" population or in the longitudinal evaluation of individual patients at the primary care site. In addition to speed and ease of testing, these devices facilitate the "mapping" of sensory loss, which may significantly augment the sensitivity of QST evaluations. Semmes-Weinstein monofilaments are perhaps the most widely used handheld QST instrument for the assessment of large diameter fiber function. [117]. A "quantitative" 64-Hz tuning fork has been used to document a treatment-related improvement in diabetic neuropathy [177]. This device takes advantage of a visual optical illusion to allow investigators to determine the intensity of residual vibration on a 0–8 scale at the point of threshold (disappearance of sensation), rather than simply the time since striking the tuning fork. Another recently developed handheld QST device, the Tactile Circumference Discriminator, assesses the perception of calibrated change in the circumference of a probe (a variant of two-point threshold) and has also proven effective in the detection of diabetic neuropathy [178]. The rapid assessment of small-fiber function has been aided by the introduction of a digital handheld thermal probe. This device uses the Peltier effect to deliver calibrated and stable thermal stimuli over a range of 40 °C [179]. By selecting an appropriate testing algorithm, an

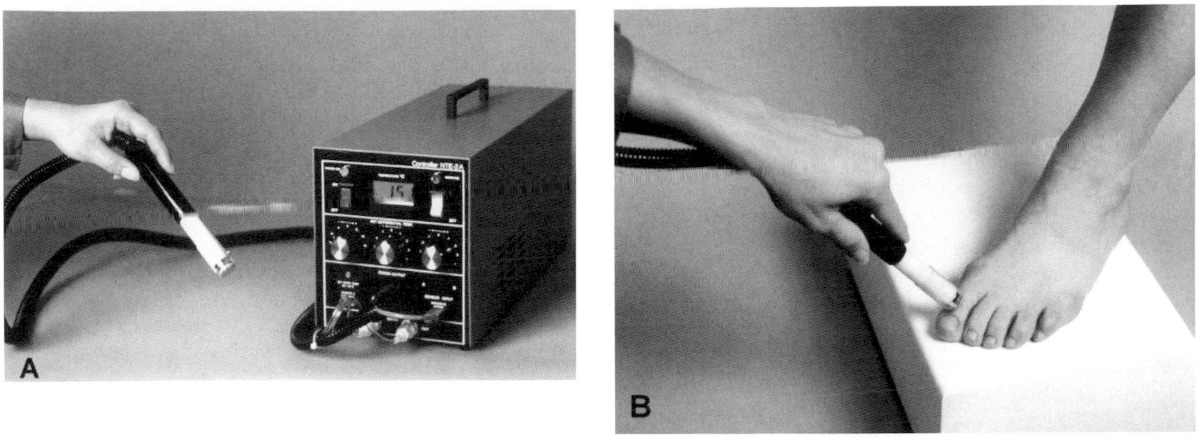

Fig. 5.**12** New handheld instrument for the assessment of thermal thresholds. **A** Temperature at the surface of the handheld probe can be digitally set and maintained over a 40 °C range. The instrument is especially valuable for mapping sensory loss on a receptor surface (e. g., **B** ventral surface of foot) or for determining changes in sensation along a distal-to-proximal gradient

investigator can evaluate both cold and warm sensation along a distal-to-proximal gradient (Fig. 5.**12**).

Epidemiologic Studies and Multicenter Clinical Trials

QST measures have been incorporated in large-scale studies of potential neuropathy sponsored by the United States Centers for Disease Control, National Institute of Occupational Safety and Health, and Environmental Protection Agency. In addition, in the past decade QST procedures have been widely used as both primary and secondary efficacy endpoints in a series of multicenter clinical trials designed to evaluate treatment of diabetic neuropathy. Positive findings in some of these studies [180,181] have been more than offset by negative results in the majority [e. g., 122]. Nonetheless, QST has provided a valuable tool for tracking changes in subjects with diabetic neuropathy and has been critical in selecting appropriate subjects, based on degree of neuropathy, for inclusion in clinical trials. These multicenter studies have demonstrated that QST procedures could be standardized across test sites and that the coefficient of variance of these measures could be reduced to levels affording reasonable statistical power. For example, vibration thresholds in a group of diabetic subjects receiving placebo in a double-blind study were significantly worse at the end of 18 months compared to their baseline values [182]. The fact that the relatively small progression of sensory loss in an untreated population of diabetic subjects over the study period was detectable is very encouraging for future intervention studies.

Limitations of QST in the Assessment of Diabetic Neuropathy

While it is clear that changes in sensory thresholds, as measured by a variety of QST procedures, are associated with the onset and progression of diabetic neuropathy, caution must be exercised in interpreting these findings. An elevated sensory threshold is not specific for peripheral neuropathy. Sensory detection reflects the integrity of the entire sensory pathway from peripheral to cortex, and altered sensory function may be due to deficits in elements beyond the peripheral nerve. For example, abnormal QST results have been reported in subjects with multiple sclerosis and in patients with isolated cortical lesions. Further, all QST procedures are based on the report of the subject, which can be influenced by psychological factors such as motivation, fatigue, and attention. Expectancy and subject bias are additional factors that can exert a powerful influence on QST findings [183,184].

QST should not be used to diagnosis diabetic neuropathy in isolation. Rather, the data from these procedures can augment the neurologic examination, provide valuable parametric information as to the nature and distribution of sensory loss, document progression or treatment related improvement in modality specific sensation, and focus available medical resources on patients at significant risk for ulceration and amputation.

Motor Function

H. Andersen and J. Jakobsen

Introduction

Motor weakness in diabetic patients has been recognized for more than a century. Before the era of insulin treatment, paresis of feet and legs was a well-known concomitant of diabetes [185]. Nowadays, the general opinion is that motor disturbances in diabetes are rare and are restricted to isolated nerve manifestations or to polyneuropathy with distal symmetric distributions in long-term patients.

There are several reasons why motor disturbances have been neglected in diabetic neuropathy. Sensory symptoms such as pain and paresthesias are bothersome and attract much attention, whereas motor impairment is silent and often unrecognized. Evaluation of sensory function is easy to perform due to the development of simple techniques to determine sensory thresholds. Sensory values also show acceptable variation and high reproducibility. In contrast, evaluation of motor performance is technically more complicated and strength varies highly between individuals depending upon sex, body weight, and physical activity. Quantitative sensory testing is recommended for evaluation of diabetic neuropathy, whereas quantitative motor assessment is not part of the diagnostic work-up [186].

The significance to the individual diabetic patient of motor weakness has not been sufficiently elucidated. It is possible that weakness of active ankle and knee movements leads to walking instability, falls, injuries, and foot ulcers. Motor weakness might, therefore, play an important role for one of the major long-term complications, the diabetic foot. In clinical studies and trials using neuropathic endpoints to register the prevalence and severity of neuropathy, quantitative evaluation of muscle strength might contribute to the overall assessment of the patients. Also, quantitative evaluation of muscle strength is relevant in patients with proximal symmetric or asymmetric muscle weakness to monitor the clinical course and the effect of treatment. Involvement of the motor system in diabetic neuropathy can, in addition, be assessed using imaging techniques such as magnetic resonance imaging, which can detect minor changes in the volume of muscles, indicating muscular atrophy [187].

This section deals with the theoretical and practical aspects of motor evaluation. Motor function relies on the activity of cortical motor areas, the corticospinal tracts, the final common pathway from the alpha motoneuron to the muscle fibers, and the contractile apparatus in the muscle. Abnormalities within any part of the motor system can lead to motor dysfunction with impairment of simple movements requiring a minimum of strength to alterations of highly complex ballistic movements.

A considerable number of quantitative techniques have been developed to evaluate the various parts of the motor system. In diabetic neuropathy, assessment of muscle strength is probably the most direct way of evaluating motor function. Also, in vivo imaging of the striated muscles is a promising technique that enables direct detection and quantification of muscular atrophy.

Muscle Strength

Evaluation of motor performance includes assessment of maximum muscle strength, which can be performed using semiquantitative and quantitative techniques. Semiquantitative techniques encompass simple functional tests and manual muscle testing whereas quantitative assessment is obtained by dynamometry.

Simple Functional Tests

Distal motor function is evaluated during the clinical examination from the ability to walk or stand on the heels and toes. In Dyck's classification of diabetic neuropathy, inability to stand on the heels defines more severe symptomatic neuropathy as the condition reflects weakness of the ankle extensors [188]. In contrast, isolated inability to stand and walk on the toes does not indicate peripheral neuropathy but rather an intraspinal disorder [189]. This may suggest a preponderance of weakness of the ankle extensors in diabetic neuropathy. However, quantitative studies have shown that a similar degree of weakness occurs in the ankle flexors [190]. Because of the higher safety factor, a greater degree of weakness of the ankle flexors can be tolerated before clinical dysfunction arises.

Evaluating the ability to stand up from a kneeling position can be used to test proximal motor function. This test is relevant in patients with severe sensorimotor polyneuropathy or with proximal diabetic neuropathy. Since functional tests are quickly and easily performed and do not require any equipment, they are suitable for large clinical studies such as epidemiologically based surveys [191]. The sensitivity and specificity of an abnormal functional test in relation to muscle weakness is, however, unclear. This is partly due to the lack of knowledge about how age, body weight, loss of proprioception, and impaired vision affect test results. Therefore, accurate quantitative information on muscle strength can not rely on functional tests.

Manual Muscle Testing

Manual muscle testing is part of the standard clinical examination but receives less attention in the evaluation of diabetic neuropathy. Several scoring systems have gained popularity, all of which apply ordinal scales, the two most commonly used being the Medical Research Council (MRC) system [192] and the motor part of the neurological impairment score (NIS) [193]. The alternative clinical scoring systems do not include manual muscle testing [194,195].

The MRC scale provides high precision for quantification of very weak muscle groups, which are rare in diabetic neuropathies. Both the NIS and the MRC scale have low sensitivity for the detection of slight to moderate degrees of symmetric weakness [196,197]. Manual muscle testing provides a quick evaluation of the muscle strength of all the major muscle groups and therefore will remain a valuable technique in diabetic neuropathy. It is less suitable for therapeutic trials as considerably more subjects are needed in order to obtain the same level of statistical significance[198].

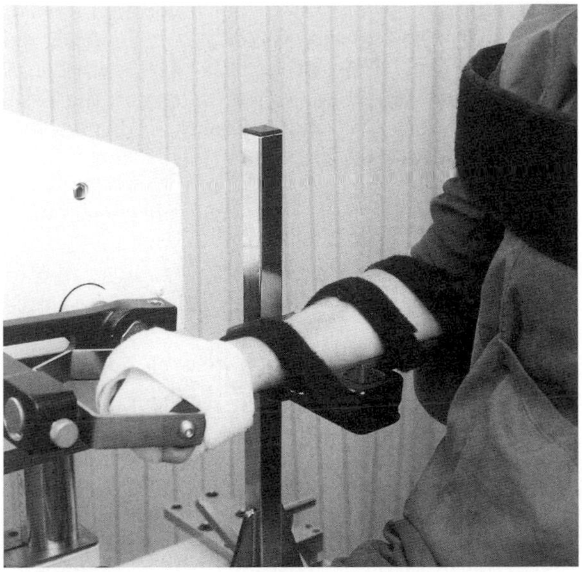

a

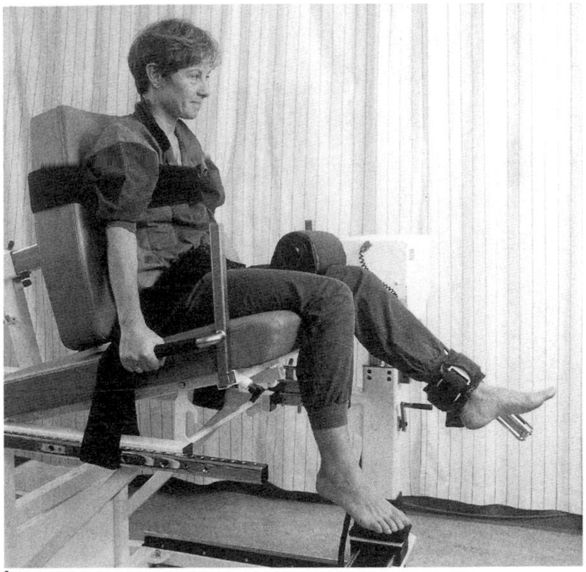

b

Fig. 5.**13** Experimental set-up for evaluation of maximum isokinetic strength of **a** the wrist flexors and extensors and **b** the knee extensors and flexors

Dynamometry

The greatest force generated by a single muscle or a muscle group can be determined quantitatively by performing dynamic or static muscle contractions. Maximum static muscle strength, i. e., isometric force, is produced at a constant length. Maximum dynamic muscle strength as reflected by isokinetic strength is the force multiplied by the lever arm length determined at a constant velocity during a concentric or eccentric contraction [199]. The concept of a muscular contraction accompanying a fixed angular velocity was first introduced in 1967 [200]. Two years later the first isokinetic dynamometer became commercially available. Since then isokinetic dynamometry has become increasingly popular in research projects and has dominated muscle testing in clinical practice, especially within the fields of rehabilitation medicine, orthopedics, and rheumatology [200]. During the testing the velocity is preset and is controlled by the accommodating resistance. In most systems, concentric isokinetic strength can be evaluated at velocities from 0 to more than 400 degrees per second. The set-up for measuring maximum strength of the extensors and flexors at the knee and wrist is shown in Figure 5.**13**. Several parameters are obtained at maximum isokinetic contraction. The most commonly used variable is peak torque, i. e., the highest torque recorded during the entire isokinetic contraction (Fig. 5.**14**). The joint position at which this occurs varies between subjects. Another parameter is the total work, defined as the area under the curve reflecting the total muscular work during the entire movement (Fig. 5.**14**).

Submaximal Performance

Measurements of maximum muscle strength assessed at voluntary contractions is useful only if recorded at a "true" maximum contraction. As in other psychophysical tests, a number of conditions may result in a "false" result. Submaximal performance leading to a "false" low strength may be due to lack of motivation or to pain, sedation, or depression. Detecting submaximal performance during supposedly maximum contractions is a major challenge to the examiner. No examination technique or isokinetic parameter enables identification of all cases of submaximal performance. In hysterical paresis, an increased variation in torque of a series of maximum contractions has been used to detect submaximal performance [202]. In dynamic muscle exercise, especially, an increased coefficient of variation is probably the best indicator of submaximal performance [203,204]. Nevertheless, depending on an increased coefficient of variation alone as an indicator is questionable [205]. Other techniques have been suggested to be more sensitive and robust, including an altered eccentric/concentric torque ratio [206], but owing to the time needed and the techniques applied this ratio will probably not come into wide used. Alternatively, suboptimal performance may be detected using the twitch superimposition technique. For this, during a "supposedly maximum contraction" external twitches can be applied to the muscle; the amount of additional torque evoked by the external twitches reflects the amount of submaximal performance. Based on the linear relation between the torque evoked and the contraction level the degree of submaximal performance can be estimated [207]. The limitations of this technique are: (1) only superficially sited muscles can be evaluated, (2) the time needed

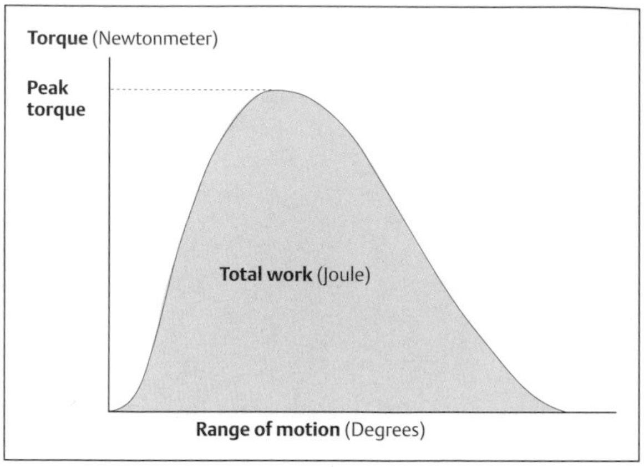

Fig. 5.14 Torque curve during an isokinetic contraction. Peak torque is defined as the highest torque obtained. Work is the total area under the curve

for a test is considerable, reducing the total number of muscles that can be evaluated, and (3) the technique is painful for the patient.

Reliability

A considerable number of studies have estimated the reliability of isokinetic and isometric strength assessments. The majority of the studies have included healthy subjects using varying test protocols which are often difficult to compare. Most authors report a high reliability; however, inadequate statistical methods are common [208,209]. In particular, there is often a lack of statistical testing except by regressional analysis [210]. Inclusion of calculations of the relative difference and coefficient of variation would allow calculation of the critical difference, reflecting the magnitude of change in strength significant in the individual patient or patient group. Despite these limitations, however, there seems to be a fairly high reliability for several muscle groups of the upper and lower extremities [209,211,212].

The technical reliability and accuracy have been found to be high in several of the commercially available isokinetic dynamometers including the Kin-Com unit [213], the Lido Digital System [214], and the Cybex II system [215]. This includes the angular velocity and the measured force compared with the expected force. Therefore, test-retest variation of maximum isokinetic muscle strength can be attributed primarily to biologic and psychophysical factors and less to technical conditions.

A great variation in investigation techniques exists between laboratories using dynamometry. Since no standardization has been done, great care must be taken in comparing strength values obtained in different studies. The relevance of publishing normal values for maximum strength of various muscle groups is also questionable. However, using standardized testing procedures, three separate clinics in the US have pooled their data on isometric strength to build a large database to predict the strength of a large number of muscle groups in the individual patient on the basis of age, gender, height, and weight [216]. Such information for isokinetic dynamometry is lacking.

Maximum Strength

Maximum isokinetic strength is inversely related to movement velocity. In patients with a reduced proportion of fast-twitch muscle fibers (type 2) the decline in strength with increasing velocity is more pronounced [200]. Muscle strength is dependent on a number of variables including the age, gender, and body surface area of the subject. Genetic factors also play an important role in the actual muscle strength, to an extent that varies between studies [217,218]. The well-known age-dependent decline in strength accelerates from the sixth decade [219], occurring earlier in females [220]. Atrophy of the muscles can only partly account for age-dependent weakness [221, 222]. Other explanations are loss of motor units [223] and a decline in the circulating testosterone level [224]. However, physical training programs can alleviate this age-dependent decline in strength [225–227]. Training programs may be effective in improving muscle strength in patients with various neuromuscular disorders [228]. In diabetic patients with neurogenic weakness, however, the effect of training with an aim to regain muscle strength is unknown. Controlled clinical trials are clearly needed to clarify this question.

The relation between muscle strength and the degree of physical activity is rather complex. In younger adults there is a direct relation between heavy work and strength [229,230]. However, in middle-aged people the relation seems to be inverse [229]. Factors without an effect on muscle strength include the number of trials before the actual test (motor learning), menstrual cycle [231], and a general warm-up period prior to the evaluation. β-Blockers and angiotensin converting enzyme inhibitors (captopril) have no effect on muscle strength, which is noteworthy as these drugs are often used in diabetic patients [232,233].

More recently there has been a growing interest in quantitative evaluation of muscle strength. Dynamic muscle function as reflected by isokinetic muscle strength is considered to be an indicator of independence and well-being in the elderly [234,235]. Long-term follow-up studies of healthy subjects have shown that strength predicts the ability to carry out activities of daily living in older age [236]. In the elderly, impaired strength increases the risk of falls and, consequently, higher morbidity and mortality [237]. These relations probably also apply to diabetic patients, further emphasizing the relevance of quantitative muscle testing.

Muscular Endurance

Dynamometry enables quantitative assessment of muscular endurance by evaluation of the degree and rate of loss of muscle strength during continuous or repetitive maximum contractions. In parallel with maximum strength, muscular endurance can be evaluated using static (isometric) or dynamic contractions (isokinetic). Another possibility is weightlifting, which includes isotonic exercise. Isometric endurance has been investigated using a number of different test protocols [232,238,239]. In isokinetic dynamometry, the relative decline in strength (peak torque) or total work during 30 or 50 maximum repetitions has been used as an index of endurance [212,240] (Fig. 5.**15**). Measurements of endurance are less reproducible than measurements of maximum muscle strength, probably due to the fact that they are expressed as an index [212]. In general, patients with neurogenic weakness due to various neuromuscular disorders are reported to have decreased endurance during isometric contractions [240].

Muscular endurance depends on the properties of the muscles involved and is of importance for activities of daily living. Endurance is related to the percentage of fatigue-resistant type 1 muscle fibers [241] and inversely related to the amount of fast-twitch fibers [242]. In contrast to maximum strength, muscular endurance is preserved during advancing age [243,244]. Somewhat surprisingly, an increased muscular endurance has been found in diabetic patients unrelated to the severity of neuropathy. No explanation for this finding has yet been found; it could be present at any level from the central command to the interaction of the contractile proteins, including impaired electromechanical efficiency and intracellular muscular processes [245].

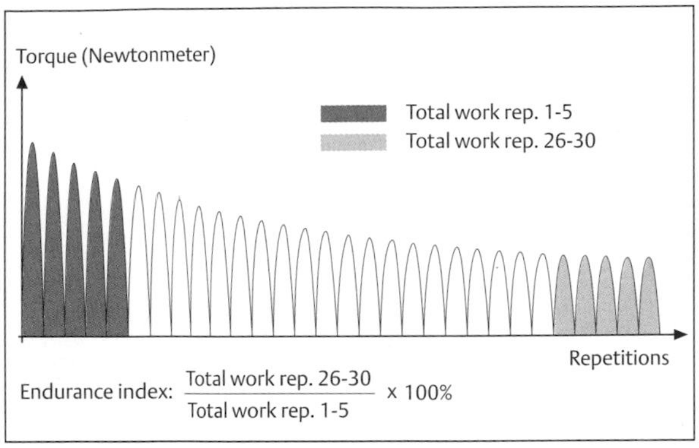

Fig. 5.**15** Torque during 30 consecutive maximum isokinetic contractions. Endurance index is calculated as the total work of repetitions 26–30 as a percentage of repetitions 1–5

Visualization and Quantification of Striated Muscle

Striated muscles may be visualized by several imaging techniques including magnetic resonance imaging (MRI), computed tomography, and ultrasonomyography [245]. In neuromuscular disorders, MRI is superior to other imaging techniques as it enables clear distinction between muscle tissues, fat, and connective tissues [245]. Thus, individual muscles and muscle groups can readily be identified using MRI. In diabetic patients MRI has been used primarily to detect infections [246] and muscular infarctions [247]. MRI can also be used to detect acute and chronic neurogenic muscle disorders, evaluating the degree and distribution of nerve injury [248].

The application of stereologic techniques enables quantification of any structure in the body [249], including unbiased estimation of the volume of any muscle or muscle group so long as the muscles can be unequivocally identified [250]. In practice, a number of cross-sectional MRI scans of a limb are performed. From a random start the images are obtained systematically, i. e., at fixed intervals. At each level the cross-sectional area of the muscles is estimated using a transparent test grid with a systematic array of test points. The number of test points hitting the muscles is counted and multiplied by the unit area per test point (Fig. 5.**16**). According to the Cavalieri principle, the muscle volume is the distance between sections multiplied by the total cross-sectional area [251]. Applying this technique in diabetic patients with neuropathy and muscle weakness, MRI of the lower part of the leg has demonstrated a substantial loss of volume of muscle tissues closely associated with the degree of weakness [191]. The atrophy occurs primarily in the distal parts of the lower leg (Fig. 5.**17**). Recently,

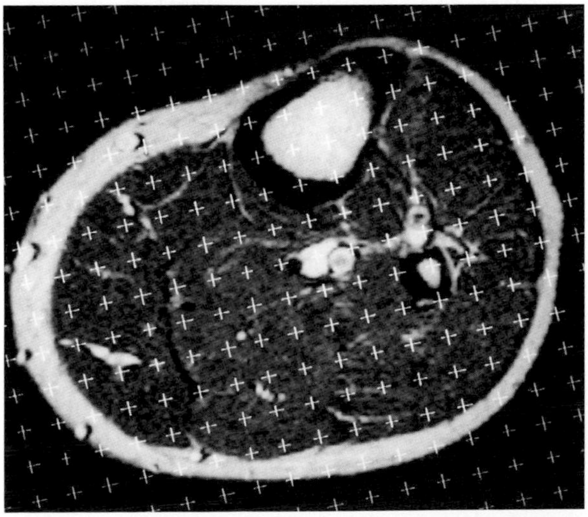

Fig. 5.**16** Transverse MRI through the lower leg (midsection) with a superimposed transparent test grid. The cross-sectional area of the striated muscles can be estimated by multiplying the area per test point by the number of test points hitting the muscle (79)

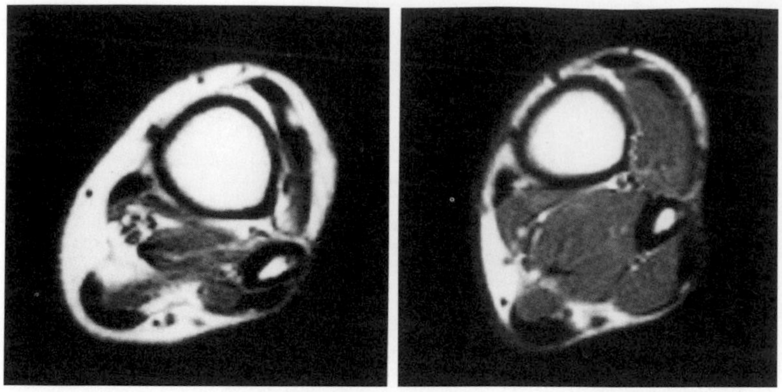

Fig. 5.17 Cross-sectional magnetic resonance images of the distal part of the lower leg in a neuropathic patient (left) and in a healthy control (right). Note the pronounced atrophy of all muscle groups in the patient

quantification of the small intrinsic foot muscles on MRI has shown atrophy in patients with early and less severe degrees of neuropathy (unpublished personal observation). There is a close relation between the degree of atrophy and the severity of neuropathy assessed clinically. These observations further demonstrate the existence of a proximal-to-distal gradient in diabetic neuropathy. In relation to muscle function, estimating the volume of the muscle groups with stereologic techniques is superior to assessing the cross-sectional muscle area or the external circumference of the leg [188].

Although MRI is superior to other visualization techniques in distinguishing between various tissues and identifying striated muscles, ultrasonomyography may in some instances be more relevant in diabetic neuropathy. Ultrasonomyography is a faster and less expensive imaging technique, and can therefore be used in larger studies such as population-based surveys. A thorough comparison including evaluation of the sensitivity and reliability of MRI and ultrasonomyography could further define the utility of these two techniques.

Conclusions

Manual muscle testing and testing of the ability to stand and walk on the toes and heels are quick and inexpensive means of evaluating muscle strength in patients with diabetic neuropathy. Dynamometry provides a more accurate and sensitive assessment of the muscle strength and endurance of the major muscle groups of the upper and lower extremities. Maximum isokinetic muscle strength is a reliable measure of motor function which can be used in clinical studies and trials. In addition, MRI of striated muscles enables detection and quantification of muscular atrophy in the foot and distal part of the leg, reflecting motor dysfunction in diabetic neuropathy. Taken together, the above techniques allow a detailed examination of the motor system which combined with sensory and autonomic examinations completes the evaluation of dysfunction in diabetic neuropathy.

Unmyelinated Nerves: Skin Biopsy and Skin Blister Methods

W.R. Kennedy and G. Wendelschafer-Crabb

Introduction

This section describes the role of skin biopsy and skin blister for evaluation of unmyelinated nerves in symmetric, predominantly sensory, diabetic neuropathy. Degeneration of unmyelinated nerve fibers occurs in several body systems, often resulting in a handicapped lifestyle. Symptoms include faulty heart rate and blood pressure regulation, gastroparesis with delayed stomach emptying, constipation, diarrhea, urinary incontinence, male impotency, poor wound healing, insensitivity to thermal or painful stimuli, and severe pain in acral regions. Early in the disease course the diagnosis is elusive. Patients hear members of the general public complain of similar symptoms and become reluctant to attach significance to their own symptoms. The neuropathy usually begins in distal nerve segments and appears to progress proximally in a "dying-back" fashion [252]. Once suspected, the diagnosis of unmyelinated nerve fiber involvement is made from the history and the presence of an increased threshold for thermal or noxious stimuli, supplemented by abnormal results from functional tests of cardiorespiratory reflexes or sweating. Morphologic verification has relied upon electron microscopic demonstration of decreased counts of unmyelinated nerve fibers in a nerve biopsy, most often of the sural or radial nerve. The invasive nature of nerve biopsy, low sensitivity to minimal unmyelinated nerve fiber loss due to the wide range of normal values, and inability to identify the function or destination of nerve fibers visualized led to a search for other methods.

Cutaneous Nerves

Skin contains sensory nerves to the epidermis, encapsulated receptors, and hair follicles, and autonomic nerves to sweat glands, arrectores pilorum, and blood vessels (Fig. 5.**18**). Attempts to analyze the terminal segments of cutaneous nerves and sensory receptors have had limited success [253]. Unmyelinated nerves were not well visualized due inadequate staining procedures. The availability of immunohistochemical methods [254] now allows clear reproducible staining of all cutaneous nerves for research and clinical practice. Skin biopsy and skin blister have emerged as methods to evaluate cutaneous unmyelinated nerves in the symmetric, predominantly sensory variety of diabetic neuropathy. The two procedures are minimally invasive, provide identification of the functional types of cutaneous nerves observed, and yield quantitative results. Protein gene product 9.5 (PGP 9.5) [255] has been the most reliable general neuronal marker for staining nerve fibers in the peripheral and central nervous systems, including dermal and epidermal nerves of man [256] and common laboratory animals [257]. Cutaneous sensory nerves are often characterized by their reactivity with antibodies to several nerve peptides including calcitonin gene-related peptide (CGRP), substance P (SP), vasoactive intestinal polypeptide (VIP), and neuropeptide tyrosine (NPY). In normal human skin CGRP and SP immunoreactive (-ir) nerves are confined to the dermis, both ending near the capillary loops in dermal papillae. Occasionally a short branch of a CGRP-ir nerve penetrates the dermal-epidermal basement membrane and ends near the basal keratinocytes. SP-ir nerves are fewer and of slightly larger diameter. SP-ir nerves are the major unmyelinated nerve component of hair follicles. Nerves to sweat glands are immunoreactive to VIP and CGRP and, rarely, to SP. Arterioles are also innervated by nerves that are immunoreactive to CGRP and NPY. The numerous nerves in the arrectores pilorum have received less attention in humans.

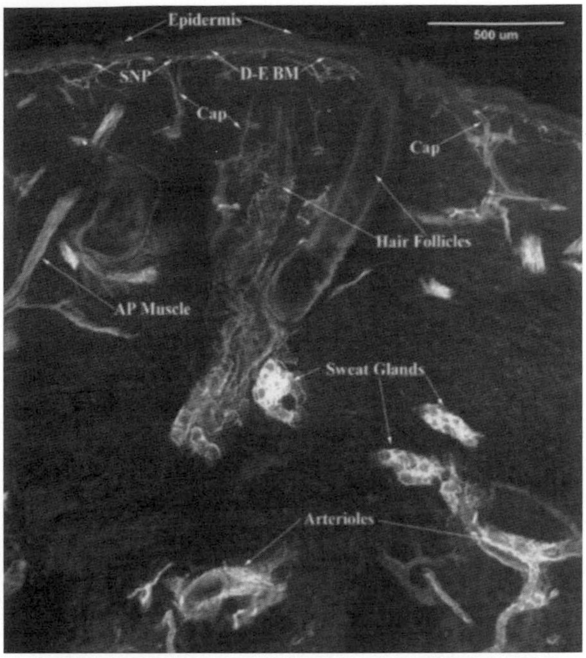

Fig. 5.**18** Typical morphology of normal human hairy skin is seen in this low-power confocal micrograph. Nerve and basement membrane immunofluorescent staining reveal arterioles, sweat glands, hair follicles, arrector pilorum muscle (AP Muscle), capillaries (Cap), the subepidermal neural plexus (SNP), the dermal-epidermal basement membrane (D-E BM), and the epidermis

Epidermal Nerve Fibers

In nonglabrous (hairy) skin the nerves innervating the epidermis are proving valuable for diagnostic purposes. Epidermal nerve fibers (ENFs) were first described over 150 years ago, yet prior to the availability of immunohistochemical methods there was debate over their existence mainly because of inconsistency of the silver and methylene blue methods [258, 259]. The morphologic features of ENFs can now be clearly shown by immunostaining for PGP 9.5 [260, 261], which has been the only reliable method by which to visualize nerves in human epidermis. The existence of ENFs has been verified by electron microscopy [262, 263].

ENFs originate in small dorsal root ganglia neurons. After entering skin they course in nerve bundles to the superficial dermis, where they make up the subepidermal neural plexus. Individual ENFs emerge from the bundles and shed their collagen collar and Schwann cell sheath as they pierce the dermal-epidermal basement membrane. They penetrate the epidermis almost to the stratum corneum (Fig. 5.**19a**). The separation into isolated nerve fibers in the epidermis facilitates counting and measurement of ENF length and branch points. The first morphologic signs of nerve degeneration in apparent length-dependent disorders like diabetic neuropathy seem to occur in ENFs, perhaps because they are the longest nerves at any given body location. This provides the potential for early diagnosis and staging of diabetic neuropathy. Through the use of immunohistochemical methods, unmyelinated nerve loss has been shown to occur in several other types of neuropathy and in a few dermatological conditions [263, 259]. In some neuropathies, e. g., Fabry disease [264], amyloidosis, and painful small-fiber neuropathy [265-267], unmyelinated nerves may be the dominant or only nerves affected. In addition to their importance in neuropathy, there is the possibility that unmyelinated cutaneous nerves could serve as a barometer of unmyelinated nerve degeneration in less accessible, internal organs of the cardiovascular and genitourinary systems and the gastrointestinal tract [268].

Biopsy/Blister Procedures, Staining, and Imaging

The standard method for sampling cutaneous nerves is with a 3-mm punch biopsy instrument. Larger

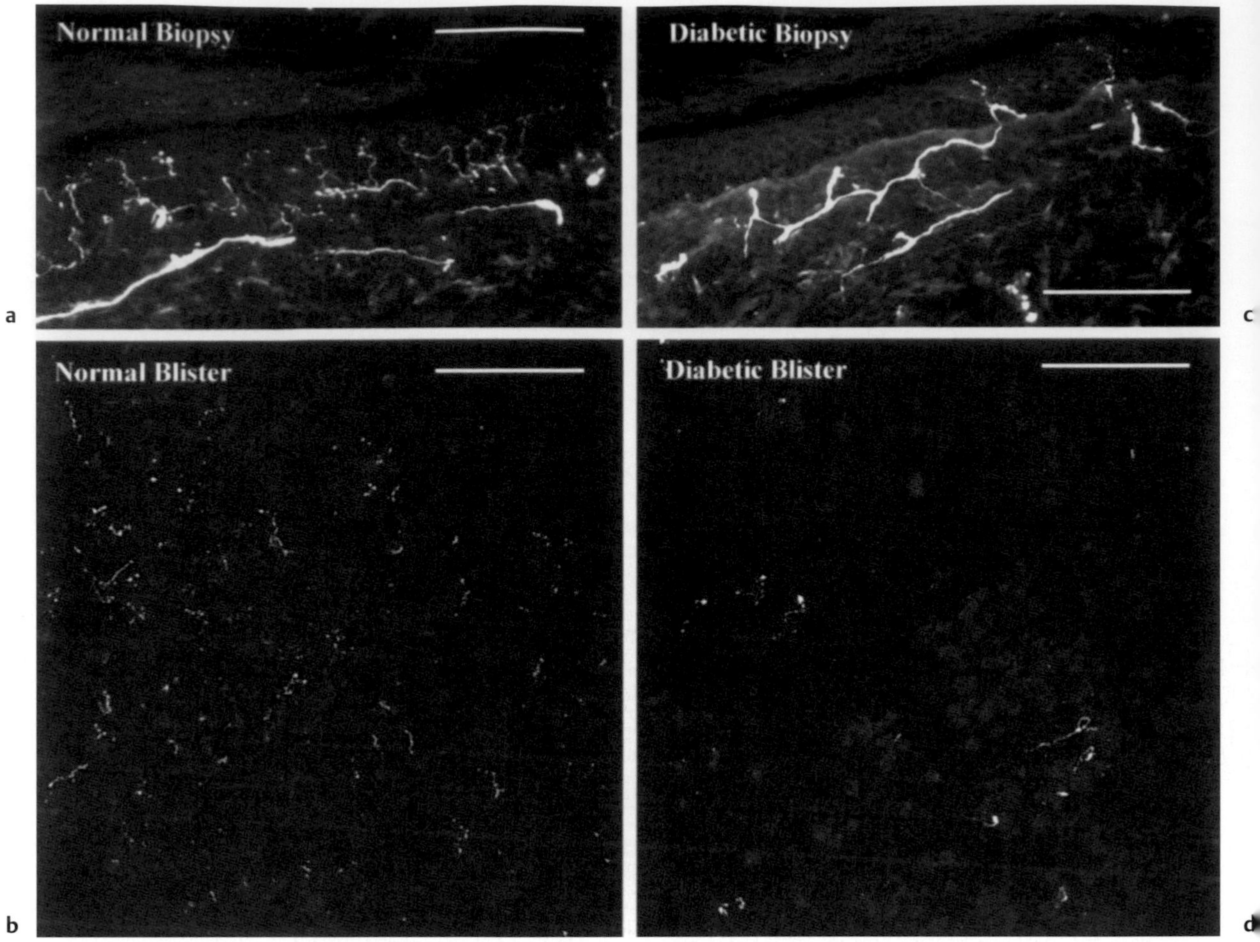

Fig. 5.**19** Confocal micrographs of skin biopsies and blisters of normal and diabetic subjects. All scale bars = 100 µm. **a** Biopsy specimen reveals many epidermal nerve fibers (ENFs) in the skin of normal subjects. **b** Blistered epidermis from normal subjects has numerous relatively evenly distributed nerve fibers. **c** Diabetic subjects have fewer ENFs and some thinning of the subepidermal neural plexus, as seen in this biopsy. **d** Few clustered nerve fibers are present in this blister from a diabetic subject

biopsies may require a suture. Biopsy specimens of normal skin always contain ENFs, autonomic nerves, blood vessels and, if deep enough, sweat glands (Fig. 5.**18**). Inclusion of arrectores pilorum and hair follicles depends upon the body location sampled, size of the biopsy, and traits of the subject biopsied.

The desirability of having a nontraumatic method of screening for onset of neuropathy led to development of the suction skin blister method [269]. Blisters are formed by application of a suction capsule to skin and evacuation to approximately 300 mmHg negative pressure. The epidermis separates from the dermis on a plane between the basement membrane and cell membrane of the basal keratinocytes. Epidermal nerves are disrupted from their proximal dermal origin where they pierce the basement membrane, leaving the full complement of ENFs within the blister roof. The result is a noninvasive, pain-free, blood-free method of tissue acquisition that does not require anesthesia. Reepithelialization occurs within three days without scarring. Reinnervation is almost complete by six weeks [270].

Biopsy and blister roof specimens are fixed overnight in cold Zamboni paraformaldehyde/picric acid fixative, then cryoprotected in buffered 20% sucrose. Frozen biopsy sections (we prefer 50- to 100-µm sections) are immunostained to detect the neuronal markers PGP 9.5, CGRP, VIP, SP, and other nerve peptides, tissue antigens, (type IV or type VII collagen or cytokeratin) and the endothelial cell-binding lectin Ulex europaeus agglutinin type I (UEA I). These markers are localized with labels that fluoresce at different wavelengths. Using this strategy, double and triple staining can be performed to help elucidate the different peptides in individual nerve fibers or the spatial relationships of nerves to other skin structures. In the blister specimens, all epidermal nerves are contained within the single thin (40–60 µm) blister roof (Fig. 5.**19b**). The specimen is immunostained en bloc in a similar manner to biopsy sections. The thick biopsy sections and blister roof are imaged in a confocal microscope which eliminates out-of-focus blur. The laser scanning confocal microscope and the newly available nonlaser confocal microscope (CARV system, ATTO instruments, Rockville, Md.) collect images of a series of thin in-focus optical sections from the thick biopsy sections or the blister roof. Both instruments have advantages. The shorter image collection time of the nonlaser microscope (approximately ten times faster) is particularly advantageous for collection of multiple image sets for quantification. The collected images can be viewed individually or projected into image sets (z series) that clearly depict the general configuration of stained structures in skin and the relationship of nerve fibers to adjacent structures in three dimensions for reconstruction of the innervation pattern. Individual ENFs can be followed for many micrometers and counted where they pierce the basement membrane.

Quantitation of Nerves in a Skin Biopsy and Blister

The confocal z series of images from the biopsy is analyzed using the Neurolucida software package (MicroBrightField, Inc., Colchester, Vt.) to determine density, length, and branching of ENFs. In our laboratory an ENF counting unit is defined as the point identified in a 2-μm optical section where an ENF pierces the basement membrane and enters the epidermis. Accurate detection of the exact point where the ENF penetrates the undulating basement membrane is important, because ENFs often branch below or above the basement membrane, so if the nerve is counted at a point above or below the basement membrane the resultant nerve total will be increased or decreased. Nerve counts are performed and normalized for 16 optical sections in a z series. Quantification data from four confocal image sets of each biopsy are averaged. Additional image sampling may be required for specimens from diabetic subjects in whom the ENFs are distributed in clusters. Most investigators express ENF counts as number per millimeter surface length of epidermis (section thickness must be specified) or per square millimeter surface area of epidermis. The clear visualization of unmyelinated nerves provided by staining for PGP 9.5-ir and imaging with the confocal microscope removes the necessity of using electron microscopy, as is necessary when counting unmyelinated nerves in a nerve biopsy.

Blisters are quantified after immunohistochemical processing. ENFs are counted in blister roofs that have been processed in toto (without sectioning) and mounted en face (bird's eye view). Changes in the pattern of nerve fiber distribution can also be evaluated from the blister preparation. The blister method avoids the time and cost of cutting, staining, and viewing multiple sections. The disadvantage is the absence of dermal nerves and structures in the specimen.

Cutaneous Nerves in Diabetic Neuropathy

Early descriptions of abnormal cutaneous nerves in diabetic patients were from immunohistochemical stained dermal (not epidermal) nerves stained for CGRP, SP, VIP, and NPY. These showed that nerve loss was greater in the patients who had clinical neuropathy. Later studies with PGP 9.5 immunostaining found that cutaneous nerves were often reduced in number in broad association with neurophysiologic test results, in some instances before abnormalities were detected by clinical or neurophysiologic examinations [271]. Improvements in staining and imaging enabled description of a reduction of epidermal nerves in patients with predominantly sensory neuropathy and in those with neuropathy associated with autoimmune deficiency syndrome [272]. Imaging of thick sections of PGP 9.5-immunostained ENFs with the confocal microscope and quantitation of their number, length, and branching with a neuron tracing system demonstrated abnormal ENFs in all stages of diabetic neuropathy [273]. Examples of ENFs in skin biopsies and skin blisters removed from a normal (Fig. 5.**19a,b**) and a diabetic subject (Fig. 5.**19c,d**) demonstrate the reduction in number of ENFs that is common in diabetic subjects. In addition to reduction in ENF number, structural changes such as nerve sprouting, increased branching, and rounded axon swellings have been described in neuropathies [273,266]. These morphologic changes occur in the subepidermal plexus and in the epidermis. They are presumed to be a harbinger of nerve degeneration. Hyperinnervation of epidermis and sweat glands is also described in the proximal limb segments of patients who have neuropathy with distal loss of ENFs. The hyperinnervation is presumed to be secondary to collateral branching as a reactive response to the distal nerve loss. Skin biopsy has been used to confirm the clinical diagnosis of truncal diabetic neuropathy [274].

Advantages of Skin Biopsy/Blister Methods

The skin biopsy is easy to perform, minimally invasive, relatively inexpensive, and has a low incidence of complications. The blister is a less invasive than skin biopsy, nontraumatic, painless, blood-free method of tissue acquisition without anesthesia. The innocuous nature of both procedures increases the probability that patients will consent to removal of one or more skin specimens for diagnosis, to follow progression of disease or to evaluate results of a therapeutic trial. Skin biopsy and blister can reveal abnormalities of nerves in diabetic patients with sensory symptoms when results of other tests are normal (unpublished observations). The syndrome of small-fiber painful neuropathy is a striking illustration of the usefulness of examining epidermal nerves. Whereas clinical examination, nerve conduction, and quantitative sensory tests are often normal, and sural nerve biopsy may not show a reduction of unmyelinated nerve fibers [275], skin biopsy can reveal a moderate to severe reduction of epidermal nerves [266,267].

When and Where to Biopsy/Blister

The time to biopsy is when the question of neuropathy first arises. Unlike nerve biopsy, the minimally invasive nature of the skin biopsy and blister techniques allows the removal of specimens from more than a single location for tissue diagnosis without harming the patient. The first biopsies should be at the site of the patient's symptoms and/or the location of abnormal sensory findings. In symmetric diabetic neuropathy a distal site—the foot or calf—will usually show a reduction of ENFs for diagnosis of neuropathy. In severe neuropathy ENFs may be absent in the foot and even in the calf. In such a case, biopsy of the thigh or an upper extremity location will usually show a reduction in number of ENFs and the morphologic abnormalities previously mentioned.

The ratio of ENF counts in proximal and distal locations has been useful for diagnosis in some cases [276]. In general, ENF loss is more severe and extends more proximally than would be predicted from the severity of symptoms or the results of electrophysiologic and sensory examinations. This distal-to-proximal gradient allows varying degrees of neuropathy in the same person to be studied simultaneously. If the patient is to be followed to detect progression or reversal of neuropathy, the aim is to remove biopsies at planned time intervals from adjacent skin locations where a definite reduction of ENFs has been demonstrated, but where a sufficient number of ENFs remain as a substrate for regeneration.

The range of normal values for the several skin locations that are commonly studied has not been generally agreed, mainly because of differences in methodology [273,276,277]. The density of ENFs in normal skin varies greatly with body location [253,278,279]. Our few observations from skin obtained from children suggest that the density of epidermal nerves is greatest in small children and decreases with increasing body size during maturation. Standardized data concerning the number and morphology of cutaneous nerves from youth to old age have not been collected, and there is so far no agreement as to whether aging results in a reduction of ENFs [276,280].

ENF Density and Sensation

Preliminary work with model systems of nerve degeneration and regeneration is showing a close correlation between nociceptive sensory deficiencies and nerves in biopsy specimens, at least in acute experiments [281,282]. The sensory examination is one of the most important part of the neurologic evaluation of the diabetic patient. Accurate quantitation of sensation is necessary to establish the diagnosis of neuropathy early, when it is presumed to be more amenable to reversal with treatment. Unfortunately, the sensory examination is time-consuming, tedious, and inescapably subjective, and the results in regard to detection and quantitation of small nerve fiber abnormality have been disappointing. It would be advantageous to have a quantitative sensory test that correlates with the ENF content in skin. Toward this end we developed a topical capsaicin model system to study ENF degeneration and correlated it with results of testing for nociceptive sensation. Short-term topical application of capsaicin causes ENF degeneration that, depending upon dosage, progresses slightly deeper than the basement membrane. Heat pain sensation is lost in parallel with ENF loss when tested with a small thermode that has a contact area of 2 or 3 mm diameter [282]. This close relationship was not found when heat pain is tested with a large thermode (900 mm^2) of the type available with commercial instruments [283]. If these findings are substantiated, the small probe thermal stimulator holds promise as a rapid noninvasive method of detecting heat pain sensation and as an indicator of ENF density in persons suspected of having diabetic neuropathy.

Conclusion

Skin biopsy and skin blister techniques are useful for detecting unmyelinated cutaneous nerve involvement in diabetic neuropathy. The techniques are attractive because they are minimally invasive, quantitative, and evaluate the terminal segments of nerves which are often the first affected in diabetic neuropathy. Further development of the immunostaining and quantitation procedures will increase specificity and sensitivity and reduce costs. We anticipate that the methods will be useful for determining progression of neuropathy or reversal with therapy, but these capabilities remain to be tested.

Diabetic Sensorimotor Neuropathy: Clinical Features

Symmetric Distal Polyneuropathy

B. Neundörfer and P.K. Thomas

Definition

Diabetic symmetric distal polyneuropathy (DSDP) is characterized by length-related, distally pronounced distribution of sensory and motor symptoms and signs in patients with manifest diabetes mellitus [284–286].

Clinical Picture

In DSDP, depression and loss of tendon reflexes, sensory loss, and disturbances of the autonomic nervous system are most prominent, but motor deficits may also be present [287–290]. Since many of the patients show involvement of the autonomic functions, it is in fact not admissible to consider DSDP and diabetic autonomic neuropathy as separate entities. However, since disturbances of the autonomic nervous system are treated elsewhere in this volume, we will focus below on describing the symptomatology and diagnosis of somatic neuropathy.

It must be assumed in type I and type 2 diabetic patients with DSDP that there has already been a disorder of glucose metabolism over a long period, mostly over several years before manifestation of neuropathic symptoms and/or deficits [285]. The time of onset of the disease is usually well defined in type 1 diabetes, so that the interval between the beginning of the disease and the first signs of DSDP can be determined relatively precisely. However, this is difficult in type 2 patients, since the diabetes may have been present for many years before diagnosis. This also explains why pathologic findings of neuropathy can already be identified in some of the cases at the time of diagnosis of diabetes mellitus. In particular, the Dyck working group [285,290] has pointed out that DSDP should only be diagnosed when other diabetic complications such as diabetic retinopathy or nephropathy can also be demonstrated. Only in exceptional cases can DSDP be diagnosed in the absence of indications of these other complications of diabetes mellitus. For this purpose, the fundus of the eye should be investigated with dilated pupils, and the total protein in 24-hour urine should be determined or microalbuminuria looked for. In the Rochester Diabetes Population Study, significant correlations of DSDP with retinopathy ($P < 0.001$) and nephropathy ($P = 0.003$) were observed. These correlations could not be demonstrated with other forms of diabetic neuropathy (e. g., diabetic amyotrophy) [290].

The diagnosis of DSDP is based on two elements: (1) on the subjective symptoms of the patients and on the signs found on clinical examination, and (2) on the detection of abnormalities in clinical neurophysiologic tests (quantitative sensory tests, electromyography and nerve conduction studies, and autonomic testing). From this, "staging" of diabetic polyneuropathy developed in which the degree of severity of polyneuropathy is described in five stages [290,291] (see also pages 170–175).

Not every DSDP patient complains of subjective symptoms, so these are not an absolute diagnostic criterion. On the other hand, they are an important indicator that DSDP may be present, especially when they are more severe distally. In a systematic survey of 2829 patients with diabetes mellitus carried out by Harris et al. [292], 30.2% of the patients with type 1 and 36% of the male and 39.5% of the female type 2 patients reported sensory manifestations, whereas these were reported by only 9.8% of the men and 11.8% of the women in a nondiabetic control group. The authors concluded from these results that about 20% of the patients with diabetes mellitus have subjective symptoms indicative of a diabetic neuropathy. In a standardized investigation of a population of diabetic subjects, the Dyck's working group [293,294] found symptomatic polyneuropathy corresponding to stages N2a and N2b in only 13%.

The fiber type affected [295] can be roughly inferred from the symptoms. In irritation of the thickly myelinated, rapidly conducting Aβ fibers which transmit touch-pressure sensitivity as well as vibration and joint position sense, the patients complain of tingling, prickling, formication, a "furry feeling," a feeling that the ends of the limb are compressed or swollen as positive symptoms, and of a feeling of numbness as a negative symptom. With dysfunction of the thinly myelinated Aδ or nonmyelinated C fibers, which conduct pain and temperature as well as autonomic impulses, patients complain of cold and warm paresthesias, most typically "burning feet" syndrome. The pain can be of the most diverse quality and quantity. Autonomic symptoms include orthostatic vertigo, faintness, diarrhea, and disorders of micturition and penile erection. Together with negative symptoms of motor function, these symptoms can be included in the neuropathy symptom score [296,297].

Amongst our own patients [288], 70 (30%) out of 230 patients complained of positive sensory irritation (symptoms), although this figure also includes the patients with an asymmetric distribution pattern. Of the 323 cases reported by Feudell [298], 93 patients (25%) also reported paresthesias. Of the 100 patients of Gibbels and Schliep [299], 49 described symptoms in terms of superficial sensitivity. It is noteworthy that the latter mainly occurred distally and that they were much more frequently in the symmetric pattern expected in DSDP. Admittedly, when there was no systematic survey, paresthesias in terms of proprioceptive sensation were reported in only 18%. Of Bischoff's 200 patients [300] with diabetic neuropathy, 67 complained of paresthesias and 68 of dysesthesia (feelings of numbness and a cotton wool feeling, "rubber soles," a furry feeling). However, no differences were shown between patients with symmetric and those with asymmetric distribution patterns.

Fifty-nine (25%) out of 230 of our own cases complained of spontaneous pain [301]. Of the 100 patients reported by Gibbels and Schliep [299], 59 patients complained of spontaneous pain, distal pain being very much more frequent than proximal pain. Amongst Bischoff's 200 patients [300], as many as 78% reported pain. Of these, 25% complained of the burning pain typical of diabetic polyneuropathy. Very divergent figures for pain are reported in the literature. These range from the 33% reported by Bonkalo [302], 49% by Feudell [298], and 78% by Daeppen [303] to the 88.7% by Gomensoro [304]. Whereas Bischoff [300] mainly reported on pain near to the trunk, most authors emphasized that pain was more severe distally in the lower limbs. Besides the typical burning pain (burning feet, burning hands), dull diffuse pain and lancinating, stabbing, boring pain may also be involved. These pains sometimes increase and subside, becoming worse at night.

As signs of an irritation of motor Aα fibers, the patients also frequently complained of positive motor symptoms. These were mainly cramps, and in some cases also myokymia and fasciculation. In our own patients [301], this was the case in 5%, as compared to 8% of Feudell's patients [298]. In response to nonsystematic questioning, 12% of the 100 patients of Gibbels and Schliep [299] reported corresponding symptoms, as did 21.5% of Bischoff's 200 patients [300]. However, Mayne [305] was unable to detect any difference in frequency in a comparison between a group of diabetic subjects and a group of nondiabetics.

In the neurologic examination, a depression or loss of the tendon reflexes of the lower limbs is one of the earliest and most frequent findings in DSDP. This finding is not uncommonly the first clue leading to diagnosis of diabetes mellitus [306]. Among our own patients, the Achilles tendon reflexes were lost in almost all cases, and they were absent in 90% of the patients of Gibbels and Schliep [299]. With one exception, the Achilles tendon reflexes were affected, the patellar tendon reflexes were reduced in 65%, and the reflexes in the arms were involved very much less often: the biceps tendon reflex in 23% and the triceps tendon reflex in 25%. Of Bischoff's 200 patients with diabetic neuropathy [300], 153 had reduced reflexes. The Achilles tendon reflexes were involved most often. The importance of the loss of the Achilles tendon reflex for the diagnosis of DSDP is also underscored by the fact that this finding was included in the minimum criteria for diagnosis of diabetic polyneuropathy by Dyck's working group [285].

Sensory disturbances in DSDP show a length-related pattern [285, 287–289,299,300,307]. They range from predominant involvement of the large fibers (large-fiber neuropathy) to predominant involvement of the small fibers (small-fiber neuropathy). Disturbances of vibration and joint position sense at the toes and of light touch sensitivity are predominantly found in the first type. When the deficits are substantial, sensory ataxia (diabetic pseudotabes) results. A predominant sensory loss mainly affecting pain and temperature sensitivity is typical of the latter type. However, usually a mixture of the two subtypes is found. Following the principle of the length-related pattern, the deficits begin in the toes, from where they spread to the rest of the feet and the lower legs, then later to the hands and forearms, to the thighs, and to the upper arms. The delimitation follows the pattern of socks, stockings, and gloves. In more severe cases the anterior midline of the abdomen is affected. The sensory loss later spreads laterally around the trunk.

In our own patients, vibration sense was affected most frequently (58%), followed by disturbances of joint position sense (40%) [301]. Amongst the 100 patients with diabetic neuropathy reported by Gibbels and Schliep [299], 78% had disturbances of superficial sensibility. The occurrence of sensory disturbances on the arms depended to a certain extent on the presence of more extensive signs in the legs, since sensory disturbances extending up to the elbow joint were observed only when in the legs they reached at least the thigh. In occasional cases, they also extended to the trunk. In Bischoff's patients [300], 124 out of 200 patients had a sensory disturbance, in most cases loss of vibration sense (52%). Other authors arrived at similar or indeed higher figures with regard to pallhypesthesia or pallanesthesia: Hirson et al. [308] found 50%, Daeppen [303] 78%, and Collens et al. [309] actually reported 93%. Bischoff [300] pointed out that sensory disturbances may also show a certain patchy distribution. Very rarely, the sensory disturbances extend all over the body [310–312].

Motor deficits are not conspicuous in DSDP [289,301,307]. Muscle weakness was found in 72% of the cases reported by Gibbels and Schliep [299]. However, muscle weakness occurred mainly in patients with asymmetric manifestations, in whom its incidence was twice as high as that of sensory disturbances. Muscle weakness was generally more pronounced distally, particularly affecting the muscles innervated by the peroneal nerves. Proximal muscles may also be affected; weakness can then be demonstrated mainly in the region of the hip flexor and knee extensor muscles [299]. Paresis in the upper limbs is rare in DSDP and then mainly involves the small muscles of the hands.

There is a close correlation between DSDP and autonomic neuropathy. The figures reported in the literature vary between 7% and 97% when abnormalities are taken on the basis of cardiovascular tests [313]. The wide divergence is explained by the number of tests required to detect involvement of the autonomic nervous system. Autonomic disorders are rarely found before DSDP becomes symptomatic [314]. In a small-scale study comprising 30 patients with diabetic nephropathy, Tackmann et al. [315] found that almost all patients with symptomatic autonomic neuropathy (16 out of 17 patients) also had somatic neuropathy, whereas in patients with sensorimotor neuropathy autonomic neuropathy was much rarer (16 out of 27 patients). However, there are reports from time to time that disorders of cardiac, vasomotor, and sudomotor function [316–319] can be detected in the absence of symptomatic polyneuropathy using sensitive laboratory tests.

For further details, especially regarding specific test methods, the reader should refer to the sections covering those specific topics. It must be emphasized that the afferent nerve fibers running parallel to the autonomic visceral fibers may also be involved. Lack of pain perception in the heart in cardiac ischemia may have appreciable consequences. For electrodiagnostic evaluation and quantitative sensory testing as well as treatment.

Differential Diagnosis

The clinical features of diabetic sensory polyneuropathy are relatively nonspecific, and as diabetes mellitus is a common disorder, the chances of a neuropathy from another cause developing coincidentally in a diabetic patient are not inconsiderable.

Amyloid neuropathy is important in the differential diagnosis of diabetic polyneuropathy, particularly since autonomic symptoms occur in both. Amyloid neuropathy usually begins with small-fiber involvement, giving rise to predominant pain and temperature sensory loss, often with spontaneous pain, accompanied by early evidence of autonomic failure. In immunoglobulin light chain (AL) amyloidosis, the amyloid is derived from monoclonal immunoglobulin light chains secondary to multiple myeloma, malignant lymphoma, or Waldenström macroglobulinemia, or to a nonmalignant immunocyte dyscrasia. Associated constitutional symptoms such as malaise, fatigue, and weight loss may be present together with purpura, peripheral edema, and hepatosplenomegaly, and symptoms related to renal or cardiovascular involvement. Of the hereditary amyloid neuropathies, only those related to mutations in the transthyretin (TTR) gene enter into the differential diagnosis. The features of the neuropathy in itself are similar to those of AL amyloidosis, but there may be a positive family history. Diagnosis can be made by sequencing the TTR gene. If there is doubt, nerve biopsy may be undertaken to look for the presence of amyloid deposits and to perform immunostaining for TTR. In both AL and hereditary amyloid neuropathy the peripheral nerves may be enlarged.

The hereditary sensory neuropathies usually develop at a younger age, but type 1 hereditary sensory and autonomic neuropathy can present in adult life. Again it begins as a predominantly small-fiber neuropathy, which may be painful, but autonomic features are only trivial. It can present with painless foot ulcers. Inheritance is autosomal dominant in pattern, but in the absence of a family history diagnosis can be difficult as confirmation by DNA analysis in individual cases is not available. The disorder has been mapped to chromosome 9q21.1-22.3 [320] but the gene has not yet been cloned.

Immune-mediated neuropathies are important in the differential diagnosis. Sjögren sensory ganglionitis is usually a large-fiber ataxic sensory disorder with xerophthalmia and xerostomia, but it can present as a generalized nonspecific sensory neuronopathy. Extractable nuclear antigen (ENA) antibodies are usually detectable, and the diagnosis can be confirmed by lip biopsy looking for inflammatory infiltrates around submucous salivary glands. Disorders giving rise to necrotizing vasculitis are commonly mainly motor in pattern, but nonsystemic vasculitis affecting the peripheral nervous system [321] can in some cases be predominantly sensory, as can neuropathy related to rheumatoid disease and systemic lupus erythematosus. The latter two disorders can be investigated by checking for inflammatory and serological markers, but autoantibodies are not usually detectable in nonsystemic vasculitis. If vasculitis is suspected, combined nerve and muscle biopsy is merited.

Paraneoplastic neuropathy can be mainly or purely sensory. If related to small-cell carcinoma of the lung, the presence of antineuronal (anti-Hu) antibodies is helpful diagnostically. Otherwise screening for underlying malignancy is required. A neuropathy related to a benign monoclonal paraprotein can be purely sensory or it can be mixed sensorimotor. In neuropathies associated with an IgM paraprotein a postural tremor is often present, less frequently in association with IgG paraproteins. In most cases patients are aged over 50 years. The neuropathy is frequently demyelinating with markedly reduced nerve conduction velocity.

Chronic inflammatory demyelinating polyneuropathy (CIDP) is probably more common in patients with diabetes [322]. This is usually a predominantly motor syndrome, but purely sensory cases are encountered. Despite this, motor nerve conduction velocity in such cases may be reduced. If the diagnosis is in doubt, nerve biopsy to look for inflammatory infiltrates and examination of the cerebrospinal fluid to check for an elevated protein concentration and the presence of oligoclonal IgG bands can be helpful.

An important diagnosis not to be missed is vitamin B_{12} deficiency. This gives rise to a purely sensory neuropathy, mainly affecting large-fiber function. Contrary to the sequence in diabetic polyneuropathy, the upper limbs may be affected initially, with numbness and paresthesias in the hands and sometimes the occurrence of Lhermitte's sign. Evidence of corticospinal tract dysfunction may also be present. Megaloblastic anemia does not always coexist, and the diagnosis is made by measuring serum vitamin B_{12} levels and uptake and checking for parietal cell or intrinsic factor antibodies.

Focal and Multifocal Neuropathies

P.K. Thomas

Although some earlier surveys led to the view that no subdivisions were possible within the totality of diabetic neuropathy [323–325], it is now clear that a variety of distinct syndromes affecting the peripheral nervous system may be encountered (see pages 175–177). A broad distinction into two groups is possible: symmetric polyneuropathies and multifocal neuropathies. This chapter will consider the latter group. It must be emphasized that mixed syndromes are not infrequent, so a patient with a symmetric sensory polyneuropathy, for example, may show a superimposed focal peripheral nerve lesion.

Cranial Neuropathies

Although there have been occasional reports of lesions affecting the lower cranial nerves in diabetic patients, their infrequency makes it difficult to determine whether these were chance associations. The cranial nerves most often affected are those to the external ocular muscles and the facial nerve, where it seems likely that there may be a definite causal relationship. Nevertheless, even for these nerves, the association has not been established by population-based or case-control studies.

Ocular Nerve Lesions

In a large series of cases, incorporating previous series by Rucker [326] and Rush and Younge [327], Richards et al. [328] assembled 4278 examples of acquired lesions of the third, fourth, and sixth cranial nerves, 103 of which were related to diabetes. Single series of cases of diabetic ophthalmoplegia have been reported by Goldstein and Cogan [329], Zorilla and Kozak [330], Teuscher and Meienberg [331], and Watanabe et al [332]. The abducens nerve appears to be the one most frequently involved, followed by the oculomotor, and lastly by the trochlear ([328] and P.J. Watkins, personal communication). The older age groups are the most commonly affected. Of the 24 patients documented by Zorilla and Kozak [330], all except three were aged over 50 years a the time of onset of symptoms. Occurrence in childhood is rare [333]. Recurrent or multiple lesions may be encountered [330,334].

The onset of symptoms is usually abrupt, with diplopia related to paresis of abduction of the eye on the affected side in sixth nerve lesions. In third nerve lesions there is accompanying ptosis and difficulty in upward, medial, and downward deviation of the eye; characteristically, there is pupillary sparing, although partial iridoplegia with pupillary dilatation occurs in a proportion of cases [329]. Complete iridoplegia is rare. The onset may be painless, but is associated with pain in about half the cases [330]. The pain may antecede the paralysis by a few days and is usually felt behind or above the eye. It is commonly aching in character, but can be intense. The pain usually clears within a few days. The prognosis for recovery of the ophthalmoplegia is good, this taking place over days or weeks. Aberrant reinnervation is rare.

The time course of the onset and recovery would be consistent with an ischemic lesion that gives rise to focal demyelination and which recovers by remyelination. In a pathologic study by Raff et al. [335] in a patient with an acute diabetic third nerve lesion, a focal lesion with demyelination and preservation of axonal integrity distal to the site of the lesion was found. This was situated between the point of entry into the nerve of two nutrient arteries. A somewhat puzzling feature is that ischemic lesions usually give rise to axonal loss rather than demyelination [336]. A possible explanation may be found in the experimental study by Nukada and McMorran [337], who showed that reperfusion injury in peripheral nerve gives rise to focal demyelination.

It has been suggested, on the basis of CT findings, that a proportion of acute isolated diabetic third nerve palsies are due to mesencephalic rather than peripheral lesions [338]. It is not certain whether the changes observed were primary or whether they could be reactive to a peripheral insult secondary to retrograde changes affecting the nucleus and surrounding glia.

Further questions are the explanation for the pain in diabetic ophthalmoplegia, discussed on pages 208–211, and pupillary sparing in third cranial nerve lesions. The latter is possibly attributable to the fact that the pupillomotor fibers in the third nerve are located superficially [339,340] and ischemia tends to affect the center of the fascicles.

Facial Nerve Lesions

In a study in Israel, Korczyn [341] found that of a series of 130 patients with an acute facial palsy, 66% showed abnormal glucose tolerance, whereas Aminoff and Miller [342] found only 6% among 70 patients with Bell palsy in London. Other series have reported intermediate values: 10.7% [343], 39% [344], 48.8% [345]. Acute facial palsy developing in diabetic subjects appears to display similar features to those seen in nondiabetic patients, although a lower rate of impairment of taste was noted by Pecket and Schattner [344]. This could indicate that the site of the lesion in diabetics is more distal, being located below the chorda tympani branch or that there is a difference in pathology, with relative sparing of the smaller nerve fibers. Takahashi and Sobue [346] considered that the prognosis for recovery was more favorable than in nondiabetic subjects.

Diabetic Truncal Radiculoneuropathy

The term "radiculoneuropathy" is employed here as it remains uncertain whether the pathology lies in the spinal nerve roots or the spinal nerves or in the nerve trunks. The condition usually presents in middle or later life and may be observed both in type 1 and type 2 diabetics. Males appear to be affected more often than females. In the series reported by Stewart [347] all seven patients were male, as were the six patients documented by Chaudhuri et al. [348], all of whom were aged over 50 years. It can be the presenting feature in type 2 diabetes. Schulz [349], Wessely and Schnaberth [350], Ellenberg [351] and Sun and Streib [352] produced early reports of such patients.

The onset is usually with pain, as was noted by Schulz [353], and was present in the cases reported by Longstreth and Newcomer [354], Child and Yates [355], and Chaudhuri et al [348]. The pain, which is characteristically worse at night, may be aching or burning in quality and felt in a girdle-like distribution. It is usually unilateral, but may be bilateral, and can also be felt in the back. There may be focal contact hyperesthesia experienced when the skin touches clothing or bedclothes. The onset may be associated with profound weight loss, sometimes as much as 30 kg [348]. In some cases there is accompanying weakness of the anterior abdominal wall, either unilateral or bilateral, which may simulate a hernia [348,356–358].

The pattern of sensory loss on examination is highly variable. None may be detectable, or it can involve combinations of several adjacent dermatomes or territories of intercostal nerves, either unilaterally or bilaterally.

The course is usually one of spontaneous recovery over some months, but recurrences are possible, sometimes as many as six [347]. There may also be evidence of an accompanying proximal lower limb neuropathy (diabetic amyotrophy), detected at the time or subsequently [359, 360].

No observations are available as to the underlying pathology, but the abrupt onset and subsequent improvement are consistent with an ischemic event. The coexistence with proximal lower limb diabetic neuropathy suggests that the underlying mechanism is the same. Electromyography shows evidence of denervation [352,361]. From the distribution of the sensory loss, Stewart [347] concluded that in some cases the lesion must be confined to the posterior primary rami of spinal nerves or sited in intercostal nerves or their branches.

Lumbosacral Radiculoplexus Neuropathy

This syndrome, originally recognized by Bruns [362] and others in the latter part of the nineteenth century, has been given a wide variety of labels, none of which is entirely satisfactory. These include "diabetic myelopathy" [363], "diabetic amyotrophy" [359], "femoral neuropathy" [364], and "proximal diabetic neuropathy" [365]. The term adopted here acknowledges the fact that the pathology affects both the spinal roots and the lumbosacral plexus, and that there is involvement of the peripheral nerve trunks.

Like diabetic truncal radiculoneuropathy, that affecting the lumbosacral plexus is commoner after the middle of life and is more frequent in males [366,367]. It can be the presenting feature in late-onset type 2 diabetes. Onset is often ushered in by pain felt proximally in the legs, the perineum, or the back. It is usually aching in quality and worse at night. This is followed by proximal muscle weakness, which may be unilateral or bilateral but asymmetric. In unilateral cases it may develop on the opposite side within a few weeks after recovery has begun on the side affected first. Distal lower limb muscles may also be affected, particularly the anterolateral group, or the weakness may be generalized ("diabetic paraplegia"). Accompanying sensory loss, usually noticed over the anterior thighs, is not prominent. Spontaneous paresthesias and contact hyperesthesia of the skin may be experienced [366].

Spontaneous improvement occurs [366], but not all patients recover fully [367]. Relapses can be encountered, occasionally after long intervals [363,364].

Muscle biopsy demonstrates evidence of denervation and reinnervation with grouped fiber atrophy and fiber type grouping. In an autopsy study, Raff et al. [335] reported the presence of multiple small infarcts in the nerves to affected muscles, but it was later realized that these were Renaut bodies, a normal structure found in peripheral nerves [368]. A single occluded vessel was detected in the epineurium, and a focal inflammatory infiltrate was present adjacent to another epineurial vessel.

In subsequent studies on patients with diabetic lumbosacral radiculoplexus neuropathy, Said et al. [369] and Llewelyn et al. [370] reported evidence of inflammatory changes, including epineurial vasculitis, in nerve biopsies from the intermediate cutaneous nerve of the thigh. Such changes were found in about one-third of the cases. There was no evidence of systemic vasculitis, and these inflammatory changes were seen in patients who showed spontaneous recovery. It is of interest that in some cases the pain unexpectedly disappeared following nerve biopsy [371]. It is also of interest that Bradley et al. [372] reported a series of six patients with painful lumbosacral plexopathy, three of whom had diabetes. In all, sural nerve biopsy, in addition to demonstrating axonal degeneration, showed epineurial perivascular inflammatory

Axonal Atrophy

The possibility that axonal atrophy could be involved in the generation of pain in diabetic neuropathy was raised by Thomas and Scadding [466] and a correlation between the presence of axonal atrophy and the occurrence of pain was reported by Britland et al. [467] in diabetic neuropathy. After nerve transection, axonal atrophy takes place central to the site of axotomy [468,469]. Following reconnection with appropriate peripheral target structures, axon diameter proximal to the site of the axotomy is restored [470], but the larger myelinated fibers regain their conduction velocity more rapidly than Aδ fibers [471]. An effect on sensation could conceivably result from an abnormal patterning of impulses. Nevertheless, Sugimura and Dyck [472] and Llewelyn et al. [458] both reported that axonal atrophy is not a feature of diabetic neuropathy.

Ephaptic Transmission

Ephaptic, i. e., nonsynaptic, electrotonic transmission between sympathetic efferent and nociceptive afferents was adduced as the explanation for the pain of causalgia following nerve injury [473] and to account for its relief by sympathectomy. It can be shown to occur as a transient phenomenon after mechanical injury [474], but it is not conspicuous at longer intervals [475]. There is electrophysiologic evidence for its occurrence between peripheral motor nerve fibers [476,477], and it probably takes place between demyelinated central nervous system fibers in the trigeminal root entry zone in trigeminal neuralgia. Currently there is no positive evidence for its occurrence in diabetic neuropathy.

Abnormal Behavior of Dorsal Root Ganglion Cells

Axotomy of peripheral sensory nerve fibers, even if undertaken distally, can result in spontaneous impulse generation by dorsal root ganglion cells of both large and small diameter [478]. In diabetic sensory polyneuropathy there is a distal degeneration of axons of a dying-back type [479], with relative preservation of dorsal root ganglion cells. Possibly, therefore, this could result in the generation of ectopic impulses by smaller ganglion cells that signal pain. On the other hand, diabetic sensory polyneuropathy may be a central-peripheral distal axonopathy with rostral degeneration of fibers entering the spinal cord as well as distal degeneration peripherally. This would mean that the dorsal root ganglion cells would be disconnected centrally and ectopic impulse generation would not be transmitted to central nervous system pathways. This caveat also applies to the question of the regenerating axonal sprouts discussed earlier.

Peripheral Blood Flow

An unexplained relationship between painful diabetic neuropathy and peripheral blood flow was uncovered by Archer et al. [480]. They compared patients with and without pain. Blood flow was increased in both groups, presumably as a consequence of autonomic neuropathy, but it could only be reduced by sympathetic stimulation in those with pain, when it was accompanied by a lessening in the severity of the pain. Reduced arteriovenous shunting was suggested as a possible explanation.

Glycemic Control

The relationship between blood glucose concentrations and pain thresholds and tolerance was examined by Morley et al. [481]. In acute experiments, subjects with diabetes displayed lower pain thresholds and lower pain tolerance than normoglycemic individuals, and glucose infusion in nondiabetic subjects reduced their pain thresholds and tolerance. Boulton et al. [482] found that continuous subcutaneous insulin infusions reduced spontaneous pain in patients with severe painful diabetic neuropathy. Hyperglycemia reduces the antinociceptive effect of morphine [483], raising the possibility of an influence of glucose on opiate receptors.

The peripheral nerves in streptozotocin-diabetic rats are hypoxic [484]. In nondiabetic rats Schneider et al. [485] found that hyperglycemic but not normoglycemic hypoxia gave rise to alterations in fast K^+ conductance and afterpotentials, related to axoplasmic acidification. Such abnormalities could give rise to positive sensory symptoms including pain through the generation of ectopic impulses.

CNS Change Secondary to Damage to the Peripheral Nervous System

A number of changes in the central nervous system resulting from peripheral nerve damage have been identified in animals and have been adduced as possibly related to the occurrence of pain in neuropathies, although these extrapolations have been subject to criticism [454].

- Surround inhibition. The activity of dorsal horn cells may be altered by afferents that have an inhibitory surround effect on the excitatory receptive field [486]. Reduced activity in such afferents would lead to reduced surround inhibition. It could explain the prominent contact hyperesthesia that is a notable feature of acute painful diabetic neuropathy [487].
- Presynaptic inhibition. Afferent volleys to the spinal cord dorsal horn cause prolonged depolarization of the terminals of the fibers transmitting the volleys, with consequent presynaptic inhibition [488]. This

effect can be abolished by nerve injury and constitutes a possible mechanism for neuropathic pain.

- Postsynaptic inhibition. This has been implicated in the dorsal horn gate control theory of pain advanced by Melzack and Wall [489]. In this theory impulses arriving in large-caliber dorsal root afferents have a facilitatory effect on substantia gelatinosa neurons that, in turn, give rise to presynaptic inhibition on a transmission pathway signaling pain. Impulses arriving in small-caliber nociceptor afferents, in contrast, inhibit the substantia gelatinosa neurons and have a facilitatory effect on the transmission neurons. The suggestion was made that activity in the large afferent fibers closed the dorsal horn gating mechanism and inhibited pain. Loss of such afference would be expected to lead to pain. Although gating clearly does take place in the dorsal horn, this theory is an oversimplification. As already pointed out, selective large-fiber neuropathies are not painful [455].

Treatment of Neuropathic Pain

D. Ziegler

Introduction

Neurogenic pain is defined as pain due to dysfunction of the peripheral or central nervous system, in the absence of nociceptor (nerve terminal) stimulation by trauma or disease [490]. Other terms used to describe some forms of neurogenic pain include "neuropathic pain," "deafferentation pain," and "central pain." Neurogenic pain is common, accounting for at least 25% of the patients attending most pain clinics. When all categories of neurogenic pain syndromes are taken into account, there are probably over 550 000 cases in the United Kingdom population at any one time, giving a prevalence of about 1%. The incidence of neurogenic pain increases with age, accounting for one-third of all pain clinic patients aged over 65 years and one-half of those aged over 70 [490].

Pain is a subjective symptom of major clinical importance as it is often this that motivates patients to seek health care. Pain is often associated with disability and is suggested as an important factor affecting quality of life [491]. The International Association for the Study of Pain defines pain as chronic if it persists for more than three months [492]. People with diabetes experience more chronic pain than the nondiabetic population. One study found that 25% of diabetic patients had chronic pain, compared to 15% of nondiabetic subjects [493]. The difference is largely attributable to pain associated with polyneuropathy. Diabetic polyneuropathy is encountered in at least one-third of the patients with diabetes mellitus [494]. Neuropathic symptoms are present in 15–20% of the diabetic patients [494,495], and 7.5% of all diabetic patients experience chronic neuropathic pain [493]. Pain associated with diabetic neuropathy exerts a substantial impact on the quality of life, particularly by causing considerable interference in sleep and enjoyment of life [496]. Despite this significant impact, one-quarter of the diabetic patients and one-fifth of the nondiabetic subjects had no treatment for their pain in a survey dating from 1990 [493].

Neuropathic Pain

According to Asbury and Fields [497] neuropathic pain may be subdivided into two types. The superficial *dysesthetic* or *deafferentation pain* is described as burning, tingling, raw, searing, crawling, drawing, and electric of variable constancy, i. e., intermittent, jabbing, lancinating, or shooting. It has been attributed to a cutaneous or subcutaneous distribution and may be linked to increased firing of damaged or abnormally excitable nociceptive fibers, particularly sprouting, regenerating fibers [497]. Dysesthetic pain is a common manifestation in diabetic polyneuropathy, particularly in those patients whose small-fiber modalities (cutaneous pin prick and temperature sensation and autonomic function) are disproportionately affected [497]. For the deep *nerve trunk pain*, descriptors such as "aching," occasionally "knifelike," and "tender" have been used. It is usually continuous, but waxes and wanes. Its hypothetical basis includes increased firing due to physiologic stimulation of endings of nociceptive afferents that innervate the nerve sheaths themselves (nervi nervorum) [497]. In addition, several other mechanisms have been proposed: (1) spontaneous activity and increased mechanosensitivity near the cell body of damaged afferents in the dorsal root ganglion; (2) loss of segmental inhibition of large myelinated fibers and small unmyelinated C fibers (modified gate control hypothesis); and (3) ectopic impulses generated from demyelinated patches of myelinated axons [498]. Examples of nerve trunk pain include spinal root compression, brachial neuritis, and neuritis of leprosy reactions. Asbury and Fields [497] emphasized that both types of pain rarely occur in pure form and that most neuropathies associated with pain will manifest some mixture of these two types of painful experience.

In a model for the treatment of chronic painful diabetic neuropathy, Pfeifer et al. [498] suggested *muscular pain* as a third type of pain that is described as a cramping, aching, muscle tenderness, or a "drawing sensation." The muscle cramping and spasms may be secondary to injury to motor nerves or attributable to a reflex loop ("Livingston's vicious circle"), where a nociceptive input activates the motoneuron within the spinal cord, leading to muscle spasm that in turn activates the muscle nociceptors and feedback to the spinal cord to sustain the spasm [498].

Regarding the origin of neuropathic pain, a recent case of typical neuropathic pain that developed 44 years after limb amputation in both the amputated and the intact limbs with the diagnosis of type 2 diabetes suggests that the origin may be rostral to peripheral nerves [499]. According to Thomas and Scadding [500], the putative mechanisms of pain in diabetic neuropathy include the following: nerve trunk pain, sensitization of nociceptor endings, active axonal degeneration, damage to Aδ and C fibers, neuroma properties (ectopic impulse generation from regenerating axon sprouts, ephaptic transmission), fiber shrinkage, ectopic impulse generation from dorsal root ganglion cells after interruption of axons signaling pain, changes in peripheral blood flow, modulation of pain threshold by the glycemic state ("hyperglycemic neuropathy"), and changes in the central nervous system secondary to peripheral nerve damage (reduced surround and presynaptic inhibition, deafferentation of dorsal horn neurons). This variety of possible underlying mechanisms of pain implies that different approaches to treatment may be required.

Clinical Features of Painful Diabetic Neuropathies

The most widely used classification of diabetic neuropathy has been proposed by Thomas [501], who differentiates between diffuse symmetric polyneuropathies on the one hand and focal and multifocal neuropathies on the other (see pages 175–177). Pain may develop in both of these forms, in which it can become one of the most unpleasant features, of variable nature and distribution.

Diffuse Polyneuropathies

The term "hyperglycemic neuropathy" has been used to describe sensory symptoms in poorly controlled diabetic patients that are rapidly reversible following institution of near-normoglycemia [501]. The most frequent form is the *distal sensory symmetric polyneuropathy*, commonly associated with autonomic involvement. The onset is insidious, and in the absence of intervention the course is chronic and progressive [502]. Persistent or episodic pain may be present in these patients, predominantly in the feet. In a recent clinical survey of 105 patients with painful polyneuropathy, the following locations of pain were most frequent: feet (96%), balls of feet (69%), toes (67%), dorsum of foot (54%), hands (39%), plantum of foot (37%), calves (37%), and heels (32%). The pain was most often described by the patients as "burning/hot," "electric," "sharp," "achy," and "tingling," and was worse at night time and when patients were tired or stressed [496]. The average pain intensity was moderate, approximately 5.75/10 on a 0–10 scale, with the "least" and "most" pain 3.6/10 and 6.9/10, respectively [496]. Allodynia (pain due to a stimulus which does not normally cause pain, e. g., stroking) may occur. The symptoms may be accompanied by sensory loss in a glove-and-stocking distribution, but patients with severe pain may have few clinical signs. Pain may persist over several years [503], causing considerable disability and impaired quality of life in some patients [496], whereas it remits partially or completely in others [504,505] despite further deterioration in small-fiber function [506]. Pain remission tends to be associated with sudden metabolic change, short duration of pain or diabetes, preceding weight loss, and less severe sensory loss [504,505].

Acute painful neuropathy has been described as a separate clinical entity [506]. The onset is associated with and preceded by precipitous and severe weight loss. The pain is of a continuous burning quality and experienced predominantly in the distal parts of the legs. Cutaneous contact discomfort (hyperalgesia) is often a troublesome feature, while motor function is preserved and sensory loss may be only slight, being greater for thermal than for vibration sensation. Depression and impotence are constant features. The weight loss has been shown to respond to adequate glycemic control, and the severe manifestations subsided within ten months in all cases. No recurrences were observed after follow-up periods of up to six years [507]. The syndrome of acute painful neuropathy seems to be equivalent to "diabetic cachexia" as described by Ellenberg [507]. It has also been described in girls with anorexia nervosa and diabetes in association with weight loss [508].

The term "insulin neuritis" was used by Caravati [509] to describe a case with precipitation of acute painful neuropathy several weeks following the institution of insulin treatment (treatment-induced neuropathy). Sural nerve biopsy shows signs of chronic neuropathy with prominent regenerative activity [510] as well as epineurial arteriovenous shunting and a fine network of vessels, resembling the new vessels of the retina, which may lead to a steal effect rendering the endoneurium ischemic [511]. This may happen in an analogous to the transient deterioration of a preexisting retinopathy following rapid improvement in glycemic control. Painful symptoms recover slowly with continued near-normoglycemic control.

Short-term changes in blood glucose do not appear to play a major role in neuropathic pain. Marked fluctuations in spontaneous neuropathic pain within several hours were not associated with significant changes in blood glucose concentrations. Furthermore, the induction of acute hyperglycemia for one hour did not alter the heat pain threshold in diabetic patients without symptomatic neuropathy [512].

Focal and Multifocal Neuropathies

Most of the focal and multifocal neuropathies tend to occur in long-term diabetic patients of middle age or older. The outlook for most of them is for recovery, either partial or complete, and for eventual resolution of the pain that frequently accompanies them. With this in mind, physicians should always maintain an optimistic outlook in dealing with patients with these afflictions [513]. Focal lesions of the third cranial nerve (diabetic ophthalmoplegia) are painful in about 50% of cases [514]. The onset is usually abrupt. The pain is felt behind and above the eye, and at times precedes the ptosis and diplopia (with sparing of pupillary function) by several days [501]. Oculomotor findings reach their nadir within a day or at most a few days, persist for several weeks, and then begin gradually to improve. Full resolution is the rule and generally takes place within three to five months [513]. Focal lesions affecting the limb nerves, most commonly the ulnar, median, radial, and peroneal, may be painful, particularly if of acute onset, as may entrapment neuropathies such as the carpal tunnel syndrome, which is associated with painful paresthesias [501].

Pain is nearly universal in the syndrome of asymmetric lower limb proximal motor neuropathy (synonyms: Bruns-Garland syndrome, diabetic amyotrophy, proximal diabetic neuropathy, diabetic lumbosacral plexopathy, ischemic mononeuropathy multiplex, femoral-sciatic neuropathy, femoral neuropathy). Characteristically, it is deep, aching, constant, and severe, invariably worse at night, and may have a burning, raw quality. It is usually not frankly dysesthetic and cutaneous. Frequently, pain is first experienced in the lower back or buttock on the affected side, or may be felt as extending from hip to knee. Although severe and tenacious, the pain of proximal motor neuropathy has a good prognosis. Concurrent distal sensory polyneuropathy is frequently present. Weight loss is also a frequently associated feature and may be as much as 16–18 kg. The weight is generally regained during the recovery phase [513].

Diabetic truncal neuropathy (thoracoabdominal neuropathy or radiculopathy) presents with an abrupt onset, with pain or dysesthesias as the heralding feature. Pain has been described as deep, aching, or boring, but also the descriptors "jabbing," "burning," "sensitive skin," or "tearing" have been used. The neuropathy is almost always unilateral or predominantly so. As a result, the pain felt in the chest or the abdomen may be confused with pain of pulmonary, cardiac, or gastrointestinal origin. Sometimes it may have a radicular or girdling quality, half encircling the trunk in a root-like distribution. Pain may be felt in one or several dermatomal distributions, and almost universally it is worst at night. Rarely, abdominal muscle herniation may occur, predominantly in middle-aged men, involving three to five adjacent nerve roots between T6 and T12 [515].The time from first symptom to the peak of the pain syndrome is often just a few days, although occasionally spread of the pain to adjacent dermatomes may continue for weeks or even months. Weight loss of 7–18 kg occurs in more than 50% of the cases. The course of truncal neuropathy is favorable, and pain subsides within months, with a maximum of 1.5–2 years [513].

Measures of Neuropathic Pain

Quantitative assessment of pain is a challenging problem. As R. Melzack has put it [516]: "Because pain is a private personal experience, it is impossible for us to know precisely what someone else's pain feels like." An important consequence of this simple statement is that there is no objective unit and no external "gold standard" for measuring clinical pain. In fact, pain is the result of a complex process involving neurophysiologic and psychologic mechanisms [517]. It has been shown that factors such as cultural variables can affect the perception of pain and its expression. Individual psychologic attitudes and communication factors can influence the description of pain and the rating of its intensity by the patient [517]. During the last 20 years, a number of reliable and valid measures for assessing chronic pain syndromes and evaluating treatment have been proposed and tested. Because of the multidisciplinary nature of the field, these measures have been derived from physiologic, psychologic (emotional, cognitive, and behavioral), sociocultural, and economic studies [518]. The following methods are being used in trials evaluating treatment effects on neuropathic pain in diabetic patients.

Visual Analog and Verbal Descriptor Scales

A visual analog scale (VAS) is a straight line, the ends of which are defined as the extreme limits of the sensation or response to be measured. It has been shown that the VAS is a satisfactory method for measuring pain or pain relief. When assessing the response to treatment, it is better to use a pain relief scale than to measure pain. With a pain relief scale, all patients start at the same baseline and all have the same amount of potential response [519].

A verbal descriptor scale (VDS) is a visual analog scale with descriptive terms placed at intervals along the line. The descriptors may assist patients in deciding the position of their scores (especially for those who have no experience of pain measurement), and make different patients more likely to record the same degree of severity in the same position. Among different types of VDSs, a horizontal type with the words spread out along the whole length of the line performed best. The failure rate was slightly lower with the VDS than with the VAS [519].

One way to ensure adequate sensitivity for analgesic trials is to test the intervention in patients who have pain of moderate to severe intensity. A recent study has shown that 85% of the patients reporting moderate pain scored greater than 30 mm (mean: 49 mm) on a 100-mm VAS, and 85% of those reporting severe pain scored greater than 54 mm (mean:

75 mm). Thus, a patient who records more than 30 mm on a VAS score would probably have recorded at least moderate pain on a 4-point VDS ("no, mild, moderate, severe pain") [520].

McGill Pain Questionnaire

The McGill Pain Questionnaire (MPQ) consists of three major classes of word descriptors: *sensory* qualities (subclasses 1–10: temporal, spatial, pressure, thermal, brightness, dullness, and miscellaneous); *affective* qualities (subclasses 11–15: tension, autonomic, fear, punishment, and miscellaneous) that are part of the pain experience; *evaluative* words (subclass 16) that describe the subjective overall intensity of the total pain experience; and supplementary qualities (subclasses 17–20). The MPQ was designed to provide quantitative measures of clinical pain that can be treated statistically. The three major measures are (1) the *pain rating index*, based on the rank values of the words, which are then added up to obtain a score for each category, and a total score for all categories; (2) the *number of words chosen*; and (3) *the present pain intensity* based on a 1–5 intensity scale [521]. It has been shown that the MPQ is a useful aid to the differential diagnosis of the painful diabetic leg [522].

Neuropathic Pain Scale

Galer and Jensen [523] have recently argued that although VAS and VDS have proven to be reliable and valid as measures of pain intensity and pain unpleasantness, these two pain dimensions do not adequately cover the domain of the neuropathic pain experience. A strength of the MPQ is that it does assess a variety of pain qualities, but although it can be scored to obtain global measures of the sensory, affective, and evaluative dimensions, it does not provide quantitation of each distinct pain quality. Another drawback of existing pain measures is that they do not identify potential subgroups of neuropathic pain that might benefit from specific therapies [523]. The Neuropathic Pain Scale (NPS) has been designed to assess distinct pain qualities associated with neuropathic pain. The NPS includes two items that assess the global dimensions of pain intensity and pain unpleasantness as well as eight items that assess specific qualities of neuropathic pain: *sharp, hot, dull, cold, sensitive, itchy, deep,* and *surface* pain. In addition, each item includes a description and other similar descriptive words for that item. Each of the 10 items has a 0–10 numerical score (0 = no, 10 = most). An eleventh item assesses the temporal sequence of pain as constant with intermittent increases, intermittent, or constant with fluctuation. Preliminary validation of the NPS suggested discriminant and predictive validity, and all but one of the NPS items were sensitive to open-label treatment [523]. However, the NPS has not yet been used in randomized clinical trials on painful diabetic neuropathy.

Quality-of-Life Measures

The concept of quality of life (QOL) has been defined in terms of three major components: functional capacity, perception of health status (or "well being"), and disease symptoms [524]. Although the impact of painful diabetic neuropathy on morbidity is increasingly recognized, there is a paucity of data related to the effects of this condition on QOL. A modified version of the interference items from the Brief Pain Inventory (BPI) has been used to demonstrate that the pain caused considerable interference in sleep and enjoyment of life and moderate interference in mobility, normal work, mood, and general, recreational, and social activities [496]. A QOL scale specific for diabetic neuropathy has been recently developed and validated [525]. Given the essential impact of neuropathic pain on QOL in diabetic patients, the use of specific measures of QOL is mandatory in evaluating the effects of pain treatments in clinical trials.

Treatment of Painful Diabetic Neuropathy

Painful symptoms in diabetic polyneuropathy may constitute a considerable management problem. Efficacy of a single therapeutic agent is not the rule, and simple analgesics are usually inadequate to control the pain. Therefore, various therapeutic schemes have been proposed, but none of them has been validated [498,526,527]. Nonetheless, there is agreement that patients should be offered the available therapies in a stepwise fashion [528,529]. Effective pain treatment aims a favorable balance between pain relief and side effects, without implying a maximum effect.

Causal Treatment Aimed at Near-Normoglycemia

There is now general agreement that long-term near-normoglycemia may prevent or slow the progression of the chronic diabetic complications including diabetic neuropathy. Six long-term prospective studies evaluated the effects of intensive diabetes therapy on the chronic diabetic complications, three of which included type 1 or type 2 diabetic patients either with mild retinopathy or without evidence of complications [530–535] (see pages 91–96). However, these studies were neither primarily designed to establish the effects of near-normoglycemia on diabetic neuropathy nor did they include sufficient numbers of patients with painful neuropathy. These trials have demonstrated convincingly in type 1 but not in type 2 diabetic patients that long-term near-normoglycemia can prevent the development of somatosensory and cardiac autonomic neuropathy. However, to a lesser degree, neuropathy also developed in the well-controlled type 1 diabetic groups, suggesting that complete prevention of this complication is difficult to achieve by the current methods of intensive insulin therapy. Other studies have shown that symptoms of diabetic neuropathy including pain may be improved and prevented by long-term near-normal glycemic control [536,537], but pain was not used as a primary inclusion criterion. Several open, uncontrolled, small-size studies in type 1 diabetic patients indicated that painful neuropathic symptoms may be significantly reduced by intensive insulin therapy [538], but no controlled trials are available to confirm these findings.

Pancreas transplantation is the most effective method of achieving long-term normoglycemia in type 1 diabetic patients, but is usually limited to patients with endstage diabetic nephropathy in combination with a renal graft. Other indications have been questioned [539]. Four long-term studies in type 1 diabetic patients with established diabetic polyneuropathy who underwent successful pancreatic transplantation have been published. Kennedy et al. [540] have shown that 42 months after transplantation the neuropathy was only slightly improved, but a significant difference was seen in the mean motor and sensory nerve conduction velocity (NCV) in the transplanted group compared with a control group who did not have functioning graft after 42 months. Improvement was more pronounced when only mild dysfunction was present initially. Solders et al. [541] found beneficial effects of combined pancreatic and renal transplantation on NCV after four years of normoglycemia. The initial improvement in motor NCV observed in these patients was also noted in diabetic patients receiving a renal transplant only, and was most likely due to the elimination of uremia. However, further improvement was seen only in the euglycemic pancreas graft recipients. None of the beneficial effects on NCV described in these studies were demonstrable after two years. Thus, periods of normoglycemia of up to about two years are presumably too short to influence established nerve conduction deficits, but longer-term normoglycemia may retard their further progression. Pancreas graft failure is associated with a deterioration in NCV to pretransplant levels after two years [542]. In contrast, controversial results have been reported regarding neuropathic symptoms. Müller-Felber et al. [543] observed a significant improvement in the Neuropathy Symptom Score (NSS) from 1.7 to 0.6 after three years in patients who underwent successful pancreas and kidney transplantation, whereas NSS did not change in those with early pancreas rejection and functioning kidney graft. However, Allen et al. [544] reported a nonsignificant decrease in the NSS from 0.43 to 0.39 in patients with combined pancreas-kidney transplants after up to eight years. None of these studies specifically evaluated the effects of normoglycemia on neuropathic pain. Thus, unequivocal evidence from appropriately designed long-term studies to support the finding from earlier uncontrolled short-term studies that intensive insulin therapy is associated with a significant reduction in neuropathic pain is still lacking. Nonetheless, intensive diabetes therapy aimed at near-normoglycemia is considered the first step in the treatment of any form and stage of diabetic neuropathy.

Treatment Based on Pathogenetic Considerations

A variety of experimental studies have provided new insights in the putative mechanisms implicated in the pathogenesis of diabetic neuropathy [545]. The following pharmacologic treatment approaches have been developed to correct the underlying putative abnormality in the diabetic nerve (Table 5.**6**):

- Aldose reductase inhibitors (ARIs) to reduce the enhanced flux through the polyol pathway [546–548]
- γ-Linolenic acid (GLA), contained in evening primrose oil, to prevent abnormalities in essential fatty acid and prostanoid metabolism [549,550]
- Antioxidants (α-lipoic acid) to reduce free radical-mediated oxidative stress [551]
- Vasodilators (ACE inhibitors, prostacyclin analogues) to increase nerve blood flow and prevent hypoxia [551,552]
- Immunosuppressants, corticosteroids, and intravenous immunoglobulins to treat the inflammatory components associated with proximal diabetic neuropathy [553–555]
- *myo*-Inositol to correct *myo*-inositol depletion [556]
- Nerve growth factor (NGF) to prevent deficits in neurotrophism and axonal transport [557,558]
- Aminoguanidine to inhibit nonenzymatic advanced glycosylation endproduct (AGE) formation [559]

Since, due to several factors, in the near future the majority of diabetic patients presumably will not achieve near-normoglycemia, the advantage of the aforementioned treatments could be that they exert favorable effects despite the presence of hyperglycemia.

Aldose Reductase Inhibitors

An increased flux through the polyol pathway resulting in multiple biochemical abnormalities in the diabetic nerve is thought to play a major role in the pathogenesis of diabetic neuropathy [545]. ARIs block the increased activity of aldose reductase, the rate-limiting enzyme that converts glucose to sorbitol. The first trials of ARIs in diabetic neuropathy were published 20 years ago. The various compounds that have been evaluated are alrestatin, sorbinil, ponalrestat, tolrestat, epalrestat, zopolrestat, zenarestat and fidarestat. Except for fidarestat, which is still being tested in clinical trials, and epalrestat, which is marketed in Japan, none of these agents could be licensed due to serious adverse events (sorbinil, tolrestat, zenarestat) or lack

Table 5.6 Treatment of diabetic neuropathy based on the putative pathogenetic mechanisms

Abnormality	Compound	Aim of treatment	Status of RCTs
Polyol pathway ↑	Aldose reductase inhibitors	Nerve sorbitol ↓	
	Sorbinil, tolrestat		Withdrawn (AE)
	Ponalrestat		Ineffective
	Zopolrestat		Withdrawn (marginal effects)
	Zenarestat		Withdrawn (AE)
	Epalrestat		Equivocal
	Fidarestat		Ongoing
myo-Inositol ↑	*myo*-Inositol	Nerve *myo*-inositol ↑	Equivocal
γ-Linolenic acid synthesis ↓	γ-Linolenic acid	EFA metabolism ↑	Withdrawn (effective: deficits)
Oxidative stress ↑	α-Lipoic acid	Oxygen free radicals ↓	Effective (symptoms, deficits)
Nerve hypoxia ↑	Vasodilators	Endoneurial blood flow ↑	
	ACE inhibitors		Effective in one RCT
	Prostaglandin analogues		Effective in one RCT
Neurotrophism ↓	Nerve growth factor (NGF)	Nerve regeneration, growth ↑	Ineffective
LCFA metabolism ↓	Acetyl-L-carnitine	LCFA accumulation ↓	Ineffective
NEG ↑	Aminoguanidine	AGE accumulation ↓	Withdrawn

NEG, nonenzymatic glycation; AGE, advanced glycation endproducts; EFA, essential fatty acids; LCFA, long-chain fatty acids; AE, adverse events; RCT, randomized clinical trial

of efficacy (ponalrestat, zopolrestat). A meta-analysis of 13 clinical trials with ARIs revealed a marginal effect on peroneal motor NCV of 1.24 m/s and an even weaker effect on median motor NCV of 0.69 m/s after one year [546]. Data of 738 subjects from three trials of tolrestat showed a benefit equal to 1 m/s in a pooled analysis of NCV in all the nerves studied [547]. The following degrees of changes in motor (M) and sensory (S) NCV that are associated with a change in the Neuropathy Impairment Score (NIS) of two points have been considered to be clinically meaningful in controlled clinical trials: median MNCV 2.5 m/s; ulnar MNCV: 4.6 m/s; peroneal MNCV: 2.2 m/s; median SNCV: 1.9 m/s; and sural SNCV: 5.6 m/s [560]. According to this suggestion the changes in NCV obtained from the ARI trials so far do not appear to reflect a meaningful magnitude of treatment effect.

Among the earlier small-size controlled trials of ARIs in painful diabetic neuropathy, the majority could not demonstrate significant pain relief [548]. Only a few large-scale trials reported the effects of ARIs on neuropathic pain. In a multicenter trial of tolrestat in 219 patients with symptomatic polyneuropathy, paresthetic symptoms but not pain were significantly improved after one year [561]. In the Sorbinil Retinopathy Trial in 497 patients, no favorable effect on the neuropathic symptoms could be detected after a median follow up of 39 months [562]. In a recent one-year trial of zenarestat in 208 patients with diabetic polyneuropathy, a dose-dependent improvement in small myelinated fiber loss and peroneal NCV was observed, but no data on neuropathic symptoms were reported [563]. In a 12-week controlled study of 196 patients, complete pain relief was noted in 48.6% of the patients receiving epalrestat compared to 22.6% of those on placebo [564]. Thus, only this single trial reported that ARI treatment is associated with pain relief. This finding requires confirmation by further trials.

γ-Linolenic Acid

Two multicenter trials have demonstrated improvement in neuropathic deficits and NCV after one year of treatment with γ-linolenic acid (GLA) in diabetic peripheral neuropathy [549,550]. However, in these studies neuropathic pain has not been assessed. In one center participating in the second trial, the three major symptoms (pain, paresthesias, and numbness) were evaluated using VASs. Paresthesias and numbness but not pain were significantly reduced after one year in the group treated with GLA but not in the placebo group [565]. Since no studies are available that examined the effects of GLA in diabetic patients with neuropathic pain as the primary inclusion criterion, it is not known whether the drug is useful in these patients.

α-Lipoic Acid (Thioctic Acid)

There is accumulating evidence suggesting that free radical-mediated oxidative stress is implicated in the pathogenesis of diabetic neuropathy, by inducing neurovascular defects that result in endoneurial hypoxia and subsequent nerve dysfunction [545]. Antioxidant treatment with α-lipoic acid has been shown to prevent these abnormalities in experimental diabetes [566], thus providing a rationale for a potential therapeutic value in diabetic patients (see pages 121, 123–128). In Germany, α-lipoic acid has been licensed and used for treatment of symptomatic diabetic neuropathy for more than 20 years. Thus far, five randomized, placebo-controlled clinical trials have been published using different study designs, durations of treatment, doses, sample sizes, and patient populations [551]. The following conclusions can be drawn from these trials:

1. Short-term treatment for 3 weeks using 600 mg α-lipoic acid i.v. per day appears to reduce the chief neuropathic symptoms, including pain, paresthesias, and numbness [567]. A three-week pilot study of 1800 mg per day indicates that the therapeutic effect may be independent of the route of administration, but this needs to be confirmed in a larger sample size [568].
2. Three-week treatment also improves neuropathic deficits [567–569].
3. Oral treatment for four to seven months tends to reduce neuropathic deficits [569] and improves cardiac autonomic neuropathy [570].
4. Preliminary data over two years indicate possible long-term improvement in motor and sensory NCV in the lower limbs [571].
5. Clinical and postmarketing surveillance studies have revealed a highly favorable safety profile of the drug [572].

In the ALADIN Study [567] the number needed to treat (NNT; see below) was 4.0 for a ≥ 30 % reduction in the total symptom score (TSS) after three weeks of intravenous infusion of 600 mg α-lipoic acid as compared with placebo (see Table 5.**8**). Thus, in the absence of significant adverse reactions, the infusion of α-lipoic acid (600 mg i.v. [30 min] over three weeks) can be recommended for the initial treatment of painful symptoms in diabetic neuropathy (Table 5.**7**). Two large multicenter trials are being conducted in North America and Europe to verify the results of the ALADIN studies (NATHAN 2 study) and to evaluate the efficacy and safety of long-term treatment with α-lipoic acid over four years for neuropathic deficits (NATHAN 1 study) [551,573].

No clinical trials in painful diabetic neuropathy are available for other antioxidants. In a preliminary study of 21 patients with symptomatic polyneuropathy, vitamin E led to an improvement in motor but not sensory NCV after six months, and it was not reported whether the neuropathic symptoms were influenced [574].

Vasodilators

Microvascular changes of the vasa nervorum and reduced endoneurial blood flow resulting in hypoxia are thought to be important factors in the pathogenesis of diabetic neuropathy [545]. Thus, there is solid theoretical background to support treatment with vasodilating drugs (see pages 115–123). In a one-year trial in 41 normotensive patients with mild neuropathy, several attributes of NCV, but not neuropathic symptoms and deficits ,were improved after one year of treatment with the ACE inhibitor trandolapril [575]. Further studies are clearly needed to define the therapeutic role of ACE inhibitors in diabetic neuropathy.

Several open-label trials from Japan reported pain relief after treatment with vasodilating agents such as the prostacyclin (PGI_2) analogues iloprost [563] or beraprost [576] and the prostaglandin derivative PGE_1.αCD [577] reported relief of pain or dysesthetic symptoms after 2,12, and 4 weeks, respectively. Due to the uncontrolled study designs these effects are uninterpretable. However, a large controlled multicenter trial including 170 patients with symptomatic polyneuropathy or foot ulcers showed a more than 50 % improvement in pain or other neuropathic symptoms in 56 % of the patients treated with an intravenous infusion of PGE_1 incorporated in lipid microspheres (lipo-PGE_1) for four weeks, compared to 28 % on placebo. In a second trial comparing lipo-PGE_1 with PGE_1-CD in 194 patients, the corresponding rates were 51 % and 35 %. Side effects were observed in 7 % of the patients treated with lipo-PGE_1 [578]. Further studies are needed to confirm these findings in a more homogeneous group with painful neuropathy.

Immunoglobulins, Immunosuppressants, and Glucocorticoids

Some patients with proximal or multifocal diabetic neuropathy show marked ischemic nerve lesions with vasculitis and inflammatory infiltration [553,554] termed *diabetic inflammatory vasculopathy*, while in others a "demyelinating neuropathy" without vascular inflammation, indistinguishable from chronic inflammatory demyelinating polyneuropathy (CIDP), may be present [555]. Thus, it is thought that treatment with intravenous immunoglobulins, immunosuppressants, or glucocorticoids may be helpful in these patients [553,555]. However, there have been no controlled studies using these agents in proximal or multifocal diabetic neuropathy. This is a critical issue, since these forms frequently tend to resolve spontaneously, and the drugs mentioned may produce significant adverse effects and are relatively expensive. In fact, some cases have recently been described who became free of pain shortly after nerve biopsy had been performed, so that additional treatment was unnecessary [554]. It has been suggested that interruption of a sensory branch of a nerve producing pain due to stimulation of sensory fibers by mediators released by inflammatory cells may decrease painful afferents and give a feeling of relief to the patient. [554]. Due to the self-limiting nature of the symptoms and the potential adverse effects, some authors are reluctant to use immunotherapy [554, 579], while others are not [553, 580]. However, there is general agreement regarding the need for future controlled studies using these agents in proximal diabetic neuropathy.

Compounds Without Evidence of Benefit from Controlled Trials

Defective metabolism of long-chain fatty acids and their accumulation in nerve may impair nerve function in diabetes by altering plasma or mitochondrial membrane integrity and disturbing intracellular metabolism and energy production [581]. Carnitine and its acetyl esters such as acetyl-L-carnitine facilitate β-oxidation of nonesterified fatty acid in the liver for energy production. A small two-week study of 20 patients with painful diabetic neuropathy showed an improvement in symptoms following acetyl-L-carnitine treatment compared to placebo [582]. However, a large multicenter one-year trial including 1345 patients failed to demonstrate any benefit of acetyl-L-carnitine on various attributes of diabetic neuropathy [583].

Nerve growth factor (NGF) promotes the survival, differentiation, and maintenance of small-fiber sensory and sympathetic neurons in the peripheral nervous system [584]. It is expressed in the skin and other target tissues of its responsive neuronal populations, binds to its high-affinity receptor (trkA) on nerve terminals, and exerts its trophic effects after being retrogradely transported back to the neuronal perikaryon [585]. A six-month phase II trial including 250 patients with symptomatic diabetic neuropathy showed an improvement of the sensory component of the neurologic examination and both cooling detection and heat as pain threshold, but no effect on neuropathic symptoms could be observed following treatment with recombinant human NGF [585]. A subsequent large phase III trial failed to demonstrate a favorable effect of recombinant human NGF on subjective and objective variables of diabetic neuropathy.

Peptides related to ACTH and MSH such as the ACTH-(4-9) analogne ORG 2766 exert a neurotrophic effect on the nervous system resulting in enhanced recovery of function after peripheral nerve damage [586]. However, two clinical trials including 62 and 124 patients, respectively, failed to demonstrate a clinically meaningful favorable effect on several attributes of diabetic polyneuropathy after one year of treatment with ORG 2766 [586,587].

myo-Inositol depletion has been suggested to be an important factor in the pathogenesis of diabetic neuropathy, but this view is controversial. Several clinical trials were unable to demonstrate unequivocally a beneficial effect of *myo*-inositol supplementation on nerve function parameters in diabetic neuropathy [556].

Aminoguanidine, an inhibitor of nonenzymatic advanced glycation endproduct (AGE) formation [559], has not been evaluated in clinical trials of diabetic neuropathy, and studies in diabetic microvascular complications have been prematurely terminated.

Controlled studies evaluating rheologic compounds have shown no effect of pentoxifylline (3 × 400 mg per day orally) over four weeks on pain in 16 patients [588], or over six months on symptoms [589] associated with diabetic neuropathy in 40 patients. The same applies to cyclandelate (1600 mg per day orally) [590,591], ginkgo biloba special extract EGb 761 [592], and sabeluzole [593]. Thus, there is no evidence to support favorable effects of rheologic remedies on symptomatic diabetic neuropathy.

Symptomatic Pharmacologic Treatment

Because there is no one therapy that is of benefit to all diabetic patients with chronic painful neuropathy, a variety of drug classes are being used to control the pain. A possible four-step rational therapeutic algorithm based on the current evidence is shown in Table 5.**7**. Prior to any decision regarding the appropriate treatment option, the diagnosis of the underlying neuropathic manifestation allowing to estimate its natural history should be established. In contrast to the agents that have been derived from the pathogenetic mechanisms of diabetic neuropathy, those used for symptomatic therapy were designed to modulate the pain, without favorably influencing the underlying neuropathy. A number of trials have been conducted to evaluate the efficacy and safety of these drugs, but only a few of them included large patient samples.

The relative benefit of an active treatment over a control in clinical trials is usually expressed as the relative risk, the relative risk reduction, or the odds ratio [594]. However, to estimate the extent of a therapeutic effect (e. g., pain relief) that can be pop popd into clinical practice, it is useful to apply a simple measure that helps the physician to select the right treatment for the individual patient. One such practical measure is the "number needed to treat" (NNT), i. e., the number of patients that need to be given a particular treatment in order to observe a clinically relevant effect or adverse event in one patient [594,595]. This measure is expressed as the reciprocal of the absolute risk reduction, i. e., the difference between the proportion of events in the control group (P_c) and the proportion of events in the intervention group (P_i): $NNT = 1/(P_c - P_i)$. The 95 % confidence interval (CI) of NNT can be obtained from the reciprocal value of the 95 % CI for the absolute risk reduction. The NNT for the individual agents used in the treatment of painful diabetic neuropathy is given in Table 5.**7**. In recent meta-analyses the NNT and NNH (number needed to harm) have been computed for several classes of drugs [596] (Table 5.**8**).

Table 5.**7** Stepwise algorithm for treatment of painful diabetic neuropathy

Step	Compound/measure	Dose per day	Remarks	NNT	Reference
I: Near-normoglycemia	Diet, insulin, OAD	Individual adaptation	Aim: $HbA_{1c} \leq 6.5\%$	–	
II: Pathogenetically oriented treatment	α-Lipoic acid (thioctic acid)	600 mg i.v. infusion 1200–1800 mg orally	Duration: 3 weeks AE rare	4.0[a]	Ziegler et al. [78]
III: Symptomatic treatment	*Tricyclic antidepressants (TCA)*				
	Amitriptyline	(10–)25–150 mg	NNMH: 15	3.0/2.0	Max et al. [606,607]
	Desipramine	(10–)25–150 mg	NNMH: 24	2.2/5.0	Max et al. [605,606]
	Imipramine	(10–)25–150 mg	CRR	1.4/1.7/3.0	Sindrup and Jensen [600,603]
	Clomipramine	(10–)25–150 mg	NNMH: 8.7	2.1	Sindrup [600]
	Nortriptyline	(10–)25–150 mg	+Fluphenazine	1.6[b]	Gomez-Perez et al. [609]
	SSRI				
	Citalopram	40 mg	Small sample	7.7	Sindrup et al. [612]
	Paroxetine	40 mg	CRR	2.9	Sindrup et al. [611]
	Ion channel blockers				
	Carbamazepine	200–800 mg	NNMH: 15	3.3	Rull et al. [615]
	Gabapentin	900–3600 mg	Fever AE	3.7	Backonja et al. [619]
	Mexiletine	675 mg	Modest effect	10.3	Oskarsson et al. [624]
	Weak opioids				
	Tramadol	50–400 mg	NNMH: 7.8	3.1	Harati et al. [640]
	Local treatment				
	Capsaicin (0.075%) cream	q.i.d. topically	Max. duration: 8 weeks	4.2[c]	McQuay and Moore [596]
IV: Pain resistant to standard pharmacotherapy	*Strong opioids*	Individual adaptation	Potential for dependence		
	Electrical spinal cord stimulation			Invasive, complications	Tesfaye et al. [673]
Complementary: Physical therapy	TENS,		No AE		Kumar et al. [670,671]
	medical gymnastics,		No AE		
	Balneotherapy, relaxation therapy,		No AE		
	Acupuncture		Uncontrolled study		Abuaisha et al. [669]

OAD, oral antidiabetic drugs; CRR, concentration-response relationship; NNMH, number needed for major harm; TENS, transcutaneous electrical nerve stimulation; AE, adverse events; SSRI, selective serotonin reuptake inhibitors

[a] ≥30% symptom relief

[b] Combined with fluphenazine

[c] Analgesic effectiveness as ascertained by the physician

Tricyclic Antidepressants

Psychotropic agents, among which antidepressants have been most extensively evaluated, have constituted an important component in the treatment of chronic pain syndromes for more than 30 years [597]. Several authors consider the tricyclic antidepressants to be the drug treatment of choice for neuropathic pain [598–603]. Putative mechanisms of pain relief by antidepressants include the inhibition of norepinephrine and/or serotonin reuptake at synapses of central descending pain control systems and antagonism of the N-methyl-D-aspartate receptor, which mediate hyperalgesia and allodynia. Imipramine, amitriptyline, and clomipramine induce balanced reuptake inhibition of both norepinephrine and serotonin, while desipramine is a relatively selective norepinephrine inhibitor [603]. The NNT (CI) for at least 50% pain relief by tricyclic antidepressants is 2.4 (2.0–3.0) [603]. The NNH is 2.8 for minor adverse events and 19 for major adverse events [596] (Table 5.**8**). Thus, among 100 diabetic patients with neuropathic pain who are treated with antidepressants, 30 will experience at least 50%

Table 5.8 Meta-analyses of medical treatments for painful diabetic neuropathy

	Antidepressants	Carbamazepine (C), phenytoin (P)	Topical capsaicin	α-Lipoic acid
Number of RCTs	13	C: 1, P: 2	4	1 (ALADIN study)
Number of patients	465	136	309	326
Outcome measure	> 50 % pain relief	> 50 % pain relief	Analgesic efficacy	≥ 30 % symptom relief
NNT (95 % CI)	2.9 (2.4–4.0)	2.5 (1.8–4.0)	4.2 (2.9–7.5)	4.0 (2.4–12.1)
NNH for minor adverse events (95 % CI)	2.8 (2.0–4.7)	3.1 (2.3–4.8)		∞
NNH for major adverse events (95 % CI)	19 (11–74)	20 (10–446)		∞

Modified after McQuay and Moore [107]
RCTs, randomized clinical trials; NNT, number needed to treat; NNH, number needed to harm

pain relief, 30 will have mild adverse events, and five will discontinue treatment due to severe adverse events [598]. The mean NNT for drugs with balanced reuptake inhibition is 2.2, while for the noradrenergic agents it is 3.6 [603].

The most frequent adverse events of tricyclic antidepressants are tiredness and dry mouth [600]. The starting dose should be 25 mg (10 mg in frail patients) taken as a single night-time dose one hour before sleep. It should be increased by 25 mg at weekly intervals until pain relief is achieved or adverse events occur. The maximum dose is usually 150 mg per day [604]. Amitriptyline is frequently the drug of first choice [604], but desipramine may be chosen as an alternative due to its less pronounced sedative and anticholinergic effects [605,606]. Comparable effects are achieved in patients with and without depression and the effects are independent of any concomitant improvement in mood. The onset of efficacy is more rapid (within two weeks) than in the treatment of depression [607]. The median dose for amitriptyline is 75 mg per day, and there is a clear dose-response relationship [608]. In two studies of imipramine, the dose was adjusted to obtain the optimum plasma concentration of 400–500 nmol/l to ensure maximum effect. The target concentration was attained in 57% of the patients [603].

Whether combined treatment with antidepressants and phenothiazines offers any advantage is not known. Nortriptyline has been evaluated in combination with fluphenazine compared to placebo [609] and carbamazepine [610]. This combination resulted in significant pain relief with a NNT of 1.6 against placebo [609] and both pain reduction and rates of adverse events similar to those for carbamazepine [610].

The notion that the character of the neuropathic pain is predictive of response, so that burning pain should be treated with antidepressants and shooting pain with anticonvulsants, is obviously unfounded [604], since both these pain qualities respond to tricyclic antidepressants [606]. Most evidence of efficacy of antidepressants comes from studies that have been conducted for only a few weeks. However, many patients continue to achieve pain relief for months to years, although this is not true for everybody [604]. Tricyclic antidepressants should be used with caution in patients with orthostatic hypotension and are contraindicated in patients with unstable angina, recent (less than six months) myocardial infarction, heart failure, history of ventricular arrhythmias, significant conduction system disease, and long QT syndrome [602].

Selective Serotonin Reuptake Inhibitors

Selective serotonin reuptake inhibitors (SSRIs) specifically inhibit presynaptic reuptake of serotonin but not norepinephrine, and unlike the tricyclics they lack the postsynaptic receptor-blocking effects and quinidine-like membrane stabilization. Three studies showed that treatment with paroxetine [611] and citalopram [612], but not fluoxetine [606] resulted in significant pain reduction. Paroxetine appeared to influence both steady and lancinating pain qualities [611]. The therapeutic effect was observed within one week and was dependent on the plasma levels, being highest at concentrations of 300–400 nmol/l. Patients who do not tolerate tricyclic antidepressants because of adverse events can be treated with SSRIs as an alternative (Table 5.7). Based on present evidence, citalopram and paroxetine (20–40 mg per day p.o.) should be given preference over fluoxetine, which should be considered only in patients with concomitant depression [606]. Besides the relatively low rates of adverse events, the advantage of the SSRIs compared to the tricyclic compounds is the markedly lower risk of death from overdose [613]. However, a recent case-control study suggested that SSRIs moderately increased the risk of upper gastrointestinal bleeding, to a degree about equivalent to low-dose ibuprofen. The concurrent use of nonsteroidal anti-inflammatory drugs or aspirin greatly increases this risk [614].

Anticonvulsants and Antiarrhythmic Agents

Carbamazepine

The successful treatment of trigeminal neuralgia with carbamazepine resulted in wider use of this anticonvulsant in painful neuropathies. Three small controlled clinical trials of carbamazepine (1–3 × 200 mg per day p.o.) in 30–40 patients have shown its superiority over placebo treatment [615–617]. In the study by Rull et al. [615] the NNT was 3.3 for pain reduction, and NNH was 1.9 for mild (somnolence, dizziness) and 15 for severe adverse events (allergic skin reactions) [618]. These relatively high rates of adverse events and the relative paucity of clinical trials somewhat limit the value of this remedy, so it should be reserved for use after the drugs mentioned earlier have proved unsuccessful (Table 5.**7**). Whether certain pain qualities (shooting or stabbing pain) respond preferentially is not known. A small four-week controlled study revealed no differences in pain relief between carbamazepine and a combination of nortriptyline and fluphenazine [610]. The pain relief by carbamazepine is presumably mediated by stabilizing neuronal membranes through an effect on sodium conductance [501].

Gabapentin

Gabapentin is an anticonvulsant structurally related to γ-aminobutyric acid (GABA), a neurotransmitter that plays a role in pain transmission and modulation. The exact mechanisms of action of this drug in neuropathic pain are not fully elucidated, but among other things involve interaction with the system L-amino acid transporter and high-affinity binding to the $\alpha^2\delta$ subunit of voltage-activated calcium channels. The antihyperalgesic properties of gabapentin are at least partially modulated through spinal cord mechanisms [619]. In an eight-week multicenter dose-escalation trial including 165 diabetic patients with painful neuropathy, 60% of the patients on gabapentin (3600 mg per day achieved in 67%) had at least moderate pain relief, compared to 33% on placebo. Furthermore, gabapentin treatment was associated with improvement in quality of life. Dizziness and somnolence were the most frequent adverse events, occurring in about 23% of the patients each [619]. A six-week study comparing the efficacy of gabapentin (1800 mg per day achieved in 65%) with those of amitriptyline showed at least moderate pain relief in 52% and 67% of the patients, respectively [620]. Thus, no significant difference was noted between the two treatments, but given the small patient sample (n = 28) the probability of a type II (β) error was high. Gabapentin has been suggested to be the preferred drug for patients in whom tricyclic antidepressants are contraindicated or who do not tolerate their adverse effects [602].

Mexiletine

Mexiletine, a class Ib antiarrhythmic agent, has been shown to be effective in a small ten-week study of 16 patients using a dose increasing from 150 mg per day to 10 mg per kilogram body weight per day p.o. [621]. However, another study over three weeks did not confirm this effect [622]. In a five-week multicenter trial using 75–225 mg t.i.d. p.o., no beneficial influence on the total pain rating index was demonstrated, but retrospective analysis indicated a favorable effect on burning and stabbing pain [623]. An oral dose of 150 mg t.i.d., well below that required for antiarrhythmic therapy (600–800 mg per day), was sufficient for this effect and did not produce any adverse events or ECG abnormalities. In contrast, in a second multicenter trial for three weeks, a dose of 675 mg per day was required to achieve a significant reduction in sleep disturbances and pain during the night. This effect had a relatively rapid onset within one week [624]. A recent review of seven controlled trials of mexiletine in painful diabetic neuropathy concluded that the drug produces a modest analgesic effect [625]. Thus, short-term treatment with mexiletine should at best be reserved for a few patients with burning or stabbing pain during the night, and who are unresponsive to a multitude of drugs such as antidepressants, anticonvulsants, or tramadol (see below); regular ECG monitoring is mandatory.

Lidocaine

In a controlled study in 15 diabetic patients with chronic painful neuropathy, a single intravenous infusion of lidocaine (5 mg per kilogram body weight over 30 minutes during continuous ECG monitoring) resulted in significant pain relief after one and eight days [626]. The effect of the single infusion was sustained for 3–21 days. The NNT for a pain reduction of more than 30% after three days was 2.2. Since lidocaine resulted in an increase in the threshold for the nociceptive flexion reflex (m. biceps femoris) in diabetic patients with painful neuropathy, it is conceivable that this compound mediates its pain-relieving effect via spinal or supraspinal mechanisms [627]. Thermal and pain thresholds are not influenced [627,628]. The onset of the analgesic effect during the intravenous infusion (500 mg in 60 minutes) is abrupt within a narrow dosage and concentration range [629].

Phenytoin (Diphenylhydantoin)

In the past, phenytoin (100 mg t.i.d. p.o.) has frequently been advocated on the basis of an open study. However, controlled trials have yielded controversial results [630,631]. Because the data for this compound are equivocal, it should not be used for treatment of painful diabetic neuropathy.

Transdermal Clonidine

A controlled six-week study using a transdermal clonidine patch (dose titration from 0.1 to 0.3 mg per day) in 24 diabetic patients has shown a nonsignificant trend towards pain relief [632]. The NNT for moderate or marked pain reduction was 5.3, while the NNH for adverse events was relatively low: 3.4 each for dry mouth and drowsiness [632]. Likewise, in a three-week trial in 41 patients no significant difference was observed between clonidine and placebo in regard to pain relief [633]. However, 12 responders were identified who experienced moderate to complete pain relief on clonidine compared to placebo patch. These patients were included in a second study using an "enriched enrollment" design (in which only patients who had been screened as responders were entered). In this study a significant 20% pain reduction compared with placebo was noted. The NNH for adverse events (dry mouth, sedation, orthostatic symptoms) was 2.0 in the responders. Thus, on the basis of these data transdermal clonidine cannot be generally recommended. The potential mechanisms for the analgesic effect of clonidine include actions at α_2-adrenergic or imidazoline receptors to cause postsynaptic inhibition of spinal cord neurons, presynaptic inhibition of nociceptive afferents, facilitation of brainstem pain-modulating systems, or peripheral or central suppression of sympathetic transmitter release [632].

Opioids

There are two extreme positions on opioid sensitivity in pain. One suggests that opioid sensitivity is a relative phenomenon and therefore that any pain can be controlled by opioids, provided that there is adequate dose escalation and control of adverse events [634]. The other extreme insists that some kinds of pain are intrinsically insensitive to opioids, and that this insensitivity can be predicted from the clinical characteristics of the pain [635]. Nociceptive pain is taught as sensitive to opioids, whereas neuropathic pain is regarded as insensitive. However, the latter view has been challenged by recent studies showing that the administration of morphine was associated with pain relief in 50% of patients with neuropathic pain of various origins [636]. Furthermore, an infusion of fentanyl induced a pain reduction by 66%, compared with 23% induced by diazepam, independent of the pain characteristics [637]. This analgesic effect is intrinsic and independent of the degree of sedation and change in mood [636–638]. Possible explanations of the overall controversial results of the studies using opioids are the multiple mechanisms involved in neuropathic pain, the use of small patient samples with selection bias, lack of individual dose titration of opioids, and the lack of a placebo group mimicking the side effects of the opioids [639]. Opioids are thought to exert their pain-relieving effect by at least two mechanisms: a presynaptic effect on small afferent C-fiber terminals and a postsynaptic hyperpolarizing effect on spinal neurons [603]. Long-term studies employing oral or transdermal administration of opioids should evaluate the risk-to-benefit ratio of these drugs in patients with pain due to diabetic neuropathy.

Tramadol acts directly via opioid receptors and indirectly via monoaminergic receptor systems. Because development of tolerance and dependence during long-term treatment with this weak opioid is uncommon and its liability to abuse appears to be low, tramadol is an alternative to strong opioids in treating neuropathic pain [603]. In painful diabetic neuropathy tramadol (up to 400 mg per day p.o., mean dose: 210 mg per day p. o.) was studied in a six-week multicenter trial including 131 patients [629]. Pain was relieved in 44% of patients on tramadol versus 12% on placebo. The most frequent adverse events were nausea and constipation. The NNH of 7.8 for drop-outs due to adverse events was relatively low, indicating significant toxicity. In a four-week study in patients with painful neuropathy of various origins, diabetes in one-third of them, tramadol significantly relieved pain (NNT: 4.3 [2.4–20]) and mechanical allodynia [641]. One conceivable mechanism for the favorable effect of tramadol could be hyperpolarization of postsynaptic neurons via postsynaptic opioid receptors. Alternatively, the reduction in central hyperexcitability by tramadol could be due to a monoaminergic or a combined opioid and monoaminergic effect [603]. Trials to assess equivalence (e. g., versus antidepressants) would clarify the relative potency and toxicity of tramadol in painful neuropathy.

Topical Capsaicin

Capsaicin (*trans*-8-methyl-N-vanillyl-6-nonenamide) is an alkaloid and the most pungent ingredient in red peppers (capsicum). It depletes tissues of substance P and reduces neurogenic plasma extravasation, the flare response, and chemically induced pain. Substance P is present in afferent neurons innervating skin, mainly in polymodal nociceptors, and is considered the primary neurotransmitter of painful stimuli from the periphery to the central nervous system [642]. Several studies have demonstrated significant pain reduction and improvement in quality of life in diabetic patients with painful neuropathy after eight weeks of treatment with capsaicin cream (0.075%) [643–649]. On the basis of a meta-analysis of four controlled trials [650], the NNT for capsaicin is 4.2 for analgesic effectiveness as ascertained by the physician [596]. However, a recent 12-week trial in painful neuropathy of different etiologies failed to demonstrate pain relief by capsaicin, and no effect on thermal perception was noted [642]. The criticism has been raised that a double-blind design is not feasible for topical capsaicin because of the transient local hyperalgesia (usually a mild burning sensation in > 50% of the cases) it may produce as a typical adverse event [501,650]. Treatment should be restricted to a maximum of eight weeks, as during this period no adverse effects on sensory function (due to the mechanism of action) were noted in diabetic patients [648]. However, a recent skin blister study in healthy subjects showed that there is a 74% decrease in the number of nerve fibers as early as three days following topical capsaicin application, suggesting that degeneration of epidermal nerve fibers may contribute to the analgesia induced by the drug [651]. This finding, which puts in doubt the safety of capsaicin in the context of an insensitive diabetic foot, limits its usefulness.

Dextromethorphan

Inhibition of N-methyl-D-aspartate (NMDA) receptor-mediated central nervous system excitation alleviates neuropathic pain in animal models, but adverse effects of dissociative anesthetic channel blockers such as ketamine limit their clinical application. It has been hypothesized that relatively high doses of low-affinity, noncompetitive channel-blocking NMDA receptor antagonists such as dextromethorphan may have a more favorable therapeutic ratio than dissociative anesthetic-like blockers [652]. In a six-week study seven out of 13 patients reported moderate or greater relief of pain during dextromethorphan treatment (mean dose: 381 mg per day) compared to none with placebo, giving a NNT of 1.9 (CI: 1.1–3.7). However, five of 31 patients who took dextromethorphan dropped out due to sedation or ataxia during dose escalation [652].

Levodopa

Levodopa is a dopamine precursor, and like dopamine agonists it may inhibit noxious input to the spinal cord or may act as a precursor to norepinephrine by modulating pain via noradrenergic mechanisms [603]. In a four-week study the NNT for levodopa (300 mg per day) was 3.4 (1.5–∞) for at least moderate pain relief. There were no side effects associated with this agent [653].

Vitamin B Complex

Because the neurotrophic constituents of the vitamin B complex exhibit antinociceptive properties when given in high doses experimentally, they are under discussion for the treatment of various pain conditions [654]. There is usually no evidence of depletion of vitamin B_1 (thiamine), B_6 (pyridoxine), and B_{12} (cyanocobalamin) in diabetic patients [655]. Hence, the putative analgesic effect rather than a substitution would appear relevant. However, the evidence for this assumption is not sufficient on the basis of the available controlled studies. Trials using vitamin B_6 for four and three months reported negative results [656,657]. Moreover, it is alarming that the intake of megadoses of vitamin B_6 (up to a maximum of 2–6 g per day p.o.) may lead to severe sensory neuropathy with ataxia [658]. The combination of vitamins B_1, B_6, and B_{12} (300/600/0.6 mg per day p.o.) administered for 18 weeks in 33 diabetic patients was not associated with an appreciable effect on painful symptoms, but resulted in an improvement in the warm and cold thresholds in the hands, though not the feet [659]. Because the bioavailability of the water-soluble B complex vitamins is low, two recent studies have employed benfotiamine, a lipid-soluble thiamine derivative with approximately 3.6-fold greater maximum bioavailability than the water-soluble thiamine [660,661]. In the first study a combination of benfotiamine, vitamin B_6, and B_{12} (120/270/0.75 mg per day p.o.) or placebo was administered to 24 patients over 12 weeks. A beneficial effect could be demonstrated in only one out of four nerve function parameters tested [660]. In the second study 40 patients were treated with 400 mg benfotiamine or placebo for three weeks. A modest, albeit statistically significant, improvement was noted on a score for symptoms and deficits, with 19% improved on benfotiamine versus 6% on placebo [661]. On the basis of these effects, which taken overall are marginal, a multicenter study has been initiated to clarify the role of benfotiamine in the treatment of symptomatic polyneuropathy.

Other Treatment Approaches

In a controlled two-week study of calcitonin treatment (100 IU per day by intranasal spray) in ten patients, three patients had complete pain relief and one experienced 50% pain relief [662].

On the basis of the idea that nucleotides may enhance nerve regeneration, uridine (300 mg t.i.d.) has been evaluated in a controlled trial studying 40 diabetic patients with peripheral neuropathy. After six months a positive effect on NCV and action potentials was noted [663]. It is unclear whether this improvement can be pop popd into favorable effects on clinical symptoms and deficits. Cerebrolysin, a peptidergic solution containing free amino acids and biologically active peptides, was infused intravenously over ten days in 20 type 2 diabetic patients with painful neuropathy. After six weeks, pain was relieved by 33% on cerebrolysin and by 12% on placebo, and no significant adverse events were observed [664].

The administration of the nonsteroidal antirheumatic agents ibuprofen (600 mg q.i.d. orally) and sulindac (200 mg b.i.d.) in an eight-week single-blind study in 18 diabetic patients was associated with an improvement in pain scores [665].

In a four-week study, OpSite, an adherent polyurethane film which is waterproof and permeable to water vapor and oxygen, has been applied to painful sites on the leg in 33 diabetic patients. OpSite dressing alleviated pain and improved patients' quality of life when compared with no treatment [666].

In Japan, goshajinkigan (herbal medicine; 2.5 g t.i.d.) has long been used to treat symptomatic diabetic neuropathy. However, possible effects on neuropathic symptoms and vibration perception threshold are rendered uninterpretable due to the uncontrolled study design [667].

Symptomatic Nonpharmacologic Treatment

Because there is no entirely satisfactory pharmacologic treatment for painful diabetic neuropathy, nonpharmacologic treatment options should always be considered.

Psychologic support: The psychology of pain should not be underestimated. An explanation to the patient that even severe pain may remit can have an effect, particularly in poorly controlled patients with acute painful neuropathy or those with painful symptoms precipitated by intensive insulin treatment. An approach addressing the concerns and anxieties of patients with neuropathic pain is essential for their successful management [668].

Physical measures: The temperature of the painful neuropathic foot may be raised by arteriovenous shunting. Cold water immersion may reduce shunt flow and relieve pain. Allodynia may be relieved by wearing silk pajamas or using a bed cradle. Patients who describe painful symptoms on walking, like "walking on pebbles," may benefit from the use of comfortable footwear [668].

Acupuncture: In a ten-week uncontrolled study in diabetic patients on standard pain therapy, 77% experienced significant pain relief after up to six courses of traditional Chinese acupuncture, without any side effects. During a follow-up period of 18–52 weeks 67% were able to stop or significantly reduce their medications and only 24% required further acupuncture treatment [669]. Controlled studies using placebo needles should be performed to confirm these findings.

Transcutaneous electrical nerve stimulation (TENS): TENS influences neuronal afferent transmission and conduction velocity, increases the nociceptive flexion reflex threshold, and changes the somatosensory evoked potentials [670]. In a four-week study of TENS applied to the lower limbs, each for 30 minutes daily, pain relief was noted in 83% of the patients compared to 38% of a sham-treated group. In patients who only marginally responded to amitriptyline, pain reduction was significantly greater following TENS given for 12 weeks as compared with sham treatment. Thus, TENS may be used as an adjunctive modality combined with pharmacotherapy to augment pain relief [671].

Electrical spinal cord stimulation (ESCS): It is generally agreed that electrical stimulation is effective in neurogenic forms of pain. Experiments indicate that electrical stimulation is followed by a decrease in the excitatory amino acids glutamate and aspartate in the dorsal horn. This effect is mediated by a GABAergic mechanism [672]. In diabetic painful neuropathy that was unresponsive to drug treatment, ESCS with electrodes implanted between T9 and T11 resulted in more than 50% pain relief in eight out of ten patients. In addition, exercise tolerance was significantly improved. Complications of ESCS included superficial wound infection in two patients, lead migration requiring reinsertion in two patients, and "late failure" after four months in a patient who experienced initial pain relief [673]. This invasive treatment option should be reserved for patients who do not respond to drug treatment.

Conclusions

Despite the recently accelerating rate of publication of controlled trials demonstrating significant pain relief with several agents, the pharmacologic treatment of chronic painful diabetic neuropathy remains a challenge for the physician. A survey of physicians experienced in treating neuropathic pain demonstrated that only a minority would judge their analgesia results as excellent or good with antidepressants (40%), anticonvulsants (35%), opioids (30%), and simple analgesics (18%) [674]. Major limiting factors are still the paucity of sufficiently large conclusive trials and the relatively high rates of adverse effects for several drug classes. Recent trials evaluating agents such as gabapentin or tramadol have included large enough patient samples, but the effect on pain was not superior to that of the tricyclic compounds which have been used for many years. Thus, individual tolerability will be a major aspect in the physician's treatment decision. There is almost no information available from controlled trials on long-term analgesic efficacy and the use of drug combinations. Combination drug use or the addition of a new drug to a therapeutic regimen may lead to increased drug toxicity or decreased efficacy. Drug interactions should be more predictable on the basis of knowledge of which compounds induce inhibition or are metabolized by specific cytochrome P450 enzymes [675]. Drug combinations might also include those aimed at symptomatic pain relief and quality of life on the one hand and improving or slowing the progression of the underlying neuropathic process on the other. Future trials should take account of these aspects in order to optimize the current treatment strategies in painful diabetic neuropathy.

Diabetic Autonomic Neuropathy

Cardiovascular System

V. Spallone, G. Menzinger, and D. Ziegler

Introduction

Cardiovascular involvement is undoubtedly the most extensively investigated aspect of diabetic autonomic neuropathy (AN). Symptomatic manifestations of cardiovascular AN, such as tachycardia or postural hypotension, occur rarely and rather late in the course of diabetes. On the other hand, the availability of simple noninvasive cardiovascular reflex tests has allowed extensive documentation of cardiovascular autonomic impairment, and these tests have become the standard diagnostic method for overall autonomic function in diabetes [676,677].

Many clinical case series and a few population-based studies using these tests have provided information on the prevalence of diabetic AN, its natural history, prognosis, clinical and pathophysiologic correlates, and relationship with other chronic diabetic complications [678]. In addition to the traditional cardiovascular autonomic reflex tests, other methods have been developed to investigate autonomic function, such as spectral analysis of heart rate variability (HRV) or assessment of the 24-hour pattern of cardiovascular autonomic indices. Despite a certain degree of complexity and limited standardization, these approaches have increased our knowledge about pathophysiological mechanisms and prognostic implications of diabetic AN.

Epidemiology, Risk Factors, and Prognosis

For the epidemiology, risk factors, and prognosis associated with diabetic AN, see Chapter 3.

Clinical Features

A *heart rate* of 90–100 bpm, unresponsive to breathing, change in posture, or mild exercise, is a characteristic finding in diabetic patients with AN. The possible occurrence of complete heart denervation with a totally fixed heart rate and denervation supersensitivity has been postulated by some authors [679] and disputed by others on the basis of 24-hour ECG monitoring and pharmacologic studies [680]. While the resting blood pressure-heart rate product is high, as a consequence of the resting tachycardia, the heart rate, blood pressure (BP), and cardiac output *responses to exercise* have been found to be significantly impaired in neuropathic patients [681,682], particularly in patients with postural hypotension [683]. Depressed left ventricular systolic function on radionuclide ventriculography and abnormal left ventricular diastolic filling have been observed in diabetic patients with AN in the absence of ischemic heart disease [684,685]. It has been suggested that the abnormalities in *contractile reserve and relaxation* observed in diabetic patients could be due to an interference of autonomic dys-function with the neural modulation of cardiovascular performance [686]. Early ventricular dysfunction, better evidenced with exercise, characterizes diabetic cardiomyopathy. The relation of AN to cardiomyopathy and the prognostic significance of the neuropathy-related ventricular dysfunction are not yet well defined [687]. However, caution is warranted against aggressive exercise programs in diabetic patients unless their autonomic function status is known.

Increased prevalence of *painless myocardial infarction* has been described in diabetic patients and attributed, on the basis of autopsy studies, to damaged afferent fibers to the myocardium [688,689]. Moreover, silent myocardial ischemia has been reported to be more prevalent in the diabetic population (10–20%) than in the nondiabetic population (1–4%) [690–692]. In the Milan Study on Atherosclerosis and Diabetes [692], abnormalities in exercise ECG test and perfusion defects shown on thallium scintigraphy were present in 12% and 6%, respectively, out of 925 type 2 diabetic patients aged 40–65 years who were free from clinical coronary artery disease. However, conclusive evidence of a higher prevalence of asymptomatic myocardial ischemia in diabetes is still lacking [693]. Discrepancies in diagnostic criteria and tests for asymptomatic myocardial ischemia, and the interference of diabetes-related factors with the sensitivity, specificity, and prognostic implications of noninvasive diagnostic tests for coronary artery disease, may partially account for this uncertainty [694]. Silent myocardial ischemia in diabetes is generally but not universally believed to be associated with neuropathy [695–698]. In particular, Ambepitiya et al. [697] studied diabetic and nondiabetic patients with angina pectoris using exercise electrocardiography and found that the delay in the perception of pain was related to the impairment in autonomic function tests. However, increasing evidence indicates a complex involvement of multiple pathogenetic mechanisms in diabetes as well as in the general population, such as the degree and extension of ischemia, localized alterations in pain threshold due to disruption of nociceptive pathways, and variations in central pain threshold as a consequence of increased levels of endorphins. The relative contribution of these putative mechanisms to asymptomatic myocardial ischemia in diabetes is not yet clear [699,700]. While a study by Langer et al. [701] suggested a link between diffuse abnormalities in sympathetic innervation assessed by a scintigraphic technique and silent myocardial ischemia (see pages 236ff), another study failed to find such a relationship in diabetic patients with coronary artery disease [702]. Nevertheless, given the high risk of cardiac events [695,703], it is undoubtedly advisable to screen for asymptomatic myocardial ischemia when neuropathy is associated with cardiovascular risk factors. Moreover, neuropathic diabetic patients with coronary artery disease should be trained to recognize and report typical anginal equivalents such as dyspnea, diaphoresis, weakness, nausea, or transient arrhythmias to avoid harmful delay in starting treatment for acute myocardial infarction.

Orthostatic Hypotension: Clinical Features

Orthostatic hypotension in diabetes has been defined as an orthostatic fall of systolic pressure of more than 30 mmHg. It occurs rarely in the diabetic population (3–6%) [704,705] and rather late in the course of AN, when reflex heart rate responses are already impaired. Interestingly, in two different population-based studies systolic orthostatic hypotension, defined as a drop of 20 mmHg or more three minutes after standing, was present in respectively 6.9% and 19% of elderly persons aged over 70 years, and was an independent predictor of all-cause mortality (relative risk 1.64) and of vascular death (relative risk 1.69) [706,707].

In diabetic patients with orthostatic hypotension, symptoms such as dizziness, weakness, and loss of consciousness are not usually present unless the fall is greater than 50 mmHg or the standing systolic BP is lower than 70 mmHg. A considerable tolerance to low BP without developing symptoms of orthostatic hypotension is present in dysautonomic patients in general and has been attributed to a shift of cerebral blood flow autoregulation to the left, in the sense that autoregulation is preserved down to systolic BP values around 60 mmHg, lower than the limit of 80 mmHg in normal subjects [708]. This change in autoregulation could be due to an adaptation to chronically low BP or to the effect of sympathetic denervation of cerebral vessels—mostly or exclusively extracerebral vessels—leading to a withdrawal of sympathetically mediated vasoconstriction and of the consequent reduction in blood flow [708].

Orthostatic hypotension fluctuates spontaneously over the years for reasons that are not always clear [709]. It can be exacerbated by exercise and many drugs, such as antihypertensives, diuretics, and psychotherapeutic agents, whereas it can be masked by fluid retention related to cardiac or renal causes. Moreover, orthostatic hypotension can be influenced by the circadian rhythm of BP and may become more severe in the morning and in the postprandial periods.

Orthostatic hypotension is mainly due to a defect in splanchnic vasoconstriction consequent to efferent vasomotor sympathetic denervation, as suggested by diminished mesenteric vasoconstriction documented by ultrasound techniques [710]. The importance of this mechanism is confirmed by the therapeutic efficacy of octreotide, which acts mainly through splanchnic vasoconstriction [711]. A minor pathogenetic role is played by the reduction in peripheral vasoconstriction and by the heart rate and cardiac output response to standing [710]. Reduced norepinephrine response to standing has also been implicated, although a hyperadrenergic variety of the orthostatic hypotension syndrome has been described in some patients with reduced intravascular volume rather than AN [710]. Other neuroendocrine abnormalities have been described in association with orthostatic hypotension but are of doubtful pathogenetic relevance, such as reduction in the renin or antidiuretic hormone (ADH) response to standing. ADH together with the atrial natriuretic peptide and the renin-angiotensin-aldosterone system is involved in the complex neuroendocrine response to orthostasis that is finalized by reducing standing natriuresis and diuresis to prevent plasma volume depletion. The role of ADH in this context is to increase free water reabsorption through activation of both renal V_2-receptors leading to an increase in water permeability of the collecting duct and renal V_1-receptors with a consequent decrease in medullary blood flow [712]. While the osmotic regulation of ADH in dysautonomias appears to be normal, the actual role of orthostatic regulation of ADH in dysautonomic and diabetic patients with orthostatic hypotension is not clear [713,714].

Recently, a possible contribution of anemia has been suggested, since treatment with erythropoietin has been shown to improve both anemia and orthostatic hypotension in dysautonomic patients [715]. Anemia with a relative deficit of erythropoietin has been described in dysautonomias [716] and in type 1 diabetic patients with both severe AN and proteinuria [717,718]. An inverse relationship between the hematocrit levels and the orthostatic fall in systolic BP has also been observed in nonproteinuric type 2 diabetic patients [719]. These observations together with the experimental evidence have led to the hypothesis of a pathogenetic role of renal denervation in these forms of erythropoietin-deficient anemia, although in most studies it was difficult to distinguish the relative contributions of renal impairment and autonomic dysfunction to the development of the hematologic defect [717,718,720]. Treatment with recombinant human erythropoietin (rHuEPO) in diabetic and nondiabetic dysautonomic patients corrected the anemia and resulted in subjective improvement [717]. From the analysis of the few studies that provide BP values [715,716] and on the basis of personal experience, this symptomatic improvement is associated with an overall increase in BP, both supine and standing, rather than with a reduction in orthostatic BP fall. The factors responsible for this symptomatic improvement are not fully known, an increase in erythrocyte mass and circulating volume, improvement in tissue oxygen delivery, or some direct hemodynamic effects of erythropoietin being all putative mechanisms [715,716]. The doses of rHuEPO shown to reverse anemia in patients with orthostatic hypotension are generally lower than those used to treat anemia in renal failure or chronic disease [715,717], and minimize the risk of increasing blood viscosity or exacerbating the supine hypertension often associated with orthostatic hypotension. In the absence of large studies that support more extensive indications, this treatment should be reserved for patients with orthostatic hypotension associated with anemia.

Finally, the cardiovascular effects of insulin deserve particular attention. In healthy subjects insulin exerts dual effects on blood flow: a vasodilator effect mediated via release of nitric oxide, and a vasoconstrictive effect mediated via activation of the sympathetic nervous system, this latter being prevalent at low physiologic concentrations [721]. In patients with autonomic failure, lacking the second mechanism, insulin exerts a hypotensive effect [710]. In a recent study, type 1 diabetic patients with AN showed a lower noradrenergic response to insulin with a marked reduction in plasma volume not accompanied by an adequate increase in peripheral vascular resistance [722]. Postprandial hyperinsulinemia probably causes splanchnic vasodila-tion that lowers BP in dysautonomic patients, because the normal compensatory sympathetic activation is lacking. This may contribute to the postprandial splanchnic vasodilation and hypotension characteristic of many autonomic disorders [723]. Finally, it must be remembered that symptoms of orthostatic hypotension may mimic a hypoglycemic crisis and therefore often require diagnostic differentiation.

Orthostatic Hypotension: Treatment

The first consideration in treatment of symptomatic orthostatic hypotension should be avoidance of situations known to exacerbate symptoms, such as prolonged standing, physical exercise early in the morning or after meals, exposure to a warm environment, prolonged hot baths or showers, stypsis, alcohol ingestion, and large carbohydrate-rich meals. Vasoactive drugs such as antihypertensives, including diuretics or nitrates, or psychiatric drugs such as tricyclic antidepressants, even in small doses, may exacerbate hypotension. Some positions and physical maneuvers are helpful in daily life, such as crossing the legs while standing, squatting, abdominal compression, bending forward, placing a foot on a chair, and stooping as if to tie shoe laces [724]. Their efficacy is due to an increase in vascular resistance and venous return. External supports to reduce blood pooling in the legs during standing have been used in the past. The most effective antigravity suits are highly uncomfortable, while elastic pressure stockings are often not accepted by the patients and provide limited benefit [708]. Raising the head of bed at night by 20° has been reported as highly effective in dysautonomic patients with orthostatic hypotension and excessive nocturnal polyuria [708], although corresponding results have not been documented in diabetic patients. Head-up tilt at night activates the neurohormonal mechanisms aimed at preventing reduction in blood volume through a reduction in nocturnal diuresis and natriuresis. In any case, in the absence of strict contraindications an adequate intake of salt and water should be ensured. Intact renal innervation appears to be essential for the kidney to express its capacity for maximum sodium reabsorption in response to a reduction in dietary sodium intake. Dysautonomic patients are unable to lower urinary sodium excretion when on a low-sodium diet, thus increasing their orthostatic hypotension [712].

If these nonpharmacologic measures are unsuccessful, fludrocortisone is the most commonly used drug. It acts by increasing vasoconstriction on standing through potentiation of the vascular response to the remaining norepinephrine and, at higher doses, by expanding the blood volume. The initial dose of 0.1 mg at bedtime can be increased every two to three weeks to a final dose of 0.4 mg, with care being taken to avoid possible side effects such as recumbent hypertension or excessive salt and water retention with marked edema. The combination of fludrocortisone (0.1 mg) with head-up tilt and a high-salt diet (150–200 mmol sodium/day) has been shown to be effective [725].

Desmopressin (DDAVP) is a vasopressin analogue with selective activation of V_2 receptors that has been used to correct nocturnal polyuria and morning orthostatic hypotension by intramuscular (2 μg/day), intranasal (5–40 μg/day), and oral administration (200 or 400 μg/day) at bedtime. Careful supervision is required to monitor hyponatremia and detect a paradoxical increase in natriuresis that occurs in some patients [708]. Various sympathomimetic vasoconstrictor agents have been used, the most studied of which has been midodrine. Midodrine is an α_1-agonist causing constriction of both arterial resistance and venous capacitance vessels. It is administered in doses of 2.5–10 mg three times daily owing to its short half-life. Side effects include piloerection, goose bumps, tingling, and pruritus in addition to urinary retention [708]. In a recent randomized, double-blind multicenter study in 171 patients with orthostatic hypotension, midodrine administered at a dose of 10 mg three times daily has been shown to be more effective than placebo in improving systolic BP and symptoms on standing, with limited side effects including pilomotor reactions, urinary retention, and supine hypertension [726]. Many other drugs have been used in the treatment of orthostatic hypotension, including β-blockers with partial agonist activity, such as pindolol, prostaglandin synthetase inhibitors, such as indomethacin

an interrelationship between the pathogenesis of obesity and disorders of the respiratory and heart rhythm-generating control centers in the brainstem [747], or the influence of mechanical factors such as intrathoracic fat deposits with consequent difficulty in lung expansion and attenuation of respiratory reflexes [687,747]. Other studies did not find any relationship in type 2 diabetes between the body mass index and autonomic function [744,748]. It is possible that differences in study populations might account for these discrepancies, and that the aggregation between obesity and AN could be limited to older patients with cardiovascular disease. In any case, the presence of marked obesity can attenuate the deep breathing stimulus and thus the heart rate response. The message is that the body mass is a confounding factor in applying autonomic function tests.

In conclusion, the recommendations of a recent consensus conference [677] to use at least three of the standard autonomic function tests for diagnostic purposes—deep breathing, Valsalva maneuver, and orthostatic hypotension—are still valid. Attention must be given to standardizing the procedure in respect of time of day, metabolic status, distance in time from meals and insulin administration, avoidance of coffee and smoking, withdrawal of interfering drugs if possible, and the patient's collaboration. In the presence of cardiovascular disease, or if drugs cannot be withdrawn, some caution is needed in interpreting the results.

Sympathetic Function Tests

A limit of the standard autonomic function tests is the relatively poor sensitivity of BP tests. In the natural course of AN, impairment of the BP response to standing or sustained handgrip generally follows that of HRV tests. The early abnormalities in sympathetic function observed when more sophisticated techniques are used, such as spectral analysis of heart rate, or when studying other functions under sympathetic control, such as sudorimotor activity, pupil function, etc., indicated a need for more sensitive and easier tests to assess cardiovascular sympathetic activity. This approach may hide an incorrect assumption. In fact, tests based on cardiovascular reflexes generally involve both parasympathetic and sympathetic pathways, although to different degrees, and thus it is an oversimplification to consider them as "pure" vagal or sympathetic tests. In any case, standing-to-lying has been proposed as a test that provides two indices evaluating parasympathetic and sympathetic function respectively, although the sympathetic index would still have a limited sensitivity [749]. The sustained handgrip has been found to be of limited sensitivity and specificity [730]. The mental arithmetic stress test (subtraction or addition of 7 or 17) has been described as more sensitive than the sustained handgrip and orthostatic tests. The cold pressor test—placing one hand in ice water—is widely used [732] but has limited specificity and a low reproducibility, particularly when testing is repeated after a short time, probably due to habituation or anticipation.

The squatting test has been recently introduced in the assessment of diabetic AN [750]. Squatting-induced bradycardia appears to be mediated by the vagus nerve, being completely abolished by atropine and not affected by propranolol. Conversely, cardioacceleration from squatting to standing is thought to represent a sympathetic activation triggered by a sustained fall in BP which takes place on standing and is abolished by propranolol. This test might give information on both parasympathetic and sympathetic function and is reported to show early simultaneous involvement of both components of the autonomic nervous system [750]. Wider use is needed to verify the practicability and real advantages of this test.

Baroreflex Sensitivity Testing

Arterial baroreflex is the key regulatory mechanism for short-term control of BP. Arterial baroreceptors of the carotid sinuses and aortic arch react to changes in arterial pressure. The afferents from these sensors through the carotid sinus nerve, the glossopharyngeal nerve, and the vagus nerve reach the nucleus tractus solitarii in the brainstem, where a complex central integration of the afferent signals occurs. The efferent pathways consist of parasympathetic fibers to the heart and sympathetic fibers to the heart and the peripheral blood vessels. As a result of the baroreflex, increases in BP lead to an increase in vagal outflow to the heart and a decrease in sympathetic outflow to the heart and the resistance vessels, with consequent readjustment of BP. Parasympathetically mediated changes in heart rate are fast, develop with almost no time lag, and provide instantaneous regulation, whereas sympathetically mediated changes in heart rate, cardiac contractility, and arteriolar vasomotor tone are slower and require a few seconds to develop [732,751].

Owing to the "closed-loop" situation in which the change in BP is both the input and the output of the baroreflex system, measurement of baroreflex sensitivity (BRS) in humans is restricted to the vagal arm of the reflex [732]. Direct information on activity of the sympathetic nerves can be provided by transcutaneous microneurographic recordings of muscle sympathetic nerve activity of peripheral nerves in the limbs, a difficult and invasive technique requiring highly trained operators. The neck chamber technique involves the application of an airtight collar round the neck, exerting a positive or negative pressure. This method provides direct stimulation to the baroreceptors of the carotid region without affecting BP and thus allows the simultaneous measurement of both heart rate and BP responses. However, this method needs the patient's collaboration, may be uncomfortable, and presents technical problems [751].

Any assessment of BRS requires a beat-to-beat measurement of arterial pressure in addition to R-R interval recording. Previously, this method required arterial cannulation, but this limitation has been overcome with the development of devices for continuous noninvasive finger measurement of BP such as the Finapres (Ohmeda 2300, Englewood, Colo., USA), which operates on the volume clamp technique described by Peňáz in 1976, or more recently the Colin tonometer (Colin Medical Instruments Corp., San Antonio, TX, USA). These are excellent techniques by which to monitor BP changes during steady state conditions and during maneuvers such as the Valsalva and orthostatic stress. Moreover, they allow accurate assessment of baroreflex function and of BP variability by means of spectral analysis [752].

BRS can be measured from the reflex heart rate response to pharmacologically induced changes in BP or by analyzing the spontaneous fluctuations of BP in steady-state conditions. The method most widely used to measure the BRS is the phenylephrine test. The rapid rise in arterial pressure induced by this α-adrenoceptor stimulant elicits a reflex bradycardia; the rise in systolic arterial pressure and the lengthening of the R-R interval are linearly related, and the slope of this relationship may be taken as a measure of BRS and expressed as milliseconds of increase in R-R interval per millimeter of mercury rise in arterial pressure [732]. Normal values range from 15 to 50 ms/mmHg for young adult subjects [753].

Spontaneous BRS can be assessed in both the time and the frequency domain by the "sequence" method or by evaluating the "α-angle". In the time domain, the sequence method is based on identifying, in a continuous recording of BP and heart rate, sequences of at least three successive beats where a progressive increase in systolic BP is associated with a progressive increase in R-R interval or vice versa. Such sequences are considered to be baroreflex-mediated, and the slope of the regression line between changes in systolic BP and subsequent changes in heart rate (regression coefficient of the sequences) is taken as an index of BRS. The frequency domain assessment involves spectral analysis enabling the linkage or cross-spectrum between the BP and R-R interval signals to be quantified in terms of amplitude or gain, phase (the time shifts between two signals), and coherence. The α-angle analyzes the gain of the baroreflex loop on the assumption that given the presence of a significant relationship between BP and heart rate, documented by the coherence function, fluctuations produced on heart rate by changes in BP are baroreflex-mediated. Thus, when applying spectral analysis to continuous BP and heart rate signals, the α-angle or α-coefficient is the ratio between R-R interval and BP spectral powers at each frequency where the powers are coherent, e. g., in the low-frequency band (around 0.1 Hz) or in the high-frequency band (around 0.25 Hz) [754]. These computer-oriented techniques have the advantage that they do not require patient cooperation and allow BRS assessment during real-life conditions, avoiding artificial laboratory conditions [751,754]. However, there are still some caveats associated with these methods, owing to such continuing problems as incomplete standardization, lack of reference values, the difficulty of measurements, and their limited availability [732].

Using both time-domain and frequency-domain methods, BRS has been found to be depressed in hypertensive patients and in the elderly. Moreover, BRS shows a circadian rhythm, with a marked increase during the night that again tends to be blunted in hypertensive subjects and in the elderly. BRS is also impaired in patients with cardiovascular diseases such as congestive heart failure and myocardial infarction [755,756].

BRS is impaired in diabetic patients, as first documented by Bennett et al. [757] using the phenylephrine test. BRS as evaluated by vasodilatory amyl nitrite inhalation and the phenylephrine test was reduced in ten type 2 diabetic patients with AN who subsequently developed hypertension, and was found to be inversely related to the degree of orthostatic hypertension [758]. BRS measured using different methods, i. e., from the relation of BP change to R-R interval lengthening during phase 4 of the Valsalva maneuver, and by the α-coefficient and the sequence method applied on resting R-R intervals and systolic BP recordings, was reduced in 30 type 1 diabetic patients without evidence of abnormal cardiovascular tests, and appeared to be related to diabetes duration, glycemic control, and increased left ventricular mass index [759,760]. Both time-domain and frequency-domain estimates of spontaneous BRS, i. e., slope of sequences and α-coefficient, were found by Frattola et al. to be quite sensitive in the early detection of autonomic cardiac neuropathy in 20 diabetic patients [761]. BRS was also reduced in 15 type 1 microalbuminuric patients without evidence of AN [762]. Thus, a reduction in baroreflex gain assessed using the sequence method and the α-angle may well prove to be more sensitive in the detection of early autonomic impairment [754]. To this end, studies are needed that assess the prevalence of autonomic dysfunction on the basis of age-related normal ranges for BRS in comparison with standard autonomic function tests.

The precise level of the defect in the baroreflex function in diabetic patients is not known and could theoretically involve any component of the reflex, from the baroreceptors, which are potentially affected by increased thickness and reduced distensibility of the carotid wall or by endothelial dysfunction, to the afferent and efferent branches of the arc. Animal studies have allowed attribution of this impairment to a selective defect in parasympathetic control of heart rate during increases in BP and, more precisely, to a defect in the activation of central parasympathetic pathways [763]. However, it is possible that baroreflex modulation is globally impaired in human diabetes. The significance of these early abnormalities, i. e., whether they are structural or functional in nature, is not completely clear [751]. Their clinical significance is also uncertain, but increasing evidence indicates that in the general population BRS has prognostic value for cardiovascular mortality, chronic heart failure, and myocardial infarction [755,756], thus indirectly suggesting that impaired BRS may also be of prognostic significance in diabetic patients [764].

QT Interval Measurement

Prolongation of the QT interval corresponding to the duration of the ventricular electrical activity has been reported in diabetic AN [765,766]. This ECG abnormality has been interpreted as the consequence of an imbalance between right and left sympathetic nerve activity and as a marker of electrical instability possibly leading to life-threatening ventricular arrhythmias. A long QT has been associated with poorer survival prognosis in diabetic patients [767], and it is still debated whether acquired prolongation of the QT interval has pathophysiologic and prognostic significance in a similar way to the congenital syndrome. There is increasing evidence of the role of genetic factors in both nondiabetic and diabetic population. QTc in diabetic twins was significantly longer in diabetic than in nondiabetic twins and correlated between them, suggesting that both genetic and environmental factors played a role [768]. In a large random sample of type 1 diabetic patients, a QT_C (corrected QT rate) greater than 440 ms (the upper limit of normal commonly used in the literature) was present in 31% of those with AN, 24% of those without, and in 8% of control subjects [769]. In the EURODIAB IDDM study many factors were associated with QT lengthening, i. e., female gender, diabetic nephropathy, ischemic heart disease, and AN, this last only in male subjects [770]. A link between insulinemia and the QT interval has been proposed in healthy subjects [771]. Physiologic hyperinsulinemia acutely prolonged the QT_C interval in a manner independent of insulin sensitivity in healthy subjects, presumably due to insulin-induced hypokalemia and adrenergic activation [772]. Acute hyperglycemia (about 15 mmol/l) produced an increase in QT_C duration and QT dispersion in healthy subjects, but these effects appeared to be independent of endogenously released insulin [773]. Thus, autonomic dysfunction does not seem to be the unique factor related to QT interval lengthening, but genetic factors, intrinsic metabolic, or electrolytic changes of heart muscle cell are probably involved. A recent meta-analysis has reassessed the role of QT_C in the diagnosis of diabetic AN, examining 17 studies that together enrolled 4584 diabetic patients. This study found that the pooled sensitivity and specificity for AN of a QT_C greater than 441 ± 8 ms were 28% and 86%, respectively, and that sensitivity was higher in men than women and in younger than older patients [774]. Thus, QT_C prolongation could be a specific albeit insensitive marker of AN. While the relationship of QT prolongation to diabetes appears to be quite complex, there is increasing evidence to support its role as an independent predictor of cardiac death in various cardiac diseases, alcoholic liver disease, dysautonomias, diabetic nephropathy, and others. In type 1 diabetic patients with overt nephropathy a prolonged QT_C was associated with an increased mortality risk independent of the presence of AN [775]. In a cohort-based prospective study in type 1 diabetic patients, QT_C prolongation was predictive of 5-year mortality (odds ratio in multivariate analysis: 24.6) [776].

In type 2 diabetes the role of QT_C as a prognostic marker of mortality is less obvious, and QT dispersion may be more important. QT dispersion (the difference between the longest and shortest QT interval from any lead of a 12-lead ECG) reflects the degree of spatial heterogeneity in recovery of excitability and is an independent marker of arrhythmogenic potential. Increased QT dispersion has been found to be a major determinant of mortality risk in type 2 diabetic patients [777], but to be more linked to structural factors and focal ischemia than to AN per se. Angiotensin converting enzyme inhibitor and angiotensin receptor antagonists have been shown to reduce QT dispersion in myocardial infarction and congestive heart failure, and physical exercise has been found to shorten the QT interval in elderly people [778].

Heart Rate Variability

Analysis of HRV has been used as a measure of cardiac autonomic control. It can be performed in two main ways, by statistical operations on R-R intervals (time-domain analysis) or by spectral analysis of a series of successive R-R intervals (frequency-domain analysis). Both can be performed on short R-R sequences or 24-hour ECG recordings.

Time-Domain Analysis

A number of time-domain indices can be obtained from R-R intervals. The standard deviation (SD) and coefficient of variation (CV) for a given R-R interval sequence are the easiest. Another approach is based on sequences of successive R-R interval differences and includes the SD and CV of these differences, and also the mean square (MSSD) or the root mean square of successive R-R interval differences (RMSSD). These two latter methods are insensitive to trends in mean R-R. Although easy to compute, time-domain indices are not clear in their meaning. SD is a measure of overall variability, including fast and slow changes, due to both parasympathetic and sympathetic influence on the heart. Moreover, the longer the R-R interval sequence, the more complex and numerous the factors influencing heart rate and its variability. The RMSSD and "counts" methods, first introduced by Ewing

[680], would be more specific for vagal activity, in that they quantitate vagal-dependent short-term variability (fast changes in heart rate), are not diminished by β-blockade, disappear following administration of atropine, and correlate with each other and with the high-frequency component of the power spectrum (see below). The "counts" method measures the number of large differences (> 50 ms or > 6%) in successive R-R intervals. R-R counts are age-related in healthy subjects, increase at night, and are almost zero in patients with diabetic AN or those with transplanted hearts [680]. This method, generally applied to 24-hour ECG recordings, is considered to be easy, relatively insensitive to artifacts, well reproducible, and more sensitive than the standard autonomic function tests for the assessment of cardiac parasympathetic function [680,779].

The widespread use of 24-hour ECG recordings in cardiology has led to a number of studies in which HRV indices were applied to the total 24-hour R-R interval sequence. These have shown the crude SD of R-R intervals and other time-domain indices to be prognostic markers for all-cause mortality, sudden deaths, and arrhythmic events following myocardial infarction [739,780]. Reduced 24-hour HRV has been interpreted as evidence of a shift in sympathovagal balance in favor of sympathetic activity which may result in an arrhythmogenic effect. A decrease in 24-hour HRV, measured by the SD of R-R intervals, SD of successive R-R interval differences, or the "counts" method, has been observed in diabetic patients, being more pronounced in those with impaired autonomic function tests [680]. However, longitudinal studies to evaluate the prognostic significance of 24-hour HRV in diabetic patients are lacking.

Frequency-Domain Analysis

The main advantage of spectral analysis is the possibility of assessing not only the amount of overall variability but also the frequency-specific oscillations, and to distinguish better than the time-domain methods the relative impact on variability of sympathetic and vagal modulations on the heart. Rhythmic oscillations have long been recognized in cardiovascular variables, such as heart rate, BP, and vasomotion. In phase with respiration and vasomotor waves, these variables appear to be under neural control, and rhythmic discharges can be detected in sympathetic and vagal outflows. The reasonable periodicity and regularity of these oscillations allow spectral analysis of the signal sequences. The hypothesis underlying this approach is that quantitative analysis of cardiovascular rhythmical oscillations allows evaluation of the complex interaction between the nervous control circuits on the basis of different time responses (faster for the vagal nerve, slower for the sympathetic system) [781]. A strong coherence exists between cardiovascular variability, assessed by spectral analysis of heart rate and BP, and efferent sympathetic muscle nerve activity variability, measured by microneurography, suggesting that common central mechanisms govern the rhythmic activity of the autonomic nervous system [782].

Two different mathematical techniques can be used for spectral analysis of R-R variability, fast Fourier transformation or an autoregressive model. The latter technique may be synthesized as follows. From continuous ECG monitoring, after analog-to-digital conversion, a computer program recognizes individual R waves and corresponding R-R intervals and inserts them in a tachogram. With an autoregressive algorithm, the computer then calculates the spectrum of R-R variability, providing a quantitative assessment of the number, frequency, and power (i. e., area) of each spectral component [783,784]. There are two main spectral components, with frequencies centered respectively between 0.03 and 0.15 Hz (low frequency, LF) and between 0.18 and 0.40 Hz (high frequency, HF). The HF component is similar in shape and center to the frequency of the respiratory signal and is generally considered a marker of vagal activity, although a sympathetic influence has been advocated on the basis of inconclusive studies using β-blockers. The LF component seems to depend on more complex mechanisms. Maneuvers enhancing the sympathetic drive or abnormal conditions associated with sympathetic hyperactivity led to a marked relative increase in the LF component [783]. Some disagreement on its relation to sympathetic tone is due to the observation that both LF and HF are reduced after administration of atropine, particularly to a subject in the supine position. Atropine increases heart rate and thus reduces overall HRV and, consequently, LF and HF, both of which constitute a fraction of HRV. The hypothesis that LF can be influenced by the vagal nerve is valid only if one evaluates LF in absolute and not in relative terms. It is therefore more appropriate to consider the relationship between LF and HF (LF/HF ratio) in terms of sympathovagal balance rather than to consider them separately as independent indices of sympathetic and vagal activity [781,783].

Both the LF and HF components are reduced in diabetic patients with AN [785]. Moreover, abnormalities in spectral parameters (particularly in the LF component) can occur before clear alterations in the standard autonomic function tests and might suggest, in addition to parasympathetic involvement, an impairment of cardiac sympathetic control relatively early in the natural history of AN. Furthermore, LF oscillations detected when applying spectral analysis to BP and peripheral flow signals suggest impaired sympathetic outflow to vessels in diabetic patients [786]. Thus, neural control of both heart rate and BP could be altered early in the course of diabetes. In patients with advanced neuropathy showing a marked decrease in HRV, a paradoxical predominance of HF over LF oscillations has been shown despite the evidence of vagal failure. This HF component synchronous with respiration is probably not autonomic in nature, but due to mechanical factors dependent on breathing acting on the atrium, similar to observations made in transplanted hearts. In these cases spectral analysis of HRV is an unreliable measure of sympathovagal balance [781].

Nonlinear Analysis

Nonlinear methods based on the chaos theory can evaluate HRV under unstable conditions, thus providing information on how the cardiovascular system reacts to real life situations. The underlying hypothesis is that the ability to generate complex HRV patterns is typical of the healthy heart and has a favorable prognostic meaning. This attribute cannot be assessed by time-domain or frequency-domain methods. Approximate entropy and fractal dimension are examples of nonlinear indices of complexity in which larger values indicate greater randomness, which have been found to be reduced in diabetic patients with AN, suggesting an impaired capacity to adapt to external stress stimuli [787]. Nonlinear parameters correlate only weakly with time-domain or frequency-domain indices, suggesting that they measure different aspects of cardiac autonomic control. Quantitative analysis of Poincaré plots of successive R-R intervals has recently been introduced as another nonlinear method of detecting patterns of heart rate dynamics, but in diabetic patients they appear to be less frequently abnormal than HRV indices [788].

Circadian Rhythm of Heart Rate and Blood Pressure

Abnormal circadian rhythms of cardiovascular parameters have been described in diabetic patients with AN. The circadian patterns studied best have been those of heart rate and BP.

Heart Rate

Twenty-four-hour ECG recordings have shown progressive flattening of the normal 24-hour heart rate pattern in diabetic patients with increasing degrees of autonomic damage, resulting in complete loss of the nocturnal fall [680]. The night-time increase in HRV is also attenuated in diabetic patients [784].

Blood Pressure

Circadian fluctuation of BP, with higher levels during the day and lower levels during the night, is well described in both healthy and hypertensive subjects. A drop from day to night by more than 10% of mean daytime BP identifies the normal pattern, the so-called "dippers," while a fall of less than 10% identifies the so-called "nondippers" [789].

Only a small number of hypertensive subjects (about 17% according to O'Brien et al. [790]), are nondippers. A reduced nocturnal BP fall can occur in association with glucocorticoid excess and hyperthyroidism, malignant hypertension or hypertension with advanced organ damage, eclampsia, congestive heart failure, sleep apnea syndrome, arteriosclerosis obliterans, and old age. Apart from these particular pathophysiologic conditions, many observations support a role of the autonomic nervous system in regulating the circadian BP rhythm. An abnormal nyctohemeral pattern has been observed in patients with primary autonomic failure, tetraplegia, diabetic or uremic AN, and in those who have undergone cardiac transplantation. It may be that an endogenous oscillator exerts its action on or by means of the autonomic nervous system [781].

A blunted or reversed circadian pattern of BP has been increasingly described in diabetic patients. This abnormality has been linked to both AN and diabetic nephropathy. We observed in both normotensive type 1 and type 2 diabetic patients that AN is the major determinant of circadian variation in BP, and that it is associated with a reduced day-night difference in BP. Moreover, in a group of type 1 and type 2 diabetic patients we found the day-to-night difference in BP gradually decreasing with increasing severity of AN [781]. Furthermore, we showed that the day-night profile of BP was related to the circadian pattern of sympathovagal balance (Fig. 5.**20**), suggesting that in diabetic patients with AN an impaired increase in vagal activity during the night could lead to an abnormal nocturnal sympathetic predominance, resulting in a blunted fall of BP and heart rate [791]. A more recent study has confirmed the strong relationship between the circadian pattern of BP and autonomic function even in the absence of diabetic nephropathy by showing a correlation between the day-night change in BP and the LF component of spectral analysis of HRV in normoalbuminuric type 1 diabetic patients [792]. Moreover, the concept that a latent hyperhydration could be responsible for the loss of nocturnal BP fall in type 1 diabetic patients with overt nephropathy has not been supported by a recent study [793]. In type 2 diabetic patients with overt nephropathy and hypertension, blunted nocturnal fall in BP was related to sympathetic activity during the night as measured by the catecholamine levels [794]. Thus, an abnormal circadian pattern of BP in patients with clinical nephropathy could be the consequence of the common association of nephropathy with AN, present in at least 50% of macroalbuminuric patients, while hyperhydration if present might play an exacerbating role.

In hypertensive patients the disruption of the normal circadian rhythm in BP has been ascribed prognostic value in relation to stroke [790], atherosclerosis, left ventricular hypertrophy [789], ectopic ventricular activity, albuminuria, and increased vascular resistance. Although the prognostic significance of nondipping with respect to the endorgan damage caused by hypertension and cardiovascular disease is being critically

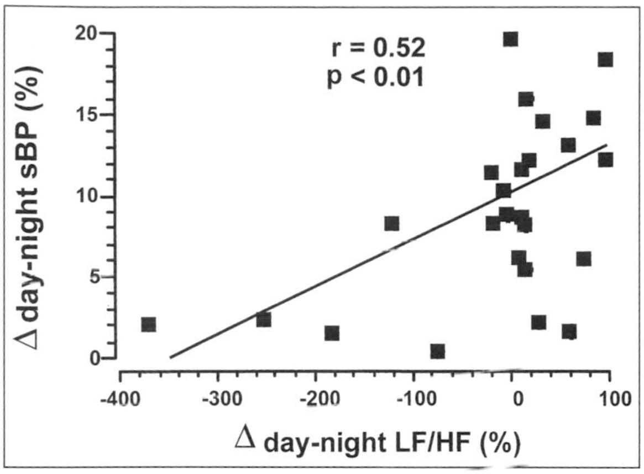

Fig. 5.20 Correlation between day–night difference (Δ day–night) of systolic BP (sBP) and day–night difference (Δ day–night) of low frequency: high frequency (LF/HF) ratio in diabetic patients, showing that the loss of nocturnal fall in BP is associated with impaired circadian variation of sympathovagal balance. (From [791], with permission)

reassessed [795], evidence is accumulating to suggest a prognostic significance of nondipping in diabetes. A higher left ventricular mass index was associated with reduced nocturnal BP fall even in normotensive diabetic patients with AN [796]. Liniger et al. [797] have shown a significantly higher incidence of fatal and severe nonfatal cardiovascular and renal events in diabetic patients with a nocturnal rise in BP. A recent 7.5-year follow-up study has confirmed a higher incidence of cardiovascular morbid events in hypertensive nondippers than in dippers, although among type 2 diabetic patients the adverse prognostic significance of the blunted nocturnal reduction in BP was limited to the female sex [798]. Recently, a longitudinal study in type 2 diabetic patients has shown that inversion of the circadian rhythm of BP has an independent predictive value for both fatal (relative risk: 11) and nonfatal vascular events (relative risk: 4) as well as hemodialysis treatment (relative risk: 16) [799,800].

Sympathovagal Activity

Using power spectral analysis of heart rate applied to 24-hour ECG recordings, a circadian rhythm of sympathovagal balance has been observed in the general population. While the LF component is predominant during the daytime, a prominent increase of the HF component occurs during the night, resulting in a marked decrease in the LF/HF ratio from day to night. This can be explained by the dominance of sympathetic activity during the day, which decreases during the night along with vagal arousal [801]. Diabetic patients with AN display an impairment in the absolute values of both HF and LF oscillations [784,791]. However, blunting of the nocturnal increase in the HF component, which expresses vagal modulation of the heart, seems to be the earliest and most prominent event. This leads to a relative predominance of sympathetic activity during the night (Fig. 5.**21**) [791].

The abnormal circadian pattern of sympathovagal balance has been shown to be related to a similar abnormality in the BP pattern [791]. These two abnormalities could be relevant to the excess cardiovascular mortality rates described in the diabetic population and in patients with AN [709,740]. A circadian behavior of cardiac and cerebrovascular events has been widely reported in the general population [802]. The morning peak of cardiovascular events has been attributed to a morning surge of some potentially triggering mechanisms [802], such as the morning rise in sympathetic activity [801]. Similarly, in diabetic patients the nocturnal predominance in sympathetic activity might predispose to, or trigger, cardiovascular events via the increase in nocturnal heart rate, BP, and vascular tone together with direct proarrhythmogenic or thrombogenic effects. Therefore, a relative predominance of sympathetic activity at night combined with higher nocturnal BP levels might represent a cardiovascular risk factor in diabetic patients. This association could also modify the circadian pattern of cardiovascular events, offering a possible explanation for the increased incidence of myocardial infarction during the night reported in diabetic patients [803].

Comparison of Methods of Assessing Changes in Heart Rate and Blood Pressure

At present, standard autonomic function tests, e.g., the modified Ewing battery, retain their utility for diagnosis of cardiac AN in diabetes. Despite the ability to detect early involvement of autonomic function, other reflex tests evaluating mainly sympathetic or baroreflex activity lack sufficient standardization and still need to be proven as valid alternatives to the widely used and better standardized autonomic function tests.

Spectral analysis of HRV seems to be a promising technique in that it allows evaluation of both components of the autonomic nervous system in steady-state conditions and can better distinguish between vagal and sympathetic modulation of heart rate than can the time-domain methods. However, since these latter methods are applicable to Holter ECG recordings, which are widely used in cardiology, they can be used as a screening approach. Generally, both the time-domain, such as R-R "counts," and frequency-domain indices of 24-hour HRV seem to be more sensitive than the standard autonomic function tests [680,784].

Although there is some degree of correlation between spectral analysis parameters and standard autonomic function tests, particularly those based on heart rate [785], it is not very close, particularly in regard to 24-hour spectral parameters [804]. This may be due to differences in the sensitivity of these

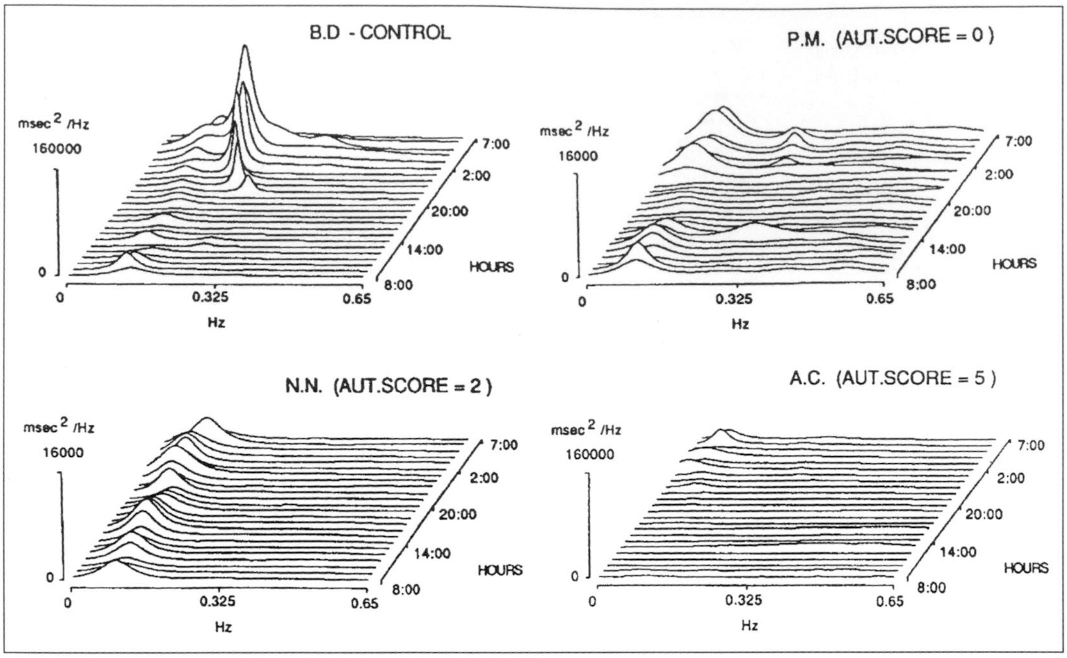

Fig. 5. **21** Examples of 24-hour pattern of LF and HF components of power spectral analysis of heart rate variability. B.D.: normal pattern in a control subject, showing the prevalence of LF during the day and the gradual increase of HF during the night; A.C.: abnormal pattern in a diabetic subject with definite AN (autonomic score = 5), showing persistence of only the sympathetic component during the night, with absence of a detectable HF component; N.N.: blunted increase in HF and LF prevalence during the night in a diabetic subject with early AN (autonomic score = 2); P.M.: presence of a normal trend in a diabetic subject with normal cardiovascular tests (autonomic score = 0), although an attenuation of HF nocturnal increase is already apparent. LF and HF are expressed in absolute units. (From [791], with permission)

techniques, but also to the fact that they express different aspects of autonomic activity.

Twenty-four-hour evaluation of HRV has some peculiarities in comparison with short-term evaluation. Its technical advantages are higher sensitivity and better intraindividual reproducibility [788,805]. Twenty-four-hour HRV values could be considered a stable individual characteristic [788,806], unless there is a significant lifestyle change with particular regard to physical exercise [779]. From a pathophysiologic point of view this approach provides data on the circadian rhythm of sympathovagal activity, and thus on autonomic control mechanisms linked to the sleep cycle, which can be affected earlier and differently from those involved in the autonomic function tests. Furthermore, the information obtained could have prognostic implications in terms of cardiovascular morbidity and mortality and offer opportunities for therapy aimed at restoring the most favorable balance throughout the 24-hour period [780]. On the other hand, there are still many problems of standardization with these methods. Different time-domain indices are being used, and there is no general consensus about the exact meaning of the frequency components of the power spectrum, leading to difficulties in comparing clinical studies. Thus, a consensus on the recording duration, measurement conditions, calculation algorithms, and age-related normal values is needed [780,806]. Normal ranges and reproducibility of different measures of 24-hour HRV have recently been provided [788]. However, the sensitivity, specificity, and predictive value of HRV assessment in relation to morbidity and mortality need to be determined in large longitudinal studies in the general and in the diabetic populations.

Cardiac Radionuclide Imaging

Difficulties in Assessing Sympathetic Dysfunction in Diabetes

During the past few decades the diagnostic assessment of cardiovascular autonomic neuropathy (CAN) has been based on heart-rate and blood-pressure responses to physical maneuvers such as deep breathing, the Valsalva maneuver, or orthostatic changes. However, these tests provide only indirect information about the integrity of the cardiovascular autonomic regulation. The heart rate changes to deep breathing at a given pace, increase and release of intrathoracic pressure, and change in body posture have been considered to represent the parasympathetic modulation of the heart. The BP response to orthostatic change (active standing or passive tilting) and to an isometric muscular contraction (sustained handgrip) were regarded as reflecting the sympathetic cardiovascular regulation [676]. It has been reported that the tests detecting sympathetic dysfunction are less sensitive than those reflecting parasympathetic alterations. On the basis of these observations, a pattern of initial parasympathetic dysfunction followed by more advanced stages of sympathetic involvement has been suggested [807]. This sequence has been interpreted as a consequence of the nerve length dependence of the neuropathic process, but on the other hand it may simply reflect a lower relative sensitivity of the tests indicating sympathetic dysfunction. Nevertheless, physiologically it does not appear useful to classify these indexes as sympathetic or parasympathetic, as has been proposed by the San Antonio conference [676], because changes in either heart rate or BP may reflect more or less activity of both systems. Moreover, the validity of the sustained handgrip test in detecting CAN has been questioned in diabetic patients, and the need for better standardization of the autonomic reflex tests has been emphasized [729]. In view of these hurdles, radionuclide imaging techniques that permit direct quantitative assessment of myocardial adrenergic dysfunction have been increasingly used in recent years to examine cardiac innervation in patients with diabetes and other diseases.

Technical Aspects

The primary neuronal structure in the ventricular myocardium is sympathetic nerve fibers. They travel in the superficial subepicardium, primarily following the coronary vessels, and as they progress from base to apex, they gradually penetrate the myocardium and innervate the endocardium by plexus terminals. By contrast, the sparse parasympathetic fibers travel along the ventricles in the subendocardium and subsequently penetrate upward to innervate the epicardium. Their respective neurotransmitters are norepinephrine and acetylcholine [808].

Early studies demonstrated that radiolabeled norepinephrine is rapidly taken up into presynaptic sympathetic nerve terminals by an energy-requiring, sodium-dependent, low-capacity, high-affinity amine uptake mechanism (uptake 1). This process is mediated by a specific membrane protein called norepinephrine transporter. Once transported into the synaptic nerve terminal, norepinephrine will be accumulated in storage vesicles by an active, reserpine-sensitive, vesicular monoamine transporter mechanism.

Hydroxyephedrine, a norepinephrine analogue, labeled with carbon-11 is a positron-emitting tracer and a highly specific marker for the norepinephrine uptake 1 and vesicular storage mechanism of the sympathetic nerve terminals, with little nonspecific binding [808,809]. Positron emission tomography (PET) using hydroxyephedrine produces high-quality images of the myocardial distribution of sympathetic nerve endings and allows in vivo quantification of tissue tracer concentration [809].

In early 1980, radioiodinated metaiodobenzylguanidine (MIBG) with a chemical structure similar to that of norepinephrine and the ganglionic blocking drug guanethidine was developed. MIBG competes with norepinephrine for uptake and granular storage mechanisms in the sympathetic nerve endings, but it is not metabolized by catechol-o-methyltransferase or monoamine oxidase. MIBG has been successfully used to study cardiac sympathetic nerve endings in both physiologic and pathophysiologic settings using single-photon emission computed tomography (SPECT), because unlike PET this method is used worldwide. MIBG using SPECT produces good-quality images of the presence and spatial distribution of sympathetic nerve terminals in the myocardial tissue and allows a qualitative and semiquantitative assessment of neuronal injury. The disadvantage of MIBG is its nonspecific uptake into nonneural tissue via a low-affinity, energy-independent diffusion mechanism in the first minutes after injection. For this reason, imaging during the first 15 minutes after intravenous injection partly reflects nonneural MIBG uptake in myocardial tissue. Late MIBG imaging between two and four hours after injection demonstrates more reliably the stable intravascular MIBG uptake in cardiac sympathetic neurons, and should be used to assess the integrity of cardiac sympathetic nerve terminals in disease. This recommendation is based on experimental studies showing that cardiac sympathetic nerve damage by stellate ganglionectomy, epicardial phenol application, or administration of 6-hydroxydopamine produces a marked decrease in myocardial MIBG uptake. Sympathetic denervation in these studies was demonstrated by biochemical or electrophysiologic techniques [810,811]. Further support is given by studies which reported that heart transplantation, transmural myocardial infarction, diabetes mellitus, and Shy-Drager syndrome produce a marked loss in MIBG uptake. These data show that myocardial MIBG uptake defects should be compared with blood flow imaging. Furthermore, the retention of MIBG in sympathetic nerve terminals is highly dependent on intact transporter systems. A variety of drugs such as tricyclic antidepressants, cocaine, reserpine, phenylephrine, labetolol, and calcium channel blockers interfere with MIBG uptake mechanisms and impair visualization.

Sympathetic Innervation Defects in Cardiac Disease

Since the sympathetic nervous system was thought to play a key role in the manifestation of many types of heart disorders, several authors have used MIBG and hydroxyephedrine to examine myocardial adrenergic innervation under physiologic and pathophysiologic conditions. Sympathetic nerve damage in denervation studies was documented by depletion of myocardial stores of norepinephrine, decreased radiolabeled norepinephrine uptake and, most specifically, by loss of electrophysiologic responses in denervated myocardium [811]. Similarly, total cardiac denervation in humans by cardiac transplantation produces a marked loss of MIBG or hydroxyephedrine uptake. Cardiac transplantation results in sympathetic denervation by surgical disruption of the sympathetic nerve fibers from their somata. In one study, no visible myocardial MIBG uptake was observed within the first year after transplantation, whereas after 1–2 years 48% of the transplanted patients developed visible MIBG uptake, which was accompanied by demonstrable transmyocardial release of norepinephrine. Thus, there was evidence for late (> 1 year) but not early (< 1 year) regional reinnervation. Similar results have been reported using the norepinephrine analogue hydroxyephedrine [808]. The success of radionuclide imaging in demonstrating cardiac sympathetic nerve damage in these conditions has resulted in studies of heart disorders such as hypertrophic cardiomyopathy, and congestive heart failure. Changes in sympathetic nerve function in these diseases are more complex and harder to interpret than in cardiac denervation. Because cardiac tracer uptake is usually less severely affected than in denervation, performing accurate quantitative studies is of great importance. In dilated cardiomyopathy, cardiac washout is accelerated compared to that seen in healthy subjects [811]. Patients with heart failure showed a decrease in hydroxyephedrine retention, and the degree of abnormality varied regionally, indicating a heterogeneous pattern of neuronal dysfunction [808].

Sympathetic Innervation Defects in Diabetic Patients

Recent studies have demonstrated decreased myocardial MIBG uptake in type 1 or type 2 diabetic patients with abnormal or normal autonomic function tests, predominantly in the left ventricular inferior and posterior segments [812,813]. Several lines of evidence suggest that MIBG scanning is more sensitive in detecting CAN than is autonomic reflex testing. Defects in MIBG uptake have been reported to correlate with reduced power spectrum of HRV, prolonged QT interval length, body mass index, systolic BP, autoantibodies to sympathetic ganglia, and abnormal left ventricular response to exercise and impaired diastolic filling [814].

Several studies in diabetic patients suggest that MIBG defects are more pronounced in the inferior, posterior, and apical segments than in the anterior, septal, and lateral regions [812–814]. However, a similar trend has also been observed in healthy subjects [815]. The putative mechanisms for this apparent heterogeneity in the distribution of MIBG uptake are several. First, there may be attenuation of MIBG uptake by the diaphragm. Second, an artifact in SPECT reconstruction caused by high uptake of MIBG in the liver has been shown in a phantom study. Third, there is evidence that myocardial MIBG uptake declines with increasing age, particularly in the inferior wall [816]. Fourth, there may be physiologic variation in that the anterior wall has predominantly sympathetic afferent innervation and vagal afferents distribute preferentially to the inferoposterior wall. A recent study has demonstrated a correlation between MIBG uptake in the inferior wall and the high-frequency power spectrum reflecting vagal activity in healthy subjects, suggesting that the heterogeneous MIBG distribution may be due to the depressor reflex mediated by the vagal fibers predominantly located in the inferoposterior wall [817]. Furthermore, it is unclear whether MIBG is also taken up by sympathetic afferents, since the sensory neurotransmitter has not yet been identified. However, it is possible that MIBG uptake indirectly reflects the innervation of afferent nerves which run through with sympathetic efferent nerves [815]. Thus, there is evidence that heterogeneous distribution of MIBG in the left ventricle may reflect a physiologic phenomenon. On the other hand, a pattern of diminished MIBG uptake predominantly in the inferior or posterior segments similar to that found in diabetic patients has been reported in the absence of coronary artery disease in patients with idiopathic ventricular tachycardia, congenital long QT syndrome predisposing to malignant arrhythmias and sudden death, and arrhythmogenic right ventricular cardiomyopathy clinically manifesting with ventricular arrhythmia. Although the exact mechanism of attenuated myocardial MIBG uptake remains to be elucidated, sympathetic denervation has been suggested as its primary underlying substrate [818]. In fact, myocardial sympathetic efferent denervation evidenced by loss of electrophysiologic responses has been shown to correlate with defects in MIBG uptake in the dog model. Patients with spontaneous ventricular tachyarrhythmias following myocardial infarction showed regions of thallium-201 uptake indicating viable perfused myocardium, with no MIBG uptake. It is possible that reduced MIBG uptake, particularly in the inferior, posterior, and apical segments, mirrors areas of denervation that might represent an arrhythmogenic substrate related to the increased mortality in diabetic patients with CAN. On the other hand, because of the complex nature of sympathetic nervous system regulation, it is difficult to determine whether a given change in sympathetic function represents a pathologic or compensatory event [811]. Studies of adequate statistical power and duration are required to evaluate whether a relationship exists between changes in MIBG uptake and mortality.

In patients with a history of sustained ventricular tachycardia or aborted episodes of sudden death, a prolonged effective ventricular refractory period was found in areas of myocardium that showed reduced retention of the norepinephrine analogue [^{11}C]hydroxyephedrine. In diabetic patients, attenuated hydroxyephedrine retention was related to the severity of CAN and was most pronounced in the inferior, apical, and lateral segments. In patients with severe CAN, the myocardial retention of hydroxyephedrine was remarkably heterogeneous, since as the extent of distal deficits increased, hydroxyephedrine retention became paradoxically increased in the proximal myocardial segments [819] which showed the highest deficits in coronary blood flow reserve [820]. This kind of proximal hyperinnervation complicating distal denervation could result in potentially life-threatening myocardial electrical instability. Thus, potential cardioprotection by β-blocking agents in these patients needs to be considered.

Recently, an impaired increase in myocardial blood flow in response to sympathetic stimulation by the cold pressor test was demonstrated in diabetic patients with reduced myocardial hydroxyephedrine uptake. Impairment in this sympathetically mediated dilation of coronary resistance vessels was significantly related to the degree of sympathetic denervation. Such an inadequate dilator response of resistance vessels could lead to myocardial ischemia or left ventricular dysfunction during periods of increased oxygen demand, even in the absence of overt coronary atherosclerosis (Fig. 5.**22**) [821].

One group reported a surprisingly high prevalence of reduced MIBG in 77 % of newly diagnosed type 1 diabetic patients [822]. It appears unlikely that these abnormalities at the time of diagnosis of type 1 diabetes reflect a myocardial denervation process. Instead, increased sympathetic activity could account for the reduced MIBG uptake. In patients with pheochromocytoma an inverse relationship between myocardial MIBG uptake and plasma norepinephrine concentration has been demonstrated. In short-term experimental diabetes a similar inverse relationship has been observed between MIBG uptake and myocardial norepinephrine levels, and myocardial sympathetic activity has been found to be increased. In contrast, post-mortem studies in long-term diabetic patients have demonstrated markedly reduced concentrations of norepinephrine in heart tissue, indicating sympathetic denervation. Thus, reduced MIBG uptake in early and longer-term type 1 diabetes may reflect different pathophysiologic events.

Sympathetic Innervation Defects in Diabetic Patients with Silent Ischemia

Anginal pain results from stimulation of the afferent fibers running through the cardiac sympathetic nerves. Hence, it is obvious to assume that CAN may interfere with the afferent cardiac sensory impulses. The association of CAN with silent coronary artery disease (CAD) is difficult to evaluate with autonomic reflex tests which mainly assess vagal control of heart rate. Studies that have addressed this issue using MIBG scintigraphy showed controversial data. While one study demonstrated a higher degree of MIBG uptake defects in diabetic patients with silent myocardial ischemia compared to those without it, two other studies found no such difference. In fact, even more pronounced MIBG defects were observed in patients with painful CAD [701,702]. This is in agreement with the finding of an association between MIBG defects and increased cardiac pain sensitivity in nondiabetic patients with recent myocardial infarction, suggesting denervation supersensitivity. Epidemiologic data suggest that increased incidence of asymptomatic myocardial infarctions, CAD, and myocardial ischemia in diabetic patients mainly reflects accelerated atherosclerosis, and that the proportion of silent CAD is not abnormally increased. Thus, despite the attractive theoretical background, there is no convincing evidence from MIBG studies for an association between CAN

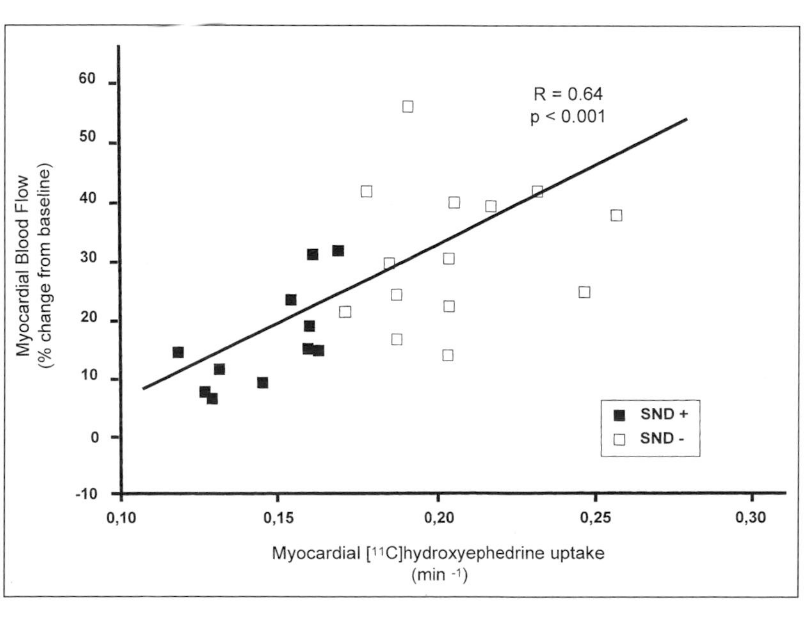

Fig. 5.**22** Scatterplot showing relation between myocardial uptake of [^{11}C]hydroxyephedrine, reflecting magnitude of cardiac sympathetic nerve dysfunction (SND), and percent change (from baseline) in myocardial blood flow in response to cold pressor test in patients with diabetes. Relation was $y = -0.201$, $x = 2.455$, $R^2 = 0.418$, SEE = 0.11, $F = 18.68$, $P < 0.001$. (From [821], with permission)

and silent ischemia [702]. The mechanisms of silent myocardial ischemia are complex, and further studies are required in this context.

Prospective Studies in Diabetic Patients

A four-year prospective study demonstrated that long-term poor glycemic control constitutes an essential determinant in the progression of left ventricular adrenergic innervation defects which may be prevented by near-normoglycemia in type 1 diabetic patients. Both global and regional MIBG defect scores in the inferior, posterior, and apical walls were increased in poorly controlled patients as compared with those who maintained near-normoglycemia over four years. In addition, the well-controlled patients showed enhanced global MIBG uptake compared with the poorly controlled group after four years [823]. Figure 5.**23** illustrates examples of a marked improvement in MIBG uptake in a patient who maintained near-normoglycemia (Fig. 5.**23a**) and a marked deterioration in a patient with poor metabolic control (Fig. 5.**23b**) during the period studied. In contrast, no such differences were noted for autonomic function testing, suggesting that direct assessment of myocardial innervation defects by MIBG scintigraphy may be more appropriate than indirect autonomic function testing for evaluating the effect of metabolic intervention in CAN. Similar results have been reported in a three-year study using hydroxyephedrine [824]. The findings of these studies challenge the notion that CAN is an irreversible complication of diabetes. Studies of the natural history of CAN have demonstrated that HRV either deteriorated at a slow rate or did not change over 4–10 years in patients with longer-term insulin-dependent and non-insulin-dependent diabetes. Given that these abnormalities evolve so slowly, any intervention aimed at near-normoglycemia appears to require many years to demonstrate a halt or slowing of progression of CAN assessed by tests based on HRV, as shown in the Diabetes Control and Complications Trial (DCCT), in which intensive insulin therapy prevented the deterioration in HRV over a mean of 6.5 years in the primary intervention cohort but not in the secondary intervention cohort [825].

Intensive insulin therapy producing stable HbA_{1c} levels for three years did not result in major changes in MIBG uptake [826]. One prospective study included 16 newly diagnosed type 1 diabetic patients who were treated by intensive insulin therapy for 1 year [827]. However, that study did not include a poorly controlled group for comparison. Despite a marked drop in mean HbA_{1c} from 11.5 % to 6.3 %, an improvement in MIBG uptake was noted only in the posterior and septal regions, and the mean global myocardial MIBG uptake score did not change at the end of one year. It is possible that less readily reversible components of cardiac sympathetic dysfunction may be present even at early stages of diabetes, but the underlying pathophysiology of these defects remains to be elucidated.

Clinical Impact

Orthostatic hypotension, reduced HRV, QT prolongation, QT dispersion, impaired baroreflex sensitivity, sympathovagal imbalance with a relative predominance of sympathetic activity during the night, and a loss of the nocturnal BP fall are all associated with both diabetic AN and increased cardiovascular morbidity. Part of the excess cardiovascular mortality in neuropathic patients (see Chapter 3) may be due to altered neural control of the cardiovascular system. Causes of death in neuropathic patients include endstage renal failure, cardiovascular disease, and some sudden unexpected deaths. The association between AN and nephropathy may in part account for the high prevalence of deaths from renal failure. A possible pathogenetic role of autonomic dysfunction in diabetic nephropathy has been suggested [828,829]. A full understanding of causes of the sudden deaths described in diabetic patients with AN is still lacking. One possible explanation has been proposed on the basis of differential sympathetic denervation of the proximal and distal parts of the left ventricle, leading to hyperexcitability of the proximal region of the ventricle [819,820]. Moreover, reduced HRV has been associated with both ischemic and nonischemic sudden death as well as ventricular tachycardia [830]. Autonomic dysfunction has been considered to explain the so-called "dead in bed" syndrome, a sudden and probably arrhythmogenic death possibly caused by nocturnal hypoglycemia. According to this hypothesis, at an early stage of AN relative sympathetic overactivity in type 1 diabetic patients would represent a favoring condition in which nocturnal hypoglycemia might further increase sympathovagal imbalance, prolong the QT_c interval via the associated hypokalemia, and thus increase the risk of ventricular arrhythmias [760].

Moreover, parasympathetic neuropathy has been found to be an independent predictor of ten-year follow-up development of stroke (odds ratio 6.7) in type 2 diabetic patients [831]. A defect of parasympathetically mediated cerebral vasodilator mechanisms that are activated during stress, such as ischemia, might be involved. Furthermore, using spectral analysis applied to transcranial Doppler signals, an autonomic modulation of cerebral blood flow has been shown to be present in healthy subjects and to be impaired in type 2 diabetic patients with AN [832]. Impaired central control of respiration leading to respiratory arrests, sleep apnea, and impaired respiratory reflexes is another possible but not proven pathogenetic mechanism of increased mortality in diabetic patients with AN.

Finally, careful monitoring of cardiorespiratory function is required during anesthesia in patients with AN, given the reports of cardiorespiratory arrests during anesthesia, increased perioperative cardiovascular instability, and abnormal cardiovascular reactions even in slightly stressful ophthalmic surgery [833].

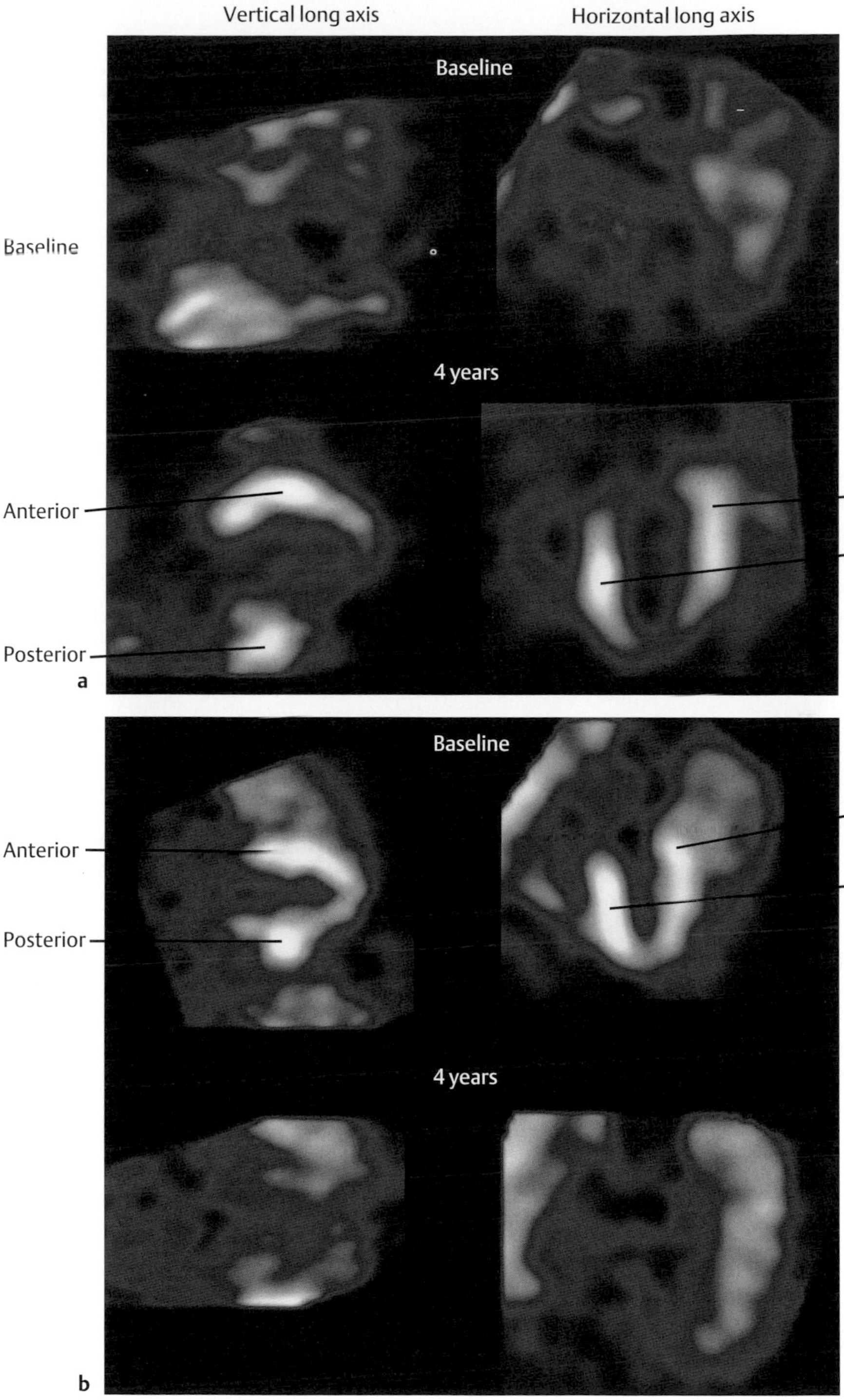

Fig. 5.**23** Examples of a marked improvement in left ventricular MIBG uptake after four years in a patient who maintained near-normoglycemia **a** and marked deterioration in left ventricular MIBG uptake in a patient who was poorly controlled over four years **b**. (From [823], with permission)

Respiratory Tract

L. Scionti and P. Bottini

Introduction

Abnormalities of respiration can be found in diabetic patients with AN, although their clinical relevance is still unknown. Diabetic patients can show changes in lung volumes and diffusing capacity. These are not related to AN, but to the duration of disease, the degree of metabolic control and, possibly, to glycation of proteins of the connective tissue [834–843].

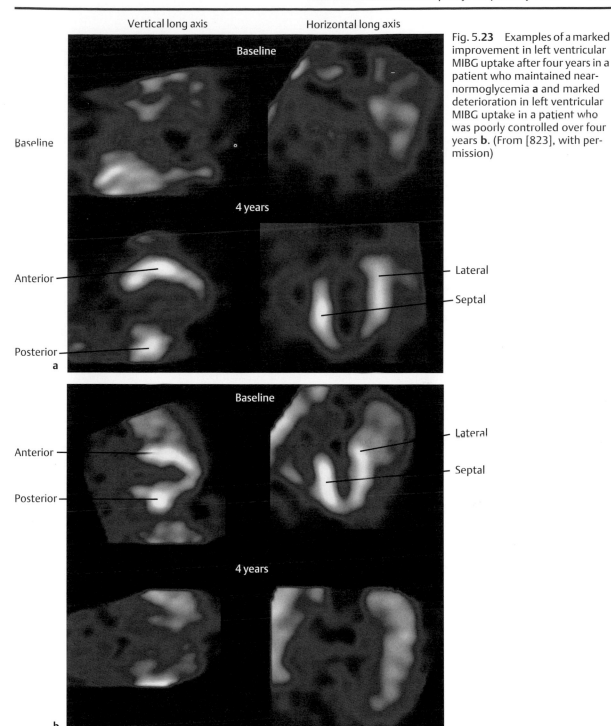

Several clinical studies have demonstrated that AN can affect (1) bronchial tone, (2) airway reactivity, (3) the pattern of breathing and ventilation during physical exercise, (4) chemical control of ventilation and, finally, (5) the control of breathing during sleep. Each of these abnormalities will be discussed below.

Abnormalities of Respiration

Bronchial Tone

For many centuries it has been recognized that the airways are innervated. Human lungs are innervated by branches from the right and left vagus nerves and the first four or five thoracic sympathetic ganglia. The parasympathetic preganglionic fibers terminate in ganglia located in the conducting airways. The ganglia contain cholinergic neurons which are responsible for the tonic activation of the smooth muscle cells of the bronchial tree. Although the autonomic nervous system influences several aspects of the airway functions (submucosal gland secretion, epithelial cell function, and bronchial vascular tone in both normal conditions and pulmonary diseases), all the studies performed in diabetic patients with AN have focused on evaluation of the bronchial tone. Because bronchial tone cannot be measured directly in human subjects, analyzing the increase in the caliber of the airways after inhalation of anticholinergic drugs is the only way to estimate this feature.

Douglas et al. [844] measured the specific airway conductance in two groups of diabetic patients, 11 with and 11 without AN, before and after inhalation of 80 μg of the anticholinergic drug ipratropium bromide. They did not find any difference in basal airway conductance between the two groups, but bronchodilation after ipratropium bromide inhalation was significantly greater in the patients without than in those with neuropathy, suggesting that airway vagal tone was reduced in the latter group.

Similar results have been obtained by our group using a greater dose of ipratropium bromide (100 μg) [845]. In our experiment the specific airway conductance (Fig. 5.**24**) and the maximum expiratory flows during a forced expiratory maneuver increased less in patients with neuropathy than in both nonneuropathic diabetic patients and healthy control subjects. No differences were found between the latter two groups.

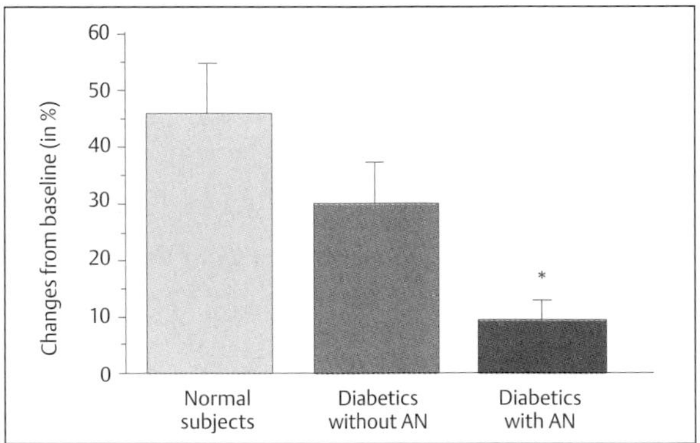

Fig. 5.**24** Changes from baseline in specific airway conductance after inhalation of 100 μg ipratropium bromide in normal subjects and in diabetic patients with and without autonomic neuropathy (AN). Bronchodilation is significantly lower in patients with AN, suggesting a decrease in the basal bronchial tone. Data are expressed as mean ± SEM. $^*P < 0.01$ versus other groups

More recently a group from Brazil [846] examined a larger group of diabetic patients with and without AN before and after atropine (1 mg) administration by aerosol. Their results did not differ from the previous ones.

Taken together, these studies show that basal bronchial tone is reduced in diabetic patients with AN in comparison to patients without this complication of diabetes. The impairment of the parasympathetic branch of the autonomic nervous system is responsible for this functional abnormality, which does not have any clinically relevant consequences.

Bronchial Reactivity

Various stimuli can induce bronchoconstriction in humans by at least three mechanisms: direct effect on the smooth muscle cells, local release of chemical mediators from mast cells, and neural reflexes. The afferent arm of the neural reflexes is made up of receptors and afferent fibers. Among others, irritant receptors have been found between superficial cells of the bronchial epithelium. These receptors respond to irritative chemical and mechanical stimuli, inducing bronchospasm and cough. It is generally accepted that all afferent nerve fibers from the receptors in the airways travel in the vagus nerve. For the above-mentioned anatomic reasons, bronchial reactivity has been studied in diabetic patients with AN using both chemical and physical stimuli to evaluate the parasympathetic nervous system of the lungs.

Heaton et al. [847] first examined the bronchial reactivity to cold air in two small groups of insulin-dependent diabetic patients with and without AN. They found that the specific airway conductance was reduced by 20% in patients with AN and by 30.8% in those without AN, demonstrating decreased bronchoconstriction in patients with neuropathy due to the vagal nerve involvement in diabetic AN.

We also studied the methacholine-induced bronchial reactivity in two groups of diabetic patients and in normal subjects [848]. We were able to demonstrate that the mean increase in the resistance of airways after a cumulative dose of 10 mg of methacholine was 55.2% in patients with neuropathy, whereas it was 149.8% and 131.6% in patients without neuropathy and in normal subjects, respectively. In this experiment we also measured the P_{100}, which is the mouth pressure generated during the first 100 milliseconds of inspiration against occluded airways and is a measure of the activity of the respiratory centers in the brain stem. We found a marked increase in P_{100} (Fig. 5.**25**) and a strong relationship between this measure and the resistance of the airways in normal subjects ($r = 0.71$, $P < 0.001$) and in patients without neuropathy ($r = 0.68$, $P < 0.001$); on the other hand, P_{100} increased to a lesser extent in

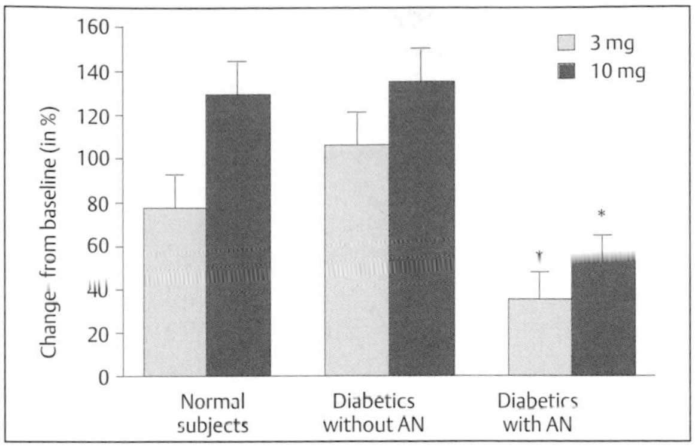

Fig. 5.**25** Changes in P_{100} after inhalation of 3 and 10 mg (cumulative doses) of methacholine in normal subjects and in diabetic patients with and without autonomic neuropathy (AN). The lower increase in P_{100} is due to a decrease of afferent vagal stimulation from the airways to respiratory centers in the brainstem. Data are expressed as mean ± SEM. *$P <$ 0.05 versus other groups

diabetic patients with AN (Fig. 5.**25**) and the above-mentioned relationship was weaker ($r = 0.44$, $P < 0.01$). These results indicate a lesser degree of afferent stimulation from the bronchial receptors to the respiratory centers due to the impaired vagal pathways.

Diminished bronchial reactivity to methacholine has also been reported by Bertherat et al. [849]. They found a negligible decrease of FEV_1 from basal value in patients with neuropathy (8 %), while it was 24 % and 22 % respectively in normal subjects and diabetics without AN. Moreover, they also found a significant relationship between the changes in FEV_1 and the degree of the autonomic impairment in their diabetic patients.

Vianna et al. [850] studied bronchial reactivity in diabetic patients by measuring the cough threshold to inhaled citric acid. They demonstrated that the cough threshold was higher in patients with neuropathy, suggesting that the vagal afferent fibers from bronchial airways mediating the cough reflex are affected in this group of diabetic patients.

In contrast with the above-reported studies, Rhind et al. [851] found an increased bronchial reactivity to histamine in diabetic patients with AN, which was ascribed to denervation hypersensitivity. However, in this study most of the subjects were smokers. This makes the conclusions of the study questionable, since the airway hyperreactivity might be due to the baseline reduction of the bronchial caliber.

It has been postulated that reduced bronchial reactivity could favor pulmonary infections [852] and, on the other hand, reduce the incidence of asthma in diabetic patients with AN. However, to our knowledge, there are no clinical studies to support this hypothesis.

Ventilation During Exercise

Diabetic patients with AN can be considered a model alternative to heart-lung-transplanted patients to study the effects of chronic autonomic denervation on ventilation during exercise. Transplanted patients show a higher ventilatory response to increasing CO_2 production and more rapid increase of respiratory rate and tidal volume at the beginning of exercise compared to normal subjects [853–855]. On the basis of these results, it has been suggested that complete pulmonary denervation modifies the level of ventilation but not the breathing pattern at the peak of exercise.

We studied the ventilatory response to exercise in 20 diabetic patients, ten with and ten without AN, and in a control group of healthy volunteers [856]. During submaximal (≥ 90 % of maximum predicted heart rate) or symptom-limited incremental exercise using a computer-driven electronically braked cycle ergometer, the minute ventilation (V_E) at corresponding values of CO_2 production (VCO_2) was significantly higher in diabetic patients with AN than in patients without neuropathy and in control subjects. The slope of the linear relationship between V_E and VCO_2 was 0.032 ± 0.002 ml/min in patients with AN and was steeper than that in diabetics without AN (0.027 ± 0.001; $P < 0.05$) and control subjects (0.025 ± 0.001; $P < 0.01$). Moreover, in our neuropathic patients higher ventilation was associated with a marked increase in respiratory rate at the end of exercise (Fig. 5.**26**). We also measured the P_{100} during exercise and found that the P_{100} was higher in both groups of diabetic patients than in control subjects at corresponding values of PCO_2, indicating an increased neural drive from the respiratory centers during effort in diabetes. Our results demonstrate that chronic autonomic denervation of the lung as can be seen in diabetic patients

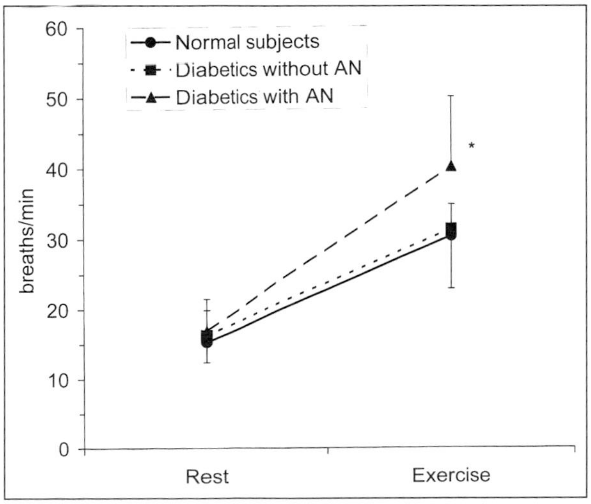

Fig. 5.**26** Respiratory rate at rest and peak of exercise in normal subjects and in diabetic patients with and without AN. The increased respiratory rate at peak of exercise indicates a change in the breathing pattern during exercise in patients with AN. Data are expressed as mean ± SEM. *$P < 0.05$ versus other groups

influences both the level of ventilation and the breathing pattern during stressful exercise. Because abnormalities in the respiratory pattern and ventilation have never been detected at rest either in studies with diabetic patients or in those with transplanted nondiabetic patients, it can be concluded that the neural control of respiration plays a role only in stressful conditions such as strenuous exercise.

Wanke et al. [857] examined another aspect of respiration during exercise: the inspiratory muscle load. Using an incremental progressive exercise test on a cycle ergometer, they demonstrated that for each level of ventilation the mechanical load on the inspiratory muscles during exercise is elevated in diabetic patients. This phenomenon, inducing inappropriately high respiratory effort, could contribute to the lower physical performance of diabetic patients. However in this study no attempts were made to correlate the results with autonomic neuropathy.

In conclusion, although changes in the breathing pattern, in the neural control of ventilation, and, possibly, in the inspiratory muscle effort can be detected during exercise in patients with AN, ventilation is still able to match the increasing demands of the body for O_2 uptake and CO_2 elimination, and it is not a limiting factor.

Chemical Control of Ventilation

Arterial blood gas tensions and pH are an important mechanism of ventilation control. Peripheral chemoreceptors in the carotid bodies monitor changes in arterial Po_2, Pco_2, and pH, whereas central chemoreceptors in the medulla detect Pco_2 variations. From the peripheral chemoreceptors afferent fibers travel to the brain stem in the glossopharyngeal nerve.

The chemical control of ventilation has been studied extensively in diabetic patients with and without AN using both hypoxic and hypercapnic stimulation. Several studies [858–862] have been performed to examine the ventilatory response to hypoxia, and in most of them [859–862] the results consistently demonstrated a blunted response in patients with AN compared with diabetic patients without AN and normal subjects. In one detailed study, Montserrat et al. [860] showed a mean increase of ventilation after transient hypoxia of 43 %, 34.7 %, and 24.7 % in normal volunteers, diabetic patients without neuropathy, and patients with AN, respectively. The reduced ventilatory response to hypoxia has been related to damage to the cholinergic fibers traveling from the carotid bodies to the brainstem.

In contrast, studies on the ventilatory response to hypercapnia of diabetic patients with AN gave highly contradictory results. A large group of diabetic patients was examined by Nishimura et al. [862], who described an increase of ventilation during hypercapnia in diabetic patients. On the other hand, Sobotka et al. [861] and Soler and Eagleton [858] were unable to detect any differences between diabetic subjects with and without AN and normal volunteers. However, Soler and Eagleton [858] reported that ventilation at a Pco_2 less than 45 mmHg was higher in patients with severe AN than in those with milder degrees of autonomic impairment. A lower-than-normal ventilation during hypercapnia has been found in other studies. In addition to the qualitative study of Williams et al. [859], Montserrat et al. [860] showed that the slope value of the regression line between ventilation and CO_2 was significantly lower in both diabetic patients with and without AN than in control subjects. Similar results were obtained by Wanke et al. [863] and Homma et al. [864], mainly at high levels of CO_2 tension. A clue to the reasons for this discrepancy has been recently proposed by Tantucci et al. [865]. They reported an increase in ventilation during hypercapnia only in diabetic patients with postural hypotension, which was considered as a marker of clinically relevant impairment of the sympathetic arm of the autonomic nervous system. This group of patients exhibited a significant increase in the slope of the linear relationship between V_E and end-tidal Pco_2 ($Petco_2$) in comparison to diabetics with neuropathy but without postural hypotension, whereas the difference in comparison to normal subjects and diabetic patients without AN was not significant. Increased ventilation was also associated with a greater-than-normal central ventilatory drive, while it was lower than normal in the other two groups of diabetic patients (Fig. 5.**27**). These results indicate that severe sympathetic system damage results in increased ventilation and increased

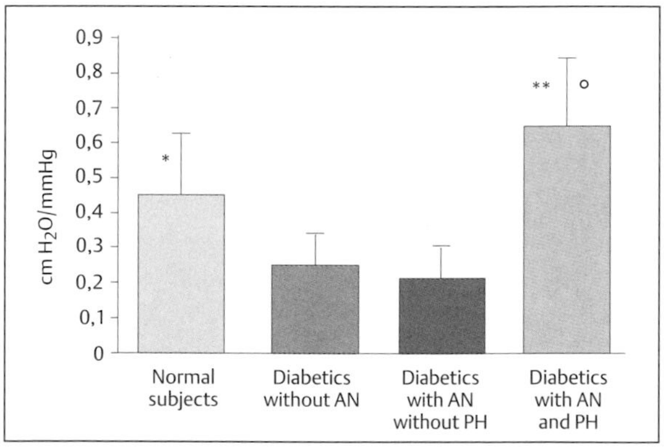

Fig. 5.**27** Values of the slopes of the linear regression analysis of P_{100} against end-tidal Pco_2 ($Petco_2$) during rebreathing in normal subjects, in diabetic patients without AN, in patients with AN without postural hypotension (PH) and in patients with AN and PH. The slope measures the rate of change in P_{100} per unit change in $Petco_2$. A clinically relevant impairment of the sympathetic system, demonstrated by the presence of PH, markedly increases the responsiveness of the respiratory centers to CO_2, otherwise reduced in diabetic patients regardless the presence of AN. Data are expressed as mean ± SD. $^*P < 0.01$ versus diabetics without AN and diabetics with AN without PH; $^{**}P < 0.05$ versus normal subjects; $^{\circ}P < 0.001$ versus other groups of diabetic patients

ventilatory drive; the opposite is true when the sympathetic system is impaired to a lesser extent and therefore does not provoke postural hypotension. Two hypothetical mechanisms have been proposed to explain these two opposite responses to hypercapnia. First, the sympathetic nervous system could directly modulate the respiratory centers in the brainstem. Experimental studies in dogs and monkeys [866] demonstrated that pulmonary sympathetic afferent fibers inhibit phrenic discharge; moreover, central noradrenergic neurons are able to inhibit ventilatory output in the absence of catecholamine-mediated peripheral effect [867,868]. Therefore, it can be hypothesized that removal of the inhibitory sympathetic activity in humans can induce higher ventilatory response during hypercapnia. On the other hand, the severely damaged sympathetic system could be unable to modulate the cerebral blood flow normally in response to hypercapnia [869,870]. Preliminary results from our group, however, do not support this hypothesis [871].

The increased central respiratory drive and ventilation during hypercapnia showed by diabetic patients with postural hypotension could play a role in inducing central apnea and/or periodic breathing during sleep, as has been demonstrated in patients with acromegaly and in other diseases [872–875].

Sleep-Related Breathing Disorders

Sleep is a crucial event for the respiratory system. Changes in central drive activity and neural control of both upper airways and ventilatory pump muscles occur in humans during sleep. Sleep apnea is defined as intermittent cessation of airflow at the nose and mouth during sleep, whereas the sleep apnea syndrome refers to a clinical disorder which arises from repeated (ten or more per hour) episodes of apnea during sleep. Sleep apnea can be classified as central (cessation of oronasal airflow without ribcage and abdominal excursions) or obstructive (cessation of oronasal airflow in the presence of ribcage and abdominal excursions). This condition is associated with several cardiac arrythmias with an increased incidence of cardiovascular morbidity, mortality, and sudden death [876]. Since diabetic patients affected by AN show a higher incidence of sudden death [877–879], several studies have been performed to explore whether or not sleep-related breathing abnormalities were responsible for these deaths.

Guilleminault et al. [880] first reported obstructive sleep apneas in two out of four subjects with AN. Rees et al. [881] also described sleep apnea in three out of eight (37 %) diabetic patients with AN, while no sleep-related breathing disorders were detected in eight diabetic subjects without AN. However, in both these studies the presence of obesity was not taken into account and the number of the examined patients was too small for conclusions to be drawn. Some years after these preliminary small studies, Mondini and Guilleminault [882] found an abnormal sleep-related breathing pattern in five out of 12 insulin-dependent diabetic patients which correlated with neuropathy. On the other hand, no significant differences between diabetic patients with and without AN in the number of sleep apneas and in other sleep-related parameters were detected in the study by Catterall et al. [883]. More recently, Ficker et al. [884] evaluated a large group of diabetic patients and reported that 26 % of patients suffering from AN had obstructive sleep apneas, whereas none of the patients without AN showed any breathing alterations. However, in some of the above-mentioned studies several patients with obstructive apneas also suffered from obesity, an important contributing factor to the occurrence of obstructive sleep apneas. Preliminary data from Bottini et al. [885], who carefully selected only nonobese insulin-treated diabetic patients, showed the occurrence of obstructive apneas in four out of 13 diabetic subjects with AN of varying severity.

Thus, there is evidence that sleep-related breathing disorders, mainly obstructive apneas, occur in diabetic patients with AN, even if oxygen desaturations are seldom lower than 80 % [886]. However, the effect of recurrent, even mild, oxygen desaturations on the cardiovascular system of patients with AN is presently unknown. The pathophysiologic mechanisms to explain the obstructive sleep events in AN are poorly understood and have so far remained speculative. Impairment of reflexes of the upper airways-dilating muscles at sleep onset [887,888] and/or damage of receptors supporting the muscle tone and patency of the upper airways [889,890] have been proposed.

Obstructive apneas were unexpected in diabetic patients with AN, because the increased central respiratory drive to CO_2 shown by diabetic patients with severe AN is known to induce periodic breathing and central apnea during slight sleep in other diseases [872–875]. However, preliminary data from Bottini et al. [885] showed that despite an increased hypercapnic central respiratory drive, diabetic patients with severe AN do not suffer from central sleep apnea, most likely because they have low peripheral chemosensitivity to CO_2, which prevents hyperventilation and hypocapnia during the waking state and, consequently, dropping of $Paco_2$ below the threshold required to stimulate the respiratory centers.

Finally, Villa et al. [891] recently described ventilatory dysfunction during sleep (central sleep apnea) in children with diabetes of short duration, with poor metabolic control, and without subclinical evidence of dysautonomia, but the mechanisms were unclear.

Gastrointestinal Tract

D. O'Donovan, M. Samsom, C. Feinle, K.L Jones, and M. Horowitz

Introduction

The outcome of recent studies has led to a redefinition of concepts relating to the prevalence, pathogenesis, and clinical significance of disordered gastrointestinal function in diabetes mellitus. Abnormal gastrointestinal function, particularly disordered motor function, occurs frequently in both type 1 and type 2 diabetes mellitus; potential sequelae include gastrointestinal symptoms, malnutrition, poor glycemic control, and delayed absorption of orally administered drugs. In patients with diabetes mellitus there is a high prevalence of gastrointestinal symptoms which affect quality of life adversely. Although both abnormal motor function and gastrointestinal symptoms have traditionally been attributed to irreversible autonomic neuropathy, it is now recognized that acute changes in blood glucose concentration affect both gastrointestinal motor function and the perception of gastrointestinal sensations.

The rapid expansion of knowledge relating to gastrointestinal motor function in diabetes over the last 15 years reflects the development of a number of techniques to quantify gastrointestinal motility in humans. There are substantial limitations in attempting to extrapolate observations made in animal models of diabetes to humans. In this section, current knowledge of the pathogenesis of disordered gut motility, the potential impact of upper gastrointestinal motility on glycemic control, and the prevalence and significance of gastrointestinal symptoms in diabetes mellitus are summarized, followed by a discussion of disordered esophageal, gastric, small intestinal, gallbladder, colonic, and anorectal motility in which diagnostic and therapeutic options are addressed.

Pathophysiology of Disordered Gut Motility

The propulsion of food and digestive products along the gut demands a complex, highly coordinated series of neuromuscular processes. The circular and longitudinal muscle layers in the gut wall are driven to contract by the interstitial cells of Cajal, which act as pacemaker cells [892]. This process is regulated by intrinsic innervation, consisting of the myenteric and Auerbach plexuses, and by an extrinsic nerve supply from the autonomic nervous system. Autonomic nerve supply consists of sympathetic and parasympathetic (vagal) efferents and sensory afferents. The neural pathways modulate gut contraction in response to stretching and other local stimuli. Smooth muscle contraction is also influenced by numerous hormones, including vasoactive intestinal polypeptide (VIP), cholecystokinin (CCK), calcitonin gene-related peptide (CGRP), and motilin [893].

The pathogenesis of disordered gut motility in diabetes mellitus is now recognized to be multifactorial; those factors which appear to be dominant—autonomic neuropathy and glycemic control—are closely related; e. g., both acute and chronic changes in the blood glucose concentration may affect autonomic function.

Autonomic Neuropathy

Putative similarities in the symptoms experienced by patients following surgical vagotomy and those with longstanding diabetes led to the assumption that disordered gut motility in patients with diabetes reflected irreversible vagal damage, occurring as part of a generalized autonomic neuropathy [894]. As there is a lack of tests to measure gastrointestinal autonomic function, evaluation of cardiovascular autonomic function has frequently been used as a surrogate marker of dysfunction of the abdominal vagus to provide information regarding the overall autonomic supply to the abdominal viscera. While the prevalence of abnormalities in gastrointestinal function amongst patients with diabetes is higher in patients with cardiovascular autonomic neuropathy than in those without [895,896], the correlation between disordered motility and abnormal autonomic function (either parasympathetic or sympathetic) is relatively weak [897,898].

In animal models of diabetes, a number of morphologic changes are evident in the autonomic nerves supplying the gut and the myenteric plexus. These include decreases in the number of myelinated axons in the vagosympathetic trunk and neurons in the dorsal root ganglia, deficiencies of neurotransmitters such as met-enkephalin, serotonin, calcitonin-related peptide, substance P, and peptide Y, and a reduced number of interstitial cells of Cajal [899]. In rodents with diabetes, there is a reduction in nitric oxide (NO) synthase expression in myenteric neurons [900], and this is associated with slower emptying; the latter is reversed by administration of insulin or the cGMP-specific phosphodiesterase sildenafil, which acts as a NO donor [901]. Although NO is an important neurotransmitter in the gut of both animals and humans, the implications for human disease are uncertain, particularly as the effects of NO on gut motility and transit differ substantially between animal and humans, [902]. In contrast to animal models, in humans there is little evidence of a fixed pathologic process in either smooth muscle or neural tissue [903]. In a recent report in a small number of patients with intractable gastroparesis, gastric smooth muscle degeneration with eosinophilic inclusion bodies was evident [904].

The less than clear-cut association between disordered gastrointestinal function in diabetes mellitus and the presence of autonomic neuropathy may in part reflect the fact that cardiac autonomic nerve function has been measured, rather than gastrointestinal autonomic function (including the enteric nervous system). Furthermore, in most studies blood glucose levels were not monitored. Despite these limitations, it appears likely that other factors, particularly hyperglycemia, are important.

Blood Glucose Concentration

Marked hyperglycemia (blood glucose concentration ~ 15 mmol/l) appears to affect every region of the gastrointestinal tract. Smaller elevations of blood glucose that are more within the normal postprandial range (8–10 mmol/l) also influence gut function and may be important in the regulation of gut motility in healthy individuals. For example, in patients with type 1 diabetes, as in healthy subjects, marked hyperglycemia (blood glucose 16–20 mmol/l) slows gastric emptying of both solids and nutrient liquids compared to euglycemia (5–8 mmol/l) [895,905]. It is not known whether the response to hyperglycemia is dependent on the rate of gastric emptying during euglycemia or previous (long-term) glycemic control. The acute effect of hyperglycemia on gastric emptying in patients with type 2 diabetes has not been specifically studied, although cross-sectional studies suggest that an inverse relationship between the rate of gastric emptying and the blood glucose concentration also exists in this group [906]. In patients with uncomplicated type 1 diabetes, gastric emptying is markedly accelerated during hypoglycemia compared to euglycemia, as in healthy subjects. Changes in blood glucose concentrations within the normal range also influence gastric emptying; emptying of solids and liquids is slower at blood glucose of 8 mmol/l than at 4 mmol/l in both healthy subjects and type 1 diabetes [907].

Changes in the blood glucose levels affect gastric emptying by modulating the underlying motor mechanisms. Acute hyperglycemia suppresses the frequency and propagation of antral pressure waves under fasting and postprandial conditions [908], relaxes the proximal stomach, and stimulates phasic pressure waves localized to the pylorus [909]. Although most evident during marked hyperglycemia (~13 mmol/l), suppression of antral motility is apparent from a threshold blood glucose concentration of as low as 8 mmol/l. This dose-response relationship is concordant with that observed between the rate of gastric emptying and the blood glucose concentration. Acute hyperglycemia also affects the gastric pacemaker which determines the frequency of antral contractions, with an increased prevalence of tachygastria in both healthy subjects [910] and patients with type 1 diabetes [911].

Effects of hyperglycemia have been observed in all regions of the gut. Acute hyperglycemia suppresses duodenal and jejunal motility [912] and slows small intestinal transit [913]. Gallbladder contraction in response to fat or intravenous cholecystokinin is dose-dependently inhibited [914a]. Both the gastrocolic and ascending component of the colonic peristaltic reflex are inhibited at a blood glucose concentration of 15 mmol/l compared to euglycemia [915], although no effects on colonic tone were evident in another study [916]. Rectal compliance has been reported to be increased [917] or unchanged [918] during hyperglycemia, while resting and maximum squeeze pressures in the anus are either decreased [917] or unchanged [918]. These latter discrepancies are likely to reflect methodologic differences.

There is relatively little information about potential mechanisms mediating the effects of the blood glucose concentration on gut motor function. In healthy subjects the secretion of pancreatic polypeptide, which is under vagal cholinergic control, is diminished during acute hyperglycemia, suggesting a reversible impairment of vagal efferent function [919]. The reduced heart rate response to standing ("30:15 ratio") in healthy volunteers during hyperglycemia when compared to euglycemia, is also indicative of transient impairment of vagal parasympathetic function [920]. Insulin does not appear to play a major role, as indicated by the effects of euglycemic hyperinsulinemia [921]. Prostaglandins may be involved in the mediation of abnormal gastric electrical rhythms during hyperglycemia [910]. Further studies are indicated to define the neural, humoral, and cellular mechanisms by which systemic glucose affects gastrointestinal motility.

Impact of Gastrointestinal Motility on Glycemic Control

Although Kassander observed in 1958 that "the retention of stomach contents in a diabetic may cause confusion as far as food intake and utilization are concerned," the potential impact of upper gastrointestinal motor function on postprandial glycemia has until recently received little attention. This is despite the recognition that there is a close association between both the development and progression of diabetic micro- (and possibly macro-)vascular complications and average glycemic control, as assessed by glycated hemoglobin. Glycated hemoglobin is influenced by both fasting and postprandial glucose levels; while their relative contributions have not been defined, it is clear that improved glycemic control can be achieved by lowering postprandial blood glucose concentrations, even at the expense of higher fasting glucose levels. Accordingly, the control of postprandial blood glucose levels represents a specific target for therapy; this forms the primary rationale for the development of short-acting forms of insulin and insulin secretagogues. It remains to be determined whether postprandial glycemia per se, including the magnitude of postprandial hyperglycemic spikes, has a distinct role in the pathogenesis of diabetic complications.

Postprandial blood glucose levels are potentially influenced by a number of factors including preprandial glucose concentrations, the glucose content of a meal, small intestinal delivery and absorption of nutrients, insulin secretion, hepatic glucose metabolism and peripheral insulin sensitivity. The relative contribution of the factors remains controversial and is likely to vary with time after a meal. The rate of gastric emptying determines the delivery of nutrients into the small intestine, which is tightly regulated as a result of feedback from small intestinal luminal receptors. It is now recognized that gastric emptying accounts for at least 35 % of the variance in peak postprandial glucose levels after oral glucose (75 g) in both healthy individuals and patients with type 2 diabetes [922]. As these were cross-sectional studies, the contribution of gastric emptying is likely to have been underestimated. In type 1 patients with gastroparesis, as would be predicted, less insulin is required to maintain euglycemia immediately after a meal compared to type 1 patients with normal gastric emptying. Although the number of formal studies is limited, it appears that much of the observed variation in the glycemic response to different food types (glycemic indices) is attributable to differences in rates of gastric emptying. The limited information that is available suggests that small intestinal motility also plays an important role in glucose absorption.

The potential for the modulation of gastric emptying to minimize postprandial glucose excursions and optimize glycemic control, either by dietary or pharmacological means, represents a novel approach to the management of diabetes which is being explored actively. Potential therapeutic strategies are discussed on pages 254–257.

Gastrointestinal Symptoms

Somewhat surprisingly, there is relatively little information about either the prevalence, determinants, or importance of gastrointestinal symptoms in patients with diabetes mellitus, and the significance of this problem remains a matter of controversy [923]. As was the case with sexual dysfunction some years ago, some clinicians do not inquire about gastrointestinal symptoms. Few population-based studies have been performed, and a number of reports relate to patients recruited from tertiary referral centers, with a high probability of selection bias [924]. In evaluating studies relating to gastrointestinal symptoms in diabetes, it should be recognized that there is a high prevalence of gastrointestinal symptoms in the community, particularly those associated with functional dyspepsia and the irritable bowel syndrome, which are known to be related to both demographic and psychologic variables. Studies should, therefore, take into account a number of factors, including age, sex, body weight, psychologic status and use of drugs (including alcohol and nicotine), as well as "diabetes-specific" variables, including the type of diabetes, acute and chronic glycemic control, diabetic complications, and usage of oral hypoglycemic medications. Cross-sectional studies are inherently associated with substantial limitations; at present there are no longitudinal studies relating to gastrointestinal symptoms in diabetes, and hence there is no information about the natural history of gastrointestinal symptoms in diabetes. It should also be recognized that in most studies symptoms were not evaluated using validated measures, and that total symptom scores, rather than the severity of individual symptoms, were quantified.

While acknowledging the caveats alluded to above, there is no doubt that the prevalence of gastrointestinal symptoms is high in both type 1 and 2 diabetes [897,923–926] (Table 5.**9**). There is, moreover, substantial support for the concept that the prevalence of gastrointestinal symptoms is also increased compared to the general population, especially in women [923,926]. For example, in a study of 110 outpatients with longstanding type 1 diabetes, Schvarcz et al. reported that the prevalence of postprandial fullness was 19 % compared to 9 % in control subjects, and that of vomiting 12 % versus 3 % [926]. A recent population-based study from Minnesota, which addressed the prevalence of gastrointestinal symptoms in 350 (predominantly type 2) diabetic subjects and their association with psychologic variables, medication intake, and symptoms of autonomic and peripheral neuropathy, found that the prevalence of most gastrointestinal tract symptoms (i. e., nausea, vomiting, dyspepsia, diarrhea, or fecal incontinence) was high, but no greater among people with type 1 and 2 diabetes than in controls of similar age and sex [927]. However, in a similar study from Australia involving subjects with type 2 diabetes, all upper and lower gastrointestinal symptoms evaluated were more common in community-dwelling people with diabetes than in controls [923]. In another US study of 483 patients with type 2 diabetes, 50 % reported one or more upper gastrointestinal symptoms, compared with 38 % in controls [928]; similar observations have also been made in Sweden [929].

The impact of gastrointestinal symptoms, as opposed to other aspects of diabetes, on "health-related quality of life" amongst patients with diabetes is poorly documented. Those studies that have been performed support an association. For example, a recent study suggests that in both type 1 and 2 diabetes, gastrointestinal symptoms impair physical functioning and general health perceptions [930].

Potential (and in many cases interrelated) determinants of gastrointestinal symptoms in people with diabetes include: disordered motility, psychologic and demographic variables, autonomic neuropathy, visceral hypersensitivity, changes in gastrointestinal myoelectrical activity, medication use, and *Helicobacter pylori* infection. Although gastrointestinal symptoms have been attributed to disordered motor function and abnormal transit, there is a relatively poor correlation between gastrointestinal symptoms

Table 5.9 Prevalence rates of gastrointestinal symptoms rated at least "often" in diabetes mellitus and controls

Symptoms	Prevalence rate %		Adjusted[a] odds ratios with 95% CI
	Controls $n = 8185$	Diabetics $n = 423$	
Abdominal pain/discomfort	10.8	13.5	1.63 (1.21–2.20)
Postprandial fullness	5.2	8.6	2.07 (1.43–3.01)
Heartburn	10.8	13.5	1.38 (1.03–1.86)
Nausea	3.5	5.2	2.31 (1.45–3.68)
Vomiting	1.1	1.7	2.51 (1.12–5.66)
Dysphagia	1.7	5.4	2.71 (1.69–4.36)
Fecal incontinence	0.8	2.6	2.74 (1.40–5.37)
Esophageal symptoms[b]	11.5	15.4	1.44 (1.09–1.91)
Upper dysmotility symptoms[c]	15.3	18.2	1.75 (1.34–2.29)
Any bowel symptom[d]	18.9	26.0	1.84 (1.46–2.33)
Diarrhea symptoms[e]	10.0	15.6	2.06 (1.56–2.74)
Constipation symptoms[f]	9.2	11.4	1.54 (1.12–2.13)

[a] Adjusted for age and gender
[b] Heartburn and/or dysphagia
[c] Any of: early satiety, postprandial fullness, bloating, nausea, or vomiting
[d] Any of: self-reported diarrhea/constipation, loose or watery stools, > 3 bowel movements each day, urgency, fecal incontinence, < 3 bowel movements each week, lumpy or hard stools, anal blockage
[e] Any of: > 3 bowel movements each day, urgency, loose or watery stools
[f] Any of: < 3 bowel movements each week, lumpy or hard stools, anal blockage
Adapted from [923]

and gastrointestinal motility; for example, some patients with marked delay in gastric emptying have few, or no, upper gastrointestinal symptoms. It should be recognized, however, that, as in patients with functional dyspepsia, total symptom scores (of a cluster of symptoms) may be insensitive; the presence of specific symptoms, such as postprandial fullness, when these are severe enough to influence normal activities, may be a more sensitive indicator. This may be the case in diabetes mellitus: in a recent study the perception of fullness/abdominal bloating (but not nausea or vomiting) was predictive of a delay in solid gastric emptying. Disordered transit is at present best regarded as a marker of gastrointestinal motor abnormality, rather than as a direct cause of symptoms, although additional studies are required.

The etiology of symptoms is likely to be multifactorial; for example, there is evidence in diabetes, as is the case in patients with functional dyspepsia, that symptoms may reflect visceral hypersensitivity and impaired gastric accommodation. Symptoms may also reflect disordered esophageal, small intestinal, or colonic motility, as well as psychiatric abnormality [925]. Uremia may contribute to nausea/anorexia and also affect gut motility. There is evidence, that, as in the case with functional disorders, the prevalence of symptoms is increased in females [926].

Studies of the impact of autonomic neuropathy on symptoms are inconsistent, but have generally shown a weak association. While it has been suggested that there is an increased prevalence of *H. pylori* infection in patients with diabetes [931], recent studies argue against this, and any association between *H. pylori* infection and upper gastrointestinal symptoms in patients with type 1 or type 2 diabetes. There are, however, no controlled studies of the effect of *H. pylori* eradication in this group. "Lower" gastrointestinal symptoms, such as diarrhea and fecal incontinence, are increased by the use of metformin (and presumably acarbose).

During euglycemia the perception of gastric distension is increased in type 1 patients with gastrointestinal symptoms [932], suggesting that, as in patients with functional dyspepsia, an increase in the sensitivity of gastrointestinal mechanoreceptors may be important in the etiology of symptoms. Acute changes in the blood glucose concentration affect the perceptions of sensations arising from the gastrointestinal tract—this issue has been studied less comprehensively than the effects of blood glucose concentration on motility. For example, in normal subjects, the perceptions of nausea and fullness produced by proximal gastric, or duodenal, distension are more intense during hyperglycemia (~15 mmol/l) compared to euglycemia [933].

In type 1 and type 2 diabetes the perception of postprandial fullness is related to the blood glucose concentrations [934]. Even elevations in blood glucose concentrations that are within the normal limits may affect the perception of gut stimuli [935]. An important role for hyperglycemia in the etiology of gastrointestinal symptoms is also supported by cross-sectional epidemiological studies [926]. The mechanisms by which hyperglycemia affects gut perception/symptoms is unknown, although changes in the activity of gastrointestinal pacemakers may play a role.

Investigation of a possible association between psychologic function and gastrointestinal symptoms in diabetes has been limited. Clouse and Lustman evaluated upper gastrointestinal symptoms, abdominal discomfort and altered bowel habit in 114 patients with diabetes, and reported that each group of symptoms was associated with affective and anxiety disorders [925]. In a recent study, a strong association between psychological distress and gastrointestinal symptoms in community subjects and outpatients with type 1 and type 2 diabetes was evident [936]. Moreover, the studies by Clouse and Lustman suggest that in patients with diabetes gastrointestinal symptoms may be more closely related to psychiatric disturbances than to autonomic neuropathy [925].

Esophagus

The most important function of the esophagus is to propel food boluses into the stomach. This is accomplished by swallow-induced peristalsis in the esophageal body and timely opening of the striated upper esophageal sphincter and smooth-muscle lower esophageal sphincter, the latter by a high-pressure zone at the esophagogastric junction, which is maintained by both the lower esophageal sphincter and the crural diaphragm. Following a swallow, the esophagus exhibits a circular contraction that is propagated in an aboral direction, a phenomenon called primary peristalsis. When the esophagus is distended, e. g., by a food bolus that was not cleared during previous peristaltic pressure waves or by an episode of gastroesophageal reflux, secondary peristaltic waves may occur. The lower esophageal sphincter not only relaxes following a swallow, but also spontaneously; these so-called transient lower esophageal sphincter relaxations constitute the major mechanism of gastroesophageal reflux in healthy subjects and in many patients with gastroesophageal reflux disease. The passage of food through the esophagus, and even gastroesophageal reflux, is usually not perceived, but the likelihood of perception becomes greater under pathologic circumstances, e. g., when transit of food is impaired. When excessive gastroesophageal reflux has led to esophagitis, heartburn occurs frequently.

The methods that have been used to evaluate esophageal motor function in diabetes, either for clinical or research purposes, can be divided into two categories: (1) measurement of esophageal transit, by scintigraphy or radiographic techniques, and (2) evaluation of the contractile activity of the esophageal body and lower esophageal sphincter function by manometry, esophageal pH recording, and endoscopy. Esophageal radionuclide transit quantifies the rate at which a solid and/or liquid bolus passes through the esophagus. While measurement of esophageal radionuclide transit is simple, noninvasive, associated with a relatively low radiation burden, and more sensitive than radiographic methods, the technique has not been standardized.

Prevalence and Pathophysiology

Disordered esophageal motility occurs frequently, perhaps in some 50% of patients with longstanding diabetes. There is, however, considerable variation in the reported prevalence reflecting, at least in part, differences in both the techniques used to evaluate esophageal motility and the population studied. Furthermore, there have not been any truly population-based studies, and no studies have been performed during euglycemia. Esophageal radionuclide transit is delayed in 30–50% of patients with longstanding diabetes [897]. For example, in a study of 87 randomly selected outpatients with diabetes (67 type 1, 20 type 2), esophageal transit of a solid bolus was delayed in 48% [937]. The relationship between esophageal transit and the rate of gastric emptying is poor, so measurement of esophageal transit cannot be used to predict gastroparesis.

The esophageal motor dysfunctions responsible for delayed transit are poorly characterized [938,939], and a spectrum of motor dysfunctions has been reported. The latter include a decreased amplitude and number of peristaltic contractions and an increased number of nonpropagated waves. In most cases delayed esophageal transit appears to result from either peristaltic failure or peristaltic waves of poor amplitude (Fig. 5.**28**). Upper esophageal function in diabetes has only been evaluated in one study, in which disordered pharyngeal function was evident in 14 of 18 patients with impaired swallowing [940].

The pathophysiologic mechanisms involved in disordered esophageal motility in diabetes mellitus have not been studied extensively. Abnormal esophageal motility is more frequent in those diabetic patients with evidence of peripheral or autonomic neuropathy [941]. De Boer et al. have reported in normal subjects that induced hyperglycemia is associated with a decrease in lower esophageal sphincter pressure and an increase in the duration and a decrease in the velocity of the esophageal peristaltic wave [914b].

Clinical Significance

Disordered esophageal motility in diabetics may potentially cause symptoms such as heartburn,

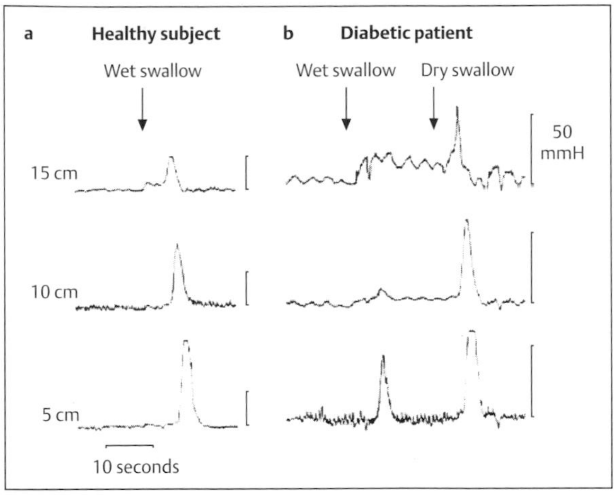

Fig. 5.**28** Wet-swallow-induced esophageal peristalsis in a healthy subject **a** and in a patient with longstanding insulin-dependent diabetes **b**. In the diabetic subject the swallow-induced peristaltic wave has insufficient force to propel the water bolus distally (failed peristalsis). Seventeen seconds later a dry swallow clears the esophagus. (Adapted from [939], with permission)

dysphagia and chest pain, and delayed transit of medications, with the consequent risks of mucosal ulceration and stricture formation. Symptoms of esophageal dysfunction are diverse. The most common is heartburn, defined as a short-lived burning sensation behind the sternum or in the epigastric region. Heartburn is a reasonably specific, but insensitive, indicator of gastroesophageal reflux disease. The most characteristic symptom of impaired esophageal transit is dysphagia. This symptom may be more likely to reflect mechanical obstruction (e. g., tumor, peptic stricture) than disordered motility of either the esophageal body or the lower esophageal sphincter.

While in some studies symptoms of esophageal dysfunction were reported to be uncommon and, when present, not usually severe, even in the presence of esophageal motor abnormalities [937,942,943], other studies suggest that symptoms occur quite frequently, especially when asked for [941]. It is clear that the relationship between symptoms and the presence or absence of delayed esophageal transit and/or abnormal esophageal motility is poor.

The prevalence of gastroesophageal reflux is almost certainly increased in diabetes [938,944]; gastroesophageal reflux may represent an underestimated cause of upper gastrointestinal symptoms in this group. For example, in a recent study of 50 type 1 patients who had no history suggestive of gastric or esophageal disease, 28 % had abnormal gastroesophageal reflux (defined as a duration in which esophageal pH was < 4 for >3.5 % of the time in a 24-hour period). In considering the motor mechanisms that may be responsible for reflux, lower esophageal sphincter pressure has been reported to be low in a number of studies [938]. The frequency of transient lower esophageal sphincter relaxations has not been evaluated. Delayed gastric emptying, particularly from the proximal stomach, may potentially contribute to gastroesophageal reflux, as has been recently suggested in patients with reflux disease unrelated to diabetes. The prevalence of esophagitis in diabetes mellitus has not been formally evaluated, but is not obviously increased.

Diagnosis

In all patients with significant esophageal symptoms, endoscopy is required to exclude organic obstruction and esophageal candidiasis; treatment of the latter with fungicidal agents usually results in rapid symptom resolution. At the present time the use of esophageal function tests (using the complementary tests of 24-hour esophageal pH monitoring, esophageal manometry, and measurement of esophageal transit) is usually reserved for symptomatic cases, with primary emphasis on the exclusion of gastroesophageal reflux, given that the treatment of esophageal motor abnormalities is often unsuccessful. It should, however, be recognized that scintigraphic measurement of esophageal bolus transit is simple and has the potential to be a useful marker of gastrointestinal involvement in diabetes.

Treatment

Patients with diabetes should routinely be advised to consume liquid after oral medication to minimize the potential for esophageal ulceration. There is limited information about the effect of drug treatment of disordered esophageal motility associated with slow transit in diabetes. Furthermore, the prognosis of disordered esophageal function in diabetes does not appear to be poor, although only one study has hitherto evaluated this issue. The effects of prokinetic drugs have been inconsistent and unconvincing. Domperidone has no effect on emptying of a solid bolus [945]. Cisapride when given acutely may improve esophageal solid bolus transit and motility [946], but neither cisapride nor metoclopramide appears to have any effect with longer-term administration. Uncontrolled observations suggest that erythromycin may be beneficial [947]. At the present time no prokinetic drug has been shown to have sustained efficacy in the treatment of disordered esophageal motility or esophageal symptoms in diabetes.

A favorable effect of fludrocortisone on esophageal emptying in diabetic patients with severe autonomic neuropathy has been reported [948] which requires confirmation. Treatment with the aldose reductase inhibitor tolrestat for one year has been reported to improve esophageal transit, and additional studies are required. Smooth-muscle relaxant drugs, such as nitrates and calcium antagonists, would not be expected to be useful. A recent report suggests that the κ-opiate agonist, fedotozine, which modifies sensory feedback from the gut, may reduce heartburn in diabetic patients with gastroparesis [949].

Stomach

Gastric emptying is a complex process involving the storage of ingesta, mixing with gastric secretions, grinding of solid food into particles 1–2 mm in diameter, and the delivery of chyme into the small intestine at a rate designed to optimize digestion and absorption. Understanding of the mechanical factors by which the stomach moves its contents into the small intestine is still limited, reflecting at least in part the technical difficulties associated with the investigation of human gastric motility. While most attention has focused on the frequency and amplitude of contractions, it is now recognized that the spatiotemporal organization of muscular activity is an important determinant of the movement of luminal content [950]. Accordingly, in many research studies a combination of methods is used. Cannon, in 1911, observed that transpyloric flow in animals is predominantly pulsatile, rather than continuous. Thus, most liquefied chyme is propelled into the duodenum as a series of small gushes [951,952]. Contrary to the earlier suggestion that one motor region could have a dominant role, the major determinant of patterns of transpyloric flow appears to be the integration of motor activity in the proximal stomach, antrum, pylorus, and proximal small intestine [953]. The proximal region of the stomach is primarily concerned with storage of ingested food. During swallowing, there is a vagally mediated transient receptive relaxation, followed by a more prolonged relaxation, known as "accommodation", so that an increase in gastric volume is not usually associated with a substantial rise in intragastric pressure [954]. The contractions of the distal stomach are controlled by electrical signals generated by a pacemaker region located on the greater curvature, which discharges at a rate of about three per minute [955]. Overall patterns of gastric emptying are dependent on the physical and chemical composition of a meal [956] so that solids, nutrient liquids, and nonnutrient liquids empty from the stomach at different rates. The major factor regulating gastric emptying of nutrients is feedback inhibition, triggered by receptors which are distributed throughout the small intestine; as a result of this inhibition, nutrient-containing liquids usually empty from the stomach at an overall rate of about 2 kcal/min.

Although other techniques, particularly ultrasound and scintigraphic breath tests, show promise [956, 957], scintigraphic measurement of gastric emptying is the most accurate and arguably the only clinically useful assessment of gastric emptying at present. Scintigraphy is relatively easy to perform and noninvasive. The radiation dose approximates that received from a single abdominal radiograph. Measurement of gastric emptying should ideally be performed during euglycemia, but at a minimum with regular blood glucose monitoring. Unfortunately, there is a lack of standardization of scintigraphic techniques, with substantial variation between different centers particularly in relation to the volume and composition of the test meal, the duration of data acquisition, and the calculation of gastric emptying rates. This makes comparisons between studies performed in different centers extremely difficult and usually means that each laboratory must have access to an appropriate control range.

Gastroparesis is usually defined as a rate of emptying that is more than two standard deviations outside a control range. In diabetes mellitus, there is a relatively poor correlation between gastric emptying of solid and liquid meal components [897,958,959], and a dual-isotope technique using different isotope markers to measure both solid and liquid emptying simultaneously (Fig. 5.**29**) is, accordingly, preferable, although this adds to the complexity of the test. If it is only feasible for a single isotope to be used, gastric emptying of solids (or semisolids) is usually measured; in this situation more prolonged observations may increase the precision of the test [960], particularly as in many patients with gastroparesis the 50% gastric emptying time is not reached for many hours. While considerable attention has been given to gastric emptying of solids, including approaches to simplify the measurements, e. g., by minimizing the duration of use of the gamma camera [960], there is little evidence that this approach offers any advantage over the use of a nutrient liquid meal (water should not be used as it does not stimulate mechanisms which retard gastric emptying). Moreover, as discussed, the rate of emptying of liquids is dependent on different mechanisms from that of solids and is frequently a major determinant of the postprandial glycemic response [958,959,961].

Scintigraphic breath tests have been used to quantify solid and/or liquid gastric emptying, most recently using stable isotopes [957]. While these tests are cheaper and simpler than external scintigraphy and, with the use of stable isotopes, avoid the use of irradiation, there is considerable debate as to the appropriate method of data analysis, and studies in patients with diabetes are limited [957,962]. Additional validation of these methods in patients with gastroparesis, particularly those in whom gastric emptying is markedly delayed, is required before their use can be advocated. It seems likely that scintigraphic breath tests will prove to be useful as a screening test for gastroparesis, and in large epidemiological studies [957].

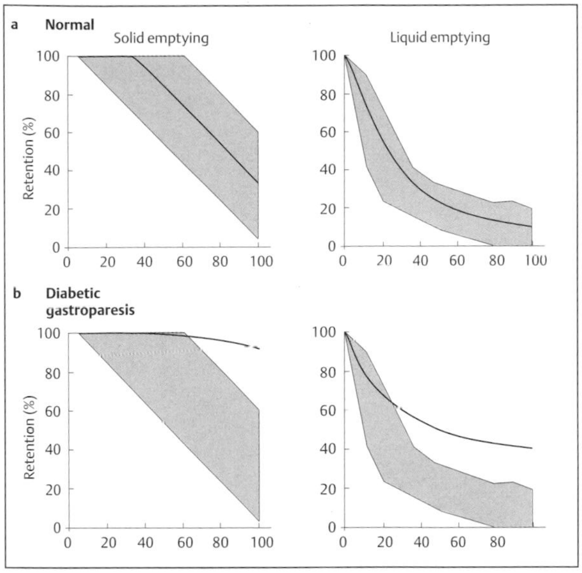

Fig. 5.**29** Gastric emptying for a mixed solid (100 g minced beef) and liquid (150 ml 10 % dextrose) meal consumed in the sitting position, measured radioisotopically in a normal subject **a** and a diabetic patient with gastroparesis **b**. The normal range (mean ± 2SD) is shown in the shaded areas. There is marked delay of solid and liquid emptying in the diabetic patient. (Adapted from [956])

Prevalence and Pathophysiology

Rundles, who in 1945 provided the first detailed description of the association between delayed gastric emptying and diabetes [894], reported that gastric emptying of barium was delayed in 5 of 35 diabetics with clinical evidence of peripheral neuropathy. In a seminal monograph, published in 1958, Kassander named the condition "gastroparesis diabeticorum" and commented that "I believe that this syndrome ... is more often overlooked than diagnosed."

Cross-sectional studies, in most cases using radionucleotide techniques to measure gastric emptying, indicate that gastric emptying of solid, or nutrient liquid, meals is delayed in 30–50 % of outpatients with longstanding type 1 [895,898,962,963] or type 2 diabetes [896,906]. The prevalence of delayed gastric emptying is greatest when gastric emptying of both solid and nutrient-containing liquids is evaluated, either simultaneously or separately [897,959]. In many cases the magnitude of the delay in gastric emptying is relatively modest, and it may be argued that a distinction should be made between "gastroparesis" and "delayed gastric emptying"; i. e., a diagnosis of gastroparesis should be restricted to those patients in whom emptying is grossly delayed. The intragastric distribution of meals is also frequently abnormal [958,964]. The prevalence of delayed gastric emptying in patients with "brittle" type 1 diabetes appears to be comparable to that in other patients with longstanding diabetes. Unlike some animal models, gastric emptying is accelerated in only a minority of patients with type 1 diabetes [897,898,965]. In contrast to longstanding type 1 or type 2 diabetes, there is evidence, albeit inconsistent, that gastric emptying in patients with "early" type 2 diabetes, particularly that of nutrient-containing liquids, is frequently more rapid than normal [959,966,967]. It has been suggested that the latter abnormality may predispose to the development of type 2 diabetes by leading to higher postprandial blood glucose concentrations [966]. The prevalence of disordered gastric emptying in patients with recently diagnosed type 1 diabetes has not been evaluated. The prevalence of delayed gastric emptying in ketoacidosis is also not known, although symptoms of nausea, abdominal discomfort, and vomiting are characteristic features that are often attributed to gastric stasis, and acute gastric dilatation is a rare complication.

It should also be recognized that there are no true population-based studies of gastric emptying in diabetes (this may prove feasible with the advent of scintigraphic breath tests), no studies have been performed during euglycemia (the prevalence of delayed emptying will presumably be less during euglycemia than hyperglycemia), and there is an absence of long-term, longitudinal studies to evaluate natural history.

In view of the incomplete understanding of the mechanisms which underlie normal gastric emptying, it is not surprising that the motor dysfunctions responsible for delayed gastric emptying in diabetes are poorly characterized. An improved understanding may allow therapy designed to accelerate gastric emptying to be targeted more effectively. It is also important to recognize that most studies in patients with diabetes have been performed either without blood glucose monitoring or during hyperglycemia, in symptomatic patients with type 1 diabetes who were assumed to have gastroparesis.

Proximal gastric function is abnormal in many patients with diabetes mellitus [932]. Antral motility has usually been evaluated as an "index" that takes into account the amplitude and frequency of pressure waves but provides no information about their organization. Both fasting (reduced phase III activity) [968] and postprandial antral hypomotility [969] occur frequently in patients with diabetic gastroparesis. In many patients there is a reduction in the number of antral waves that are temporally associated with duodenal waves; this abnormality may be a major factor contributing to slow gastric emptying [968,969]. An increase in both fasting and postprandial antral waves, as assessed by ultrasound, has been demonstrated and is of uncertain significance. Increased pyloric motility does not appear to be a major factor contributing to gastroparesis, at least during euglycemia [969]. Abnormal proximal small intestinal motor function is frequently present in patients with diabetes but has been poorly characterized [970]. In most patients the activity of the gastric pacemaker is normal during euglycemia [911]; earlier reports of an increased prevalence of gastric arrhythmias, particularly tachygastria, as assessed by cutaneous electrogastrography are likely to be due to hyperglycemia [971].

Clinical Significance

Disordered gastric motility may, at least theoretically, be associated with upper gastrointestinal symptoms, changes in oral drug absorption, and alterations in glycemic control. The potential impact of gastric emptying on glycemic control has been discussed above (pages 247–248). Postprandial hypotension, leading to syncope and falls, is an important clinical problem, particularly in the elderly and patients with autonomic dysfunction (usually diabetes mellitus). The demonstration that the magnitude of the postprandial fall in blood pressure after an oral glucose load in type 2 diabetes is related to the rate of gastric emptying has potential implications for the treatment of this condition [972].

A significant proportion of patients with disordered gastric motility suffer from severe symptoms, such as nausea, early satiation, and postprandial fullness, which can lead to life-threatening electrolyte imbalances and nutritional deficiencies. While it has been assumed that upper gastrointestinal symptoms are a direct result of delay in gastric emptying, this concept is now recognized to be overly simplistic. The relationship between upper gastrointestinal symptoms and the rate of gastric emptying is generally considered to be weak [956,973] (Fig. 5.**30**).

Gastric emptying is an important determinant of oral drug absorption; most orally administered drugs (including alcohol) are absorbed more slowly from the stomach than from the small intestine, because the latter has a much greater surface area. Thus, delayed gastric emptying (particularly of tablets or capsules, which are not degraded easily in the stomach) may potentially lead to fluctuations in the serum concentrations of orally administered drugs.

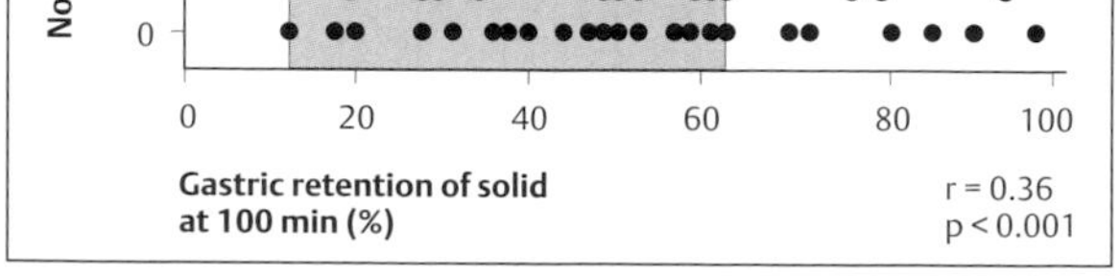

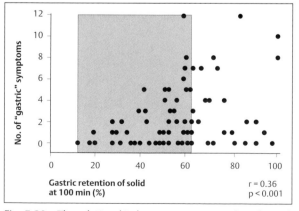

Fig. 5.**30** The relationship between symptoms (total score) referable to delayed gastric emptying and gastric emptying of a solid (minced beef) meal. The normal range for gastric emptying is shown in the shaded area. (From [897], with permission)

Diagnosis

Deciding when to evaluate diabetic patients for disordered gastric motility is not always easy. In any patient who presents with upper gastrointestinal symptoms and suspected delay in gastric emptying, a comprehensive history and examination should be performed, followed by appropriate investigation to identify other causes of gastroparesis, particularly those that may be reversible, such as a drug effect, electrolyte abnormality, or hypothyroidism. It should be recognized that there are many causes of gastroparesis (Table 5.**10**), which may be either acute or chronic. For example, gastric emptying of solids is delayed in 30–50 % of patients with functional dyspepsia. Chronic gastroparesis is a common accompaniment of diseases which cause motor dysfunction throughout the gastrointestinal tract.

Modulation of Gastric Emptying to Improve Glycemic Control

The concept that modulation of gastric emptying could be used to optimize glycemic control represents a new and exciting therapeutic option for the management of diabetes [935]. The underlying strategies are, however, likely to differ fundamentally between type 1 and type 2 diabetes – in type 1 diabetes interventions that improve the coordination between nutrient absorption and the action of exogenous insulin are likely to be beneficial, i. e., by accelerating or slowing gastric emptying so that the rate of nutrient absorption is more predictable. In contrast, in type 2 diabetes it may be anticipated that slowing of the absorption of nutrients would be desirable, as insulin release is both diminished and delayed even in those patients who have slow gastric emptying. Such permutations need to take into account the differential rate of gastric emptying of various meal components, e. g., acceleration of gastric emptying of high-carbohydrate liquid components of a meal may potentially have a greater impact on postprandial blood glucose than that of solids.

Nonpharmacologic Approaches

In the treatment of type 2 diabetes mellitus, dietary modifications potentially represent a more attractive and cost-effective approach than drugs. A number of dietary strategies may result in slower glucose absorption; in patients with type 2 diabetes, it has recently been confirmed that an increase in dietary fiber improves glycemic control. The magnitude of the improvement, which is likely to be due to soluble, rather

Table 5.10 Causes of gastroparesis

Transient delayed gastric emptying:
Drugs: e. g., morphine, anticholinergics, nicotine, dopaminergics
Postoperative ileus
Viral gastroenteritis
Electrolyte abnormalities: hyperglycemia, hypokalemia, hypomagnesemia
Hypothyroidism, hyperthyroidism, hypopituitarism, Addison disease
Herpes zoster
Critical illness
Pregnancy
Chronic gastric stasis:
Diabetes mellitus
Idiopathic/functional dyspepsia
Postsurgical: e. g., vagotomy
Gastroesophageal reflux
Atrophic gastritis
Progressive systemic sclerosis
Chronic idiopathic intestinal pseudo-obstruction
Myotonia dystrophica
Dermatomyositis/polymyositis
Systemic lupus erythematosus
Duchenne muscular dystrophy
Amyloidosis
Autonomic degeneration
Spinal cord disease
Tumor-associated
Anorexia nervosa and bulimia nervosa
Central nervous system disease, brainstem lesions, Parkinson disease
Postirradiation
HIV infection
Porphyria
Liver disease

than insoluble, fiber, is comparable to that achieved by oral hypoglycemic agents [974]. Slowing of gastric emptying is likely to be important in mediating this effect. Fat, depending on its chain length and saturation, is a potent dietary constituent in slowing gastric emptying, and there is a potential role for relatively small quantities of fat given immediately before consumption of or with a meal to have a marked effect on gastric emptying and minimize the postprandial rises in blood glucose and insulin [975]. In the broadest sense, the glycemic response to a meal is also likely to be critically dependent on whether food from the previous meal is still in the stomach and/or small intestine at the time of its ingestion, so that glucose tolerance may be expected to be worse in the fasted state than after a meal. The observation that the nonabsorbable polysaccharide guar gum improves second-meal tolerance to glucose in healthy subjects by decreasing glucose absorption is consistent with this concept [976].

Pharmacologic Approaches

A number of pharmacologic agents that modify gastric emptying have been shown to affect glycemic control in patients with diabetes; these include prokinetic drugs (e. g., erythromycin, cisapride, levosulpiride) and agents which slow gastric emptying (e. g., the amylin agonist pramlintide and the glucagon-like peptide GLP-1). In patients with type 1 diabetes and delayed gastric emptying, both the rate of emptying and the glycated hemoglobin improved after six months' treatment with the prokinetic drug levosulpiride, a D_2-dopamine receptor antagonist [977]. Conversely, when gastric emptying was increased with cisapride, postprandial blood glucose levels increased [961]; glycated hemoglobin was unchanged after eight weeks of treatment, possibly because the acceleration of gastric emptying was modest. The best characterized of the drugs to slow gastric emptying is pramlintide, which is administered by subcutaneous injection and slows gastric emptying in both type 1 and type 2 diabetes. In the longer term, administration of pramlintide results in a modest improvement in glycemic control, as assessed by glycated hemoglobin, without apparently increasing the risk of hypoglycemia [978]. The use of pramlintide is intuitively attractive as type 1 patients (and some type 2 patients) are by definition amylin-deficient. Pramlintide also suppresses postprandial glucagon secretion and causes weight loss, which may contribute to a reduction in postprandial blood glucose concentrations.

The use of GLP-1 represents another potential strategy for patients with type 2 diabetes. As an incretin hormone it augments the postprandial insulin response as well as suppressing both glucagon secretion and, probably, food intake. However, its predominant effect on postprandial glucose excursions is almost certainly mediated through the slowing of gastric emptying. The short half-life (only a few seconds as a result of inactivation of the protease dipeptidyl peptidase) of GLP-1 limits its potential therapeutic use, and longer-acting analogues are currently in development. One of these, exendin-4, which is produced by the salivary glands of the Gila monster lizard, is structurally similar to GLP-1 and shares several biologic properties, but may be a more potent insulinotropic agent than GLP-1. Exendin has been shown to reduce postprandial glycemia in type 2 patients after subcutaneous administration [979]. Interestingly, it has recently been demonstrated that α-galactosidase inhibitors, such as acarbose, stimulate GLP-1 secretion. Though all these agents present exciting possibilities for the management of diabetes in the future, large-scale prospective studies are required to demonstrate sustained effects on glycemic control before they can be widely applied in therapeutic management.

Treatment of Gastroparesis Associated with Gastrointestinal Symptoms

Management of symptomatic diabetic gastroparesis/disordered gastric motility is often challenging. Paradoxically, delay in gastric emptying per se does not appear to be associated with a poor prognosis [980]. In any patient who presents with upper gastrointestinal symptoms and suspected delay in gastric emptying/disordered gastroduodenal motility, a comprehensive history and examination should be performed, followed by appropriate investigations to identify (particularly reversible) causes of gastroparesis, such as a drug side effect or electrolyte abnormality. It should, however, be recognized that in some patients it may not be feasible or appropriate to withdraw medication that could slow gastric emptying, including drugs used in the treatment of peripheral neuropathy. Gastric candidiasis is increasingly prevalent. Gastric bezoars are usually responsive to mechanical or chemical dissolution performed endoscopically. As with esophageal symptoms, upper gastrointestinal endoscopy is usually required, in this case primarily to exclude gastric outlet, or proximal, small intestinal obstruction, as well as mucosal disorders. As discussed, evidence of reflux esophagitis does not exclude concurrent gastroparesis. When these investigations are unremarkable, gastric emptying should be measured by scintigraphy (and possibly, in the future, by a scintigraphic breath test), as this enables therapy to be targeted. Because of the uncertain predictive value of symptoms, objective measurement is required for the diagnosis of gastroparesis; nonspecific terminology such as "gastropathy" and "gastroparesis symptoms," while intuitively appealing, should probably be avoided. Despite these considerations, it is reasonable to give an empirical trial of prokinetic therapy for about four weeks, while recognizing that there is a substantial placebo response. Gastric emptying should be measured if symptoms fail to improve or recur following the cessation of therapy and in all patients who have had previous gastric surgery. Rigorous attempts should be made to optimize glycemic control [935], although there are no persuasive data to support this approach [981]; it may be necessary to maintain blood glucose levels close to the euglycemic range to facilitate symptomatic improvement.

The identification and correction of malnutrition represents an important component of therapy. While it is appropriate, and logical, to support a dietary intake of small, low-fiber and low-fat meals with homogenized solid foods and increased nutrient liquids, there is surprisingly little evidence to suggest that such an approach is useful. Elemental diets have been used to facilitate an adequate oral intake. The acute gastric dilatation of ketoacidosis characteristically responds to nasogastric intubation and correction of hyperglycemia and electrolyte abnormalities. In patients with severe nausea, antiemetics may be of benefit.

At present the use of prokinetic drugs (mainly cisapride, domperidone, metoclopramide, and erythromycin) forms the mainstay of therapy, and most patients will require drug treatment. In general, these drugs all provide dose-related improvements in gastric emptying, although their mechanisms of action differ (Table 5.**11**), involving simulation of 5-HT_4 receptors (cisapride and metoclopramide), dopamine receptor blockade (domperidone and metoclopramide) [956,982], and stimulation of motilin receptors (erythromycin) [982,983]. The response to prokinetic therapy (change in gastric emptying) tends to be greater when gastric emptying is more delayed. There are relatively few controlled studies which have evaluated the effects of prolonged (> 8 weeks) prokinetic therapy.

With the possible exception of erythromycin, all of these drugs have been shown to improve symptoms [946,984,985]. A beneficial effect on quality of life has also been evident in some studies, although this issue has not been evaluated widely [985,986]. In general, there is poor correlation between effects on symptoms and gastric emptying; furthermore, there is little information as to whether the symptomatic response differs in patients with and without delayed emptying-patients with normal gastric emptying may also respond [986]. There is some evidence that tolerance may develop to the gastrokinetic effects of metoclopramide [987], domperidone [984], and erythromycin [988]. The mechanical effects of prokinetic drugs which are responsible for faster gastric emptying are poorly defined; the dominant effect is likely to relate to a change in the organization of antroduodenal contractions to an expulsive pattern [935,970,989], although proximal stomach motility is also affected.

Erythromycin is the most potent drug when given intravenously (in doses below 3 mg/kg) [983] and may be particularly useful in the initial phase of management [990]. When used orally, erythromycin may have greater efficacy when given as a suspension rather than as a tablet, but is probably less effective than

Table 5.**11** Prokinetic drugs used in the treatment of gastroparesis

Drug	Mechanism of action	Route of administration	Oral dose
Cisapride	5-HT_4 receptor agonist	Oral	10–20 mg t.i.d.
Domperidone	Dopamine D_2 receptor antagonist	Oral	10–20 mg b.d.–q.i.d.
Metoclopramide	5-HT_4 receptor agonist, D_2 antagonist	Oral, subcutaneous, intramuscular, intravenous	10 mg t.i.d.
Erythromycin	Motilin receptor agonist	Oral or intravenous	250–500 mg t.i.d.

Adapted from [982]

when given intravenously [988]. The gastric motor response to erythromycin is also critically dependent on the dosage [989]. It has also recently been demonstrated, in both healthy subjects [991] and patients with diabetes [992], that the gastric motor response to erythromycin is markedly attenuated during hyperglycemia; this effect is likely to be evident with other prokinetic drugs. Variations in the blood glucose concentration may accordingly account for the negative outcome of some studies relating to the effect of prokinetic therapies on gastric emptying in diabetes [993–995].

The drug of first choice for oral administration is probably cisapride, which appears to have the most diffuse gastrointestinal effects [946,963,993]. While cisapride has been well tolerated in clinical trials, there have been recent reports of cardiac arrhythmias, including deaths [996]. It has now been established that cisapride has the potential to induce cardiac adverse effects as a result of prolongation of the cardiac action potential (leading to lengthening of the electrocardiographic Q–T interval and torsades de pointes), which are probably related to class III antiarrthymic properties rather than 5-HT_4 receptor activation [996]). Other substituted benzamides, including metoclopramide, do not have class III antiarrhythmic effects. The clinical relevance of the cardiac effects of cisapride is still uncertain, particularly as the majority of patients who have died while taking cisapride had other risk factors for cardiac disease and were taking the drug in relatively high dosage (~80 mg/day) although concerns about this issue have led to restrictions in its use in a number of countries. However, the potential for cardiotoxicity dictates that the use of cisapride should be more circumspect than previously recommended. Drugs that inhibit cisapride metabolism, such as ketoconazole and erythromycin, or that may prolong the Q–T interval, should ideally not be used concurrently, and before initiating therapy with cisapride it is appropriate to perform an electrocardiogram. The risk/benefit ratio may be difficult to calculate in patients with diabetes mellitus, particularly in those with severe symptoms given the high prevalence of symptomatic and asymptomatic cardiac disease, and there is little information to guide the clinician.

Metoclopramide appears to be less effective than cisapride, although it has the advantage of being available for parenteral (including subcutaneous) use and having central antiemetic properties. Some 20% of patients taking metoclopramide experience central nervous system side effects [997]. It would not be surprising if the use of domperidone, which has been shown to improve quality of life in diabetic patients with upper gastrointestinal symptoms, and is better tolerated than metoclopramide because of the reduced risk of central nervous system side effects, increases [986,998].

Treatment of symptomatic gastroparesis is certainly not uniformly satisfactory. If symptoms are refractory to prokinetic therapy, placement of a feeding jejunostomy may be required to maintain nutrition. In most cases surgery is to be avoided, as this may be associated with deterioration. If surgery is performed, it should be in specialized centers. There may be a place for small intestinal manometry in the evaluation of such patients, although it has not been established that the presence of severe small intestinal motor abnormalities represents an additional contraindication to subtotal gastrectomy. There are uncontrolled data to suggest that pancreatic transplantation may improve both gastric emptying and symptoms [999].

There is a need for novel therapeutic options. Dopamine antagonists, such as levosulpiride [977], and 5-HT_4 agonists which do not affect cardiac function, such as tegaserod [1000], are currently in development. There may be therapeutic advantages in combining drugs that have different mechanisms of action, the most logical being cisapride and domperidone (the combination of cisapride with erythromycin is contraindicated). Drugs designed to modulate sensory feedback from the gastrointestinal tract, such as 5-HT_3 antagonists and κ-opiate agonists, may have a therapeutic role. However, a recent study which evaluated the effects of the κ-opiate agonist fedotozine yielded disappointing results [949]. Since administration of erythromycin is associated with the risk of long-term antibiotic use and, possibly, diminished efficacy, potent motilides which lack antibiotic activity have been developed; the outcome of a study of one of these drugs in diabetic patients with upper gastrointestinal symptoms was, however, disappointing [1001].

There is also renewed interest in the potential role of gastric electrical stimulation as a therapy—either using neural electrical stimulation at a high frequency (which probably stimulates vagal sensory nerves and may suppress the vomiting center) or gastric electrical pacing, in which electrical stimulation of cholinergic motor neurons approximates the physiologic frequency (~3 cycles/min). While there are observations to suggest that both approaches may be beneficial, controlled trials are required.

Small Intestine

The contractile patterns of the small intestinal muscle layers are primarily determined by the enteric nervous system comprising the submucosal and myenteric plexuses. Interstitial cells of Cajal are associated closely with the myenteric plexus and probably play a role in the generation of pacemaker activity [892]. During fasting, a distally migrating motor sequence termed the migrating motor complex (MMC) sweeps from the antropyloroduodenal region along the gut in a cyclical fashion, each cycle lasting for ~100 minutes. The MMC consists of a period of motor quiescence (phase I ~40 minutes) followed by a period of irregular contractile activity (phase II ~50 minutes), culminating in a short burst of regular phasic contraction (phase III ~5–10 minutes). The role of the MMC is unclear, but phase III contractile activity appears to propel food residue and secretions in an aboral direction–accordingly it is sometimes described as the "housekeeper" of the gut. In the postprandial state the MMC pattern is disrupted and replaced by irregular contractions which appear to have a mixing function, allowing contact of digestive enzymes with intraluminal content.

Evaluation of small intestinal (orocecal) transit can be performed noninvasively using a number of commercially available breath tests, including the H_2-lactulose breath test. However, the simplicity and low cost of such tests is often offset by limitations in reproducibility and/or interpretation. For example, the lactulose breath test evaluates only the arrival of the "head" of the meal at the cecum, which may not correlate closely with transit of the remainder of the meal, and is influenced by the rate of gastric emptying. The development of perfused tube manometry using multilumen assemblies has allowed improved definition of disordered small intestinal motility. While only available in specialized centers, this technique has now made its way from the physiology laboratory into the clinical setting.

Prevalence and Pathophysiology

Small intestinal motility is frequently abnormal in patients with diabetes mellitus. The motor dysfunctions are heterogeneous and include a decreased amplitude and frequency of contractions, reduced or absent phase III activity, prolongation of phase II, and simultaneous and nonpropagated contractions. These abnormalities have been attributed to both parasympathetic and sympathetic denervation [1002,1003]. Both normal, rapid, and slow small intestinal transit have been reported, probably partly reflecting differences in subject selection and the methodology used to evaluate small intestinal transit. Diabetic diarrhea may potentially be attributable either to more rapid transit with a diminished time available for absorption, or to delayed transit predisposing to bacterial overgrowth.

Although the pathogenesis of diarrhea in patients with diabetes is multifactorial, it is considered to result primarily from small intestinal dysfunction. Impaired α-adrenergic control of intestinal secretion may also be important [1004]. Acute changes in the blood glucose concentration affect small intestinal motility; in normal subjects small intestinal transit is slower during marked hyperglycemia [917]. Abnormal small intestinal motility in diabetes may have implications for intestinal glucose absorption.

Clinical Significance

Diarrhea occurs in up to 20% of diabetic patients, most often those with longstanding, poorly controlled type 1 diabetes [924], and is typically a chronic disorder. Although classically nocturnal, diarrhea can occur at any time of day and is often experienced soon after eating. Fecal urgency and incontinence may be associated. Diarrhea is not infrequently intermittent, alternating with periods of normal bowel habit or even constipation. It may be precipitated by enteral nutrients introduced for nutritional support. Body weight is usually maintained; marked weight loss should suggest an alternative diagnosis. It is not known whether disordered small intestinal motor/sensory function contributes to other gastrointestinal symptoms in patients with diabetes, such as abdominal bloating.

Diagnosis

The diagnosis of diabetic diarrhea is one of exclusion. A detailed history should be taken to determine the frequency and consistency of stool and the presence of any fecal urgency or incontinence. A detailed drug history is essential, particularly relating to the use of antibiotics, antacids, alcohol, and sorbitol. Previous abdominal surgery, sexual behavior, travel, and a history of lactose intolerance may also be relevant.

As the treatment of "diabetic diarrhea" is largely empirical, investigation should be directed at the exclusion of other conditions including small intestinal bacterial overgrowth, pancreatic insufficiency, celiac disease, and anorectal dysfunction. Physical examination should exclude systemic disorders and provide evidence of autonomic neuropathy. A three-day stool collection to assess fecal weight, fat, and bile acids may be useful, though not always easy to perform. Tests for malabsorption, jejunal biopsy, and barium studies of the small and large bowel are indicated in many cases, though the results are often unremarkable. Serologic screening for celiac disease is indicated in the majority of cases, in view of the strong association with diabetes. Bacterial overgrowth is suggested by a premature rise in breath H_2 after oral lactulose administration and confirmed by jejunal aspirate. When no obvious cause can be elicited, dysmotility of the small (and large) intestine is likely to be important in the etiology of diarrhea. Consideration should be given to measurements of small intestinal transit and small bowel manometry.

Treatment

The overall aim of treatment of "diabetic diarrhea" is to slow small intestinal and colonic transit. The effect of optimization of blood glucose control has not been evaluated. First-line agents include opiate-like antidiarrheal agents such as loperamide and codeine phosphate [1005]. Rapid intestinal transit sufficient to cause diarrhea is often associated with bile acid malabsorption. Treatment with the bile acid-binding resin cholestyramine given in association with loperamide is effective in some cases. However cholestyramine must be taken half an hour before a meal as bile acids are released with a meal, and compliance is often poor. The use of α_2-adrenergic agents such as clonidine has also been advocated. Clonidine restores sympathetic tone, enhancing water and salt absorption and reducing propulsive contractions [1005]. Octreotide has also been shown to be useful in the management of intractable diabetic diarrhea, probably by decreasing intestinal, pancreatic, and gallbladder secretions and stimulating phase III-like motor activity in the small intestine while slowing intestinal transit [1006]. If a diagnosis of bacterial overgrowth is suspected or established, a short therapeutic trial of a broad-spectrum antibiotic should be undertaken. In such patients intermittent use of antibiotics (with or without a prokinetic) may be necessary in the longer term. When all measures fail, intravenous hyperalimentation may be required to maintain nutrition.

Gallbladder

The gallbladder serves as a bile reservoir, allowing the concentration of bile by absorbing water. It responds to stimulation by CCK by contracting strongly and releasing bile into the duodenum.

Prevalence and Pathophysiology

Diabetes mellitus is associated with an increased incidence of cholelithiasis and cholecystitis. The pathogenesis may be related to decreased motility, sphincter of Oddi dyskinesia, and/or a lithogenic bile composition. Increased volume of the gallbladder during fasting and poor contraction following stimulation with a fatty meal or CCK is well recognized in diabetic patients [1007]. While autonomic neuropathy was considered to be the dominant etiologic factor, acute hyperglycemia has been shown to reduce gallbladder contraction in response to CCK stimulation [914].

Diagnosis

Gallbladder dysmotility is usually a chance finding made during cholecystography or ultrasonography. Ultrasonography is highly reliable in the detection of stones in the gallbladder, but has a lower sensitivity for detection of stones in the common bile duct. Dynamic ultrasonography can be used for detection of sphincter of Oddi dyskinesia. An increase in the common bile duct diameter of 1 mm or more in response to CCK or a fatty meal is suggestive of sphincter of Oddi dyskinesia.

Treatment

Although the incidence of biliary tract complications may be increased in diabetic patients, asymptomatic gallstones should not in general be treated. When surgery is required, laparoscopic techniques are suitable.

Colon

Every day the colon receives approximately 1 l effluent from the small intestine consisting of unabsorbed carbohydrate, protein, and fat as well as water, fiber, bile salts, and digestive enzymes. Most of this is absorbed during colonic transit, so that no more than 100 g feces containing indigestible fiber and bacterial cells are excreted. Functionally the colon can be divided into three components: a proximal portion which is involved in fermentation, a more distal portion where salt and water are absorbed and colonic contents are concentrated and solidified, and the rectum, which is specialized for defecation.

Ring-like haustral contractions gently mix colonic contents with secretions and bacteria and thereby facilitate their exposure to the mucosal surface and distal propagation of contents at rates compatible with efficient absorption of fluid, electrolytes, and the products of bacterial degradation [1008]. The circular muscle of the sigmoid colon is usually tonically contracted and probably functions as a valve, restricting the entry of colonic contents into the rectum, from where they are expelled [1009]. Transit and absorption of colonic contents are controlled via the autonomic and enteric nervous systems. Postganglionic sympathetic nerves reach the colon along the mesenteric arteries and inhibit smooth-muscle contractility, with the exception of the internal sphincter where the effect is stimulatory. Parasympathetic nerves arising from the dorsal motor nucleus of the vagus supply the proximal colon, whereas the distal colon is innervated via the sacral plexus. Parasympathetic nerves supply the colon with both excitatory cholinergic nerves and inhibitory noradrenergic nerves. At certain times, characteristically early in the morning, the colon assumes a propulsive mode of activity, with a reduction in haustral contractions and the presence of powerful contractions, so-called "great migrating contractions" which sweep down the colon propelling feces into the rectum. This type of propulsive motor activity is produced by stimulation of the parasympathetic nervous system.

Colonic transit can be evaluated using radiopaque studies (the most common technique) or scintigraphy; these tests can potentially discriminate between transit in the right and left semicolon and rectosigmoid regions. Colonic manometry should at present be considered primarily as a research tool.

Prevalence and Pathophysiology

Data relating to the prevalence of symptoms relating to altered colonic function are limited and inconsistent. Constipation, diarrhea, and abdominal pain have been reported in up to 60% of diabetic patients attending a tertiary referral center [924], suggesting that it is the most common gastrointestinal complaint associated with diabetes; however, in a population-based study of type 1 patients there was no increase in lower

important implications for therapy. Anal sphincter injury occurring as a result of birth trauma or hemorrhoidectomy should be excluded, as these are potentially remediable by surgery. Further investigations may include anorectal manometry, endoanal ultrasonography, X-ray defecography, and colonic transit. Using anorectal manometry, basal and squeeze pressures along with sensory and rectal internal and external anal sphincter (IAS, EAS) pressure responses to graded rectal distension can be recorded. Unstable oscillations of IAS tone and electrical activity occur more frequently in diabetic patients than in healthy subjects [1015]. Anorectal manometry is also useful to identify short-segment Hirschsprung disease, spinal lesions such as a prolapsed lumbar disk, cervical spondylosis, or syringomyelia, and to demonstrate the paradoxical sphincter contraction during attempts to defecate evident in patients with idiopathic constipation.

Defecography can assess the degree of perineal descent and reveal the presence of partial rectal prolapse and rectal intussusception, either of which can be associated with rectal seepage or indeed cause obstruction. Endoanal ultrasonography is the only technique that satisfactorily identifies the presence of a defect in the sphincter ring caused by obstetric trauma, and should be carried out in all women with fecal incontinence who have undergone vaginal deliveries and have low sphincter pressures.

Treatment

Treatment of disordered anorectal motility is largely symptomatic. As discussed, the first step in the management of fecal incontinence is to treat the underlying diarrhea. It is also logical to optimize glycemic control. Biofeedback training is now being used increasingly for the treatment of incontinence of all types. It is thought to be effective by increasing external sphincter strength and rectal sensations, and improving coordination between rectal perception and external sphincter contraction. Sphincter activity during conscious contraction is displayed visually to the patient, who then makes a conscious effort to improve these responses. While impressive responses to biofeedback training have been reported in patients with idiopathic fecal incontinence, when attempts were made to control for the active principle by not offering any feedback patients still did well. This latter observation suggests that the beneficial effects of biofeedback may originate from the establishment of confidence through the nature of the relationship between the patient and therapist. While biofeedback represents a promising treatment option for diabetic patients with fecal incontinence, its position has not yet been fully established. If instability of the internal anal sphincter proves to have a major role in the etiology of incontinence, therapy with α-adrenergic agonists may prove to be useful.

Conclusion

Disordered gastrointestinal motility occurs frequently in patients with diabetes and is generally underestimated as a cause of morbidity. While the etiology of gastrointestinal symptoms, presumed to arise primarily as a result of abnormal gastrointestinal motor function, is still poorly understood, there have been significant advances in both the understanding of the pathophysiology and treatment. It is clear that reversible abnormalities in gastrointestinal motility may occur as a result of either an increase or a decrease in the blood glucose concentration and, conversely, that gastric (and perhaps small intestinal) motility is a major factor in glycemic control.

■ Urogenital System

C.G. Stief and D. Ziegler

Introduction

In addition to nephropathy, retinopathy, and angiopathy, erectile dysfunction and micturition disorders have been well recognized as complications of diabetes for over a century. Disturbances of bladder emptying and/or urine storage are often asymptomatic to the patient, especially in the early stages of this diabetic complication. Sexual dysfunctions, by contrast, are readily perceived by the patient. Sexual dysfunctions such as erectile or ejaculatory dysfunction and infertility are frequently found in the male diabetic compared to the nondiabetic population. Although these sexual dysfunctions often have a dramatic negative impact on the psychosocial life and self-esteem of the diabetic patient, they remain unacknowledged in most instances. Owing to shame and embarrassment on the part of the patient, or unawareness or old-fashioned neglect of the problem by the physician, they fail to attract either medical attention or, as a consequence, the possibility of treatment. A detailed review of 428 charts of male diabetic patients from ten general practices in the UK revealed a 53% prevalence of erectile dysfunction, with 39% of these suffering from the problem all the time. However, this complication was documented in only 8% of the cases, and in only 1% was the patient told about possible treatment options. The authors concluded, that "erectile dysfunction is the most neglected complication of diabetes mellitus" [1016].

Since both impairment of bladder storage and emptying and sexual dysfunction may have severe organic and psychosocial consequences, their existence (often unapparent to the patient) should be systematically screened for in the routine diabetes clinic.

Erectile Dysfunction

Male erectile dysfunction (ED), defined as "the inability to achieve or maintain an erection sufficient for sexual intercourse" [1017], is one of the most common sexual dysfunctions in men. ED is more common with advancing age, and since the aged population is increasing, its prevalence will continue to rise [1018]. Diabetes mellitus is the most frequent organic cause of ED, the onset of which is about 15 years earlier in the diabetic than in the nondiabetic population. In the Massachusetts Male Aging Study (MMAS), the age-adjusted prevalences of minimal, moderate, or complete ED were 17 %, 25 %, and 10 %, respectively, among 1238 nondiabetic men, and 8 %, 30 %, and 25 % among 52 treated diabetic men [1019]. Thus, although the number of diabetic subjects in the MMAS was low, this population-based study showed an increased prevalence particularly of complete ED among men with diabetes. The crude incidence of ED in the MMAS was 26 cases per 1000 man-years in 847 men aged 40–69 without ED at baseline who were followed for an average of 8.8 years [1020]. Population projections for men in this age group suggest an estimate of 617 715 new cases of ED per year for the United States. The age-adjusted risk of ED was higher for men with lower education, diabetes, heart disease, and hypertension. The incidence of ED in diabetic men was twice as high, with 50 cases per 1000 man years. In a population-based study from southern Wisconsin the prevalence of ED among 365 type 1 diabetic patients increased with age, from 1.1 % in those aged 21–30 years to 47.1 % in those aged 43 years or older, and with increasing duration of diabetes [1021]. In a recent study from Italy of 9868 men with diabetes, 45.5 % of those aged above 59 years reported ED. Risk factors and clinical correlates included the following (odds ratio [95 % confidence interval]): autonomic neuropathy (5.0 [3.9–6.4]), diabetic foot (4.0 [2.9–5.5]), peripheral neuropathy (3.3 [2.9–3.8]), peripheral arterial disease (2.8 [2.4–3.3]), nephropathy (2.3 [1.9–2.8]), poor glycemic control (2.3 [2.0–2.6]), retinopathy (2.2 [2.0–2.4]), hypertension (2.1 [1.6–2.9]), and diabetes duration (2.0 [1.8–2.2]) [1022]. In another survey from Italy the combination of diabetes and hypertension was the major risk factor for ED, giving an OR (95 %CI) of 8.1 (1.2–55.0) compared with diabetes without hypertension 4.6 (1.6–13.7), hypertension without diabetes 1.4 (0.7–3.2), current smoking 1.7 (1.2–2.4), and previous smoking (now ceased) 1.6 (1.1–2.3) [1023]. However, even when neuropathic complications are present, psychiatric illness such as generalized anxiety disorder or depression may be important contributors to ED in men with diabetes [1024]. Overall, erectile dysfunction affects around one-third to one-half of diabetic men, independent of the type of diabetes.

Physiology of Erection

Although the active role of the cavernous tissue was shown over a hundred years ago, the phenomenon of erection was viewed rather mechanistically, being regarded as the result of an increase in cavernous arterial inflow and a reduction in cavernous venous outflow. The arterial supply of the cavernous bodies emerges from the internal iliac arteries, then runs via the pudendal artery to the branching of the penile arteries, the dorsal and cavernous arteries. This "classic" penile arterial supply varies considerably, thus constituting a pitfall for the interpretation of selective arteriograms. Since the mid-1980s, the crucial role of the cavernous smooth muscle tone has been widely recognized, with the arterial and venous changes being only a secondary phenomenon to changes in the smooth muscle tone. During flaccidity, the cavernous smooth muscles are in a state between full contraction and full relaxation. During erection they relax, resulting in wide sinusoids with a low peripheral resistance and a consequent increase in inflow; venous restriction is brought about by passive compression of the venules between the tunica albuginea and the expanding cavernous tissue. During elevated alpha tone (stress, anxiety, cold), cavernous smooth muscles contract fully; an elevated alpha tone may inhibit erections in an otherwise healthy man (e. g., psychogenic impotence evoked by performance anxiety). Electron microscopic and histomorphologic studies have shown cavernous smooth muscle degeneration to be a major cause of erectile dysfunction. The smooth muscle tone is regulated by autonomic input from the sympathetic and parasympathetic system. The sympathetic spinal cord center is situated in the thoracolumbar region and the parasympathetic in the sacral region. The peripheral parasympathetic fibers emerging from S2 to S4 course over the lateral and anterior aspect of the rectum to form the cavernous nerves, running dorsolaterally adjacent to the prostate [1025–1033].

Penile erection is a neurovascular event modulated by psychologic factors and hormonal status and depending on appropriate trabecular smooth muscle and arterial relaxation in the corpus cavernosum. Upon sexual stimulation, nerve impulses cause the release of cholinergic and noncholinergic nonadrenergic (NANC) neurotransmitters that mediate erectile function by relaxing the smooth muscle of the corpus cavernosum. A principal neural mediator of erection is nitric oxide (NO), which activates guanyl cyclase to form intracellular cyclic guanosine monophosphate (GMP), a potent second messenger for smooth muscle relaxation. Cyclic GMP in turn activates a specific protein kinase, which phosphorylates certain proteins and ion channels, resulting in a drop in cytosolic calcium concentrations and relaxation of the smooth muscle. During the return to the flaccid state, cyclic GMP is hydrolyzed to GMP by phosphodiesterase type 5 (PDE5) [1018,1034]. Four PDE isoforms have been identified in the corpus cavernosum (types 2, 3, 4, and 5), but PDE5 is the predominant one; the others do not appear to play an important role in erection [1034].

Pathophysiology

The pathogenesis of ED in diabetes is thought to be multifactorial as it may be linked to neuropathy, accelerated atherosclerosis, or alterations in the corporal erectile tissue. Such alterations may include smooth muscle degeneration, abnormal collagen deposition, and endothelial cell dysfunction [1035]. If irreversible, these corporal degenerative changes can limit the success of any drug therapy. Advanced glycation endproducts (AGEs) have been shown to quench NO and to be elevated in human diabetic penile tissue. It has been hypothesized that AGEs may mediate ED via upregulation of inducible nitric oxide synthase (iNOS) and down-regulation of endothelial NOS (eNOS) [1036]. Furthermore, protein kinase C activation in diabetes may reduce NOS activity [1037].

In vivo studies of isolated corpus cavernosum tissue from diabetic men have shown functional impairment in neurogenic and endothelium-dependent relaxation of corpus cavernosum smooth muscle [1038]. In diabetic rats, endothelium-dependent NO-mediated relaxation in response to acetylcholine and NANC stimulation is reduced by 40% after four to eight weeks [1039]. These alterations were prevented by administration of the antioxidant α-lipoic acid, suggesting an involvement of increased oxidative stress. By contrast, endothelium-independent relaxation in response to the NO donor sodium nitroprusside is not impaired in diabetes [1039]. Increased penile endothelial and total NOS activity was found after two to three months in diabetic rats [1040]. After four to eight months, however, reduced penile total (endothelial and neuronal) NOS activity and neuronal NOS levels were observed in type 1 and type 2 diabetic rats. [1041]. Thus, diabetes-induced changes in NOS activity may be biphasic, with an initial increase followed by a decrease. Finally, an increased rate of apoptosis in corpus cavernosum was recently described in diabetic rats [1526].

It has been shown in rats that diabetes induces hypogonadism and a reduction in size of androgen-sensitive organs. In diabetic men, however, the incidence of hypogonadism is comparable to that in the nondiabetic population (approx. 5–8%).

Electron microscopic studies have shown cavernous autonomic neuropathy and cavernous smooth muscle degeneration to be major etiologic factors of diabetic erectile dysfunction. This correlates well with clinical findings, where approximately 60% of the diabetic patients with erectile dysfunction showed significantly irregular cavernous electric activity, thus being highly suggestive of cavernous autonomic neuropathy and/or cavernous smooth muscle degeneration.

Similarly, electron microscopic findings revealed microangiopathy to be a major etiologic factor of diabetic erectile dysfunction. These morphologic findings are again substantiated by clinical studies showing significantly impaired arterial flow velocity within the cavernous arteries. Peak systolic flow rates were significantly lower in diabetic subjects than in healthy men (mean 23.9 ± 5.2 cm/s versus 29.3 ± 6.6 cm/s for PGE1). In men and animals, disturbances of the peripheral neurotransmitter pool have been reported in diabetes. Endothelial alterations followed by an impaired NO pathway have been described.

Although most diabetic patients develop their erectile dysfunction on the basis of organic etiologies, the psychoreactive component present in most patients must not be overlooked.

Diagnosis

The high incidence of erectile dysfunction and the dramatic impact this dysfunction has on the patient and his psychosocial life warrant the inclusion of questions about sexuality in the screening procedure of a routine diabetic check. Libido, the quality and duration of the erection, and the ability for penetration and intercourse should be specifically addressed. The ability to ejaculate and to experience orgasm should then be mentioned.

The International Index of Erectile Function (IIEF) [1527], a brief and reliable measure of erectile function that is cross-culturally valid and psychometrically sound, can be used to address the relevant domains of male sexual function (that is, erectile function, orgasmic function, sexual desire, intercourse satisfaction, and overall satisfaction). It is psychometrically sound and has been linguistically validated in ten languages. This questionnaire is readily self-administered in clinical settings or research. The IIEF demonstrates sensitivity and specificity for detecting treatment-related changes in patients with erectile dysfunction.

For many patients examination can be limited to the regular monitoring of diabetes and its risk factors and complications together with examination of the genitalia. Patients should be informed about the advantages and disadvantages of each treatment and given advice on treatment outcome and ease of use. If erectile dysfunction is suspected or found to exist, a rationalized but comprehensive work-up should be done. A stepwise diagnostic procedure is advisable (Table 5.**11a**).

The first, noninvasive diagnostic step should uncover any psychogenic etiology or severe underlying organogenic factors of the erectile dysfunction. It includes a detailed case history, physical examination, blood laboratory tests (including testosterone), and a psychologic evaluation with a specifically sexual case history. It is important to establish the nature of the erectile problem and to distinguish it from other forms of sexual difficulty such as penile curvature or premature ejaculation. An interview with the partner is advisable and will confirm the problem but may also reveal other causes of the difficulties, e. g., vaginal

INTERNATIONAL INDEX OF ERECTILE FUNCTION

Patient Questionnaire

These questions ask about the effects that your erection problems have had on your sex life over the last four weeks. Please try to answer the questions as honestly and as clearly as you are able. Your answers will help your doctor to choose the most effective treatment suited to your condition. In answering the questions, the following definitions apply:

- **sexual activity** includes intercourse, caressing, foreplay & masturbation
- **sexual intercourse** is defined as sexual penetration of your partner
- **sexual stimulation** includes situation such as foreplay, erotic pictures etc.
- **ejaculation** is the ejection of semen from the penis (or the feeling of this)
- **orgasm** is the fulfilment or climax following sexual stimulation or intercourse

---

	Over the past 4 weeks:	*Please check* ***one*** *box only*
☐ **Q1**	**How often were you able to get an erection during sexual activity?**	0 No sexual activity 1 Almost never or never 2 A few times (less than half the time) 3 Sometimes (about half the time) 4 Most times (more than half the time) 5 Almost always or always
☐ **Q2**	**When you had erections with sexual stimulation, how often were your erections hard enough for penetration?**	0 No sexual activity 1 Almost never or never 2 A few times (less than half the time) 3 Sometimes (about half the time) 4 Most times (more than half the time) 5 Almost always or always
☐ **Q3**	**When you attempted intercourse, how often were you able to penetrate (enter) your partner?**	0 Did not attempt intercourse 1 Almost never or never 2 A few times (less than half the time) 3 Sometimes (about half the time) 4 Most times (more than half the time) 5 Almost always or always
☐ **Q4**	**During sexual intercourse, how often were you able to maintain your erection after you had penetrated (entered) your partner?**	0 Did not attempt intercourse 1 Almost never or never 2 A few times (less than half the time) 3 Sometimes (about half the time) 4 Most times (more than half the time) 5 Almost always or always
☐ **Q5**	**During sexual intercourse, how difficult was it to maintain your erection to completion of intercourse?**	0 Did not attempt intercourse 1 Extremely difficult 2 Very difficult 3 Difficult 4 Slightly difficult 5 Not difficult

☐ Q6	How many times have you attempted sexual intercourse?	0 No attempts 1 One to two attempts 2 Three to four attempts 3 Five to six attempts 4 Seven to ten attempts 5 Eleven or more attempts
☐ Q7	When you attempted sexual intercourse, how often was it satisfactory for you?	0 Did not attempt intercourse 1 Almost never or never 2 A few times (less than half the time) 3 Sometimes (about half the time) 4 Most times (more than half the time) 5 Almost always or always
☐ Q8	How much have you enjoyed sexual intercourse?	0 No intercourse 1 No enjoyment at all 2 Not very enjoyable 3 Fairly enjoyable 4 Highly enjoyable 5 Very highly enjoyable
☐ Q9	When you had sexual stimulation <u>or</u> intercourse, how often did you ejaculate?	0 No sexual stimulation or intercourse 1 Almost never or never 2 A few times (less than half the time) 3 Sometimes (about half the time) 4 Most times (more than half the time) 5 Almost always or always
☐ Q10	When you had sexual stimulation <u>or</u> intercourse, how often did you have the feeling of orgasm or climax?	1 Almost never or never 2 A few times (less than half the time) 3 Sometimes (about half the time) 4 Most times (more than half the time) 5 Almost always or always
☐ Q11	How often have you felt sexual desire?	1 Almost never or never 2 A few times (less than half the time) 3 Sometimes (about half the time) 4 Most times (more than half the time) 5 Almost always or always
☐ Q12	How would you rate your level of sexual desire?	1 Very low or none at all 2 Low 3 Moderate 4 High 5 Very high
☐ Q13	How satisfied have you been with your <u>overall sex life</u>?	1 Very dissatisfied 2 Moderately dissatisfied 3 Equally satisfied & dissatisfied 4 Moderately satisfied 5 Very satisfied
☐ Q14	How satisfied have you been with your <u>sexual relationship</u> with your partner?	1 Very dissatisfied 2 Moderately dissatisfied 3 Equally satisfied & dissatisfied 4 Moderately satisfied 5 Very satisfied
☐ Q15	How do you rate your <u>confidence</u> that you could get and keep an erection?	1 Very low 2 Low 3 Moderate 4 High 5 Very high

dryness. Drugs which may be associated with ED include tranquilizers (phenothiazines, benzodiazepines), antidepressants (tricyclics, selective serotonin reuptake inhibitors), and antihypertensives (β-blockers, vasodilators, central sympathomimetics, ganglion blockers, diuretics).

The second, semi-invasive diagnostic step aims to differentiate between various organogenic etiologies. The most important issues in relation to therapeutic consequences are cavernous competence (or, more precisely, cavernous smooth muscle competence) and cavernous autonomic integrity. The diagnostic screening method for overall cavernous competence is the standardized intracavernous injection of vasoactive drugs (pharmacotesting). The cavernous EMG (CC-EMG) provides information on the integrity of the autonomic supply and of the cavernous smooth muscle cell itself (Fig. 5.**31**).

Table 5.**11a** Organization of comprehensive approach for erectile dysfunction

1. Basic diagnosis (mandatory for all patients): Case history Physical examination Blood chemistry, blood pressure, pulse, ECG Sexual case history
2. Specific andrologic approach (advisable for diabetic patients in whom a therapeutic trial with sildenafil has failed) Pharmacotesting CC-EMG Duplex ultrasonography
3. Invasive extended diagnostics (limited to specific cases) Pharmacoangiography Pharmacocavernosometry and cavernosography Comprehensive neurologic examinations

Table 5.**11b** Stepwise protocol for treatment of erectile dysfunction

General management: control of risk factors and diabetes; sexual counseling	
Pharmacologic treatment	Dose range
First-line therapy:	
Sildenafil (Viagra)	50–100 mg
[Tadalafil][a]	10–20 mg
[Vardenafil][a]	10–20 mg
Apomorphine (Uprima, Ixense)[b]	2–4 mg s.l.
Oral therapy inappropriate:	
Transurethral alprostadil (MUSE)	500–1000 μg
Intracavernosal injection therapy:	
Alprostadil (Caverject)	5–20 μg
Papaverine/phentolamine (Androskat)	
Thymoxamine (Erecnos)	10–20 mg
VIP/phentolamine (Invicorp)	
Papaverine/phentolamine//alprostadil (Trimix)	
Surgery and mechanical treatments	
Pharmacologic therapy inappropriate:	
Vacuum devices	
Arterial/venous surgery	
Penile prostheses	

[a] Market approval expected in 2002
[b] Only marginally effective in unselected diabetic patients

Noninvasive diagnostic assessment of the penile arterial supply has seen significant improvements in recent years. The Doppler examination has mostly been replaced by duplex or color-coded duplex ultrasonography, allowing precise and functional evaluation of the peripheral cavernous arterial supply (Fig. 5.**32**).

The third, invasive diagnostic step is mainly limited to patients who would, if the diagnosis is positive, undergo surgery. Patients must be carefully selected before they are subjected to radiologic procedures that can have severe complications, either related to the procedure itself or to the contrast medium employed. Selective penile angiography should only be done when penile reconstructive procedures are planned; another indication may be legal cases.

Other Sexual Problems in Men

Diminution or absence of testicular pain has been described as an early sign of autonomic neuropathy. Retrograde ejaculation from the prostatic urethra into the bladder may occasionally occur and follows loss of sympathetic innervation of the internal sphincter, which normally contracts during ejaculation. Complete loss of ejaculation probably indicates widespread pelvic sympathetic involvement and, like retrograde ejaculation, causes infertility, which may be treated by insemination [1528].

Female Sexual Dysfunction

Scientific knowledge about sexual dysfunction in women with diabetes is rudimentary. Problems affecting sexuality in diabetic women are fatigue, changes in perimenstrual blood glucose control, vaginitis, decreased sexual desire, decreased vaginal lubrication, and an increased time taken to reach orgasm. Even minor episodes of depression, which is twice more frequent in women than in men, can result in a loss of libido. To what extent these symptoms are related to autonomic neuropathy has been examined in a few studies, with contradictory results. The examination of a diabetic woman with sexual dysfunction should cover the duration of symptoms, psychologic state, concomitant medications, presence of vaginitis, cystitis, and other infections, frequency of intercourse, blood pressure, body mass index, retinal status, pelvic examination, presence of discharge, and glycemic control [1529].

Therapy

Initially, the patient should be advised to reduce possible risk factors and to optimize glycemic control. However, no studies are available to show that improvement in glycemic control will exert a favorable effect on ED. In fact, a recent study failed to demonstrate an effect on ED of intensive diabetes therapy maintained for two years in type 2 diabetic men [1530]. Even if the cause is organic, almost all men

sildenafil (25–100 mg), the percentages of those giving the maximum score for the six questions in the erectile function domain of the IIEF were 61.3% among 69 type 1 and 60.8% among 399 type 2 diabetic men on sildenafil as compared to 39.3% among 452 diabetic men on placebo [1544].

Side effects consist mainly of headache (18%), facial flushing (15%), and dyspepsia (2%). A mild and transient disturbance of color vision and also increased blurred vision or sensitivity to light has been found in 4.5% of diabetic men [1543]. Concerns have been expressed regarding an increased number of deaths associated with sildenafil as compared with other treatments for ED [1545]. However, after an average follow-up of six months the Prescription Event Monitoring (PEM) Study including 5601 sildenafil users from England showed an expected mortality rate of 28.9 per 1000/year for ischemic heart disease/myocardial infarctions. The comparison rate in the general population of England in 1998 was 73.9 per 1000/year [1546]. The prevalence of diabetes in the cohort was 15%, which is similar to the 16% prevalence in the clinical trials of sildenafil, but much higher than the 3.3% prevalence of men with diabetes in England in 1998. Although these results are reassuring, further follow-up of this study and other pharmacoepidemiologic research is needed for confirmation. In men with severe stenosis of at least one coronary artery, acute administration of sildenafil (100 mg) did not result in adverse hemodynamic effects on coronary blood flow or vascular resistance, but coronary flow reserve was improved [1547].

Apart from its effect on ED, favorable effects of sildenafil have recently been reported in pilot studies of various disorders including primary pulmonary hypertension, achalasia, and endothelial dysfunction. The endothelium modulates the vascular tone, the antithrombotic and antiadhesive properties of the vessel wall, vascular wall architecture, and vascular permeability. Endothelial dysfunction is regarded as an early key event in the development of atherosclerosis, both of which are accelerated in diabetes. It has recently been demonstrated that erectile and endothelial dysfunction are associated in type 2 diabetic patients. Plasma concentrations of markers of endothelial dysfunction such as soluble thrombomodulin, P-selectin, and intercellular cell adhesion molecules-1 (ICAM-1) were significantly elevated in type 2 diabetic patients with ED compared to those without ED and were inversely related to the IIEF [1548]. Endothelium-dependent flow-mediated dilatation induced by five-minute occlusion of the brachial artery measured by ultrasound imaging is a reliable index of endothelial function that is impaired in diabetic patients. In a recent controlled crossover trial acute (25 mg) and chronic (25 mg/day for 2 weeks) administration of sildenafil (25 mg) improved endothelial function compared with placebo in type 2 diabetic patients, suggesting that PDE5 inhibition may exert favorable cardiovascular effects [1549]. Likewise, in patients with heart failure who frequently show endothelial dysfunction, the latter was improved after single-dose administration of 25 or 50 mg sildenafil [1550]. These findings require further confirmation in larger studies.

According to the recommendations of the American Heart Association, sildenafil is contraindicated in men taking nitrates, due to the risk of hypotension, and in those with severe cardiovascular disease. Treadmill testing may be indicated before sildenafil is prescribed in men with heart disease, to assess the risk of cardiac ischemia occurring during sexual intercourse. Initial monitoring of blood pressure after the administration of sildenafil may be indicated in men with congestive heart disease who have borderline low blood pressure and low volume status, and in men being treated with complicated multidrug antihypertensive regimens [1551].

Because sildenafil treatment is costly and ED is not a life-threatening illness, the appropriateness of insurance coverage for sildenafil has been questioned. However, recent cost-effectiveness studies using cost per quality-adjusted life-year (QALY) gained as outcome measures have shown that sildenafil treatment compared favorably with intracavernosal injection therapy [1552] or with accepted therapies for other medical conditions [1553].

In a 12-week multicenter trial including 216 diabetic men (91% type 2), but excluding nonresponders to sildenafil), the rates of men with improved erections were 64% with 20 mg *tadalafil* (Cialis), 56% with 10 mg tadalafil, and 25% on placebo [1554]. Tadalafil 10 mg and 20 mg were both superior to placebo in improving penetration ability (IIEF question 3) and ability to maintain an erection during intercourse. Thus, although nonresponders to sildenafil were excluded, the effect of tadalafil was not superior to that of sildenafil. Treatment-related adverse events (> 5%) on 20 mg, 10 mg, and placebo were dyspepsia (8.3%, 11.0%, and 0%) and headache (6.9%, 8.2%, and 1.4%).

In a recent large 12-week multicenter trial including 439 diabetic men (88% type 2) that excluded sildenafil nonresponders, the rates of men with improved erections were 72% with 20 mg *vardenafil* (Nuviva), 57% with 10 mg vardenafil, and 13% on placebo [1555]. Vardenafil 10 mg and 20 mg were both superior to placebo in improving the IIEF erectile function domain score (questions 1–5, 15). As with tadalafil, despite the exclusion of nonresponders to sildenafil the effect of vardenafil was comparable to that reported previously for sildenafil. Treatment-related adverse events (> 5%) on 20 mg, 10 mg, and placebo were headache (10%, 9%, and 2%), flushing (10%, 9%, and < 1%), and headache (6%, 3%, and 0%).

Phentolamine

The nonselective α-receptor-blocking agent phentolamine (Vasomax) was evaluated for a possible beneficial effect on the erectile behavior. In prospective, randomized, double-blind studies, a beneficial effect of orally administered fast-resolving phentolamine on the erectile capacity of men with erectile dysfunction was shown. These beneficial effects were more pronounced in elderly men. The side effect profile of this drug, introduced decades ago for other indications, seems to be safe, with stuffy nose and some hypotension being the most frequent complaints. However, published data are minimal so a thorough evaluation is not possible for the moment [1556].

Future Perspectives

Since more drugs with various modes of action and different modes of application are being developed at the moment, future pharmacologic treatments will allow a more refined approach towards an individually adapted regimen. To improve patient care we also need more prospective comparative multicenter studies including different drugs and well-defined patient subgroups, since although one drug may be superior to another in inducing fully rigid erections, some of our patients seem to prefer a more physiologic situation. They like a pharmacologically induced tumescence that turns into a full rigid erection on additional sexual stimulation. Others may prefer a drug with a maximum safety profile.

Local Pharmacotherapy

Local pharmacotherapy of erectile dysfunction comprises intracavernous injection and intraurethral administration of smooth muscle relaxant drugs. This mode of application allows high drug concentrations within the cavernous tissue in the presence of low or even no cardiovascular side effects. For this reason, this therapeutic option may be recommended to patients with cardiovascular risk factors, those in whom other treatment options are contraindicated, those who are afraid of the cardiovascular side effects of some oral agents, and those who do not respond to oral agents.

Intracavernosal Pharmacotherapy

The introduction of intracavernous injection of vasoactive drugs has revolutionized the treatment of erectile dysfunction. After extensive worldwide experience, prostaglandin E_1 (PGE1) has today come to represent the gold standard for locally administered drugs [1533]. Systemic side effects are extremely rare and are usually mild due to the small doses of PGE1 used (in most centers, less than 20 µg). Intracavernousal therapy requires some specialist knowledge and the ability to treat priapism should it occur. Patients need to be taught how to perform self-injection, and the dose needs to be chosen carefully to avoid prolonged erections or priapism. Some patients find it helpful to use one of the many autoinjector devices available. The erection occurs after ten minutes and may be enhanced by sexual stimulation. The incidence of complications varies with the different pharmacologic agents. Some pain is not uncommon, but long-term problems are limited to priapism or penile fibrosis.

Alprostadil (PGE1) is the most widely used agent [1557,1558]. It is effective in more than 80% of patients with different etiologies of ED and has a low incidence of side effects. In a recent comparative study of intracavernosal versus intraurethral administration of alprostadil, the rates of erections sufficient for sexual intercourse were 82.5% versus 53.0%, respectively [1558]. Patient and partner satisfaction was higher with intracavernosal injection, and more patients preferred this therapy. Penile pain occurs in 15–50% of patients, but is not often troublesome. The dose range is 5–20 µg, but some physicians will increase it further or combine it with papaverine and phentolamine. Priapism occurs in about 1% of patients. The cumulative incidence of penile fibrosis was 11.7% after a period of four years, and the risk of irreversible fibrotic alterations was 5% [1559]. About half of the cases with fibrosis resolved spontaneously. Other, less frequently used agents include thymoxamine (moxisylyte hydrochloride [Erecnos]), papaverine/phentolamine mixtures (Androskat), papaverine/phentolamine/alprostadil mixtures (Trimix), and VIP/phentolamine (Invicorp).

Intraurethral Instillation of PGE1

Although the intracavernous injection of drugs proved to be very effective in inducing rigid erections in a high percentage of patients, many patients refuse these injections for a variety of reasons. In such patients, the intraurethral application of PGE1 (MUSE: *m*edical *u*rethral *s*ystem for *e*rection) [1560] offers a significant advantage by combining the advantages of local pharmacotherapy with ease of administration by a well-designed applicator. This drug has been incorporated into a pellet that can be given by intraurethral application. In contrast to sildenafil, it initiates the relaxation of cavernous smooth muscle to bring about erection. Patients need to be instructed in the use of MUSE, in which the drug is introduced into the urethra with a disposable applicator. First the patient passes urine to act as a lubricant to facilitate the passage of the applicator and the absorption of the drug. Drug absorption is also facilitated by the patient's rolling his penis between the palms of his hands. Some patients find that a constrictive ring around the base of the penis enhances the efficacy. The erection takes about ten minutes to develop and the dose range varies between 125 and 1000 µg; the majority of patients require 500 or 1000 µg. The use of MUSE is contraindicated without a condom when the partner is pregnant or likely to conceive.

In the US and European multicenter trials, about 65% of men with ED of different causes who tried MUSE had erections sufficient for intercourse during in-clinic testing [1560,1561]. About one-half of the treatments at home were successful, but the drop-out rate after 15 months was 75%, the main reason being lack of efficacy [1561]. The most common side effects are penile pain (30%), urethral burning (12%), or minor urethral bleeding (5%) [1562]. Systemic side effects (such as hypotension or even syncope) were usually uncommon but help to highlight the role of the physician in administering the first supervised dose. Disappointing results have recently been reported in a study conducted in a urology practice setting, in which adequate rigidity scores were achieved in only 13% and 30% of the patients using 500 and 1000 µg, respectively. Pain, discomfort, or burning in the penis were observed in 18%, but orthostatic hypotension (defined as a decrease in systolic/diastolic blood pressure by 20/10 mmHg or orthostatic symptoms) was present in 41% of the patients. The discontinuation rate was very high, achieving 81% after 2–3 months [1563].

Vacuum Devices

Although they have been known for over a hundred years in the treatment of erectile dysfunction, vacuum devices have only recently been gaining the attention of physicians. The vacuum device induces its erectile effect by venous pooling within the cavernous bodies by means of subatmospheric pressure; the pooled venous blood is then trapped in the cavernous bodies by an external ring placed at the base of the penis after the suction procedure. The disadvantages are that some degree of dexterity is required in handling the device, and applying it takes some time. Vacuum devices should only be used for 30 minutes at a time, and require the willing cooperation of the partner. There are few side effects, although there is some degree of discomfort and the penis feels cold. Ejaculation is usually blocked and some men find this makes orgasm less satisfactory. Bruising can occur in 10–15% of men. Vacuum devices are particularly useful in older men in stable relationships and when other treatment options are ineffective. They may also be used to augment the result of pharmacotherapy. Some men find that the constrictive ring is a useful aid in itself for maintaining the erection, without the use of a vacuum device. However, the long-term drop-out rates among users of vacuum constriction devices are relatively high. A recent study showed an overall drop-out rate over three years for the ErecAid system of 65%: 100% among men with mild ED, 56% among those with moderate ED, and 70% among those with complete ED. The main reasons for stopping use were that the device was ineffective (57%), too cumbersome (24%), and too painful (20%) [1564].

Penile Reconstructive Surgery

The enthusiasm for penile reconstructive procedures has seen waves of high peaks and deep troughs. The disappointing results are not due to general non-functioning of the surgical procedures but to inadequate preselection of the patients. The surgical principle of penile revascularization is bypassing the inferior epigastric artery to a dorsal penile artery; the physiologic effect is thought to be an increase in cavernous arterial inflow. Due to the high incidence of other coetiologies of erectile dysfunction in diabetic patients, such as autonomic neuropathy and smooth muscle degeneration, diabetic patients should not undergo arterial reconstructive procedures.

The surgical principle of penile venous surgery is ligation and/or resection of veins draining the cavernous bodies. The physiologic effect is thought to be normalization of the cavernous drainage in patients with venous leakage. Because excessive cavernous drainage ("venous leakage") may be caused by either impaired cavernous smooth muscle function ("myopathy" or "neurotransmissiopathy") or by a localized malfunction of the cavernous occlusive system, diabetic patients should not undergo these procedures except in very carefully selected cases.

Prosthetic Surgery

The first reliable treatment for organogenic erectile dysfunction was penile prosthesis implantation. Although prosthetic implantation has become the last treatment option to be offered to a patient, since it definitively defunctionalizes the cavernous tissue, it still has a place in the therapy of impotence. If a patient is selected for penile prosthesis implantation, he should be informed of the different types of prosthesis, the possible complications, and possible implications for his lifestyle. Today, two main different types of prosthesis are available, the semirigid and the inflatable, each with a wide array of manufacturers and particular modifications. Each type has its specific advantages and disadvantages, which should be explained to the patient and his partner. When the selection criteria are adequate and the patient and his partner well informed, long-term satisfaction with penile prostheses is good.

Bladder Dysfunction

Physiology of Micturition

In the adult, the storage capacity of the urinary bladder is 300–600 ml. Until the final volume is reached, only a minimal intravesical pressure increase is observed, and involuntary spinal reflexes avoid uninhibited contractions. During the filling phase, afferent impulses from the bladder are suppressed by both intraspinal and cerebral mechanisms, and the sphincter apparatus is activated. When the maximum storage capacity is reached, afferent impulses transmit this information to the conscious level. Then, efferent motor activity from the pontine micturition center via the intermediolateral nuclei of the spinal micturition centers at the T10–L2 and S2–4 levels initiate micturition. These impulses are transmitted to the secondary cholinergic neuron within the pelvic plexus. Peripherally, micturition is initiated by relaxation of the extrinsic striated sphincter muscle and contraction of the smooth muscles of the bladder wall. In the absence of relevant anatomic subvesical obstruction, complete bladder emptying occurs in the presence of quite low intravesical pressures.

Pathophysiology and Clinical Symptomatology of the Diabetic Bladder

In the rat with experimentally induced diabetes, micturition disturbances start with degeneration of the afferent myelinated fibers [1565]. In man, "diabetic bladder" refers to a syndrome of reduced awareness of bladder filling, followed by increased bladder storage capacity and decreased bladder contractility. The reduction of sensation of a filled bladder (caused by the degeneration of the afferent myelinated fibers) is rapidly followed by degeneration of the nonmyelinated efferent fibers, with resulting detrusor hypocontractility. This hypocontractility pop pops clinically into reduced urinary flow, incomplete bladder emptying, recurrent urinary tract infections and, as end-stage disease, into bladder desensitization and acontractility with overflow incontinence.

In contrast to this classical scenario of a diabetic bladder, autonomic neuropathy may cause irritative symptoms as urge, pollakiuria, nocturia, or incontinence in the presence of other urologic diseases [1566–1568].

Diagnostic Approach for Micturition Disturbances

In 40–80 % of urologically asymptomatic diabetic patients, abnormal findings were obtained in a detailed urodynamic work-up. Many of these patients became aware of their abnormal micturition patterns only in structured questioning. However, these often asymptomatic micturition disturbances may have deleterious consequences for the upper urinary tract, with significant renal impairment or even end-stage renal disease. This low incidence of symptoms in the presence of possible severe consequences makes it necessary to include specific questions regarding micturition patterns in the routine annual diabetic check-up. Frequency, sensation of incomplete bladder emptying, urinary tract infections, urge symptoms, dysuria, nocturia, incontinence, and the need for abdominal strain to empty the bladder should be specifically addressed. Where the situation is unclear, keeping a micturition record for three consecutive days and nights may be helpful. A urinary laboratory analysis completes the routine urinary bladder function check.

If the history indicates that there may be micturition disorders or recurrent urinary tract infections, a noninvasive urological work-up comprising uroflometry and a postvoid ultrasonography of the bladder should be initiated. A full urological work-up with formal urodynamics and radiologic imaging of the urinary tract is needed in the presence of recurrent urinary tract infections or abnormal noninvasive findings. Diagnostic endoscopy will be carried out depending on the findings of the aforementioned diagnostics. Depending on the treatment planned, further and mostly highly specialized diagnostic procedures are needed, e. g., placing "temporary wires" as time-limited percutaneous testing of the effect of neurostimulation or instruction in self-catheterization before surgical construction of a catheterizable neobladder (see specific procedures) [1569].

Therapeutic Options for Micturition Disturbances

The need to treat micturition disorders is determined by the subjective and objective severity of the impairment, its etiology, any urologic (nondiabetic) comorbidities, any secondary negative impact on the upper urinary tract, and the intellectual capacity and manual dexterity of the patient. Although autonomic neuropathy will most likely be a reason for voiding dysfunctions in a patient with diabetes, other cofactors or coetiologies such as hormone deficiency, obstructive prostatic hyperplasia, or urethral and meatal stenosis may play an important role and must be taken into account when treatment options are being considered and discussed with the patient. To determine these individual variables, the aforementioned rationalized urologic approach is mandatory before treatment.

The majority of diabetic voiding dysfunctions can be safely managed conservatively. However, close follow-up of the patient may be necessary in order to detect any treatment failure early and avoid secondary complications.

Treatment of a *large-capacity bladder* may start with regular voiding intervals (during the day, three-hour intervals are often appropriate). In addition, the patient is advised to take his time in voiding and to try to relax his pelvic floor during micturition. A hypocontractile or even acontractile bladder may benefit from pharmacotherapy with parasympathomimetics. If mild to moderate infravesical prostatic obstruction is present, an α-receptor-blocking drug can be additionally prescribed. If recurrent urinary tract infections occur despite these measures and residual postvoid urine is significantly over 100 ml, either clean intermittent self-catheterization (4–5 times daily) should be started or a suprapubic catheter be placed. Surgical reduction of the bladder's capacity has not been very successful in the past; the ability of neuromodulation or neurostimulation to restore bladder emptying in these patients (in the presence of autonomic neuropathy) also seems very limited [1569–1572].

Anatomic *infravesical obstruction* is mostly seen in elderly male patients, although urethral strictures are a frequent cause of recurrent urinary tract infection in females. Significant bladder outlet obstruction by benign prostatic hyperplasia should be treated by ablative procedures (transurethral resection, laser vaporization, thermoablation, open surgery). Urethral or meatal strictures warrant endoscopic or formal repair [1573].

Stress *incontinence* caused by descent of the pelvic floor and sphincteral insufficiency is a frequent finding in elderly female diabetic subjects. Depending on the severity of symptoms and the individual's preference, various approaches may be chosen. In mild to moderate cases, conservative options such as functional rehabilitation by regular pelvic floor exercises, local or systemic hormonal replacement, or vaginal electrostimulation give good results. However, these treatment modalities must be carried out regularly and require a well-motivated patient. The principle of surgical correction of stress incontinence is elevation of the pelvic floor by various procedures. Success rates of minimally invasive sling procedures (Raz, Stamey) are approximately 50 % (or less) after five years, whereas formal surgical repair (fascial sling, Burch) achieves an 80 % rate of dryness after five years. Implantation of an artificial sphincter for correction of urinary stress incontinence in an elderly diabetic should be viewed with caution and remain as a last resort when all other approaches have failed, since it is accompanied by a higher rate of prosthesis infection in diabetic than in nondiabetic subjects.

Pollakiuria, dysuria, *urge*, or incontinence symptoms may be caused by neurogenic bladder hyperreflexia in the diabetic patient. Compared to stress incontinence, most of these symptoms respond well to conservative treatment. The mainstays of pharmacotherapy are antimuscarinic or spasmolytic (direct smooth muscle relaxant) agents; however, since these drugs have very limited or no bladder selectivity, their individual effectivity is often limited. Nonpharmacologic approaches to the urge symptom complex include vaginal electrostimulation as well as neuromodulation (electrical stimulation of sacral nerves).

■ Sudomotor Function

P.A. Low

Normal Sweat Response

There are two types of sweat glands, eccrine and apocrine [1042]. The eccrine sweat gland is a simple tubular gland that extends down from the epidermis to the lower dermis. The lower portion is a tightly coiled secretory apparatus consisting of two types of cells. One is a dark basophilic cell that secretes mucous material, and the other a light acidophilic cell that is responsible for the passage of water and electrolytes. Surrounding the secretory cells are myoepithelial cells whose contraction is thought to aid the expulsion of sweat. These glands receive a rich supply of blood vessels and sympathetic nerve fibers but are unusual in that sympathetic innervation is cholinergic. The full complement of eccrine glands develops in the embryonic state [1042]. No new glands develop after birth.

The distribution of eccrine glands shows area differences [1043], with the greatest density in the palms and soles. The glands vary in density from 400/mm^2 on the palm to about 80/cm^2 on the thighs and upper arm. The total numbers are approximately 2–5 million [1043].

In addition to the spinothalamic tract, afferent pathways ascend as multisynaptic fibers diffusely in lateral spinal cord, to reticular formation of brainstem and finally to hypothalamus and thalamus. The major thermoreceptors are present in the preoptic-anterior hypothalamus area. Other inputs derive from skin, viscera, midbrain, medulla, and spinal cord [1044]. There are two types of thermoreceptors, warm- and cold-sensitive ones, the former predominating. Skin thermoreceptors play little role in thermoregulation but are important in moment-to-moment responses to changes in ambient temperature. Other brain centers can cause a resetting of the set point, as occurs during sleep, exercise, and fever.

In addition to thermoreceptors, thermoregulation is also affected by changes in fluid volume and electrolyte concentrations. Dehydration results in central hyperosmolarity [1045], which inhibits the firing of "warm" neurons in the preoptic-anterior hypothalamus area [1046] and reduces heat-dissipating responses. It has also been demonstrated that hyper- and hypovolemia without changes in osmolarity cause respectively a rise and a fall in body temperature [1047].

A number of hypothalamic neuropeptides have been reported to play a significant role in thermoregulation. A number of peptides are thermolytic. These include arginine vasopressin [1048], ACTH, melanocyte stimulating hormone (α-MSH) [1049], and thyrotrophin releasing hormone (TRH) [1050]. In man, intravenous TRH causes cutaneous vasodilation and sweating, resulting in a drop of core temperature [1050]. Bombesin is inhibitory, causing a poikilothermic state [1051]. Other peptides with effects on thermo-regulation include neurotensin [1052], vasoactive intestinal peptide (VIP) [1053], cholecystokinin octapeptide (CCK-8), and somatostatin. Endogenous opioids, such as β-endorphin and met-enkephalin, exhibit various thermoregulatory effects in different species, environments, and doses and with or without restraint, and may participate in changes in body temperature with stress [1049].

Thermoreceptors in the preoptic-anterior hypothalamus area function as detectors of core temperature and integrate thermal information. These signals

Table 5.**12** Methods to measure sweat output in human subjects

Method	Principle	Reference
Minor's	Iodine-alcohol-castor oil application; sweat droplets → violet black	List and Peet [1056]
Sweat imprint	Soft impression mold showing sweat imprint	Kennedy et al. [1057]
Guttmann	Indicator powder → purple when wet	Guttmann [1058]
Tannic acid	Sweat droplet seen as a brown dot	Silverman and Powell [1059]
Starch paper and iodine paint	Hard copy of Minor's method	Randall [1060]
Starch-iodine paper	Iodine impregnated starch paper	MacMillan and Spalding [1061]
Bromophenol blue soaked filter paper	Sweating turns bromophenol blue from light tan to dark	Herrmann et al. [1062]
Skin resistance or potential recordings	Sweating causes reduction in skin resistance or generates skin potential	Richter [1063] Shahani et al. [1064]
Prism method	Sweat droplets seen through prism	Netsky [1065]
Conductivity change	Humidity increase changes conductivity of silk fiber coated with a salt	Darrow [1066]
Capacitance hygrometry	Capacitance changes with change in moisture content	Ogawa et al. [1067] Lang et al. [1068]
Sudorometer	Change in humidity or thermal mass	Low et al. [1069] Adams et al. [1070]

are integrated, and a set point is established. The posterior hypothalamus has been ascribed the role of setting the set point, although recent evidence suggests a more limited role [1054].

Tests of Sudomotor Function

Numerous tests of sudomotor function have been devised and differ in the nature of the stimulus and the methods used to monitor the sweat response [1055]. A summary of tests of sudomotor function with references that detail methodology is shown in Table 5.**12**. Significant work has been done using four tests: thermoregulatory sweat test, QSART, imprint method, and skin potential recordings.

Thermoregulatory Sweat Test

The thermoregulatory sweat test (TST) is a sensitive qualitative test of sudomotor function that provides important information on the pattern and distribution of sweat loss. The original method by Guttmann [1058] involved the application of quinizarin indicator onto dry skin. The presence of sweating causes a change in the indicator from brown to a violet color. Quinizarin is not readily available and is allergenic, but alizarin red may be substituted [1071], and skin reactions are rare. Thermal stimulation using heat cradles or sweat cabinets can be used. Fealey [1072] made several important contributions in the clinical application of thermoregulatory sweat testing. He has developed a set of recommendations on the standardization of the performance of the TST in the clinical laboratory, especially in terms of patient preparation, the sweat cabinet, and TST endpoint. The commonly used endpoint of a rise in oral temperature of 1 °C is satisfactory only if (a) the resting core temperature is above 36.5 °C, and (b) the subject is not dehydrated. It is essential that the subject has not taken anticholinergic agents, including antihistamine, antidepressant, and some antiparkinsonian drugs, for 48 hours before the test. There are several distinctive abnormal sweat patterns [1072]. Fealey has also developed a semiquantitative method of evaluating the severity of anhidrosis, in which the percentage of anterior body surface anhidrosis is derived from the sweat pattern. Certain sweat patterns are recognizable and are well exemplified in a study by Fealey et al. on human diabetic neuropathy [1073]. Of 51 patients suspected of having neuropathy on the basis of a clinical examination, 48 (94%) had unequivocal abnormalities on the TST. Pathologic loss of sweating occurred distally in 65%, segmentally in 25%, and only in isolated dermatomes in 25%; 78% of patients had a combination of two or more patterns. Global anhidrosis was noted in eight patients (16%), all of whom had profound autonomic neuropathy, and in the entire group, the percentage of body surface anhidrosis correlated with the degree of clinical dysautonomia (rank correlation coefficient = 0.77; $P < 0.01$).

Major advantages of the method are its simplicity, sensitivity, the ability to recognize patterns of anhidrosis, including mixed patterns, and its semiquantitative nature. The disadvantages are its inability to distinguish between postganglionic, preganglionic, and central lesions, the discomfort, the qualitative nature of the information obtained, and the staining of

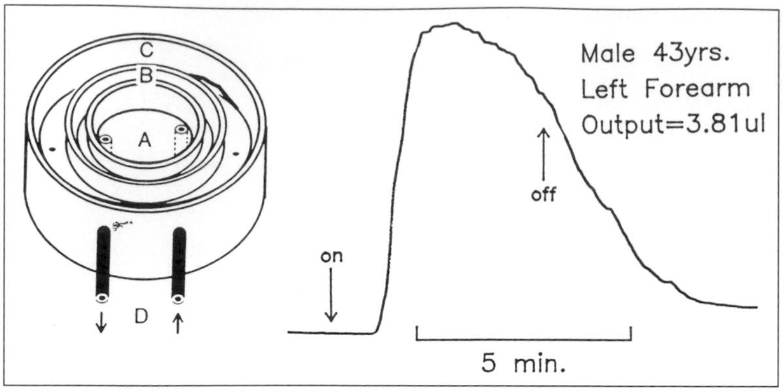

Fig. 5.**33** QSART sweat cell (left) and QSART response (right). The sweat response in compartment A is evoked in response to acetylcholine iontophoresis in compartment C. Compartment B is an air gap. Sweating causes a change in thermal mass of the nitrogen stream (D), which is sensed by the sudorometer and displayed (right). (Reproduced from [1074], with permission)

clothing. Certain characteristic patterns are described below.

Quantitative Sudomotor Axon Reflex Test

QSART, the quantitative sudomotor axon reflex test, is a routine test of autonomic function and is a component of the autonomic reflex screen [1075]. Because autonomic tests are significantly affected by many confounding variables, standardization, the recognition of pitfalls, and patient preparation are critically important. The patient should take no food for three hours before testing, and the antecedent meal should be a light breakfast or lunch. Anticholinergic and diuretic medication should be stopped at least 48 hours, preferably four days, before testing. The patient should be comfortable and pain-free (the bladder recently emptied), the room should be warm and quiet and the personnel quiet.

Physiologic Basis

The principle of the test can be surmised from Figure 5.**33**. The neural pathway consists of an axon "reflex" mediated by the postganglionic sympathetic sudomotor axon. The axon terminal is activated by acetylcholine. The impulse travels antidromically, reaches a branchpoint, then travels orthodromically to release acetylcholine from nerve terminal. Acetylcholine traverses the neuroglandular junction and binds to M_3 muscarinic receptors on eccrine sweat glands [1060] to evoke the sweat response. Acetylcholinesterase in subcutaneous tissue cleaves acetylcholine to acetate and choline, resulting in its inactivation and cessation of the sweat response.

Physiologic Setup

Dehumidified gas or air is piped through to the sudorometer, then to a multicompartmental sweat capsule attached to skin, and returns to the sudorometer. The stimulus is acetylcholine applied by iontophoresis using a constant current generator. An alternative stimulus is carbachol, which is not broken down by acetylcholinesterase and hence has a longer duration of action [1075]. The resultant axon-reflex-mediated sweat response is recorded from a second population of sweat glands using a sudorometer and a multicompartmental sweat cell. Output from the sudorometer is displayed and analyzed on a computer console.

A key component of QSART is the multicompartmental sweat cell comprising an outside stimulus compartment surrounding a central recording compartment, the two compartments being separated from each other by an air gap. The stimulus compartment is loaded with acetylcholine via a cannula. The stimulus compartment is connected to the anode of a constant current generator. The stimulus is a constant current of 2 mA applied for five minutes, and the sweat response is recorded during the stimulus and for five subsequent minutes. The solution consists of 10% acetylcholine loaded into the outer compartment (C in Fig. 5.**33**).

Reproducibility

The tests are sensitive and reproducible in controls [1069] and in patients with diabetic neuropathy [1076]. Tests repeated on two different days regress with a high coefficient of regression. Tests repeated daily to the identical site may evoke local skin alterations, possibly to the sweat duct after about the third or fourth repetition, but this "tolerance" is highly variable. The coefficient of variation is ≤ 20%.

Recording Sites

The recordings are symmetric, so that in normal individuals the left side is not significantly different to the right [1055]. We routinely record from the left but will study the right side when clinically warranted, e.g., following left sural nerve biopsy or with unilateral symptoms. Standard recording sites are over the distal forearm and three lower extremity sites.

Normative Data

Normative data were available on 357 subjects. A consistent gender difference was found, with females having approximately one-half the sweat volume of males. A series of equations are provided in Table 5.**13** that describe the normative data by age and gender. The mean, 5th, and 95th percentile values for ages 20, 40, and 60 years and older are given in Table 5.**14** for males and Table 5.**15** for females.

Abnormal QSART

There are now several recognized abnormal QSART patterns. The response may be: (1) normal, (2) reduced, (3) absent, (4) excessive, or (5) persistent. In diabetic neuropathy, the forearm site can be excessively large, while the foot site is reduced or absent. Short latencies are common with patterns 4 and 5. Pattern 5, consisting of persistent sweat response when the stimulus ceases, is often seen in patients with hyperalgesia, such as painful diabetic and other neuropathies, in mild neuropathies, and in florid reflex sympathetic dystrophy. QSART recordings have been done in many neuropathies, including diabetic neuropathy [1069,1076].

Interpretation

A normal test indicates integrity of the postganglionic sympathetic sudomotor axon. An absent response indicates a lesion of the axon, providing iontophoresis is successful and eccrine sweat glands are present. Since the axonal segment mediating the axon is likely to be short, the test probably evaluates relatively distal function. A reduced or absent sweat response indicates postganglionic sympathetic sudomotor failure.

Skin Potential Recordings

The electrical activity that originates from sweat glands and adjacent tissues is known as electrodermal activity. Sympathetic skin response (SSR) is the term commonly used to refer to the evoked electrodermal activity [1077]. Shahani et al. [1064] suggested that the response can be adapted to electrophysiologic equipment used in many EMG laboratories. The measurement of SSR has been proposed as a simple and sensitive test of autonomic function. In this section, we will briefly review the underlying origins and generators of the SSR and critically assess the clinical utility of SSR in the evaluation of autonomic function.

Spontaneous electrodermal activity is recorded with macroelectrodes applied to the skin. The resulting electrical activity reflects the complex interactions of surface potentials arising from the sweat glands and

Table 5.**13** Regression of QSART (left side) sweat volumes with age for males and females for standard sites in human subjects: based on a normative database of 357 normal subjects evenly distributed by age and gender

Variable	Intercept		Gender		Age		Gender × age	
	B_0	*P*	*b1*	*P*	*b2*	*P*	*b3*	*P*
Forearm	4.5291	0.0001	−1.6188	0.0001	−0.0072	0.5752	0.0020	0.7989
Proximal leg	4.0209	0.0001	−1.0076	0.0026	−0.0163	0.1410	0.0011	0.8724
Distal leg	5.5929	0.0001	−1.5921	0.0001	−0.0437	0.0002	0.0075	0.3049
Proximal foot	4.5174	0.0001	−1.5171	0.0001	0.0310	0.0066	0.0101	0.1548

Table 5.**14** Male QSART responses: mean, 5th, and 95th percentile values

Sites	**20 Years**			**40 Years**			**≥ 60 Years**		
	Mean	**5th**	**95th**	**Mean**	**5th**	**95th**	**Mean**	**5th**	**95th**
Forearm	2.67	0.76	5.06	2.67	0.76	5.06	2.67	0.76	5.06
Proximal leg	2.67	1.27	4.54	2.32	0.93	4.19	1.97	0.58	3.84
Distal leg	3.28	1.37	5.27	2.55	0.98	4.55	1.83	0.59	3.82
Proximal foot	2.58	0.87	4.48	2.17	0.78	4.07	1.75	0.68	3.65

Table 5.**15** Female QSART responses: mean, 5th, and 95th percentile values

Sites	**20 Years**			**40 Years**			**≥ 60 Years**		
	Mean	**5th**	**95th**	**Mean**	**5th**	**95th**	**Mean**	**5th**	**95th**
Forearm	1.15	0.20	2.78	1.15	0.20	2.78	1.15	0.20	2.78
Proximal leg	1.48	0.36	3.17	1.48	0.36	3.17	1.48	0.36	3.17
Distal leg	1.83	0.61	2.85	1.26	0.39	2.28	0.68	0.18	1.70
Proximal foot	1.27	0.23	3.07	1.05	0.18	2.85	0.84	0.12	2.64

adjacent epidermal tissues, modulated by central nervous system structures. The central areas implicated in animal models include the posterior hypothalamus, ventrolateral brainstem reticular formation, and cervical spinal cord [1078,1079].

Different techniques have been reported to obtain an evoked electrodermal activity [1064,1080]. The most commonly used technique involves brief electrical stimulation of peripheral nerve afferents (i.e., median nerve). The recording electrodes are placed in the palmar and plantar surfaces of the hands and feet. The response is generally biphasic, with an initial negativity followed by a positive deflection. A late negative component may be observed in some patients. SSR habituates with a repetitive stimulus, so stimuli are usually given at irregular intervals greater than 30 s. A summary of reported latencies and amplitudes in different studies has been given elsewhere [1077]. Due to the extreme variability of the SSR, most investigators consider the SSR to be abnormal only when it is absent. Yokota et al. [1081] have suggested the additional criterion of 50% reduction between ipsilateral and contralateral limb as a useful measure. SSR is abnormal in several types of peripheral neuropathies [1064,1082–1086] and in central nervous system disease such as primary autonomic failure [1087] and multiple sclerosis [1081,1088]. Most of these studies have shown that SSR is abnormal in the context of peripheral neuropathy, but it is not a reliable index of sudomotor dysfunction.

In summary, SSR is relatively simple to record and is abnormal in many conditions ranging from axonal neuropathies to multiple sclerosis. Its clinical utility is hampered by the high variability, habituation, and lack of specificity.

Pupillary Function

R.H. Straub

Introduction

The pupil of the eye has for many years been recognized as a perfect object for the study of the autonomic nervous system in diabetic subjects [1089–1095]. Quantitative and reproducible stimuli can be easily applied to the pupil, and with the different techniques of today the pupillary responses can be measured very precisely. Since the iris is innervated with autonomic nervous fibers from both the parasympathetic and the sympathetic nervous system [1096], an imbalance of these two parts of the autonomic nervous system can be easily detected. Abnormalities of the steady-state pupil size (responses during continuous illumination, light intensity-adapted), of dynamic pupillary reflexes (latency time, contraction and dilation velocity), and of pharmacological responses have been reported in patients with diabetes mellitus [1089–1095,1097]. However, pupillary dysfunction is not only seen in diabetic subjects, and sometimes more than one lesion underlies pupillary abnormalities (Table 5.**16**).

This section summarizes aspects of anatomy and physiology of pupillary reflex pathways, provides methods of measuring pupillary function in normal and diabetic patients, gives age-related normal values of pupillary function, lists the symptoms of diabetic pupillary dysfunction, provides data about its prevalence, and addresses the questions of its significance and treatment.

Anatomy and Physiology

The iris of the eye is centrally perforated by an opening, the pupil. The main function of the iris is to regulate the amount of light reaching the retina. This is done by continuously adjusting the size of the pupil. The pupil size is regulated by a muscle system with a circular part, the sphincter pupillae (with

Table 5.**16** Neuro-ophthalmologic lesions with pupillary abnormalities [1098]

Type of lesion	Pupillary response
Lesions of the afferent pupillary pathways:	
Failure of retinal function	Diminished
Optic nerve lesions	Diminished
Optic chiasm lesions	Pupillary hemiakinesia
Optic tract lesion	Pupillary hemiakinesia
Lesion of the upper visual pathway	Diminished or increased
Lesions of the midbrain involving the pretecto-oculomotor tract:	
Tumors (e.g., pinealoma)	Mydriasis, loss of response
Tabes, Argyll Robertson pupil	Spastic miosis, irregular, loss of response
Lesions of the efferent pupillary pathways:	
Parasympathetic, first neuron, preganglionic	Diminished
Parasympathetic, second neuron, postganglionic	Absolute pupillary akinesia, tonic pupil
Sympathetic, Horner syndrome, first, second, and third neuron	Miosis, ptosis, enophthalmus

predominantly parasympathetic innervation), and a radial part, the dilator pupillae (with predominantly sympathetic innervation). The parasympathetic innervation of the sphincter pupillae consists of two neurons: the Edinger-Westphal nucleus and the ciliary ganglion (Fig. 5.**34**). Supranuclear inhibition, rather than sympathetic outflow, leads to relaxation of the sphincter pupillae during pupillary dilation [1098]. The sympathetic innervation of the iris consists of three neurons. The fibers of the first neuron come from the hypothalamus and pass the ciliospinal center located in the lateral part of the anterior horns of the spinal cord (Fig. 5.**34**). From neurons in the anterior horns (second neuron), fibers arise which end in the cervical sympathetic trunk. The third neuron is located in the superior cervical ganglion, traveling from there through the carotid plexus to the first division of the trigeminal nerve and the long ciliary nerves to the eye.

The pupillary light reflex is maintained not only by the above-mentioned efferent parasympathetic and sympathetic pathways, but also by an afferent pathway, which consists of the retina, the optic nerve, mesencephalic centers, and the cortex. These regulatory elements are closely interrelated, as is demonstrated in the regulatory circuit shown in Figure 5.**34**. It is obvious that central tonic inhibition is the important factor for regulation of the sphincter pupillae, whereas central and peripheral stimulation is the fundamental factor in the regulation of the dilator pupillae (Fig. 5.**34**). Most anatomic parts of the reflex loop (> 80 %) are located in the central nervous system (Fig. 5.**34**). A small part of the parasympathetic portion (along with the third cranial nerve) and a larger part of the sympathetic portion (sympathetic trunk–superior cervical ganglion-carotid plexus-long ciliary nerves) are outside the central nervous system and belong to the peripheral autonomic nervous system. In particular, the sympathetic portion of the reflex loop is more prone to lesions related to diabetes mellitus. Thus, the pupillary light reflex involves many central nervous structures, including the afferent pathways (e. g., retina, optic nerve), and is therefore significantly different to other autonomic reflexes.

Measurement

Several methods have been used to assess pupillary abnormalities. Methods using direct observation are

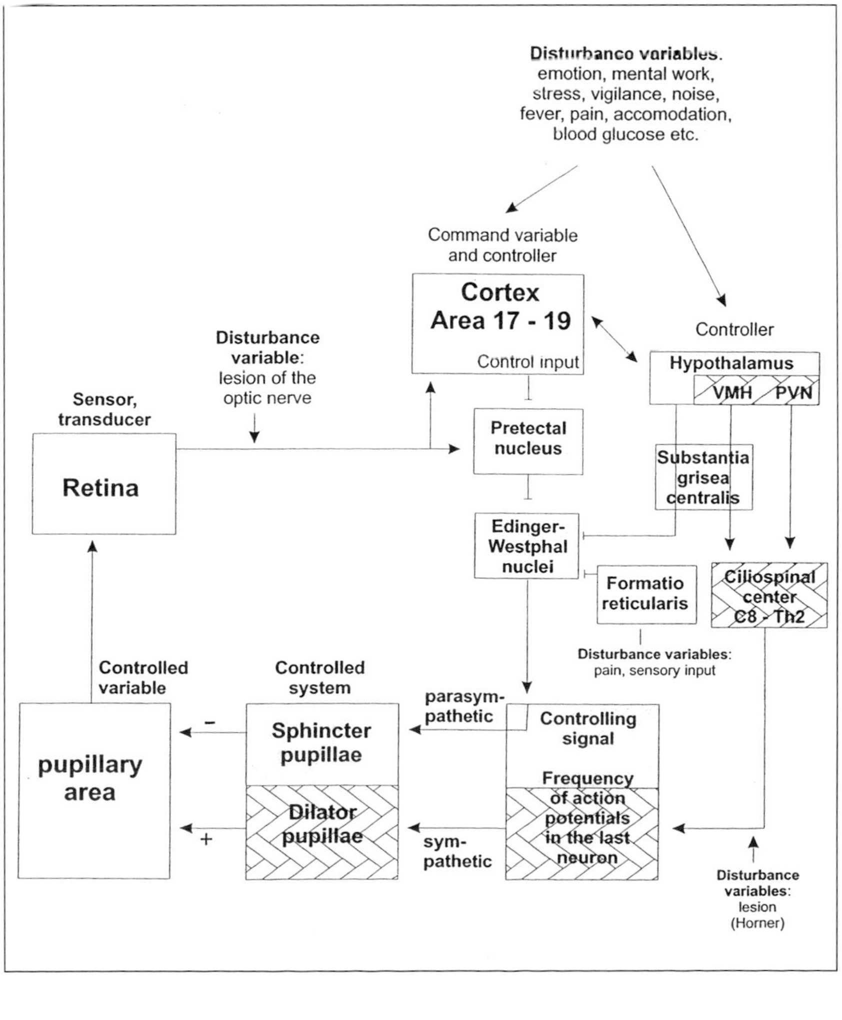

Fig. 5.**34** Regulatory circuit of the pupillary light reflex. Light illuminates the retina, which is the sensor in the regulatory circuit. The incoming signals pass through the optic nerve and modulate the pretectal nuclei. These nuclei have an inhibitory influence on the Edinger-Westphal nucleus. In the Edinger-Westphal nucleus, parasympathetic fibers arise which travel through the third cranial nerve to the iris to modulate the sphincter pupillae and the pupillary area (controlled variable). The sympathetic portion of the regulatory circuit has its origin in the hypothalamus (VMH, ventromedial nuclei of the hypothalamus; PVN, paraventricular nuclei of the hypothalamus). From there nerve fibers arise and travel to the ciliospinal center in the spinal cord C8–T2. From there nerve fibers travel to the sympathetic trunk and the superior cervical ganglion, which is the last neuron of this pathway. The controlling signal is the frequency of action potentials in this last neuron which modulates the dilator pupillae and the pupillary area (controlled variable). At several levels, disturbance variables may influence the regulatory circuit. Gray area, parasympathetic parts of the regulatory circuit; hatched area, sympathetic parts of the regulatory circuit

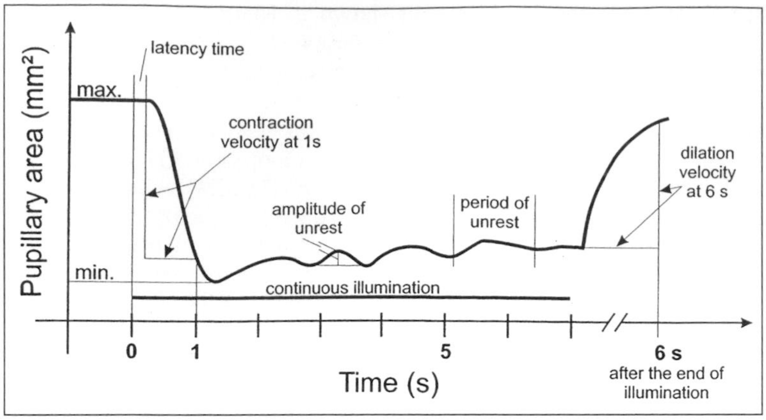

Fig. 5.**35** Typical pupillogram during pupillary stimulation with light. The various pupillary reflex parameters are demonstrated. The velocities are calculated as the ratio between the change in pupillary area and time elapsed. Max., maximal pupillary area; min., minimal pupillary area.

suitable for routine observation of the pupil size in a comparison with standard scales [1098]. A simple device is the Haab scale, which has a series of black circles, graduated in size, that are compared with the patient's pupil [1098]. By these simple techniques, pupil diameter can be determined with an accuracy of ± 0.2 mm. A disadvantage of direct observation is that pupil size cannot be measured in darkness. To overcome this problem, photographic methods with infrared or Polaroid films have been used [1099]; infrared reflex pupillography was first introduced in the 1950s [1096,1098, 1100]. This technique has been refined in the last 40 years, making use of videopupillometry [1101,1102]. By using these techniques, steady state and functional parameters can be determined. A continuous record of the phasic pupillary light reflex, called the pupillogram, is shown in Figure 5.**35**. This diagram demonstrates several parameters that can be assessed using videopupillometry (Fig. 5.**35**). The most often used are maximum pupillary area, latency time, maximum contraction velocity (similar to the 1s contraction velocity), and dilation velocity. The disadvantage of videopupillometry is the time resolution of 40 ms, which is dependent on the video technique (25 images per second).

Table 5.**17** Requirements for the investigation of pupillary parameters in subjects with diabetes mellitus

Be careful when interpreting data of
- Patients with a visual acuity for distance and proximity < 0.5 (retinopathy ?)
- Patients with drugs that influence the autonomic nervous system (e. g., β-blocker)
- Patients with other causes of autonomic nervous dysfunction
- Patients with sleep reduction during the night before the investigation
- Patients after extreme physical and emotional stress
- Patients suffering from painful diseases (e. g., sensorimotor neuropathy)
- Patients who smoked prior to the investigation (10 hours before)
- Patients who are used to drinking a lot of coffee or alcohol

However, this time resolution allows accurate measurement of most parameters of pupillary function.

With respect to the diabetic patient, investigation of the pupillary light reflex requires several considerations to be borne in mind, which are listed in Table 5.**17**. To qualify the findings of pupillary function analysis, it is important to know the status of retinal abnormalities in a diabetic patient (funduscopy). For routine measurements, it is best to investigate subjects between the hours of 1000 and 1200 to exclude strong daily variations. Before measuring pupillary function parameters, subjects should rest in an upright position for 10 minutes in darkness (less than 1 lux). Dark adaptation is necessary to obtain maximum dilation of the pupil. The pupillary light reflex depends on the state of dark adaptation of the retina, the intensity and wavelength of the light stimulus, and its magnitude and duration [1098]. Thus, using different types of pupillographs results in a significant variation of the numerical value of pupillary parameters except for the maximum pupillary area in darkness. For each individual pupillograph, it is absolutely necessary to set up a database of pupillary function parameters in normal subjects of different ages.

Pharmacologic testing of the pupil is not described here because anisocoria is a rare disorder in diabetic pupillary autonomic neuropathy. The interested reader should refer to the specialist literature [1098,1103].

Age-Related Normal Values

The age-related normal values given here were obtained with a closed-loop pupillometer [1102]. Using this apparatus, the subjects look at an illuminated area 5 cm × 6 cm (30 cm^2) from a distance of about 16 cm. This means an angle of 8.9° upward and downward and an angle of 10.6° toward the nose and the lateral side. The light intensity measured at that distance was 175 lux, which is significantly above the threshold value. The wavelength of the light was 680 nm ($x = 0.725$ and $y = 0.265$ on the DIN 5033 standard color scale). After dark adaptation for 10 minutes, a video recorder was started to record the images of the pupil (time

Table 5.**18** Correlation coefficient for the relationship between age and numerical value of a pupillary function parameter determined in 103 normal subjects [1104,1105]

Diameter of the iris	−0.142 (n. s.)
100 × maximum pupillary diameter/diameter of the iris	−0.615 ($P < 0.001$)
Maximum pupillary area	−0.609 ($P < 0.001$)
Maximum contraction velocity	−0.414 ($P < 0.001$)
Contraction velocity at 1 s	−0.638 ($P < 0.001$)
Dilation velocity at 6 s	−0.613 ($P < 0.001$)
Latency time of the pupillary light reflex	0.419 ($P < 0.001$)
Amplitude of the pupillary unrest	−0.283 ($P = 0.004$)
Period of the pupillary unrest	0.044 (n. s.)

point 0). After ten seconds, the light stimulus was given at an intensity of 175 lux. After another ten seconds, illumination ended (20th second) and the dilation of the pupil was recorded for further 20 seconds. Using this technique, most of the pupillary function parameters were found to be age-dependent (Table 5.**18**). Since no real gold standard of age-related pupillary autonomic nervous function is available, the 5th percentile can be used as a cut-off value to distinguish the normal range from hyperreflexia or hyporeflexia (Fig. 5.**36**). By definition, autonomic pupillary dysfunction is present when the numerical value of a parameter is below the 5th percentile (hyporeflexia). In a previous study, we demonstrated how to calculate the percentile value of a given parameter of a patient when statistical values from a database of measurements in normal subjects are available [1104].

Most of the pupillary function parameters correlated closely to each other [1105]. This was particularly true for maximum pupillary area, contraction velocity, minimum pupillary area, and dilation velocity. Using factor analysis and partial correlation, one can reduce the different pupillary parameters to three independent factors (Table 5.**19**). Factor 1 represents a test group of static and simple dynamic parameters, factor 2 represents pupillary unrest parameters, and factor 3 second-order dynamic parameters (Table 5.**19**). To reduce the factors to one meaningful test, the strongly correlating parameters of the independent factors must be eliminated to obtain the one test which is easiest to perform. In an earlier study, we proposed the maximum pupillary area (sympathetic portion of the

Table 5.**19** Independent factors of pupillary function analysis [1105]

Factor 1	Factor 2	Factor 3
Maximum pupillary area	Amplitude of unrest	Latency time
Contraction velocity at 1 s	Area under the unrest curve	
Dilation velocity at 6 s	Period of unrest	
Minimum pupillary area		

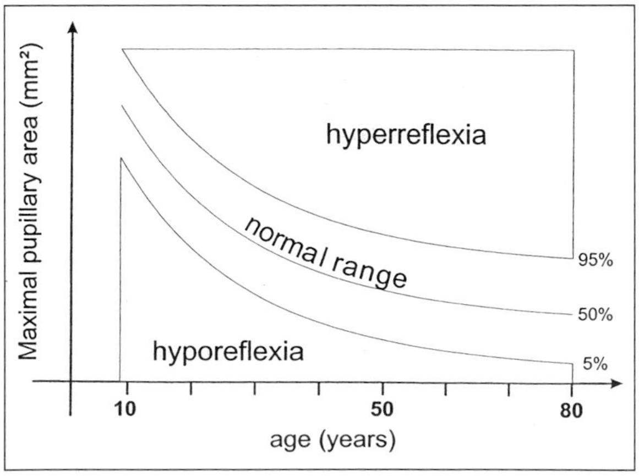

Fig. 5.**36** Definition of pupillary hyporeflexia and pupillary hyperreflexia. The gray areas demonstrate the areas below and above the 5th percentile and 95th percentile, respectively. The normal range lies between the 5th and the 95th percentiles

Table 5.**20** Fifth percentile of the most important pupillary parameters [1104,1105]

Age range (years)	Maximum pupillary diameter (mm)	Maximum pupillary area (mm^2)	Latency time (ms)
15–19	5.9	27.3	290
20–24	5.8	26.4	295
25–29	5.6	24.6	298
30–34	5.4	22.9	301
35–39	5.2	21.2	304
40–44	5.0	19.6	308
45–49	4.9	18.9	312
50–54	4.6	16.6	315
55–59	4.4	15.2	319
60–64	4.1	13.2	323
65–69	3.9	11.9	327

By definition, hyporeflexia is present if the value of a patient is below the given value for the maximum pupillary diameter or the maximum pupillary area or above the given value for the latency time of the pupillary light reflex pupillary light reflex) and the latency time (parasympathetic portion of the pupillary light reflex) as valid parameters by which to measure pupillary function [1105]. Interestingly, these two were the most significant parameters with respect to both normal and diabetic subjects [1105]. Parameters of pupillary unrest were not useful because they do not discriminate between normal subjects and diabetic patients. Table 5.**20** gives the 5th percentile values for maximum pupillary diameter, maximum pupillary area, and the latency time of the pupillary light reflex. These cut-off values can be used for pupillary function examination in diabetic subjects.

It should be mentioned that day-to-day variation is often large in neurophysiologic function examinations. With respect to maximum pupillary area and latency time, a relative day-to-day variation coefficient of up to 10% was found [1106].

Pupillary Autonomic Dysfunction in Diabetic Neuropathy

Symptoms

The most prominent symptom of pupillary dysfunction is the small and sometimes nearly spastic pupil. This is a typical sign of severe involvement of the pupillary regulatory circuit. However, most often a small contraction of the pupil is still visible in diabetic patients. Sometimes diabetic patients have an amaurotic pupillary akinesia when retinal function is completely abolished (blindness). When retinal function is disturbed, the pupils are of equal size before and during the light reflex (isocoria). The severity of the disturbance of the light reflex corresponds to the severity of the retinal dysfunction. Thus, prior investigation of the retinal status is very important in patients with long-standing diabetes mellitus. Moreover, retinal dysfunction is not the only thing that leads to alterations of the light reflex; a conduction disturbance central to the retina (optic nerve and upper visual pathways) also does so. The hallmark of efferent pupillary defects is anisocoria (a lesion of the efferent pathway on one side). However, this type of symptom is very rare in diabetic patients, and most often has another cause than diabetes mellitus.

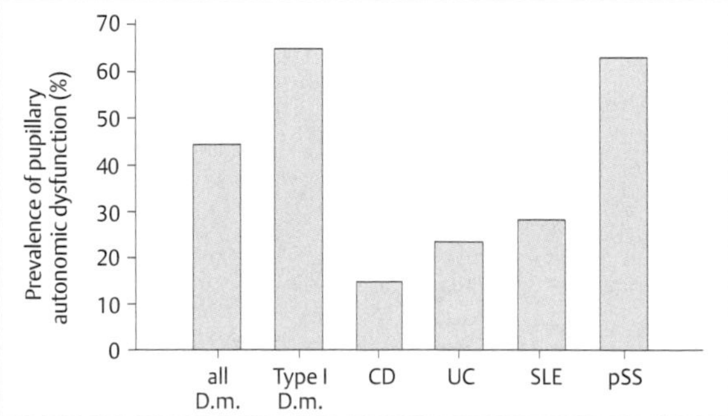

Fig. 5.**37** Comparison of prevalence rates between different diseases using the same pupillometric technique and definition. All D.m., all patients with diabetes mellitus; Type I D.m., type I diabetes mellitus; CD, Crohn disease; UC, ulcerative colitis; SLE, systemic lupus erythematosus; pSS, progressive systemic sclerosis

Prevalence

Assessments of prevalence are very dependent on the number of normal and diabetic subjects investigated, the age-related control group, the considerations included in the investigation of pupillary parameters (see Table 5.**17**), the parameters investigated, the cut-off value for the different parameters, accompanying retinopathy, and the disease duration of diabetes mellitus. Thus, very different prevalence rates have been cited in the literature (Table 5.**21**). In our opinion, it is sufficient to use the maximum pupillary area and pupillary light reflex latency time for the function examination [1107]. If one or both parameters were below the 5th percentile of those of age-related normal subjects, at least one part of the pupillary autonomic nervous system is altered and pupillary autonomic neuropathy is present [1107]. Using this rather simple definition, prevalence of pupillary autonomic neuropathy is dependent on disease duration irrespective of age [1108]. In a recent study using the same technique, we were able to compare the prevalence of pupillary autonomic neuropathy in different diseases [1109]. Patients with type I diabetes mellitus had pupillary autonomic dysfunction significantly more often than did those with Crohn disease, ulcerative colitis, or systemic lupus erythematosus, but a comparable rate to patients with progressive systemic sclerosis (Fig. 5.**37**). In this comparative study, maximum pupillary area was more severely disturbed than pupillary light reflex latency time, which was more obvious in patients with diabetes mellitus than in the other diseases [1109]. Furthermore, in the patients with chronic inflammatory diseases, pupillary autonomic hyperreflexia (shown by a numerical value above the 95th percentile, Fig. 5.**36**) was frequently present. Pupillary

Table 5.**21** Prevalence of pupillary autonomic neuropathy in patients with diabetes mellitus

	Number of patients	Prevalence (%)
Smith et al. [1089]	36	38.8
Namba et al. [1116]	24	29.0
Smith et al. [1117]	66	10.0
Clark [1118]	28	88.5
De Vos et al. [1119]	18	78.0
Neil et al. [1099]	175	22.9
Straub et al. [1094]	77	30.0
Straub et al. [1107]	119	39.0
Straub et al. [1108]	166	23–59[a]

[a] The prevalence rate depends on the disease duration

hyperreflexia seems to depend on the inflammatory state in these diseases [1110,1111]. Thus, hyperreflexia may be a central nervous read-out for basal overactivity of the pupillary autonomic nervous system.

Changes in Pupillary Function During the Course of the Disease

Several studies have addressed this subject and found a significant increase of pupillary autonomic nervous dysfunction during the course of the disease [1106, 1108, 1112–1115]. The deterioration of pupillary autonomic nervous function is related to the degree of retinopathy [1108] and glycemic control [1115]. Thus, pupillary autonomic nervous function examination is a useful way to study retinal function longitudinally, as was demonstrated earlier [1098].

Significance and Treatment

Since pupillary autonomic nervous function deteriorates in parallel with retinal function, pupillary examination can be used as a method to study retinal changes longitudinally (pupilloperimetry). However, pupillary function examination can never replace direct retinal observation by an ophthalmologist. In addition, examination of pupillary autonomic nervous function can be used to study changes of the optic nerve and upper visual pathways longitudinally [1098]. It can also be used to study more central aspects of the sympathetic and parasympathetic autonomic nervous system in diabetes mellitus. This can be particularly interesting with respect to hyperreflexia, which is rare in diabetic patients. In our view at present, pupillary dysfunction is not an indicator for higher mortality in patients with diabetes mellitus as has been shown for cardiac autonomic neuropathy. In fact, the significance of pupillary dysfunction in relation to upcoming problems in diabetic patients is unknown. No specific treatment other than improving glycemic control [1113] is available to treat pupillary autonomic dysfunction. It would be very important to start longitudinal studies that would shed light on the implications of pupillary autonomic dysfunction for future problems in patients with diabetes mellitus. It may be that pupillary function examination will help to define patients at risk of certain late complications of diabetes.

Endocrine Regulation in Response to Physiologic Maneuvers

J. Hilsted and M. Taskiran

Diabetic neuropathy profoundly effects the adaptation to physical maneuvers in diabetic patients. This is to be expected, since coordinated changes in the activity of both the autonomic and the somatic nervous system are essential for physiologic adaptation to physical activity in man. Diabetic neuropathy affects all parts of the peripheral nervous system, and so varying degrees of maladaptation to physical maneuvers follow from the existence of diabetic neuropathy.

Physical Exercise

Changes in the activity of the autonomic nervous system are essential for physiologic adaptation to exercise in man. Cardiac muscle must be able to increase in contractility if cardiac output is to be increased in response to exercise. Finally, striated muscle performance is the basis of locomotion. All these functions may be affected in diabetic neuropathy, either by way of altered nerve function or by indirect changes in innervated organs and muscles. Thus, diabetic neuropathy is the main cause of physical inability in patients with long-term diabetes.

Exercise Capacity

Maximum exercise capacity in the upright position is significantly reduced in type 1 diabetic patients with neuropathy compared to those without neuropathy [1120–1123]. This has been documented by experiments in which the maximum tolerable workload was reduced, along with a decrease in maximum oxygen uptake, in type 1 diabetic patients with autonomic neuropathy. In these experiments, exhaustion was documented by lack of increase in oxygen uptake at maximum exercise intensity, as well as by profound increments in blood concentration of markers of anaerobic glycolysis (i. e., lactate). In patients with long-term type 1 diabetes without neuropathy, exercise capacity is comparable to that of healthy control subjects matched for age and sex [1124]. At submaximum workload, diabetic patients with autonomic neuropathy have a normal ventilatory anaerobic threshold and normal rates of increment in oxygen uptake [1125], suggesting important roles for non-neurogenic mechanisms in the regulation of circulatory control and performance at low exercise intensity (Table 5.**22**). Indeed, neuromuscular and ventila-tory outputs in relation to increasing $\dot{V}CO_2$ were progressively higher in patients with diabetic autonomic neuropathy compared with patients without neuropathy and control patients [1126]. This may suggest that pulmonary autonomic denervation affects ventilatory response to exercise by excessively increasing respiratory rate and alveolar ventilation [1126].

The relationship between diabetic neuropathy and exercise capacity has been studied less in type 2 patients. Apparently, diabetic microangiopathy (nephropathy and retinopathy) are associated with reduced exercise performance, whereas diabetic neuropathy

Table 5.22 Physiologic responses to exercise in type 1 diabetic autonomic neuropathy and in diabetic patients without neuropathy

	Exercise capacity	$\dot{V}_E$	Plasma volume	Heart rate	Blood pressure	Plasma norepinephrine	Plasma epinephrine	Splanchnic vasoconstriction
Diabetic neuropathy	↓	↑	→	↓	↓	↓	↓	↓
Diabetes, no neuropathy	→	→	→	→	→	→	(↓)	→

↑, →, and ↓, increased, normal and decreased responses, respectively, in comparison with findings in healthy subjects

was not [1127]. However, type 2 patients with severe neuropathy did show impaired cardiovascular adaptation to exercise, although cardiovascular neuropathy scores did not correlate with exercise capacity in a large type 2 diabetic population [1128].

Intravascular Volume

In normal man, plasma volume decreases during exercise, mainly due to the effect of circulating catecholamines on the vasculature. During exercise, plasma volume decreased to a similar, normal extent in diabetic patients without neuropathy [1129]. Furthermore, atrial natriuretic factor increased to a similar extent in diabetic patients with and without autonomic neuropathy [1130]. Thus, abnormalities in plasma volume changes during exercise do not contribute to the decrease in exercise capacity in diabetic neuropathy.

Cardiac Function

Heart rate responses to exercise in diabetic patients with autonomic neuropathy are affected in a way that is compatible with combined parasympathetic and sympathetic dysfunction. At low exercise intensities, the normal increase in heart rate is due to withdrawal of vagal tone, resulting in an abrupt increase in heart rate. This phenomenon does not exist in patients with diabetic autonomic neuropathy [1131]. Instead, heart rate does not increase at low exercise levels with these patients. Furthermore, maximum heart rate is reduced in diabetic neuropathy [1120–1123], probably due to diminished sympathetic stimulation of the heart.

Blood pressure responses to exercise are lower in patients with autonomic neuropathy than in control patients [1131]. Indeed, in severe neuropathy including orthostatic hypotension, blood pressure actually decreases during exercise [1129]. The inability to maintain a normal blood pressure during exercise is probably due to both impaired increments in cardiac output and deficient innervation of splanchnic vascular resistance vessels. This is in accordance with anatomic studies in diabetic patients with autonomic neuropathy, in whom morphologic evidence of splanchnic denervation has been reported [1132].

Cardiac output increases during exercise due to the combined effect of a rise in stroke volume and an increase in heart rate. The increase in cardiac output during exercise is subnormal in diabetic patients with autonomic neuropathy, because both heart rate responses and stroke volume responses to exercise are blunted [1129,1133]. The stroke volume changes during exercise may be due to deficient sympathetic innervation or to cardiomyopathy, or both.

Even in type 1 diabetic patients without cardiac symptoms, diastolic function is frequently abnormal, and in patients with other diabetic complications both systolic and diastolic function are abnormal [1134], suggesting a definite role for diabetic cardiomyopathy in the defective cardiac response to exercise in diabetic autonomic neuropathy.

Resistance Vessel Function

During exercise, total peripheral vascular resistance decreases in order to allow an increase in perfusion of working muscle [1135]. To counterbalance this very large increase in vascular conductance, vascular resistance increases in other areas, i. e., the splanchnic vascular bed [1135]. This vasoconstriction did not occur to a significant extent in diabetic patients with autonomic neuropathy [1129]. The combined effect of this lack of vasoconstriction and of a diminished increase in cardiac output is most likely responsible for the blunted blood pressure response to exercise in diabetic autonomic neuropathy.

Hormonal Responses

During exercise, plasma norepinephrine and epinephrine concentrations increase due to activation of sympathetic nerves innervating heart and resistance vessels as well as the adrenal medulla [1136]. Consistent with the physiologic changes described above, plasma concentrations of catecholamines were diminished in diabetic patients with autonomic neuropathy compared with those in patients without neuropathy [1122,1123,1137,1138]. The catecholamine response to exercise in diabetic autonomic neuropathy was somewhat less affected compared with that in patients with autonomic neuropathy of other etiologies (familiar amyloid polyneuropathy and pure autonomic failure). In the latter groups, severe blood pressure falls were encountered during exercise, reflecting a more severe state of autonomic denervation in these patients than in the diabetic patients [1139]. Findings from recent experiments suggest that low catecholamine responses are associated with a high rate of cardiac and cerebrovascular events in patients with type 2 diabetes [1140]. The exercise-induced increases in plasma glucagon, growth hormone, and cortisol found in healthy subjects were significantly blunted in patients with diabetic autonomic neuropathy [1137]. Growth hormone and cortisol responses to exercise are to a large extent mediated by impulses through afferent nerves [1136]. It is possible that the impaired growth hormone and cortisol responses to exercise in diabetic patients with autonomic neuropathy are also due to afferent nerve damage.

Physical Training

Physical training increases parasympathetic tone on the heart and may increase maximum oxygen uptake by conditioning of striated muscles [1136]. Since these physiologic mechanisms are hampered in diabetic neuropathy, it is a reasonable assumption that physical training may improve some of the defects encountered during exercise in diabetic neuropathy. Regular physical training in type 1 diabetic patients with autonomic neuropathy was, however, associated with reduced maximum oxygen uptake [1141], like the findings in untrained diabetic patients with autonomic neuropathy [1130].

Orthostatic Hypotension

Orthostatic hypotension, i. e., a drop in blood pressure of 30 mmHg or more during the transition from supine to standing, is a disabling complication in diabetic neuropathy. It affects a comparatively small proportion of diabetic patients, occurring only in those with severe long-term neuropathy [1141,1142]. The symptoms involved may vary from a light postural dizziness to, in a few patients, fainting and inability to maintain erect position.

Intravascular Volume

Postural hypotension may be caused by a reduction in intravascular volume, as for example in Addison disease or anemia [1131]. In some diabetic patients postural hypotension is reported to be associated with few signs of neuropathy and with exaggerated heart rate responses to standing (and enhanced catecholamine responses): hyperadrenergic orthostatic hypotension [1143]. In these patients, the physiologic basis of orthostatic hypotension is found to be a decrease in intravascular volume rather than diabetic neuropathy.

In patients with a hypoadrenergic orthostatic hypotension (patients with severe neuropathy and orthostatic hypotension associated with blunted catecholamine responses to standing), intravascular volume was normal and decreased in a normal fashion on standing up [1144] (Table 5.**23**). Thus, in these patients, orthostatic hypotension was not caused by intravascular volume contraction. However, in a recent study in type 2 diabetes mellitus, patients with orthostatic hypotension had a 10% decrease in plasma volume [1145]. Subnormal responses of arginine vasopressin, atrial natriuretic polypeptide, and aldosterone to standing may in some cases contribute to standing hypotension [1146].

Cardiac Output

In autonomic neuropathy of other etiology, the postural hypotension is associated with blunted heart rate responses to standing. In diabetic patients with orthostatic hypotension, the heart rate response to standing is generally preserved to some extent; yet in some pa-

Table 5.**23** Physiological responses to study in three district subtypes of orthostatic hypotension in diabetic patients

	Blood pressure	Heart rate	Intra-vascular volume	Cardiac output	Splanchnic vaso-contriction	Sympathetic venomotor function	Plasma norepi-nephrine
Hypoadrenergic orthostatic hypotension	↓	→ (↓)	→	→	↓	→ (↓)	↓
Hyperadrenergic orthostatic hypotension	↓	↑	↓	→	↑	→	↑
POTS (Postural tachycardia syndrome)	↓	↑	→	↓	↑	↓	↑

↑, →, and ↓, increased, normal, and decreased responses, respectively, in comparison with findings in healthy subjects tients with extensive orthostatic hypotension, heart rate responses may be absent [1131]. The cardiac response to standing is not considered of major importance for maintenance of a normal blood pressure in the erect position. This is because pharmacologic blockade of the cardiac responses does not play an important role in the adaptation to upright posture. Moreover, patients with cardiac transplant cannot increase heart rate in the upright position, but do not develop orthostatic hypotension [1147].

Cardiac output decreases in normal man upon standing are due to the venous pooling of blood. In diabetic orthostatic hypotension, cardiac output decreases to a similar extent to that seen in patients without neuropathy. Abnormal cardiac function is therefore not a major cause of hypotension in diabetic orthostatic hypotension [1144].

Resistance Vessel Function

Standing up causes pooling of blood in the lower extremities and splanchnic vascular bed due to gravity. The healthy organism compensates by increasing peripheral vascular resistance, notably in splanchnic vascular bed and in striated muscle and skin. This normal compensatory mechanism is defective in patients with diabetic orthostatic hypotension, i. e., these patients do not increase their vascular resistance in the splanchnic vascular bed to any greater extent, nor does vasoconstriction occur to any major extent in the skin [1144]. The effect of standing up on resistance vessel function in muscle has not been studied in diabetic patients. In some patients with mild autonomic neuropathy, postural hypotension is due to a deficiency in sympathetic vasomotor function (selectively impaired) while postural arteriolar function remains relatively intact (postural tachycardia syndrome) [1148]. Lack of splanchnic vasoconstriction in response to standing occurred in diabetic patients with and without autonomic neuropathy, whereas healthy control subjects had an increase in vascular resistance [1149]. This may indicate that splanchnic denervation may also occur in diabetic patients without neuropathy.

Catecholamine Responses

Plasma catecholamines (notably norepinephrine) increase in response to standing up [1131]. This is due to sympathetic activation of heart and resistance vessels. In diabetic orthostatic hypotension, plasma norepinephrine responses are absent or blunted, in accordance with a lack of sympathetic activation. However, in some patients with mild orthostatic hypotension, plasma norepinephrine may be near normal [1142, 1144]. It has been suggested that plasma norepinephrine may not be an accurate reflection of sympathetic neural activity in such patients. This might be so since norepinephrine is cleared from blood to some extent by sympathetic neurons, possibly with a neuropathic defect in the neuronal reuptake mechanism. However, whole-body plasma clearance of norepinephrine was similar in diabetic patients with and without autonomic neuropathy [1150].

Treatment

Treatment of diabetic orthostatic hypotension is difficult since most of the patients have supine hypotension because of concomitant diabetic nephropathy. The rational approach to the treatment of orthostatic hypotension is to increase blood pressure, a concept which obviously is harmful in the long term in diabetic patients. The treatment principles include intervascular volume expansion with mineralocorticoids or erythroproteins as well as sodium chloride administration. Head-up tilt at night may increase sodium retention and may be useful in some cases. β-Blockers have been said to be efficient in a case report, but the effect is doubtful in double-blind randomized studies [1151].

Final Remarks

Diabetic neuropathy is the major source of physical incapacity in long-term diabetes. Since the neuropathic process is largely irreversible, preventing the development of neuropathy by tight metabolic control is at the moment the only valid approach to the condition [1152].

■ Response to Hypoglycemia

G.B. Bolli, C.G. Fanelli, F. Porcellati, and S. Pampanelli

Introduction

Traditionally, diabetic autonomic neuropathy has been regarded as constituting a risk condition for hypoglycemia while at the same time reducing perception of hypoglycemia symptoms, a condition presently referred to as "hypoglycemia unawareness." Until recently, therefore, the dominant view has been that the presence of autonomic neuropathy is a contraindication to intensified insulin therapy aiming at near-normoglycemia in type 1 diabetes mellitus. Reversing this reasoning, autonomic neuropathy has been pointed to as causing the loss of symptoms of hypoglycemia (hypoglycemia unawareness) and/or loss of responses of counterregulatory hormones to hypoglycemia, primarily epinephrine [1153]. Even loss of glucagon response to hypoglycemia was initially attributed to autonomic neuropathy [1154], a hypothesis that has recently regained consideration based on some animal data [1155].

On the other hand, over recent years it has become evident that recurrent iatrogenic hypoglycemia in patients with type 1 diabetes mellitus can induce loss of symptoms of hypoglycemia and blunt counterregulatory hormone responses, reproducing closely what occurs in type 1 diabetes with autonomic neuropathy [1156]. However, because hypoglycemia unawareness and loss of epinephrine responses may well occur even in patients with type 1 diabetes of very short duration, and because these defects are rapidly reversible provided that hypoglycemia is meticulously prevented [1157], autonomic neuropathy cannot be invoked as a factor. For this reason, the whole story of autonomic neuropathy as cause of loss of epinephrine responses and symptoms in response to hypoglycemia is now in need of critical reassessment. In particular, the relative roles of "structural" factors (i. e., autonomic neuropathy) versus "functional" factors (i. e., recurrent antecedent hypoglycemia) in causing loss of symptoms and epinephrine responses need to be discussed.

Physiology of Responses to Hypoglycemia

Tissues such as muscle and liver can easily switch from oxidation of glucose to other nonglucose fuels, e. g., nonesterified free fatty acids , ketones, and lactate. In contrast, from a practical point of view, the brain can utilize only glucose as a source of energy. In fact, although in theory the brain can oxidize ketones [1158,1159] and lactate [1159,1160], this occurs in humans only under experimental hypoglycemia conditions where supraphysiologic concentrations of these substrates are produced in plasma by exogenous infusion. During insulin-induced hypoglycemia closely mimicking the spontaneous condition of insulin-treated type 1 diabetes, the plasma ketone concentration decreases, and lactate concentration does not increase substantially [1161]. Thus, these substrates cannot compensate the condition of neuroglycopenia which follows hypoglycemia. One notable exception might be the hypoglycemia in the postprandial condition [1162], where the increase in plasma lactate concentration might in part replace glucose for use by the brain [1163]. Because the brain cannot operate gluconeogenesis, or store any large amount of glucose in the form of glycogen, the brain is very dependent on continuous glucose delivery from the circulation for its metabolism and function.

Since maintenance of the plasma glucose concentration above a given threshold is crucial for brain function (and the survival of the whole body), it is no surprise that multiple mechanisms cooperate to prevent hypoglycemia in mammals. The homeostatic mechanisms include, first, release of counterregulatory hormones [1164] and, second, the generation of specific symptoms. The latter include the autonomic (anxiety, palpitations, hunger, sweating, irritability, tremor) and the neuroglycopenic (dizziness, tingling, blurred vision, difficulty in thinking, faintness). An important concept which has evolved during the last few years is that the brain responses to hypoglycemia are hierarchical [1165]. During progressive falls in plasma glucose concentrations, the release of counterregulatory hormones starts *before* the symptoms of hypoglycemia are generated [1166]. The counterregulatory hormones glucagon, epinephrine, cortisol, and growth hormone are released at an (arterial) plasma glucose concentration of approximately 70–65 mg/dl (~ 3.9–3.5 mmol/l). Symptoms (both autonomic and neuroglycopenic) appear when plasma glucose drops to about 55 mg/dl (~ 3.0 mmol/l). If plasma glucose continues to decrease below about 50 mg/dl (~ 2.7 mmol/l), cognitive function deteriorates [1166].

Definition of Hypoglycemia

Hypoglycemia has traditionally been defined by a plasma glucose concentration below 55–50 mg/dl (~ 3.0–2.7 mmol/l). However, in normal humans the counterregulatory hormone responses—primarily suppression of endogenous insulin secretion—start already at a notably modest drop in plasma glucose in the order of around 10 mg/dl (~ 0.5 mmol/l) below the normal fasting values of 90 mg/dl (5.0 mmol/l), and are fully evident already at plasma glucose concentration of about 70 mg/dl (~ 4.0 mmol/l). Therefore, a more meaningful plasma glucose threshold for the definition of hypoglycemia is about 70 mg/dl (~ 4.0 mmol/l).

Pathophysiology of Hypoglycemia in Type 1 Diabetes

Inappropriate hyperinsulinemia, either absolute or relative, is the initiating cause of hypoglycemia in type 1 diabetes. However, when type 1 diabetes patients and nondiabetic subjects are exposed to similar conditions of hyperinsulinemia, hypoglycemia is more severe and prolonged in the former because of their impaired defenses against hypoglycemia [1167]. The most common and apparently unavoidable defect is loss of glucagon response to hypoglycemia [1168]. When the glucagon responses are deficient, the defense against hypoglycemia relies almost exclusively on responses of epinephrine [1169]. Under these conditions, if for any reason plasma epinephrine fails to increase appropriately, severe hypoglycemia may supervene. This occurs in the experimental condition in adrenalectomized patients [1170], and in the real lives of people with type 1 diabetes and hypoglycemia unawareness [1156,1157] and/or autonomic neuropathy [1171].

Glycemic Control and Glucose Thresholds of Brain Responses to Hypoglycemia

One of the major findings over the last few years has been that the glycemic thresholds for responses to hypoglycemia given above are not fixed, but may shift upward or downward depending on the preceding glycemic control. For example, chronic hypoglycemia in insulinoma patients [1172] and recurrent hypoglycemia in type 1 diabetes [1173] are associated with high thresholds (i. e., responses occur at lower than normal plasma glucose) of responses of counterregulatory hormones and symptoms to hypoglycemia. On the other hand, chronic hyperglycemia in diabetes is associated with low thresholds (i. e., responses occur at higher than normal plasma glucose levels) [1173,1174]. The importance of this observation lies in the fact that, in daily life, patients with type 1 diabetes may experience normal, subnormal, or even no symptoms of hypoglycemia, depending on whether they have recently been experiencing recurrent hypoglycemia.

Hypoglycemia and Cognitive Function

Brain function becomes impaired when plasma glucose concentration drops below about 50 mg/dl (~2.7 mmol/l). In patients with a history of chronic [1172] or recurrent hypoglycemia [1157,1175,1176], brain function is "protected," i. e., the onset of cognitive dysfunction occurs at a lower than normal plasma glucose concentration. However, in type 1 diabetic patients with hypoglycemia unawareness, the loss of symptoms may be so severe that they are unable to perceive hypoglycemia during the progressive fall in blood glucose before the onset of cognitive dysfunction supervenes. In such cases, cognitive dysfunction may be so severe that the patients are unable to take measures to correct the hypoglycemia. Recent data indicate that the rate at which blood glucose falls may play a role: if the rate of fall to the level of hypoglycemia level is fast, like the fall after a subcutaneous injection of a short-acting insulin analogue at a meal time, the impairment in cognitive function is greater than in a situation where the rate of fall is slower [1162].

Preceding Hypoglycemia as Primary Cause of Loss of Responses of Epinephrine to Hypoglycemia

Loss of responses of epinephrine (as well as other counterregulatory hormones, symptoms, and onset of cognitive dysfunction) in type 1 diabetes is largely, although not entirely, the result of frequent preceding hypoglycemia.

The first line of evidence comes from studies in which hypoglycemia has been either cured or prevented. The observation in insulinoma patients [1172] that cure of hypoglycemia after surgical resection of the tumor is followed by full recovery of appropriate epinephrine responses (as well as other counterregulatory hormone responses, symptoms, and onset of cognitive dysfunction) has prompted similar observations in type 1 diabetes. Fanelli et al. [1157] were the first to report that meticulous prevention of hypoglycemia in type 1 diabetes patients who had previously experienced nearly one episode of hypoglycemia per day is followed by rapid recovery of symptoms (both autonomic and neuroglycopenic) and counterregulatory responses (Figs. 5.**38**, 5.**39**). These results have subsequently been confirmed [1175,1177,1178].

The second line of evidence derives from experimental studies in normal human volunteers, in whom two episodes of mild, brief insulin-induced hypoglycemia [1179] or a single episode of nocturnal hypoglycemia [1180] blunts the responses to an episode of hypoglycemia induced next day. Similar observations have been made in patients with type 1 diabetes [1181–1183]. Taken together, these observations indicate that frequent hypoglycemia in type 1 diabetes, caused by inappropriate treatment and/or impaired counterregulation, rapidly induces loss of symptoms and blunts the release of counterregulatory hormones in response to hypoglycemia.

Importantly, a therapeutic strategy which prevents hypoglycemia [1184] reverses, largely if not fully, unawareness of and improves counterregulation of hypoglycemia. However, the effect of prevention of hypoglycemia on epinephrine responses is stronger in diabetes of short duration than in diabetes of long duration [1175].

Mechanisms of Hypoglycemia Unawareness and Loss of Epinephrine Responses to Hypoglycemia in Type 1 Diabetes

In rats, chronic hypoglycemia increases [1185], whereas chronic hyperglycemia decreases [1186], glucose transport to the brain. In humans, prolonged hypoglycemia increases fractional extraction of glucose from blood [1187]. In type 1 diabetic patients with low values of glycosylated hemoglobin owing to frequent preceding hypoglycemia, fractional extraction of glucose does not increase during hypoglycemia as it does in nondiabetic subjects and type 1 diabetic patients with no preceding episodes of hypoglycemia [1188]. Taken together, these observations support the view that brain glucose transport is influenced by the preceding prevailing plasma glucose concentration. Hypoglycemia accelerates delivery of glucose to the brain, so that during subsequent hypoglycemia the brain is less neuroglycopenic than normal, and does not necessarily need to generate the counterregulatory responses and the autonomic symptoms to defend the subject and give early warning of impending hypoglycemia.

However, recent studies using positron emission tomography (PET) to assess cerebral glucose metabolism have indicated that the rate of glucose transport is not decreased in type 1 diabetes patients with long-term hyperglycemia [1189], and that 24-hour hypoglycemia in normal, nondiabetic subjects does not result in an increased rate of glucose transport to the brain [1190]. To the extent to which the PET technique can reliably measure the rate of brain glucose transport,

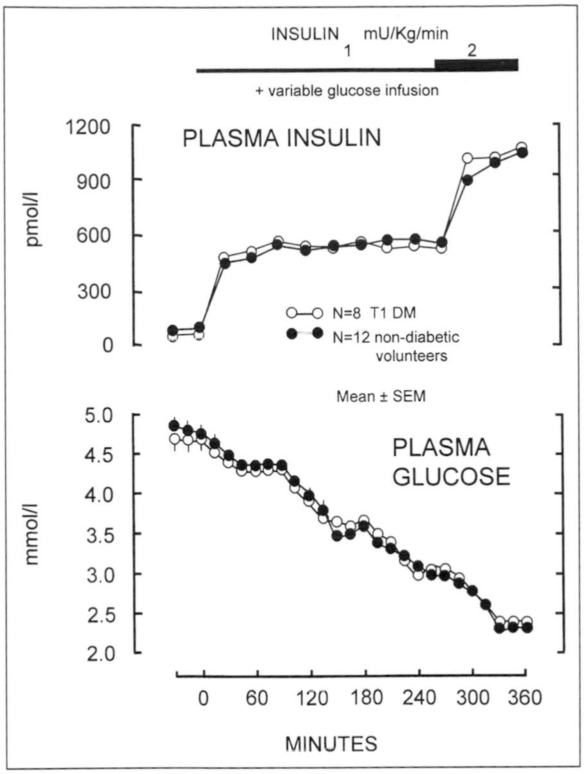

Fig. 5.**38** Hyperinsulinemic-hypoglycemic glucose clamp technique to study responses to hypoglycemia. In the setting of hyperinsulinemia, glucose is infused at variable rate to produce stepwise glycemic plateaus during which plasma concentration of counterregulatory hormones, symptoms, and cognitive function are measured in normal nondiabetic subjects and patients with type 1 diabetes. (From [1157], with permission)

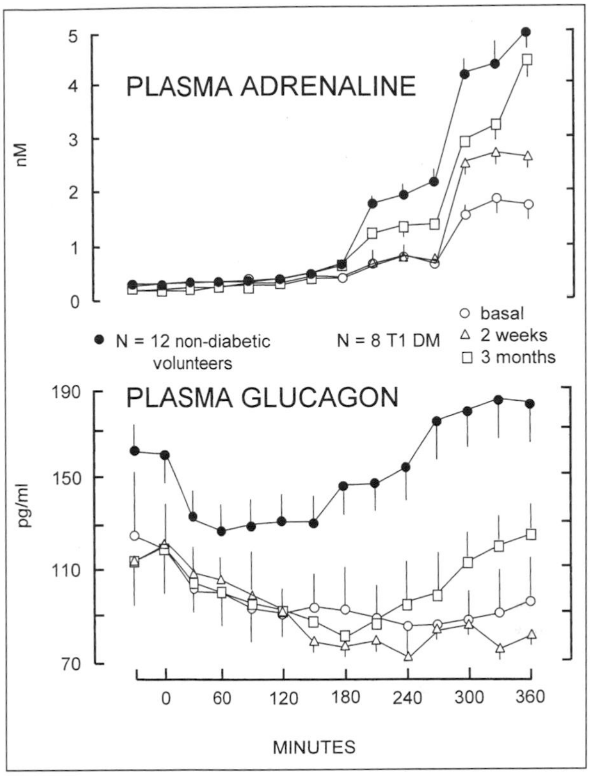

Fig. 5.**39** Plasma norepinephrine and glucagon responses to the experimental hypoglycemia represented in Fig. 5.**38**, before, two weeks, and three months after meticulous prevention of hypoglycemia in a group of type 1 diabetic patients. (From [1157], with permission)

these data do not support the concept that recurrent preceding hypoglycemia induces unawareness and loss of epinephrine responses by increasing the rate of glucose transport to the brain. Alternatively, it is possible that there are regional differences in the rate of glucose transport to the brain. For example, if the increase in the rate of glucose transport following hypoglycemia were restricted to the hypothalamus area, a region that makes a modest contribution to the glucose uptake of the whole brain, this would clearly have major impact on counterregulatory hormone release during subsequent hypoglycemia, but would not necessarily be detected by measurement of the overall rate of brain glucose transport. Thus, at present, the role of the rate of brain glucose transport in the pathogenesis of hypoglycemia unawareness and loss of epinephrine responses remains in dispute.

An additional possible mechanism of hypoglycemia unawareness is the response of plasma cortisol, which blunts the autonomic responses to subsequent hypoglycemia [1191]. In particular, the overall autonomic discharge in response to hypoglycemia, i. e., responses of epinephrine and those of muscle sympathetic activity, are reduced by preceding infusion of cortisol to mimic the response of cortisol during hypoglycemia, in the absence of preceding hypoglycemia. Thus, cortisol appears an important mediator, although possibly not the only one, of preceding recurrent hypoglycemia in inducing loss of autonomic responses to subsequent hypoglycemia. The mechanism by which an increase in plasma cortisol blunts autonomic responses is not clearly understood, but is probably related to the suppressive effects of cortisol on the hypothalamus area [1192]. Indirect evidence for an important role of cortisol response to preceding hypoglycemia derives from a study in normal, nondiabetic humans, in whom blockade of cortisol responses to preceding hypoglycemia prevented most losses of autonomic responses to subsequent hypoglycemia [1193]. Taken together, these studies indicate an important role for cortisol response in the pathogenesis of hypoglycemia unawareness and blunted autonomic responses to hypoglycemia. Whether this is the sole mechanism or is perhaps associated with other mechanisms, such as for example an increased rate of brain glucose transport, remains to be established.

Recurrent Hypoglycemia—Loss of Epinephrine Response: The Vicious Circle

Intensive insulin therapy aims at near-normoglycemia [1184]. Because subcutaneous insulin replacement is imperfect, despite the modern techniques of continuous subcutaneous infusion by a minipump and/or injections of insulin analogues [1194], mild hypoglycemia is inevitably induced from time to time. If hypoglycemia occurs frequently, e. g., once a day, the mechanisms for induction of hypoglycemia unawareness and loss of epinephrine responses are activated, whether they be increased rate of brain glucose transport and/or increased cortisol responses. Thus, a vicious circle is initiated in which loss of symptoms favors recurrent hypoglycemia simply because episodes are not recognized and corrected early by taking glucose. In turn, the associated loss of epinephrine response, in the setting of an absent glucagon response, substantially compromises the defenses against hypoglycemia. Ultimately, the combination of loss of symptoms and epinephrine responses promotes the risk of severe hypoglycemia (Fig. 5.**40**).

It is important to emphasize that the modern definition of hypoglycemia is a decrease in blood glucose below 72 mg/dl (4.0 mmol/l). Therefore, even modest decreases in blood glucose just below the normal, nondiabetic blood glucose values may well induce hypoglycemia unawareness and loss of epinephrine responses to hypoglycemia. It is therefore important that in the daily life of diabetic patients even minor episodes of hypoglycemia are prevented, in order to avoid hypoglycemia unawareness and loss of epinephrine responses.

Role of Recurrent Preceding Hypoglycemia in Responses to Hypoglycemia in Diabetic Autonomic Neuropathy

As studies of reversibility of hypoglycemia unawareness have moved from patients with type 1 diabetes of short duration [1157] to those with type 1 diabetes of long duration [1175,1177,1178], heterogeneous results have been obtained. In short-term type 1 diabetes, recovery from symptoms and recovery of epinephrine responses is nearly complete after meticulous prevention of hypoglycemia [1157]. In contrast, in long-term type 1 diabetes, recovery of symptoms and recovery of epinephrine responses [1175] is only partial, or symptoms improve but epinephrine responses do not [1178]. Clearly, factors in addition to recent preceding hypoglycemia play a role in the pathogenesis of hypoglycemia unawareness and impaired hormonal counterregulation of patients with type 1 diabetes of long duration.

One important question is to establish the role of "structural" factors, i. e., autonomic neuropathy, in loss of epinephrine responses to hypoglycemia and hypoglycemia unawareness, and to distinguish this from the "functional" factor of recurrent preceding hypoglycemia discussed above.

In the study by Fanelli et al. [1171], when patients with type 1 diabetes with and without autonomic neuropathy were examined at baseline (i. e., after recurrent preceding hypoglycemia), there was a marked impairment in responses of epinephrine in terms of both glycemic thresholds and maximum responses. Although the impairment in responses was also observed in the group with similarly long diabetes duration (~ 20 years) but without autonomic neuropathy (Fig. 5.**41**), the responses were more suppressed in the group with autonomic neuropathy. Interestingly, the

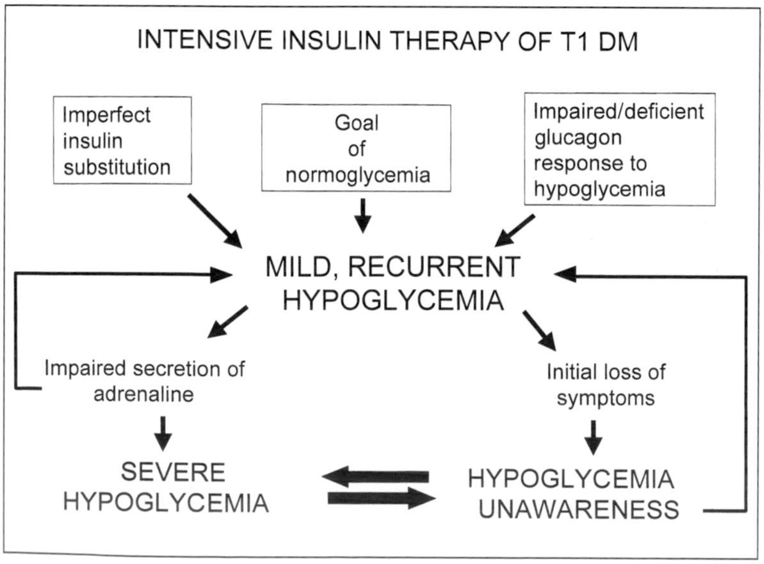

Fig. 5.**40** Vicious circle in which recurrent mild hypoglycemia induces loss of symptoms and epinephrine response to subsequent hypoglycemia. In turn, hypoglycemia unawareness favors more frequent hypoglycemia episodes, ultimately increasing the risk of severe hypoglycemia

impairment was similar in the subgroup with and that without postural hypotension (Fig. 5.**41**). When patients were restudied after six months of meticulous prevention of hypoglycemia, plasma epinephrine responses improved in patients without autonomic neuropathy and only marginally in those with autonomic neuropathy but without postural hypotension. In patients with autonomic neuropathy who did have postural hypotension, the recovery was barely appreciable. The responses of plasma pancreatic polypeptide, a marker of parasympathetic activity [1153], paralleled those of plasma epinephrine both before and after six months of meticulous prevention of hypoglycemia (Fig. 5.**42**). The responses of both autonomic and neuroglycopenic symptoms were reduced in all groups as compared to nondiabetic subjects (Fig. 5.**43**). After prevention of hypoglycemia, the responses of autonomic symptoms improved in all groups, although they did not normalize. However, these responses remained lower in patients with autonomic neuropathy and postural hypotension than in those with autonomic neuropathy but no postural hypotension. In contrast, the neuroglycopenic symptoms normalized in all groups.

From these studies it appears that the characteristics of hypoglycemia unawareness and impaired epinephrine response are similar in patients with and those without autonomic neuropathy, but that the responses of epinephrine and pancreatic polypeptide are suppressed more in the latter than in the former group, and more in patients with than in those without postural hypotension. These studies indicate that unawareness of hypoglycemia in diabetic autonomic neuropathy is largely the result of preceding recurrent hypoglycemia, and is therefore reversible, at least in part, after meticulous prevention of hypoglycemia. In contrast, the loss of epinephrine responses is only partly reversible in autonomic neuropathy, especially in patients with postural hypotension, in whom the reversibility is lacking. The intriguing finding that autonomic symptoms recover better than epinephrine response is not limited to patients with autonomic neuropathy, but also occurs in patients without who have a similarly long duration of diabetes. Thus, there is something in duration as a factor of type 1 diabetes which accounts for incomplete recovery of autonomic symptoms and, more importantly, epinephrine responses. The fact that the responses of pancreatic polypeptide parallel those of epinephrine in all groups suggests that the reduced epinephrine responses are "structural." This conclusion also applies to patients without autonomic neuropathy, who may possibly suffer from a subclinical, latent autonomic neuropathy owing to long duration of type 1 diabetes. Thus, it is likely that autonomic neuropathy, even if subclinical, plays a role in long-term type 1 diabetes and accounts for reduced epinephrine responses as well as symptoms of hypoglycemia. In the real life of patients, however, the "structural" factor of autonomic neuropathy combines with the "functional" factor of recurrent hypoglycemia, leading to the patient characteristics found by Fanelli et al. at entry to the study [1171]. Unlike autonomic symptoms, recovery of neuroglycopenic symptoms was complete after long-term

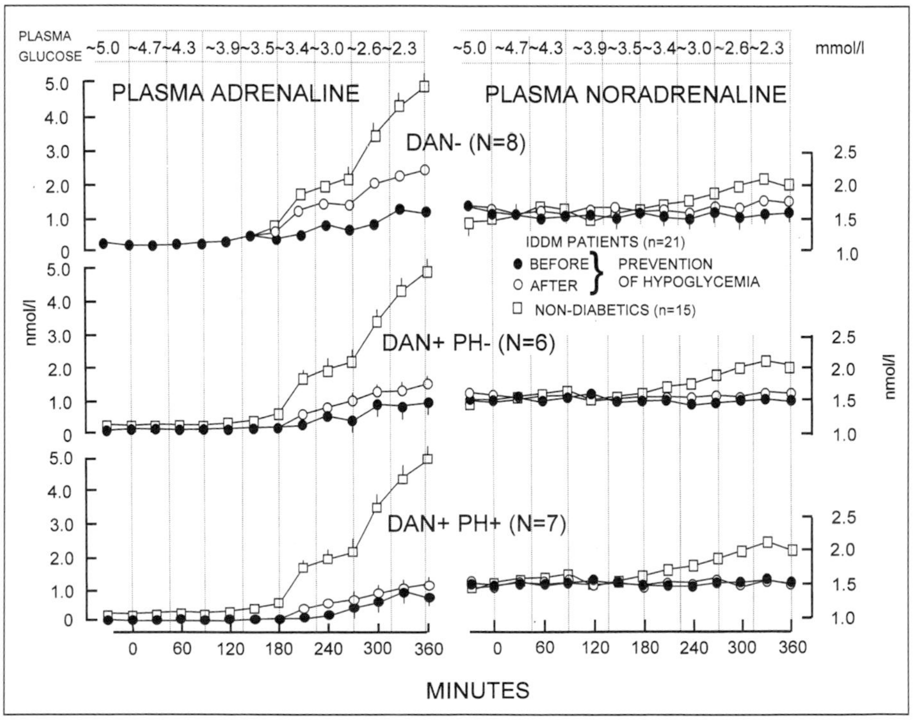

Fig. 5.**41** Plasma epinephrine and norepinephrine responses to hypoglycemia in type 1 diabetic patients before and after six months of meticulous prevention of hypoglycemia. DAN–, diabetic patients without autonomic neuropathy; DAN+PH–, patients with autonomic neuropathy but without postural hypotension; DAN+PH+, patients with autonomic neuropathy and postural hypotension. (From [1171], with permission)

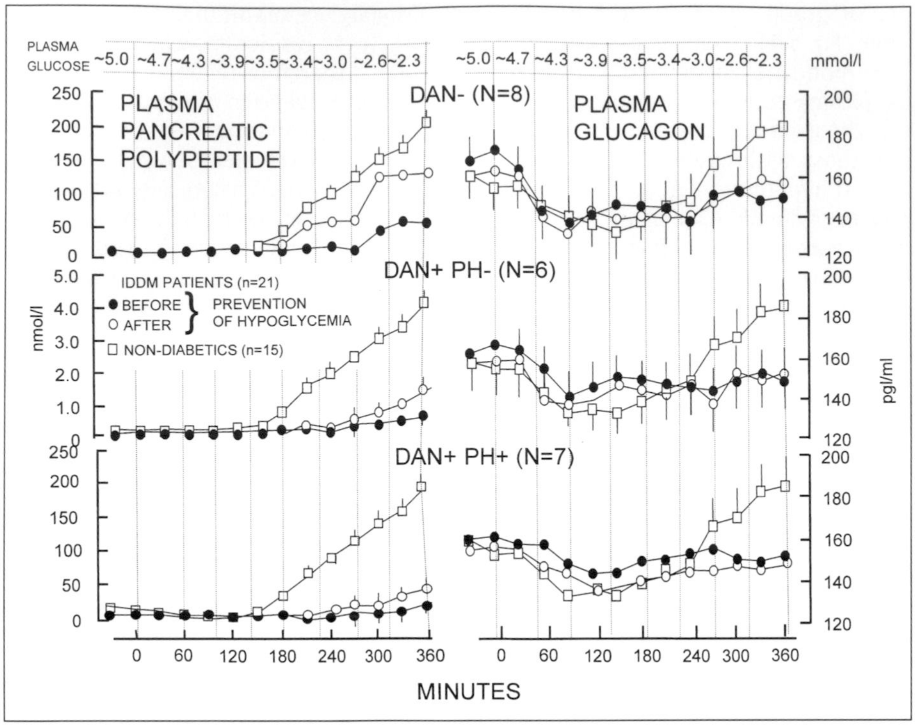

Fig. 5.**42** Plasma pancreatic polypeptide and glucagon responses to hypoglycemia in type 1 diabetic patients before and after six months of meticulous prevention of hypoglycemia. (From [1171], with permission)

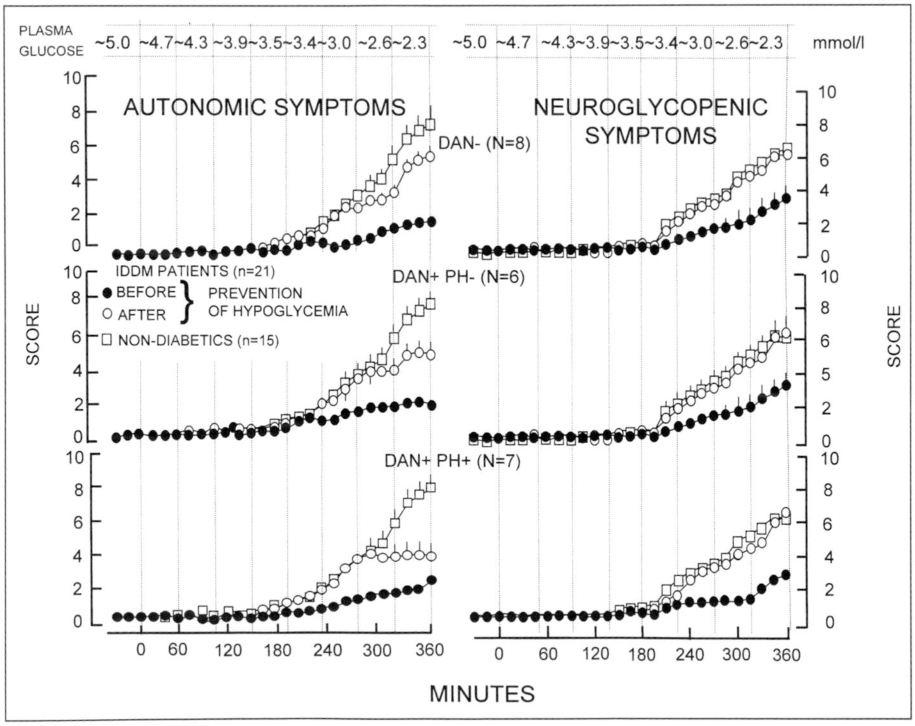

Fig. 5.**43** Responses of autonomic and neuroglycopenic symptoms to hypoglycemia in normal nondiabetic subjects and type 1 diabetic patients before and after six months of meticulous prevention of hypoglycemia. (From [1171], with permission)

prevention of hypoglycemia in all groups of patients. Although autonomic symptoms are more specific for early awareness of hypoglycemia, it is important that patients with long-term type 1 diabetes are educated also to use neuroglycopenic symptoms for recognition of hypoglycemia *before* cognitive dysfunction supervenes.

In another study, by Kendall et al. [1195], responses to hypoglycemia were examined in a group of type 1 diabetes patients with autonomic neuropathy after pancreas transplantation, a model of nearly absolute prevention of hypoglycemia. The findings of better epinephrine responses observed by Kendall et al. [1195] as compared to the study by Fanelli et al. [1171]

are difficult to interpret because of the difference in study design (cross-sectional versus longitudinal). An additional difference between the two studies is that in the study by Kendall et al. [1195] patients were submitted to long-term corticosteroid and immunosuppressive therapy, which might have influenced the responses observed. However, in the study by Kendall et al. the epinephrine responses remained subnormal despite absolute prevention of hypoglycemia. Taken together, the observations by Kendall et al. [1195] and Fanelli et al. [1171] concordantly indicate that autonomic neuropathy per se, irrespective of preceding hypoglycemia, is a factor in subnormal epinephrine response to hypoglycemia.

The intriguing observation of several studies [1175,1178,1195] that in long-term type 1 diabetes the recovery of symptoms is complete or nearly complete after meticulous prevention of hypoglycemia, whereas the epinephrine response remains largely subnormal, remains to be explained. One possible explanation is that the improved epinephrine and overall autonomic response, albeit modest, after prevention of hypoglycemia or pancreas transplantation, might be associated with increased sensitivity of autonomic receptors to the released neurotransmitters, thereby generating normal [1175,1178,1195,1196] or near-normal [1171] autonomic symptoms.

Contribution of Diabetic Autonomic Neuropathy Per Se to Reduced Plasma Epinephrine Responses to Hypoglycemia in Type 1 Diabetes

From the above considerations, it follows that one important question is to establish the contribution of autonomic neuropathy to reduced responses of epinephrine to hypoglycemia in type 1 diabetes. Several studies support an association between blunted epinephrine responses to hypoglycemia and autonomic neuropathy [1153,1168,1197], but others do not [1182]. Of course one confounding factor is that, in many studies, preceding recurrent hypoglycemia was not prevented.

The study by Bottini et al. [1198] examined whether autonomic neuropathy per se, i. e., independent of recent hypoglycemia, contributes to reduced plasma epinephrine responses to hypoglycemia, and assessed the selectivity of the hypoglycemic stimulus as compared to other stimuli such as exercise. After long-term meticulous prevention of hypoglycemia, patients with type 1 diabetes of long duration (~20 years), with or without autonomic neuropathy, were studied during a hyperinsulinemic-hypoglycemic clamp and 30-minute steady-state exercise at 55% $\dot{V}O_2$ max. In response to hypoglycemia, the plasma epinephrine was reduced both in patients without and, to a greater extent, those with autonomic neuropathy (Fig. 5.**44**), and this was paralleled by responses to exercise (Fig. 5.**45**). This study shows that, first, long-term type 1 diabetes is associated with reduced epinephrine responses; second, autonomic neuropathy contributes to reduced responses of epinephrine to hypoglycemia; and, third, this epinephrine defect is not selective for hypoglycemia, suggesting the existence of "structural" damage. An intriguing observation in these studies is that autonomic neuropathy in the stage of predominantly parasympathetic involvement (patients without postural hypotension) is already associated with marked deficiency of epinephrine responses to hypoglycemia. This defect appears to be as severe as that in patients with more severe autonomic neuropathy (patients with postural hypotension).

Conclusions

Loss of autonomic symptoms and epinephrine responses to hypoglycemia are part of the natural history of type 1 diabetes. When advanced, these losses pop pop into the clinical syndromes of impaired counterregulation and hypoglycemia unawareness. Under these conditions, if recurrent hypoglycemia is not prevented, a vicious circle is established with increased risk of severe hypoglycemia (see Fig. 5.**41**). Preceding recurrent iatrogenic hypoglycemia plays an important role in the pathogenesis of syndromes of hypoglycemia unawareness and loss of epinephrine responses at all stages of type 1 diabetes, as demonstrated by recovery of these syndromes upon prevention of hypoglycemia. However, once diabetes duration increases beyond 15–20 years, additional factors play a role in the pathogenesis of hypoglycemia unawareness and impaired counterregulation. These factors are clinically overt autonomic neuropathy and, probably, a subclinical form of autonomic neuropathy not detected by currently available cardiovascular tests. If the clinically overt expression is only the "tip of the iceberg" of a more common condition of autonomic neuropathy, it is well possible that responses of epinephrine to hypoglycemia are a more sensitive test by which to detect latent autonomic neuropathy, likewise hemodynamic responses to hyperinsulinemia [1197]. Autonomic neuropathy results in an irreversible loss of epinephrine response to hypoglycemia and major impairment of autonomic symptoms.

Prevention of hypoglycemia is always important in the insulin treatment of type 1 diabetes, but it becomes crucial in patients with autonomic neuropathy. If hypoglycemia is prevented, the partial recovery of epinephrine responses is accompanied by near-normal symptoms of hypoglycemia. This allows early recognition and treatment of hypoglycemia and the prevention of a more severe fall in blood glucose. Strategies to prevent hypoglycemia have been discussed extensively [1184]. A special point to emphasize in patients with autonomic neuropathy is the elevated insulin sensitivity they have, which pop pops into quite low insulin requirements in terms of daily units. These

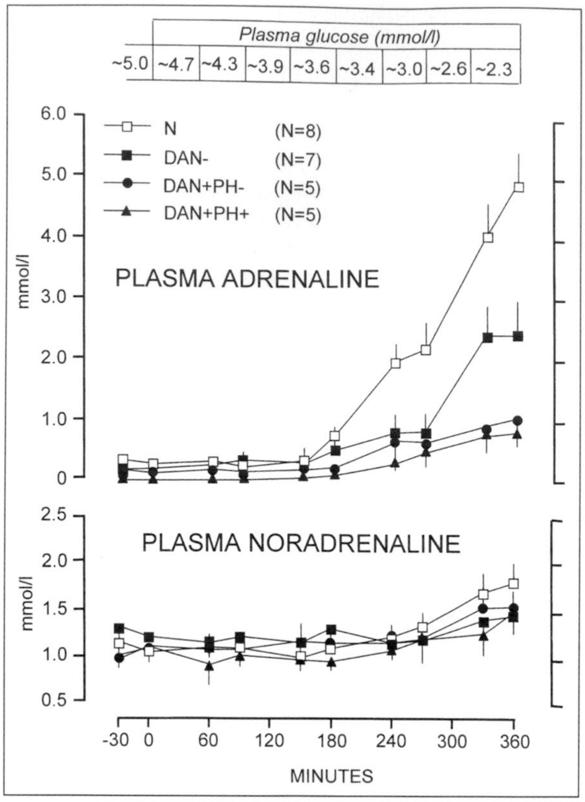

Fig. 5.**44** Plasma epinephrine and norepinephrine responses during the hyperinsulinemic-hypoglycemic clamp in the four groups of subjects studied. N, nondiabetic normal subjects; DAN–, type 1 diabetic patients without autonomic neuropathy; DAN+PH–, type 1 diabetic patients with autonomic neuropathy without postural hypotension; DAN+PH+, type 1 diabetic patients with autonomic neuropathy and postural hypotension. (From [1198], with permission)

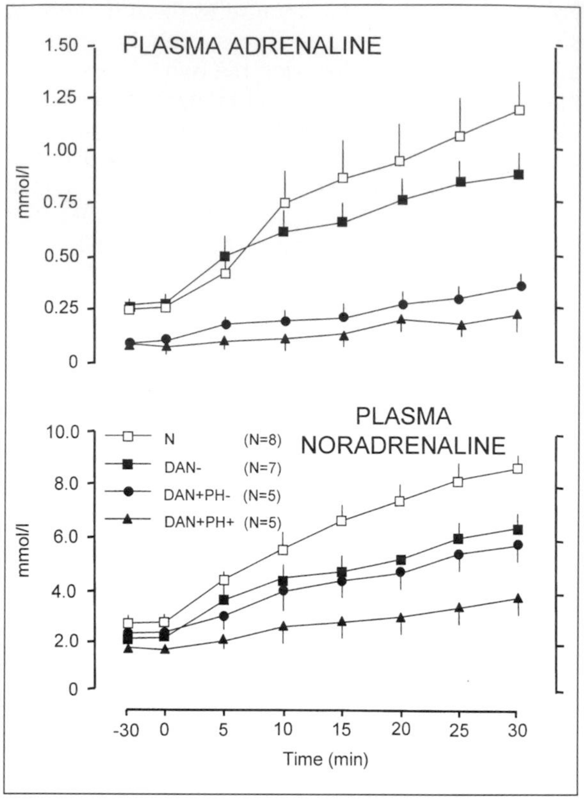

Fig. 5.**45** Plasma epinephrine and norepinephrine responses during the steady-state exercise at 55% $\dot{V}O_2$ max in the four groups of subjects studied. (From [1198], with permission)

units of insulin should be given as small boluses every four to six hours as combinations of short-acting and intermediate-acting insulin at meal times (or after meals in cases of gastroparesis), and NPH at bedtime [1184,1194]. Continuous subcutaneous insulin infusion is the gold standard in this condition, but is limited because it requires cooperative and intelligent patients, is expensive, and is not always judged to be convenient. An additional possibility to be explored in the future is the use of the long-acting insulin glargine [1199], which should result in better prevention of hypoglycemia, especially at night [1200].

In a recent cross-sectional study in type 1 diabetic patients with seven years of disease duration, who had been on intensive therapy since diabetes onset, epinephrine responses to hypoglycemia have been found to be normal [1201]. It will be interesting to assess this population longitudinally and establish whether the response of epinephrine to hypoglycemia will remain normal with longer duration of diabetes and optimal glycemic control by intensive therapy. If so, intensive control from the onset of type 1 diabetes will be proven to prevent counterregulatory failure due to reduced epinephrine response, thus improving the prospect of type 1 diabetes treatment.

The Diabetic Foot

A.J.M. Boulton

Introduction

The global term "diabetic foot" is used to refer to a variety of pathologic conditions that may affect the feet of people with diabetes. Neuropathy is a major contributory factor in the etiopathogenesis of foot ulceration and of Charcot neuroarthropathy, and all too often can be implicated in the causal chain ultimately resulting in amputation. A number of facts attest to the importance of diabetic foot disease:

1. Foot ulceration is common, affecting 15% of diabetic patients during their lifetime [1202,1203].
2. Over 80% of lower limb amputations are preceded by foot ulcers, and diabetes remains the commonest cause of nontraumatic amputation in western countries [1202].
3. Foot ulceration is generally preventable, and relatively simple interventions can reduce amputations by up to 80% [1204].
4. Foot ulcers are the commonest reason for hospitalization of diabetic patients in western countries, and carry a significant morbidity and mortality [1205,1206].
5. Diabetes is now the commonest cause of Charcot neuroarthropathy in western countries [1207].

Despite the obvious importance of diabetic foot disease, the research and evidence base for management remains poor: of 2348 randomized trials on clinical diabetes management reported by the Cochrane diabetes group, only 3% were concerned with the diabetic foot [1208].

In this section, the epidemiology and cost of diabetic foot disease will be discussed, followed by the role of somatic and autonomic neuropathy in the causation of foot lesions. The potential for prevention of these late sequelae of neuropathy will be discussed, followed by a description of Charcot neuroarthropathy. Finally, management of foot ulcers will be described. Throughout, emphasis will be placed on neuropathic foot problems, although other etiological factors such as peripheral vascular disease and abnormalities of pressures and loads under the feet will be mentioned.

Epidemiology and Economic Aspects

Foot ulceration is common in both main types of diabetes and occurs in every part of the world [1209] (Table 5.**24**). It is much more common in neuropathic patients: the annual incidence rises from less than 1% in non-neuropathic patients to more than 7% in those with established sensory loss [1210,1211]. The most recent epidemiological data are from the western USA, where the cumulative incidence of foot ulcers in a population of nearly 9000 diabetic patients was 5.8% over three years of observation [1205].

The attributable cost of a 65-year-old male with a new foot ulcer was almost $28 000 for the two years after diagnosis. Another US study from a database of 7 million people estimated the total expenditure on lower extremity ulcers over a two-year period to be $16 million [1212]. European data from Sweden estimated a total cost of care over three years to be $26 700 for patients with both foot ulcers and critical limb ischemia, whereas the cost of ulcers without critical ischemia was reported to be $16 100 [1213]. All these figures must, however be treated with caution and

Table 5.**24** Epidemiological data on the prevalence/incidence of diabetic foot ulcers and amputations around the world: population-based studies unless otherwise stated

Country/reference	*n*	Prevalence (%)		Incidence (%)		Risk factors for foot ulcers (%)
		Ulcers	Amp	Ulcers	Amp	
Netherlands, 1993[a]	300 000	–	–	0.8	0.4	
UK, 1994[a]	811	1.4	–	–	–	41.6
UK, 1996[a]	9710	4.8	1.4	–	–	67
Slovakia, 1997[a]	1205	2.5	0.9	0.6	0.2	58.4
Algeria, 1998[a,b]	865	11.9	6.7	–	–	
USA 1999 [1205]	8905	–	–	1.9	0.3	41.6

[a] For original reference see [1209]
[b] Clinic-based study

probably underestimate the true costs as the assessment of the economic burden of foot ulcers is still hindered by the lack of accurate population-based studies. Moreover, most studies have centered on estimations of the direct health care costs of diabetic foot lesions (costs of services involved in identification, treatment, and care), and have failed to take into account indirect costs resulting from loss of function (or life) that results from the condition, and the loss of services or benefits to society that inevitably follow. These indirect costs are high in diabetes, possibly up to 50% of the total costs of the disease.

Suffice it to say, in summary, that diabetic foot disease is common and results in a huge cost to the health care system.

Etiopathogenesis of Diabetic Foot Lesions

If we are to succeed in reducing the incidence of foot ulceration and amputation in diabetes, then a clear understanding of the various factors that interact to result in ulceration is essential. It is important to understand that the diabetic neuropathic foot does not spontaneously ulcerate: neuropathy is simply a component cause or permissive feature, and it is the addition of trauma (e. g., foreign body in shoe, tight shoes, callus plus high pressure, etc.) that results in tissue destruction and ulceration [1214]. Other factors such as psychosocial problems [1215] and abnormalities of pressures and loads under the feet have also been implicated.

Diabetic foot problems can be divided into three clinical entities: neuropathic, neuroischemic, and ischemic (see Fig. 5.**46**). It is estimated that, of 100 diabetic foot lesions presenting to a diabetologist, neuropathy is implicated in up to 90%, with neuropathic and neuroischemic lesions seen in similar numbers. The ischemic foot will not be considered further in this chapter. Individual component causes that interact to result in ulceration will now be considered in detail.

Sensorimotor Neuropathy

As outlined elsewhere in this text, diabetic sensory neuropathy is very common in diabetic patients; it has been estimated that up to 50% of older type 2 diabetic patients have evidence of sensory loss on clinical examination and must therefore be considered at risk of insensitive foot injury. Patients with acute painful sensory neuropathy rarely have significant sensory loss, and as they recover within a year they are not considered to be at increased risk of foot ulceration. It is those with the common chronic, insidious, sensorimotor neuropathy who develop sensory loss, and who, on examination, usually manifest a sensory deficit in a stocking distribution to all modalities: evidence of small muscle wasting is also often present. While some patients may have a history of typical neuropathic symptoms (burning pain, paresthesias, dysesthesias, stabbing pain, all with nocturnal exacerbation), others may develop sensory loss with no history of any symptoms. Another particularly dangerous situation is the patient who complains bitterly of severe neuropathic discomfort, and yet, on examination, has severe small- and large-fiber sensory deficits: such patients are at great risk of painless injury to their feet (the "painful-painless" leg).

It should, therefore, be clear that there is a spectrum of symptomatic severity, with some patients experiencing severe pain with no signs while others have pain and sensory loss. Perhaps the most challenging patients are those who develop sensory loss with no symptoms, who are difficult to convince that they are at risk of foot ulcer and are consequently difficult to motivate to regular self foot care [1214,1215].

The important message is that *neuropathic symptoms correlate poorly with sensory loss, and their absence must never be equated with lack of foot ulcer risk. Thus, assessment of foot ulcer risk MUST ALWAYS include a careful foot exam after removal of shoes and socks, whatever the neuropathic history* [1216].

Autonomic Neuropathy

Sympathetic autonomic neuropathy in the lower limb results not only in reduced sweating and therefore dry skin that is prone to crack and fissure, but also to increased blood flow, in the absence of large-vessel peripheral vascular disease. This latter abnormality is a consequence of an increase in arteriovenous shunting and results from a warm foot, with distended dorsal foot veins, both useful physical signs of an "at risk" foot.

There are now strong prospective data to support the role of both small- and large-fiber neurologic deficits in the etiopathogenesis of ulceration in diabetic patients [1202,1210,1211,1217,1218]. Indeed, in a recent study assessing pathways to ulceration, neuropathy was the single most important component cause [1219].

Other Risk Factors

Of the other risk factors for ulceration (Table 5.**25**), one of the most important is a past history of similar

Table 5.**25** Factors increasing risk of diabetic foot ulceration

Peripheral neuropathy
Somatic
Autonomic
Peripheral vascular disease
Past history of foot ulceration
Other long-term complications
Plantar callus
Foot deformity
Edema
Ethnic background
Poor social background

The most important factors are in **boldface**

problems. In many series this is associated with a 50% annual risk of reulceration.

Other long-term complications: Patients with other late complications, particularly nephropathy, have been reported to have an increased foot ulcer risk. Retinopathy, with impaired vision, is a major risk in those in whom laser therapy has restricted peripheral and dark vision. There have been reports of frequent minor trauma in such patients, whose stability is further impaired by a proprioceptive deficit secondary to neuropathy. Postural instability is increasingly being recognized as a neuropathic symptom due to large-fiber sensory loss [1220].

Plantar callus: Callus forms under weight-bearing areas as a consequence of dry skin (autonomic dysfunction), insensitivity, and repetitive moderate stress from high foot pressures. It acts as a foreign body and causes ulceration [1221]. The presence of callus in an insensate foot should alert the physician that this patient is at high risk of ulceration, and callus should be removed by a podiatrist or other trained health care professional.

Elevated foot pressures: Numerous studies have confirmed the contributory role that abnormal plantar pressures play in the pathogenesis of foot ulcers [1202,1214,1222].

Foot deformity: A combination of motor neuropathy, cheiroarthropathy, and altered gait patterns are thought to result in the "high risk" neuropathic foot with clawing of toes, prominent metatarsal heads, high arch, and small muscle wasting (Fig. 5.**47**).

Ethnicity: There are data to suggest that foot ulceration is more common in Europids than other ethnic groups such as Asians, although amputations seem to be more common among Hispanics and Blacks [1202].

Pathway to Ulceration

Complex Causality

As shown in Figure 5.**46**, the pathway to ulceration is complex and involves a complicated interaction of numerous factors. Reiber et al. recently studied the causal pathways that result in diabetic foot ulcers and applied the Rothman model of causation [1219]. Component factors are not sufficient by themselves to result in an ulcer, but the interaction of a number of component causes may result in a sufficient cause for ulceration (Fig. 5.**48**). The commonest component causes interacting to result in ulceration in this study [1219] were neuropathy, deformity, and trauma: this triad was present in 63% of the 150 patients studied.

A typical scenario is thus a patient with insensitive feet who buys shoes too small that traumatize the feet at maximum pressure points caused by the tight fit. Reiber et al. reported that neuropathy was the commonest component cause (present in almost 80% of

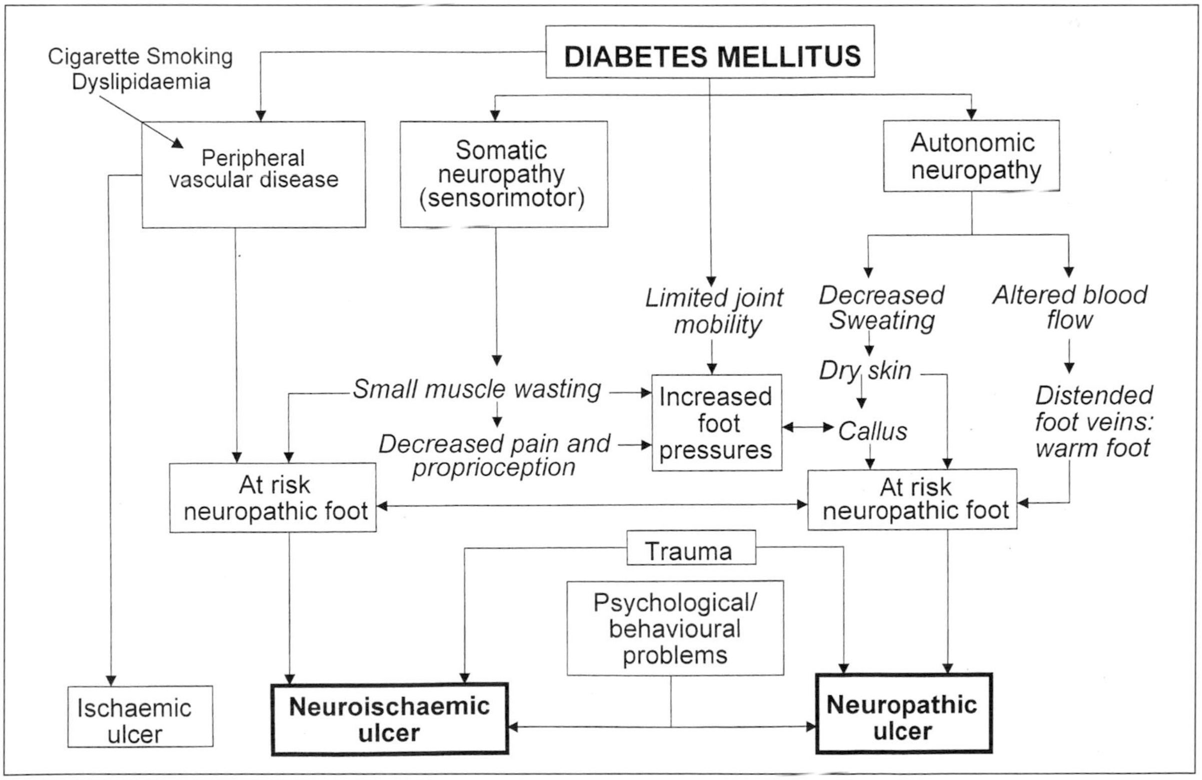

Fig. 5.**46** Pathways to diabetic foot ulceration. (Reproduced from [1222a], with permission)

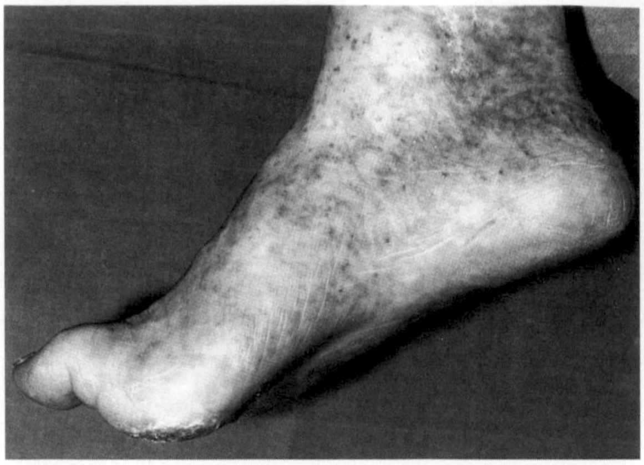

Fig. 5.**47** A typical high risk neuropathic foot showing clawing of the toes, prominence metatarsal heads, and callus under the first metatarsal head

ulcers), and that ischemia was a component cause in 35% of ulcers. The vast majority of ulcers in this series were deemed to have been potentially preventable.

The Patient with Sensory Loss

It should now be possible to achieve a significant reduction in foot ulcers and amputations in diabetes as much of the pathogenesis and pathways to ulceration are described and understood. International guidelines for the diagnosis and management of neuropathy [1216] and foot ulceration [1223] are now published, and there is an increasing understanding of the complex psychosocial issues that surround neuropathy and ulceration [1215].

However, a reduction in neuropathic foot problems will only be achieved if we remember that patients with insensitive feet have lost their warning signal – the pain that ordinarily brings the patients to their doctors. It is pain that leads to many medical consultations: our training in health care is orientated around the causes and relief of pain and other symptoms. Thus, the care of the patient with no pain sensation or other peripheral sensations is a new challenge for which we have little training. It is difficult for us to understand, for example, that an intelligent patient would buy and wear a pair of shoes three sizes too small, and come to our clinic with an extensive shoe-induced ulcer. The explanation, however, is simple: with reduced sensation, a very tight fit stimulates the remaining pressure nerve endings and this is interpreted as a normal fit. Hence the common complaint when patients are provided with custom-designed shoes: "These are too loose." We have learned much about the diagnosis and management of the patients with sensory loss from the treatment of patients with leprosy: if we are to succeed, we must realize that with loss of pain there is also diminished motivation in the healing of and prevention of injury.

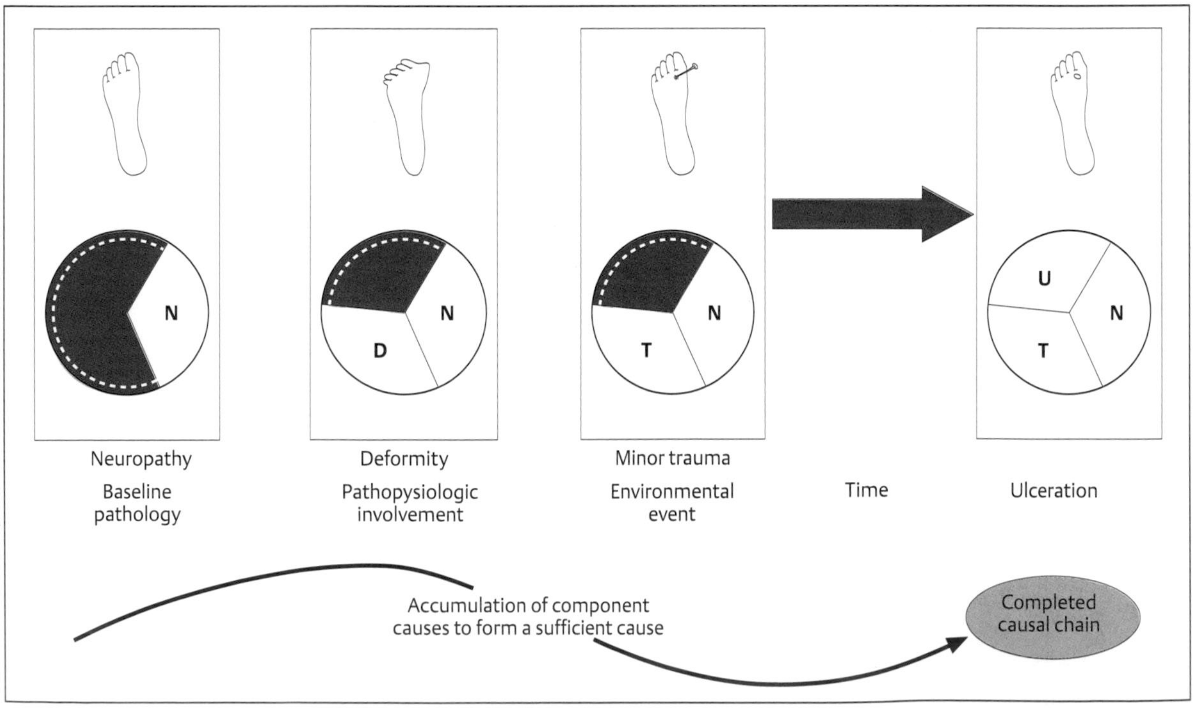

Fig. 5.**48** The commonest pathway to neuropathic foot ulcerations. (Reproduced from [1219], with permission)

Prevention of Diabetic Foot Ulcers

Screening

As stated above, it has been estimated that more than 80% of ulcers are potentially preventable, and the first step in prevention is the identification of the "at risk" population. Many countries have now adopted the principle of the "annual review" for patients with diabetes, whereby every patient is screened at least annually for evidence of diabetic complications. Such a review can be carried out in either a primary care center or a hospital clinic [1216,1223].

The at risk foot can easily be identified in a brief clinical exam without the need for any expensive equipment. The most important step is the removal of the patient's shoes and socks, followed by a careful inspection of the feet. The exam should include:

Inspection:

- Evidence of past or present ulcers? (Check between toes)
- Foot shape?
  - Charcot deformity
  - Prominent metatarsal heads/claw toes
  - Hallux valgus
  - Muscle wasting
- Callus?
- Areas of erythema – from shoe rub?
- Skin color – evidence of ischemia?

Neurologic:

- Ankle reflexes
- Pain or temperature sensation
- Vibration perception

Vascular:

- Skin temperature
- Foot pulses palpable?

A recent prospective study [1223a] has shown that the best predictor of foot ulceration in the follow-up of nearly 10 000 patients was a simplified neuropathy disability score that was based on the above simple exam [1224]. However, a number of simple quantitative sensory tests may also aid in the identification of the high risk diabetic foot.

Semmes-Weinstein Monofilaments

Semmes-Weinstein filaments are available in a number of variable diameters which, when applied to the skin surface with sufficient force to buckle, impart a pressure sensation that can be felt by the patient. The 10 g (5.07) monofilament has been shown to be a useful measure of foot ulcer risk in several studies [1202]. It has even been suggested that patients may be given filaments in order to self-monitor for sensory loss.

Vibration Perception Threshold and Thermal Threshold

Many large diabetic clinics have portable instruments to test for vibration perception, such as the Biothesiometer (Biomedical Instrument Company Inc., Newbury, Ohio, USA). Loss of vibration perception has been shown in several studies to be highly predictive of foot ulcer risk [1201,1210,1211,1222]. Loss of thermal perception has also been equated with foot ulcer risk [1218].

A number of other techniques have been proposed to screen for neuropathy, such as tactile discrimination or use of the graduated tuning fork, but these have yet to be tested prospectively [1217].

Interventions for High Risk Patients

Having identified a patient as being at risk of foot ulceration, the question of appropriate interventions to reduce the future risk of ulceration then arises. Potential interventions will now be discussed under a number of headings, the most important being education.

Education

Previous studies have suggested that patients with foot ulcer risk lack knowledge and skills, and consequently are unable to provide appropriate self foot care [1217]. Patients need to be informed of the risk of having neuropathic feet, the need for regular self-inspection, foot hygiene, and chiropody/podiatry treatment as required, and they must be told what action to take in the event of injury or the discovery of a foot ulcer [1204,1217]. However, recent studies summarized by Vileikyte [1215] suggest that patients often have distorted beliefs about neuropathy, thinking that it is a circulatory problem, and link neuropathy directly to amputation. Thus, an education program that focuses on reducing foot ulcers will be doomed to failure if patients do not believe that foot ulcers precede amputation. It is clear that much work is required in this area if appropriate education is to succeed in reducing foot ulcers and consequently amputations.

There have been a small number of reports that assessed educational interventions, but these have mostly been single-center studies. Although they generally suggested a benefit of education, it is often difficult to assess the direct impact of the educational component when there have been more frequent visits to the clinic, telephone prompts by healthcare staff to encourage regular foot inspection, and so on.

In one interesting randomized study, although the intervention group (who entered a foot protection program) did not develop fewer ulcers than the control group, there was a significant reduction in amputations [1225].

a

b

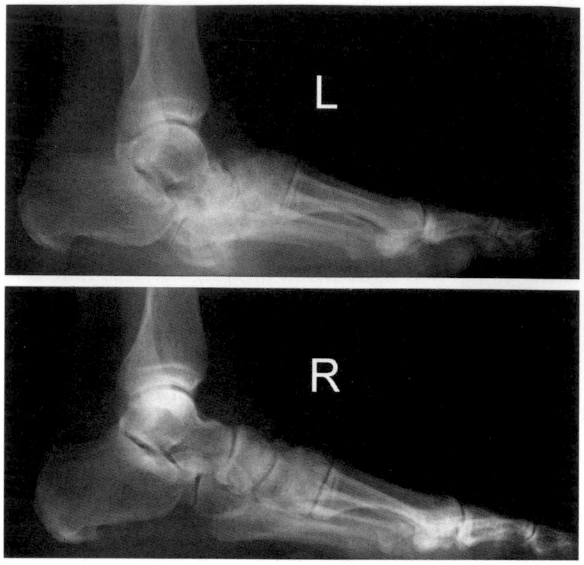

Fig. 5.**51** Lateral radiographs from a patient with a left Charcot foot. The right foot is shown below for contrast (note the calcaneal spur on the right foot). The Charcot process in the left foot involves the subtalar and talonavicular joints as well as the mid-tarsal bone. There is complete disruption in this area, collapse of the arch ,with downward dislocation of the cuboid bone which forms a bony prominence just distal to the calcaneum

Table 5.**26** Traditional Meggitt–Wagner ulcer classification system

Grade 0:	No ulcer, but high risk foot (bony prominences, callus, claw toes, etc.)
Grade 1:	Superficial full-thickness ulcer
Grade 2:	Deep ulcer, may involve tendons. No bone involvement
Grade 3:	Deep ulcer with bone involvement: osteomyelitis
Grade 4:	Localized gangrene, e. g., toes
Grade 5:	Gangrene of whole foot

Modified from the original Meggitt-Wagner classification [1231]

Table 5.**27** San Antonio wound classification system

Stage	Grade			
	0	1	2	3
A	Prepost-ulcerlesion, no skin break	Superficial ulcer	Deep ulcer to tendon/capsule	Wound penetrating bone/joint
B	+Infection	+Infection	+Infection	+Infection
C	+Ischemia	+Ischemia	+Ischemia	+Ischemia
D	+Infection and ischemia	+Infection and ischemia	+Infection and ischemia	+Infection and ischemia

Modified from Armstrong et al. [1232]

[1231,1232]. Classification systems may include the presumed etiology, the location, size or depth of the lesion, together with the vascular and infection status. However, the most widely used foot ulcer classification system in use at the time of writing is the Meggitt–Wagner grading, as shown in Table 5.**26** [1231]. A problem with this system is that it is not possible to assess the degree of ischemia in grade 1–3 wounds, although it has been shown to give an accurate prediction of amputation risk and has generally been regarded as the "gold standard."

The new San Antonio wound classification system (Table 5.**27**) is based on the Meggitt-Wagner system, but stages each grade of ulcer according to the presence or absence of infection and/or ischemia. The system has been validated in a longitudinal study, and it has been shown that outcomes deteriorate with increasing stage and grade of wounds [1232]. It is likely that this system will be adopted as the standard in many countries, as it is simple, predicts outcome, is helpful as a guide to therapy, and should ease communications across specialties [1203].

Wound Healing in Diabetes

The biology of wound healing is an area of active research. Normal wound healing can be described as a succession of four distinct phases, each with characteristic cellular and physiologic components [1203, 1233]. Chronic wounds lack such an orderly and progressive healing process [1203]: they appear to "stick" in the inflammatory/proliferative stage. A key question is, therefore: Is there a fundamental impairment of wound healing in diabetes, and, if so, what are the molecular/cellular impairments and are they specific to chronic wounds? Limited data suggest that there is inhibition of fibroblast proliferation in diabetic foot ulcers and that there may be a lack of insulin-like growth factor 1 in the basal keratinocyte layer of diabetic foot ulcers [1234,1235]. There are also differences between chronic diabetic and venous ulceration, with small-vessel disease and reduced epidermal cell migration in diabetic foot ulcers [1236].

It seems, therefore, that chronic diabetic wounds may exhibit biology that is different from the classical description of acute wound healing. The role of various cytokines and growth factors in diabetic wound healing is an area of ongoing investigation which is pivotal to the development of novel foot ulcer therapies.

Off-Loading

The key to successful management of neuropathic foot ulcers is the relief of pressure on the wound. In the absence of pain, patients with plantar neuropathic foot ulcers will walk without a limp or any difficulty as there is no sensory input to inform them of the presence of the lesion. The ulcer pictured in Figure 5.**52** would be classified as Wagner grade 1, or

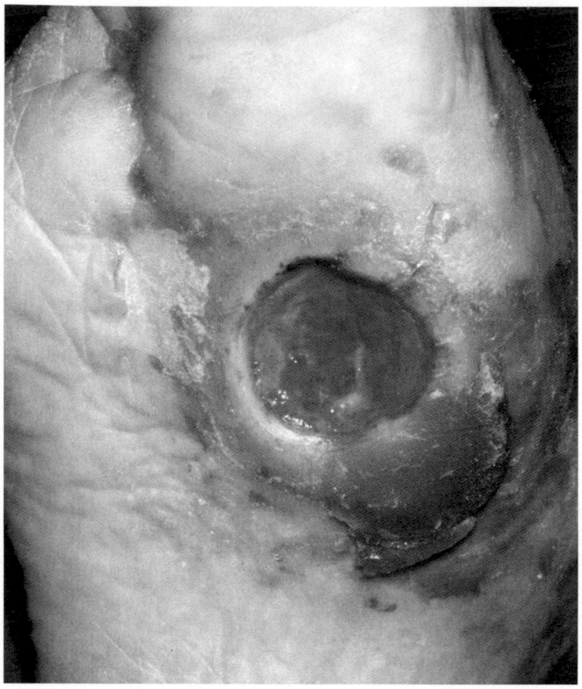

Fig. 5.52 Wagner grade 1/San Antonio 1A ulcer showing surrounding callus and no clinical evidence of infection. This ulcer occurs under a high pressure metatarsal head area

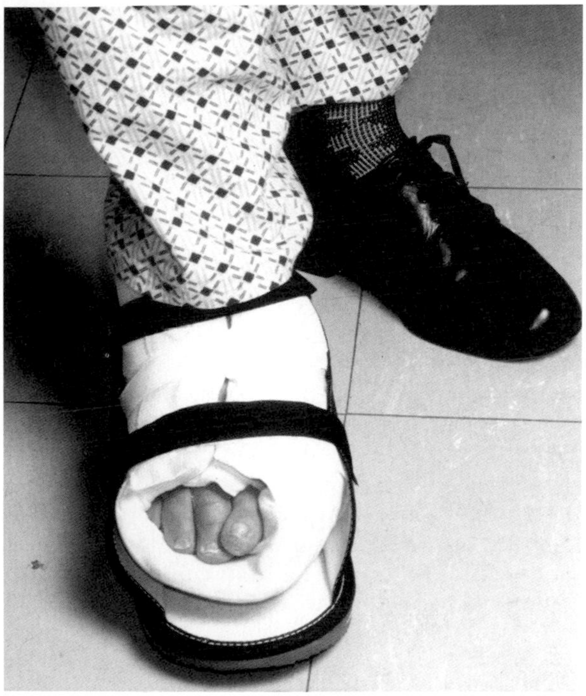

Fig. 5.53 Scotchcast boot specially made to off-load ulcer under metatarsal head region of a patient with a diabetic neuropathic foot ulcer grade 1

San Antonio 1A, as foot pulses were palpable and there was no clinical evidence of infection. It is plantar ulcers such as this that require some of off-loading, which can be defined as avoidance of all mechanical stress on the injured extremity [1203]. There is supportive evidence for the efficacy of total contact casting (TCC) as a means of achieving off-loading [1203,1237], although the cast has the disadvantage of being nonremovable and there have been reports of TCCs causing injury to bony prominences such as the malleoli. Other, removable casts are often used in Europe, although these have not been tested in randomized trials: one example, the removable Scotchcast boot, is shown in Figure 5.**53**. Off-loading should be continued until the wound is healed, and should probably be continued for another week or two to permit wound maturation. Special footwear or extra-depth shoes with appropriate insoles should then be introduced gradually, with great care, to ensure that there is no suggestion of any pressure or rubbing.

Dressings

The danger of dressings and bandages is that some healthcare professionals may draw from them a false sense of security, believing that by dressing an ulcer they are curing it. Nothing could be further from the truth for a neuropathic ulcer. The three most important factors in the healing of a diabetic foot ulcer are: freedom from pressure, freedom from infection, and good vascularity. The purpose of dressings is to protect the wound from local trauma, minimize the risk of infection, and optimize the wound environment, which should be moist in most cases. The evidence base to help in the choice of dressings is woefully inadequate, with the few trials generally hampered by small numbers, inappropriate comparators, or poor study design [1237]. There is little evidence that any specific dressing type has a major impact on the rate of wound healing.

Management of Infection

One of the first steps in the management of a foot ulcer is to determine whether infection is present: remember that all foot ulcers are colonized with potentially pathogenic organisms, and most authors suggest that the absence of inflammatory findings implies the absence of infection [1238]. Thus, the presence of signs such as a purulent discharge, erythema, local warmth, and swelling would suggest infection requiring appropriate therapy.

Clinically Noninfected Ulcers

Where ulcers are not infected (Wagner grades 1, 2; San Antonio 1A, 2A), the use of antibiotics may be withheld, as Chantelau et al. [1239] have shown that with appropriate dressings and off-loading, patients do equally as well with or without systemic antibiotics. However, frequent review, debridement, and callus removal are essential, and should signs of infection develop antibiotics may be needed. For ulcers with ischemia (San Antonio 1C), antibiotics should probably be given in most cases. In all cases, great care should be taken in the choice of antibiotics, remembering the increasing prevalence of resistant organisms [1230,1231].

Clinically Infected Ulcers

Non-limb-threatening infected foot ulcers (Wagner grades 1,2; San Antonio 1B,1D, 2B, 2D) can generally be treated on an outpatient basis, and oral broad-spectrum antibiotics can be used, remembering also the need to off-load the ulcer. Commonly used antibiotics include clindamycin or amoxycillin/clavulanate [1238, 1239]. Radiographs should be taken to exclude osteomyelitis. The duration of antibiotic therapy is also controversial, with no data from controlled trials to guide us in the length of treatment. In cases of infected neuropathic ulcers, treatment is usually continued until the ulcer is clinically noninfected.

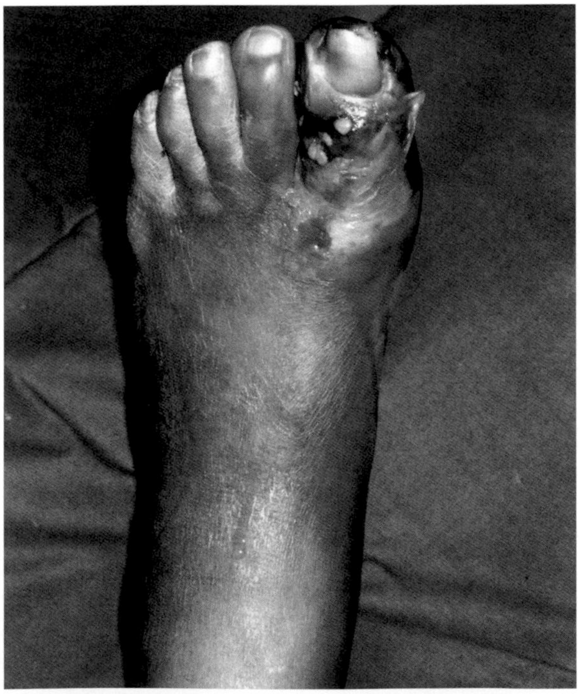

Fig. 5.**54** A supposed case of pyrexia of unknown origin. This patient was referred to the diabetes team because of unexplained pyrexia. The patient was on dialysis and had had numerous investigations to investigate the pyrexia, but nobody had removed the dressing from his great toe. On examination gross evidence of infection was seen, and radiographs confirmed osteomyelitis which was the cause of the pyrexia. Wagner grade 3/San Antonio 3B. The patient had a good peripheral circulation, the infection was treated with broad-spectrum antibiotics, and the toe was removed. This demonstrates the essential requirement that all patients should have their feet examined in great detail with any dressings or other coverings removed

Limb-Threatening Infections

Patients with limb-threatening infection usually have systemic symptoms and signs, and require hospitalization with parenteral antibiotics. Deep wound and blood cultures should be taken, the circulation assessed with noninvasive studies initially, and metabolic control is usually achieved by intravenous insulin infusion [1203,1238,1240]. Early surgical debridement is often indicated in such cases, and initial antibiotic regimens should be broad-spectrum until sensitivities are determined from the microbiological cultures. Examples of initial antibiotic regimens include: clindamycin and ciprofloxacin, or flucloxacillin, ampicillin, and metronidazole.

Osteomyelitis

The diagnosis of osteomyelitis (Fig. 5.**54**) is a controversial topic, and several diagnostic tests have been recommended. Amongst these, "probing to bone" has been shown to have a high predictive value, plain radiographs are insensitive early in the natural history of osteomyelitis, and the indium-labeled white cell scan can be useful [1238]. Contrary to traditional teaching, some cases of localized osteomyelitis can be managed by long-term (10–12 weeks) antibiotic therapy that should cover *Staphylococcus aureus*, which remains the commonest etiological organism. However, localized bony resection after appropriate antibiotic therapy remains a common approach (Fig. 5.**54**).

Other Therapies

A number of new approaches to treating diabetic neuropathic foot ulcers have been described in the past decade.

Growth Factors

These can be applied topically with the aim of speeding the wound healing process. rhPDGF, or becaplermin, is a recombinant platelet-derived growth factor which is now available in most western countries. A number of controlled trials suggest that becaplermin is efficacious in promoting more rapid wound healing, remembering that the appropriate off-loading, dressing, and good wound care is also essential [1237,1242]. Wieman et al., in a study of 382 neuropathic foot ulcer patients, demonstrated a significant improvement in healing rates in those subjects randomized to receive topical rhPDGF versus placebo [1242].

Cultured Human Dermis

In vitro cultured human neonatal dermal fibroblasts, grown on a bioabsorbable mesh, produce a living metabolically active tissue producing dermal matrix proteins and cytokines. Studies suggest that the use of this product can increase wound healing rates, although cost is a major concern [1237].

Hyperbaric Oxygen

Despite the widespread use of hyperbaric oxygen (HBO) in the management of neuroischemic and ischemic ulcers in certain countries, particularly the USA, there is no good controlled evidence to support its use [1203,1237]. Controlled studies should help to clarify the use of HBO in the diabetic foot: in the meantime, its use should be restricted to predominantly ischemic ulcers that are resistant to other therapies.

Larval Therapy

The use of sterile maggots, the larvae of the common green bottle fly, is not new: indeed, early observations of the efficacy of maggots on wound healing were made by one of Napoleon's surgeons, who noted that maggot-infested battle wounds did not become infected and healed faster! Today, sterile maggots are useful in the desloughing of wounds that are resistant to surgical debridement. It is believed that they secrete a broad spectrum of powerful enzymes that break down dead tissue: limited evidence also suggests that they do not harm healthy tissue as the enzymes are inactivated by inhibitors present in normal skin [1243]. A number of reports, predominantly case series, support their use in certain sloughy diabetic foot ulcers [1243].

Granulocyte-Colony Stimulating Factor (G-CSF)

Granulocyte-colony stimulating factor (G-CSF) increases both the production and the release of neutrophils from the bone marrow, enhancing neutrophil function in fighting infection. Recombinant G-CSF has mainly been used in neutropenic patients during chemotherapy, but a small, controlled study in diabetic patients with severe foot infections from Gough et al. suggested that patients with severe cellulitis who received intravenous G-CSF responded faster to antibiotic therapy, required shorter courses of intravenous antibiotics, and had shorter hospital admissions [1244]. Clearly larger trials of this promising, though expensive, treatment are required in severe foot infection [1237].

Prediction of Outcome

As stated above, appropriate classification of a foot ulcer should help in the prediction of outcome: a San Antonio 3D lesion is much more likely, for example, to end up in a major amputation than a 2B ulcer. In a retrospective cohort study, Pittet et al. recently reported on the outcome of 105 patients with diabetic foot ulcers admitted to a Swiss teaching hospital [1245]. Two-thirds of these patients were successfully managed with conservative therapy: factors associated with poor outcome (e. g., amputation) included higher Wagner grading, severity of vascular status, and renal impairment. It therefore seems that prolonged antibiotic therapy and regular wound debridement, control of diabetes, etc., can be successfully employed in the majority of patients hospitalized for diabetic foot ulceration. Similarly, Adler et al. report that a low transcutaneous oxygen tension is associated with delayed healing and increased risk of amputation [1246]. It is therefore quite clear that neuropathic foot lesions generally carry a good prognosis, whereas those with a significant ischemic component are more likely to require the input of the vascular surgeon.

The Team Approach

It should be clear that the spectrum of diabetic foot problems requires the involvement of individuals from many specialties. The diabetic foot cannot be regarded as the responsibility of the diabetologist alone, and a number of reports in the last two decades have promoted the benefits of a multidisciplinary approach to diabetic foot care [1204]. The team approach, involving diabetologists, surgeons (both orthopedic and vascular), specialist nurses, podiatrists, orthotists, and often many other specialist healthcare professionals, has been shown to improve the outlook for patients with diabetic foot ulcers. Although many regard the specialist nurse as the key team participant [1247], most agree that it is the high risk or foot ulcer patients themselves that must be regarded as the conductor of the diabetic foot orchestra. Without their willing participation, there is little that the other team members can achieve to improve the overall outlook for the diabetic foot in the twenty-first century.

Special Syndromes

■ Insulin, Hypoglycemia, and Peripheral Neuropathy

S.E.M. Eaton and S. Tesfaye

Introduction

A complete understanding of the pathogenesis of diabetic polyneuropathy remains elusive, although a variety of metabolic and vascular hypotheses have been put forward, each centered on hyperglycemia [1248]. There is growing evidence, however, that peripheral nerve dysfunction may also result as a consequence of hypoglycemia and insulin therapy [1249]. In many textbooks of diabetes this area is overlooked, but there are a number of reasons why the issue may be important. As a general principle, consideration of different aspects of a disease process often yields important lessons, in this case in the understanding of the pathophysiology of neuronal function. Furthermore, hypoglycemia is often encountered in pursuit of optimal glycemic control in diabetes, and therefore a detrimental effect of insulin treatment and/or hypoglycemia on the nerve may have important implications to clinical practice.

In this section we review the evidence from both animal and human studies that hypoglycemia may cause peripheral nerve dysfunction. We also discuss the nature and pathogenesis of insulin neuritis, an acute painful neuropathy associated with institution of glycemic control, and the potential role of insulin and hypoglycemia. We conclude by discussing the potential implications of these issues for diabetic polyneuropathy and the management of diabetes in general.

Hypoglycemic Neuropathy

Animal Studies

Hypoglycemia and Peripheral Nerve Function

Unlike the brain, the peripheral nerve is able to utilize energy substrates other than glucose in times of hypoglycemia [1250]. Experimental studies of prolonged hypoglycemia would suggest that these alternative substrates are exhaustible, however, and nerve fiber degeneration will eventually result [1251,1252]. The degree of neurologic deficit is determined by the severity and length of hypoglycemic insult. Acute, nonsustained hypoglycemia does not cause any measurable structural abnormality; indeed, Yasaki and Dyck showed that severe hypoglycemic conditions (glucose levels around 1.4 mmol/l) can be tolerated for 12 hours before axonal degeneration occurred [1251], while Sidenius and Jakobsen demonstrated that milder degrees of hypoglycemia (less than 2.5 mmol/l) could be tolerated for at least 72 hours [1252]. However, the latter authors have also shown that individual functional elements of the nerve may be more susceptible to glucose deprivation, with a significant slowing of anterograde axonal transport in acute hypoglycemia [1253]. Pretreatment with insulin abolished this effect, and diabetes itself was at least partially protective, suggesting that the diabetic nerve may respond differently to hypoglycemia. More recently, Mohseni et al. have shown abnormalities in nerve end terminals in diabetic rats treated with insulin implants, which manifested predominately in muscle rather than skin [1254].

Mechanism of Hypoglycemia-Related Damage

The mechanism by which hypoglycemia induces neuronal damage is not clear. The nerve may be damaged directly by glucose deprivation or via other consequences, such as hypothermia [1255,1256]. Alternatively, there is evidence for an important role of nerve blood flow and hypoxia, factors which are strongly implicated in the pathogenesis of hyperglycemia-related neuropathy [1257,1258]. Similarities exist between experimental studies of microvascular occlusion [1259,1260] and acute hypoglycemia [1261] in the spatial distribution of axonal degeneration, with both predominating in the central fascicular region of the nerve, the watershed areas of poorest perfusion. However, structural microvascular disease, prominent in hyperglycemia-related neuropathy [1262], does not appear to be present in hypoglycemic neuropathy [1263], suggesting a more acute, dynamic effect. This possibility has been confirmed by studies showing reductions in nerve blood flow with acute hypoglycemia [1264,1265], an effect which may be related to adrenergic activation with the counterregulatory response [1266]. In an effort to maintain neuronal blood flow, there is also evidence of release of vasodilator substances, including nitric oxide, which might actually counterbalance this [1267].

Hypoglycemia or Hyperinsulinemia?

One of the clear benefits of experimental studies is the ability to design protocols aiming to differentiate between the individual effects of hypoglycemia and hyperinsulinemia. This distinction is vital in understanding the pathogenic mechanisms at hand, although the limited studies thus far have had contradictory results. In their experiments, Sidenius and Jakobsen demonstrated that anterograde axonal transport slowing was due to hypoglycemia rather than hyperinsulinemia [1253]. Conversely, Kihara et al. have studied the effects of insulin infusion in nonhypoglycemic conditions and showed a dose-dependent reduction in endoneurial oxygen tension in nondiabetic rats [1268]. Diabetic rats appeared to be resistant, although susceptibility to endoneurial hypoxia returned with glycemic control. This effect was felt to be due to an insulin-induced opening of arteriovenous shunts causing a reduction in nutritive blood flow. Whilst this is certainly an interesting finding, it should not necessarily be taken as strong evidence of a deleterious effect of insulin. Indeed, insulin has been shown to have a vasodilatory effect in skeletal muscle, probably through nitric oxide release [1269]. Furthermore, insulin undoubtedly has a beneficial effect in diabetic rats, reversing deficits in neuronal blood flow caused by hyperglycemia [1270].

Human Studies

Peripheral Neuropathy in Patients with Insulinoma

The majority of evidence implicating hypoglycemia in the development of peripheral neuropathy in humans is based on anecdotal reports in chronic, persistent hypoglycemia due to insulinoma. Although neurologic symptoms are extremely common with insulinoma, they usually relate to cognitive dysfunction, and peripheral neuropathy is relatively rare with just 32 reported cases [1263,1271–1275]. The presentation tends to be of a symmetric sensorimotor peripheral neuropathy, although there are distinct differences from hyperglycemia-related neuropathy (Table 5.**28**). Motor symptoms and signs usually predominate, and weakness is often more severe in the upper limbs, characteristically associated with wasting of the small muscles of the hands. Tendon reflexes are usually, but not invariably, absent or diminished. Sensory symptoms are often reported as mild though may be masked by concomitant cerebral dysfunction. Motor and sensory nerve conduction velocities can be normal but are usually reduced to some degree, and action potential amplitudes are reduced or absent. Nerve biopsy reveals axonal degeneration and myelinated fiber loss, similar to that found in hyperglycemia-related neuropathy although without any structural microvascular disease. Electromyography indicates denervation, which is also suggested by the finding of fiber atrophy on muscle biopsy. Removal of the insulinoma tends to result in an improvement of the neurologic deficit, although muscle wasting and weakness may persist [1274,1275].

The exact mechanism of peripheral neuropathy associated with insulinoma is not known, and there is the possibility of a paraneoplastic influence. However, the strong association of peripheral neuropathy with other manifestations of hypoglycemia-related damage, particularly cerebral dysfunction, suggests a hypoglycemic etiology [1272].

Insulin Shock Therapy

Induction of hypoglycemia in order to cause loss of consciousness has been extensively used in the treatment of psychiatric conditions. A number of neurologic sequelae have been reported and are often quoted as further evidence for hypoglycemia inducing nerve damage [1276,1277]. However, the majority of these reports relate to cerebral and cognitive dysfunction or transient peripheral symptoms; there are very few reports of persisting peripheral neuropathy.

Table 5.**28** Clinical features of hyperglycemia-related (diabetic) and hypoglycemia-related peripheral neuropathy

	Hyperglycemia-related peripheral neuropathy	**Hypoglycemia-related peripheral neuropathy**
Prevalence	**Common**	**Rare**
Symptoms:		
Sensory	Common	Mild (masked by cognitive dysfunction?)
Motor	Subclinical until later stages	Common, especially in the upper limbs
Related to diabetes	Common complication of diabetes	Never reported in association with diabetes
Associations with ...	Other diabetic complications (retinopathy, nephropathy)	Other signs of hypoglycemia-related damage (esp. cognitive)
Relation to glycemia	Related to prolonged hyperglycemia	Related to hypoglycemia (prolonged or acute?)
Other pathogenic factors	Combination of vascular and metabolic factors	Unclear; vascular factors may be important
Prognosis	Progressive; may benefit from improvements in glycemic control	Often improves with avoidance of hypoglycemia (removal of insulinoma)
Nerve biopsy	Axonal loss Myelinated fiber loss Microvascular disease is prominent	Axonal loss Myelinated fiber loss No microvascular disease

Hypoglycemia in the Treatment of Diabetes

Hypoglycemia may often be encountered in the treatment of diabetes mellitus, especially in the context of achieving good glycemic control [1278]. However, there have been no published case reports of the development of a peripheral neuropathy in diabetes mellitus that can be attributed solely to hypoglycemia [1279]. This may reflect a natural tendency to ascribe any problems to the more frequently encountered hyperglycemia-related neuropathy or different neuronal responses to hypoglycemia in diabetic nerves. It is also possible that hypoglycemia encountered in the treatment of diabetes is rarely severe or persistent enough to produce neuronal dysfunction.

Insulin Neuritis (Acute Painful Neuropathy of Rapid Glycemic Control)

Clinical Features

Whilst good glycemic control in diabetes does not seem to be associated with the development of hypoglycemic peripheral neuropathy there is strong evidence that an acute painful neuropathy may occasionally develop. This has been termed "insulin neuritis" and although the pathogenesis is unclear, a potential role of insulin and/or hypoglycemia has been suggested. This phenomenon was first described by Caravati [1280] and has subsequently been reported by several other groups [1281–1288]. Each describe neuropathic symptoms developing within a few weeks of institution of good glycemic control, usually with insulin. This has a distinct presentation and outlook from the painful symptoms of chronic diabetic distal symmetrical polyneuropathy. Invariably the patient has painful symptoms that may be confined to the feet but can extend into a glove and stocking distribution [1289]. These are often extremely distressing and difficult to treat and frequently interfere with day-to-day activities including ability to work and sleep. However, they are usually associated with little objective evidence of peripheral nerve dysfunction, certainly compared to the extreme nature of the symptoms, with normal or near-normal nerve conduction and sensory testing [1289]. In some cases no signs of sensory loss may be apparent at all and there is rarely any evidence of motor deficit. Fortunately the prognosis is good in that complete resolution of the symptoms can be expected within 10 months and recurrence is very rare [1290].

Pathogenesis of Insulin Neuritis

The pathogenesis of insulin neuritis has been relatively understudied and remains unclear. The proximity of the symptoms to the institution of insulin therapy has led to the suggestion that it may be due to a direct toxic effect of insulin. However, several features suggest that this may not be the case. First, the symptoms will resolve if good glycemic control is maintained by continuing insulin treatment. Furthermore, Ward et al. demonstrated an improvement of nerve conduction on initiation of insulin at diagnosis in type 1 diabetes [1291]. Similarly, recent large prospective studies, in both type 1 and 2 diabetes, have produced unequivocal evidence that good glycemic control (in most cases with insulin therapy) has beneficial effects on neuronal function [1278,1292]. Finally, a similar picture can be seen when good control is attained on oral hypoglycemic agents, suggesting that exogenous insulin may not have a direct role [1285]. Indeed, the term "insulin neuritis" is a misnomer as it implies the underlying pathology is inflammation, which is not the case. A different descriptive term, "acute painful neuropathy of rapid glycemic control," has therefore been recommended [1288].

Initiation of insulin therapy may well result in episodes of hypoglycemia as the glycemic control improves. However, there is no strong evidence to implicate hypoglycemia in the pathogenesis of acute painful neuropathy of rapid glycemic control. Indeed, a similar acute painful neuropathy can be associated with poor glycemic control which is actually ameliorated by improving control, usually with insulin. Initially described as "neuropathic cachexia" by Ellenberg [1293], a more recent description of the natural history has been published by Archer and colleagues [1294]. The presentation is remarkably comparable to acute painful neuropathy of rapid glycemic control, with severe painful symptoms out of keeping with the relatively minor sensory deficit and complete resolution of symptoms in less than a year. However, this condition is paradoxically associated with extremely poor diabetic control associated with precipitous weight loss that resolves once tight glycemic control has been initiated and weight starts to increase. It has therefore been suggested that the painful symptoms of both syndromes may relate more to fluctuations of glycemia rather than to the overall level of control [1295].

Other factors may well be important in the pathogenesis of acute painful neuropathy of rapid glycemic control. The acute onset associated with fluctuations in glycemia led many to believe there was a purely metabolic cause. However, we have reported a case series in which the microvascular status of the sural nerve was assessed with the use of nerve photography and fluorescein angiography. Even in this acute setting we demonstrated gross abnormalities [1288]. Epineurial nutrient vessels demonstrated vessel tortuosity, arteriolar attenuation, venous distention, and extensive arteriovenous shunting, similar to that seen in chronic diabetic polyneuropathy [1296]. A new finding was the presence of neovascularization on the surface of the nerve, similar to that observed in the retina, in three of the five subjects (Fig. 5.**55**). This may represent a "steal" effect, rendering the endoneurium hypoxic, which may be an important step in the genesis

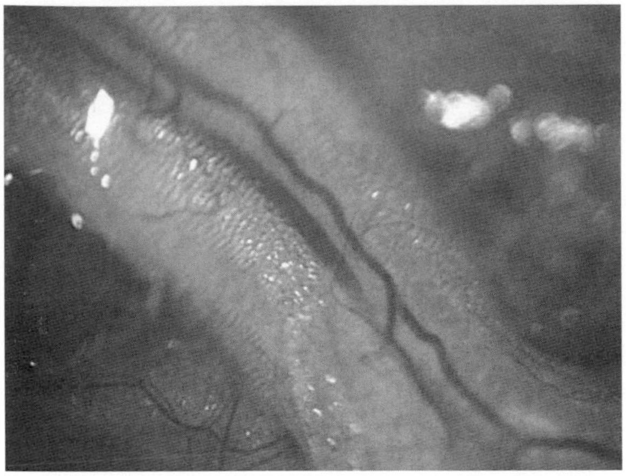

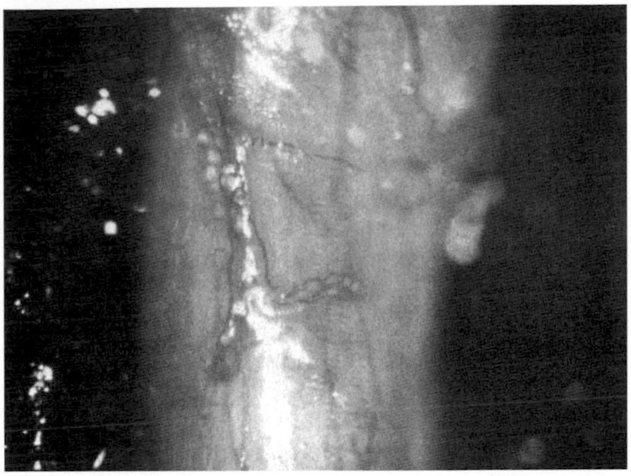

Fig. 5.55 Neural "new vessels" in acute insulin neuritis. **a** Normal, **b** acute insulin neuritis

of pain [1288]. The demonstration of acute arterio-venous shunting with infusion of insulin by Kihara et al. is further evidence that this may be the case [1268].

More recently, we have studied the role of vascular factors in chronic painful neuropathy and have paradoxically demonstrated increased blood flow and higher oxygen saturation in those subjects with pain than in those without [1297]. However, the techniques used (microlightguided spectrophotometry and fluorescein angiography) primarily measure the epineurium, and it is therefore not clear whether this represents a generalized hyperperfusion of the nerve or shunting from the endoneurium. Clarification of these issues will provide vital insights into the pathogenesis of the painful symptoms of neuropathy.

The factors that drive these changes in blood flow and/or shunting are not clear. Growth factors may be important and are strongly implicated in proliferative retinopathy, which also has a vascular base and shows a tendency to deteriorate aggressively and acutely with tight control [1298–1300]. Indeed, a temporal relationship has been demonstrated between tightening of glycemic control with subcutaneous insulin infusion, a rise in growth factor levels, and onset of proliferative retinopathy [1301].

Implications for Diabetic Neuropathy

The evidence from animal studies would suggest that the peripheral nerve is susceptible to glucose deprivation, leading to functional and structural abnormalities. This is very rarely significant in humans, however, being mainly reported in patients with insulinoma. To date, there have been no reports of such a problem relating to the treatment of diabetes. However, rapid improvements in glycemic control may precipitate an acute painful neuropathy, perhaps due to a combination of metabolic and vascular factors. This is an issue that should be considered when treating poor glycemic control and may suggest that aiming for gradual improvements would be sensible.

Vascular factors and hypoxia are strongly implicated in hyperglycemia-related peripheral neuropathy, and there is considerable evidence that they may be important in nerve damage relating to hypoglycemia and fluctuations of glycemic control. Whilst the mechanisms causing the hypoxia may vary considerably, the strong implication is that the oxygen status of the nerve is a key factor for nerve function and survival. Thus, a further understanding of the mechanisms of nerve hypoxia and the development of interventions to maintain oxygenation or increase resistance to hypoxia may be vital in the treatment of these conditions.

The thrust of diabetes management is to aim at good glycemic control wherever possible, especially in the presence of early microvascular complications. Perhaps, therefore, the most important issue relating to this section of the volume is whether hypoglycemia suffered as consequence of good glycemic control in diabetes causes any further insult to the nerve–a particularly important consideration in the circumstance of the already compromised nerve in early diabetic neuropathy. On balance there does not seem to be any strong evidence that it does, although this topic has not been specifically studied and therefore the possibility cannot be excluded. The diabetes physician should therefore remain vigilant to the possibility whilst continuing to pursue the goal of glycemic control.

■ Ketosis-Related Neuropathy

R.A. Malik

Introduction

Ketoacidosis may account for up to 8% of all hospital admissions amongst diabetic patients [1302] and may be associated with a 5–10% mortality [1303]. Absolute or relative deficiency of insulin results in diabetic ketoacidosis and is commonly precipitated by infections, but may also occur secondary to trauma, surgery, and thromboembolic events such as stroke and myocardial infarction [1304]. In a minority of cases extreme dehydration and the ensuing hypercoagulable state results in a number of potentially life-threatening complications secondary to arterial and venous thrombosis. Whilst deep venous thrombosis is the most common, cerebral [1305] and hepatic [1306] infarction have also been reported. Cardiorespiratory problems include acute myocardial infarction, pulmonary embolism, and pleuropericardial effusions. Gastrointestinal problems include a raised serum amylase concentration which may be mistaken for pancreatitis, and frank hematemesis, which may occur in up to 10% of patients due to erosive esophagitis, gastritis, or duodenitis [1307].

Other complications include cerebral and pulmonary edema, though these are most often related to the treatment employed to correct the metabolic acidosis.

Diabetic Ketoacidosis-Associated Neuropathy

In a large prospective study of 3250 type 1 diabetic patients, multiple logistic regression analysis demonstrated that severe diabetic ketoacidosis carried a significantly increased standardized relative risk for the development of neuropathy [1308] (Fig. 5.**56**). The authors postulated that this was further supportive evidence for a vascular basis of diabetic neuropathy. It is more likely that this relationship simply reflects a generally poor glycemic control, which results both in more frequent ketoacidosis and in neuropathy, as opposed to any direct relationship between diabetic ketoacidosis and neuropathy. However, neuropathy related to diabetic ketoacidosis is a completely different entity from chronic sensorimotor neuropathy. It is acute in onset, has both peripheral and central manifestations, and may resolve completely with treatment

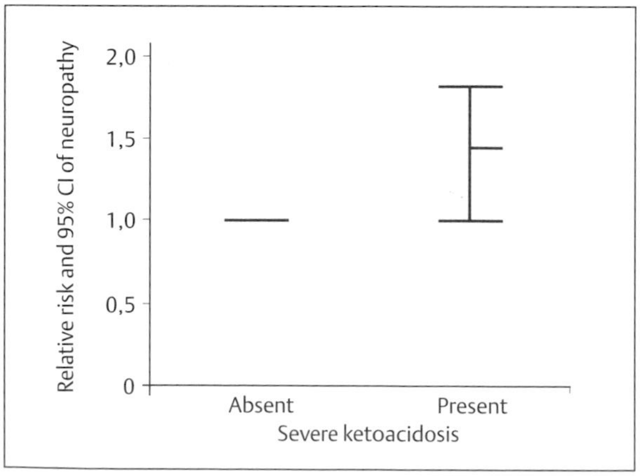

Fig.5.**56** Incidence of diabetic ketoacidosis and neuropathy in the EURODIAB study [1311]

of the ketoacidosis. Because of its rare occurrence, there is a limited understanding of the clinical features, underlying pathophysiology, and appropriate treatment of this condition. However, several factors may be important determinants in the onset, severity, and outcome of diabetic ketoacidosis-associated neuropathy (DKAAN). Patients who develop ketoacidosis are more likely to have poorer metabolic control and therefore will already have an underlying peripheral sensorimotor neuropathy [1308], and hence any added insult to an already diseased peripheral nerve will result in significant neurologic deficit. Conversely, a prospective population-based study has also shown that ketoacidosis is more likely to develop in diabetic patients who already have the microvascular complications of diabetes [1309], although, a recent study has shown that following the withdrawal of insulin, type 1 diabetic patients with autonomic neuropathy show a less rapid rise in plasma fatty acids and ketone bodies, apparently affording them protection from developing ketoacidosis [1310].

Clinical Features

The neurologic manifestations of diabetic ketoacidosis may be complex, with a combination of upper and lower motoneuron signs. The commonest presentation is a reduction in conscious level, resulting in precoma and coma. Although this has been attributed to metabolic derangement, the exact mechanisms of this clinical presentation are not precisely understood as its severity is related to neither the degree of hyperglycemia or acidosis. One of the clearest insights into the grave consequences of severe diabetic ketoacidosis was most clearly illustrated in a detailed report describing the postmortem pathology of six fatally ill diabetic patients ranging from a three-month-old infant to a 68-year-old woman with type 2 diabetes [1311]. In summary, macroscopic examination showed cerebral edema with intravascular thrombi in medium- and large-sized vessels in the meninges, and in deeper structures including the pons, cerebellum, and cerebral cortex. Neuronal involvement included necrosis and vacuolation of neurons and glial cells along with perivascular foci of demyelination in the brain [1311]. Thrombosis was widespread involving other vital organs including the kidney, liver, lungs, myocardium, and pancreas in three out of six patients. This was accompanied by diffuse superficial hemorrhage on the surface of the frontal and parietal lobes, with numerous petechial hemorrhages in the pons and hypothalamus in a further two patients. Other sites of hemorrhage included the duodenum and upper jejunum, which in one case was sufficient to cause frank hematemesis [1311]. In combination, thrombosis with hemorrhage implies a state of disseminated intravascular coagulation (DIC) in severe diabetic ketoacidosis. Less severe presentations of ketoacidosis appear to have less serious clinical manifestations. Thus, three cases of newly presenting patients with diabetic ketoacidosis were initially treated as neurosurgical emergencies [1312]. A 62-year-old woman with type 2 diabetes became semicomatose following a road traffic accident and was believed to have a subdural hematoma. However, active treatment of her ketoacidosis resulted in complete resolution of her reduced conscious level. Similarly, a 59-year-old woman presented in a semiconscious state associated with convulsions and a left hemiparesis with left homonymous hemianopia, which was thought to be secondary to a cerebral tumor. Again, correction of her metabolic state resulted in near-complete resolution of her focal neurologic signs. A 37-year-old woman with bilateral otitis media presented in an unconscious state with dense left hemiparesis suggestive of a cerebral abscess. However, this patient died, despite adequate treatment of ketoacidosis.

Thus, there is a wide spectrum of clinical presentations and a wide degree of potential recovery of what initially appear to be profound neurologic deficits associated with diabetic ketoacidosis. This clearly reflects varying degrees of severity of the DIC which occurs with ketoacidosis [1311–1313]. Many of the neurologic manifestations of diabetic ketoacidosis are of upper motoneuron origin. However, lower motoneuron, peripheral nerve involvement may also occur, but, unlike chronic sensorimotor neuropathy, the onset of neuropathy is usually acute, predominantly motor in nature, and may be associated with cranial nerve deficits. In the majority of cases neurologic improvement occurs either immediately or within weeks of recovery from ketoacidosis [1314]. Five patients have been reported, of whom four had sensory symptoms, including aching and cramping sensations in the thighs and calves, which occurred four to six weeks after presentation and treatment of the underlying diabetic ketoacidosis. All symptoms and signs resolved within a further four weeks [1315]. In one patient profound symmetric motor weakness of the lower limbs developed and was associated clinically with DIC. However, the patient made a complete recovery upon treatment of the ketoacidosis [1315]. Sural nerve biopsy demonstrated fibrin deposition, degenerate endothelial cells, and pericytes as well as endothelial cell hyperplasia sufficient to cause luminal occlusion [1315] (Fig. 5.**57**). Neurologic deficits may also develop in type 2 diabetic patients who develop hyperosmolar nonketotic coma. The clinical presentation ranges from upper motoneuron deficits of hemianopia and hemiparesis to lower motoneuron signs such as abnormal muscle tone, myoclonic twitches [1316], and a progressive ascending, predominantly motor neuropathy [1317]. The patient in the latter case report made a complete recovery 15 days after commencing insulin therapy [1317].

The development of the microvascular complications of diabetes in the setting of a ketoacidosis is, however, not limited to neuropathy alone, as

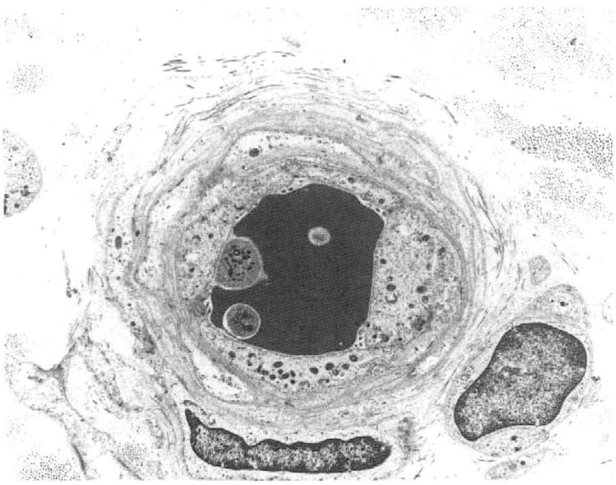

Fig.5.**57** Sural nerve endoneurial capillary with a thrombus and platelet plug in a patient with an acute neuropathy precipitated by diabetic ketoacidosis

proliferative retinopathy and nephropathy have also been shown to accompany an autonomic neuropathy in patients with severe diabetic ketoacidosis [1318]. The converse situation also exists: a 19-year-old type 1 diabetic patient developed a severe peripheral and autonomic neuropathy that led to recurrent vomiting and weight loss and resulted in ketoacidosis [1319]. High-dose cisapride as a prokinetic agent along with strict glycemic control terminated both the vomiting and the ketoacidosis. More permanent neurologic deficits have also been described in a young child with newly diagnosed diabetes and ketoacidosis and have been attributed to thrombosis of the vasa nervorum and resultant ischemic neuronal damage secondary to DIC [1320], similar to the previous reports of Timperley et al. [1311].

Pathogenetic Factors

The neurologic manifestations of DKAAN probably represent a spectrum of deficits that reflect the severity of dysmetabolism and associated DIC. A prothrombotic state has been described in patients with diabetic ketoacidosis [1311]. The acute onset of symptoms and motor involvement in DKAAN suggests an ischemic basis. However, it is difficult to reconcile ischemia and, presumably, nerve infarction with the rapid improvement in clinical deficits that can be observed upon improvement of the metabolic state and resolution of the ketoacidosis in the majority of patients. Therefore, in patients who make a full recovery, the underlying pathophysiology is likely to be of a transient hemodynamic or perhaps purely metabolic nature, which may explain the acute onset of neuropathy and may also explain the equally fast recovery. Additionally, patients with diabetic ketoacidosis demonstrate a raised plasma angiotensin II concentration, compared to patients with hyperosmolar nonketotic coma, which is independent of the degree of hydration, although the rise in angiotensin II is greater in patients without chronic microvascular complications of diabetes [1321]. Consistent with these findings is the demonstration of elevated plasma renin and aldosterone levels in patients with diabetic ketoacidosis, although overall there is a down-regulation in its production with the development of the microvascular complications of diabetes [1322]. Other associated metabolic abnormalities include the development of gross hyperlipoproteinemia, which can lead to the development of a severe peripheral neuropathy [1323].

Models of Ketoacidotic Neuropathy

Animal models of neuropathy secondary to ketoacidosis are not readily available. One might argue that the streptozotocin-induced diabetic rat is probably in a mild state of ketoacidosis in most of the studies reported in the literature. Thus, the reduction in nerve conduction velocity and blood flow may simply reflect a degree of acidosis, lower blood pressure, and functional deficits but do not have any significant structural pathology of either the nerve fibers or the endoneurial capillaries [1324]. Transient but debilitating neurologic signs have been described in two diabetic cats characterized by flinching and head tilt, both of which disappeared after correction of the ketoacidosis [1325].

The rat poison Vacor (N-3-pyridylmethyl-N′-p-nitrophenyl urea) antagonizes nicotinamide metabolism and acts in a similar way to streptozotocin. When ingested it causes widespread B cell damage with resultant insulinopenia and diabetic ketoacidosis [1326]. A toxic neuropathy characterized by orthostatic hypotension, gastrointestinal hypomotility, and peripheral sensory loss has been described. Neurologic deficits appear to be independent of its primary mode of action since the neuropathy progresses despite nicotinamide administration, which counteracts the direct neurotoxic effects of Vacor. Full recovery is uncommon and the orthostatic hypotension tends to persist [1327]. Its direct neurotoxic effects have been studied in detail in Wistar rats, six hours after ingestion of 100 mg/kg of Vacor [1328]. Interestingly, the primary site of damage was the central nervous system, with focal hemorrhage, edema, spongy degeneration, and demyelination in the white matter, which is in many ways reminiscent of the changes described in diabetic patients by Timperley et al. [1311]. The peripheral nerve appeared to be spared as detailed electron microscopy of the sciatic nerve showed minimal degenerative changes and sparing of the vagus nerve [1328]. Other potential models of ketoacidosis-related neuropathy include the organoacidopathies, which cause episodic ketoacidosis and may result in severe peripheral and central neurologic deficits [1329].

In conclusion, a comprehensive understanding of the basic pathophysiology of neuropathy related to ketoacidosis is at present poor, as information is limited to case reports. There may be several different clinical entities at extreme ends of the spectrum. Patients may present with minimal neurologic deficits which may be related primarily to a metabolic or possibly neurohumoral abnormality, which when corrected results in resolution of the neurologic deficits. However, there may be a more severe form, which involves central and peripheral neurons secondary to more permanent damage as a consequence of tissue ischemia and infarction, which clearly does not lead to recovery.

Because of the rarity of the syndrome it is difficult to advocate a standard therapeutic approach to the management of DKAAN, such as anticoagulation, thrombolysis, or other measures to counteract DIC in a bid to prevent tissue thrombosis and infarction. The most important step in management is probably early recognition and correction of the diabetic ketoacidosis using standard measures including correction of hypovolemia, hyperglycemia, and acidosis.

■ Diabetic Acute Motor Neuropathy

Phillip A. Low

Introduction

Although diabetic neuropathy is primarily a distal and sensory neuropathy, there are a number of well-recognized neuropathies that reflect microvascular and macrovascular involvement, resulting in mononeuropathy and mononeuropathy multiplex. Whether the entity of diabetic motor neuropathy, and in particular acute motor neuropathy, truly exists is controversial. Some cases of acute motor neuropathy, such as Guillain-Barré syndrome, may occur in a diabetic patient and the relationship might be fortuitous. It is pragmatically useful nevertheless to consider a number of entities where motor deficits predominate.

Acute or Subacute Distal Motor Neuropathy

Acute and severe hypoglycemia can cause neuropathy [1330,1331]. Hypoglycemic neuropathy is sensorimotor, although sometimes it can be a predominantly motor and distal motor neuropathy, affecting both upper and lower extremities. Atrophy of the small muscles of the hands is characteristic. Pathologically this is an axonal neuropathy; insulin can cause endoneurial hypoxia by the opening up of arteriovenous channels [1332]. Recovery has been described in cases that are secondary to insulinomas, following resection of the tumors [1333].

Subacute or chronically progressive distal diabetic neuropathy is another uncommon diabetic motor neuropathy [1334,1335]. One variety consists of progressive distal motor neuropathy, with significant demyelination on nerve conduction studies and inflammatory demyelination on sural nerve biopsy. There is more axonal degeneration in these nerves than is usually seen in chronic inflammatory demyelinating polyneuropathy [1334]. The relevance of recognizing this entity is the potential of this neuropathy to respond to immunotherapy [1336]. In some patients progressive distal motor neuropathy is associated with pathologic features of advanced microvascular disease. Changes include plugging of the vascular lumen by degenerate cellular material and vascular occlusion, suggesting that the neuropathy, at least in part, relates to multiple small infarcts [1335].

Diabetic Proximal Motor Neuropathy

This entity, more accurately designated lumbosacral radiculoplexopathy [1337], is covered elsewhere (see pages 203–204). It is of subacute onset and typically affects motor, sensory, and autonomic fibers [1338]. However, a subset of cases can be predominantly or completely motor [1339]. Patients have a subacute onset of severe proximal weakness and atrophy, followed by recovery over the next three to 18 months. The pathophysiology of the condition is likely to be a combination of autoimmune attack on nerve and microvasculitis [1337]. Immunotherapy could be efficacious but is unproven at this time.

Diabetic Motor Mononeuropathies

These are described in other chapters and will be mentioned here for completeness. A number of mononeuropathies can occur which have a mainly or completely motor presentation. These include the oculomotor nerve, abducens, and facial nerves. Limb nerves affected can also be predominantly motor. For instance, peroneal neuropathy can present with a footdrop.

Truncal and especially abdominal radiculopathy can pose diagnostic problems. For instance, abdominal radiculopathy can be painless and present as an abdominal bulge. When painful, the condition can lead to unnecessary investigation of visceral pathology [1340].

Evaluation of Drug Effects

D. Luft and D. Ziegler

Introduction

In addition to metabolic control, drug treatment of both incipient and clinically manifest diabetic neuropathy will be necessary for years to come because, first, it is not possible today to achieve near-normoglycemic control in all type 1 diabetic patients with currently available methods of treatment that have been proved to be effective in reducing the incidence of diabetic neuropathy; and, secondly, type 2 diabetes mellitus is sometimes only diagnosed when neuropathy is the presenting complication. Moreover, we are far from reaching normoglycemic control in most patients with type 2 diabetes. Since 1–2 % of the whole population in western societies (20–40 % of all diabetic patients) may be affected by diabetic neuropathy, the search for effective drug treatment is not only a very important goal for the patient suffering from the neuropathy and for the practicing physician, but also an economic task for both the healthcare systems and the pharmaceutical companies.

During the last 30 years a variety of drugs have been evaluated for treatment based on the various pathogenetic hypotheses that have been proposed (Table 5.**29**). Assessing the quality of studies for drug treatment for diabetic neuropathy, Cavaliere et al. [1341] stated that in general their quality was poor. Problems most frequently identified were (1) the randomization method was not specified, (2) no a priori estimation was carried out of the number of patients necessary to obtain significant differences, and (3) there was almost no power calculation. For these reasons, most studies were unable to prove the effect of a given treatment—which, of course, does not mean that it would not have been shown to be effective had it been investigated properly. Other problems often encountered were short treatment periods, the unknown clinical relevance of the endpoints studied, and the inclusion of patients with advanced stages of neuropathy who may perhaps not respond to any treatment.

Table 5.**29** Treatment options for diabetic polyneuropathy based on pathogenetic considerations. Agents in parentheses have been withdrawn for various reasons (because apparently ineffective or causing severe side effects)

1. Near-normal glycemic control
2. Aldose reductase inhibitors
3. α-Lipoic acid
4. (γ-Linolenic acid)
5. Vasodilators , e.g., prostaglandins, ACE inhibitors
6. Nucleosides
7. Vitamin mixtures B_1,(B_6, B_{12})
8. (Nerve growth factor)
9. (*myo*-Inositol)
10. (Gangliosides)
11. (Aminoguanidine)
12. (Acetyl-L-carnitine)
13. C peptide
14. PKC β inhibitor

These disappointing results, therefore, do not allow any conclusion as to whether the lack of success was due to inefficacy of the drug tested or to the inappropriate study design. In recent years, several reviews have been published dealing with these methodologic problems, which must be solved before any judgment about the efficacy of a study drug is possible [1342–1345]. This section will summarize some of the most important problems in designing, conducting, and evaluating clinical trials.

Classification, Diagnosis, and Staging

Diabetic neuropathy has been defined as a demonstrable disorder, either clinically evident or subclinical, that occurs in the setting of diabetes mellitus in the absence of other causes of peripheral neuropathy [1346]. To date no pathogenetically based classification has been possible, so classification remains along clinical criteria that include localization, symmetry, symptoms, natural course, predominant involvement of either sensory, motor, or autonomic fibers, and time of onset during the course of diabetes (Table 5.**30**). Overlaps between different syndromes have prevented the formulation of a generally accepted classification. For drug treatment, the chronic syndromes (in contrast to rapidly reversible, probably functional deficits) are the target of intervention [1347]. The most common of these syndromes, symmetric sensorimotor polyneuropathy, including distal predominantly sensory and autonomic involvement, is the form for which treatment is most important, because it is associated not only with impaired quality of life, but also with high morbidity (development of diabetic foot syndrome, devastating symptoms like pain and paresthesia) and increased mortality [1348,1349].

Conceptually, nerve damage may develop through biochemical alterations induced by hyperglycemia leading first to functional disturbances, either within the neural structures like the Schwann cell, the myelin sheath, or the axons, or within the neural nutritional vasculature, leading to oxidative stress and hypoxia and thus inducing further damage. Over time, functional deviations may lead to structural changes which may not then be reversible and—in diabetic patients—may not be restored as easily as other nerve lesions, e. g., traumatic changes in metabolically healthy organisms. For treatment purposes, therefore, distal symmetric sensorimotor polyneuropathy may be subdivided into a clinical and a subclinical form, the first in patients with no demonstrable symptoms or signs and the second in patients with symptoms, signs, or both (Table 5.**31**). Given the variability of clinical presentations and the variety of classification approaches, the clinical diagnosis should be supplemented with easily measurable, reproducible, noninvasive (or at least only minimally invasive) measures to standardize patient selection for clinical studies. The Consensus Development Conference on Standardized Measures in Diabetic Neuropathy [1346] recommended the following five measures for characterization: clinical measures, morphologic and biochemical analyses, electrodiagnostic assessment, quantitative sensory testing, and autonomic nervous system testing. Clinically applicable and repeatable scoring systems have been proposed by Dyck and coworkers, who use the Neuropathy Symptom Score (NSS), the Neuropathy Impairment Score (NIS), nerve conduction velocities, quantitative sensory testing including vibration or cold/warm detection thresholds, and autonomic function tests, e. g., R–R variation during deep breathing or the Valsalva maneuver. Minimum criteria may then be defined for the diagnosis of neuropathy and hence for inclusion in a treatment study [1350].

Patients included in a therapeutic trial should not vary with regard to the form and stage of neuropathy they are suffering from, because pathogenesis, age at manifestation, correlations with metabolic control, concomitant complications, diabetes duration, gender distribution, natural course, prognosis and, most importantly, the potential for improvement may differ considerably [1346]. Since there is uncertainty as to

Table 5.**30** Criteria for the definition of nerve involvement in diabetes. Criteria in *italics* are of critical importance in defining the various forms of neuropathy which differ in pathogenesis, clinical picture, natural history, and prognosis

Acute	–	*Chronic*
Symmetric	–	Asymmetric
Distal	–	Proximal
Sensory	–	Motor
Symptomatic	–	Asymptomatic
Painful	–	Painless

Table 5.**31** Definition of different stages of severity of diabetic distal sensorimotor polyneuropathy according to clinical signs, symptoms, and electrophysiologic tests

Stage	Symptoms and deficits	Electrophysiology
0	0	0
1	0	Abnormal
2	Chronic painful Acute painful Painless with complete or partial loss of sensitivity Amyotrophy	Abnormal
3	Foot lesions Deformity Nontraumatic amputation	Abnormal

whether nerve lesions in type 1 and type 2 diabetes are different, careful selection of the diabetes type seems warranted. Studies in elderly type 2 diabetic patients may be more difficult since concomitant effects of age, macroangiopathy, and drugs on nerves have to be taken into account. Only patients suffering from stage 1 neuropathy (no symptoms, but clinical or electrophysiologic signs) or early stage 2 neuropathy (symptoms with or without clinical or electrophysiologic signs) (Table 5.**31**) should be included. Stage 3 includes late complications (e.g., diabetic foot syndrome, amputation) and is not considered suitable for the investigation of new treatment modalities since the disease process—analogously to end-stage nephropathy or proliferative retinopathy—may be too advanced to allow reversibility or even improvement [1342]. The duration of symptoms should be comparable in all patients, because newly developing symptoms may tend to reverse at a much faster rate than chronic manifestations. Type 1 diabetic patients suffering from symptoms of diabetic neuropathy with a very short duration of the disease should be excluded, since they may be suffering from acutely developing diabetic neuropathies, e.g., "insulin neuritis," which may be rapidly reversible. This form of neuropathy would add bias to any evaluation of treatment effects. This is particularly true in trials of pain treatment, since mixing acute and chronic painful neuropathies may lead to erroneous conclusions. For this reason, trials dealing with painful neuropathies should include only patients whose symptoms last for longer than six months [1351].

Relevant Outcome Measures in Controlled Clinical Trials

Problems Related to the Use of Surrogate Variables

Measures employed in the diagnosis and staging of diabetic neuropathy are frequently used to quantitate drug effects in clinical trials. These are, however, surrogate variables for relevant clinical endpoints. Surrogate endpoints are defined as laboratory measurements or physical signs used as a substitute measured rapidly, with good precision, sensitivity, and specificity, which reflect a clinically meaningful endpoint that measures directly how a patient feels, functions, or survives [1352]. Changes in a surrogate endpoint induced by a certain treatment are expected to reflect changes of a meaningful clinical endpoint in the same direction and to the same extent. However, this may only apply in monocausal pathogenetic sequences in which the reversal of a certain biochemical defect at which the treatment is targeted is assumed to be effective at any given stage of a disease. To be a reliable surrogate variable for a clinical outcome, the effect of the intervention on the surrogate must predict with sufficient certainty the clinical outcome and the correlation must be causal and not merely statistical [1353]. Models for a more rational approach for the use of surrogate variables have been proposed by Boissel et al. [1354]. Surrogate markers may not specifically define diabetic neuropathy, and at least among older patients a significant number may develop impaired tendon reflexes due to other causes besides diabetes [1355]. Due to their better reproducibility, the advantages of these surrogate markers are the smaller number of patients required and the shorter duration of treatment needed to observe significant differences. However, it is possible for incorrect conclusions to be drawn, because there are only a few studies indicating that certain surrogate markers have a clinical or prognostic meaning for the development of stage 3 diabetic polyneuropathy. Young et al. [1356] have demonstrated that the cumulative incidence of neuropathic foot ulcers over four years was 20% in patients with a vibration perception threshold (VPT) above 25 V compared to those with lower thresholds (4% for a VPT between 15 and 25 V and 3% for a VPT lower than 15 V). In a one-year study of 1035 diabetic patients with polyneuropathy, VPT, age, and the Michigan diabetic polyneuropathy score for muscle strength and reflexes were significant independent predictors for first foot ulceration, which developed at an incidence of 7.2% [1357]. Since proven prognostic importance of a symptom, sign, measurement, etc., does not necessarily imply that modifying this symptom, etc., may influence the long-term rate of complications, at least one decisive study such as the DCCT [1358] should define the predictive value of the various surrogate markers for ultimate clinical endpoints such as neuropathic ulcers or amputations. Reliance on surrogate endpoints, based on deductive conclusions, was shown to harm the patients treated, e.g., suppressing ventricular premature beats with antiarrhythmic drugs such as flecainide (CAST trial) and D-sotalol (SWORD trial) [1359,1360]), increasing vitamin concentrations with high doses of vitamins, e.g., vitamin E [1361] or β-carotene [1362] to prevent lung cancer, or increasing bone density with sodium fluoride to prevent fractures [1363].

Surrogate endpoints may be useful in phase II proof-of-concept trials to identify agents that are biologically active, thus facilitating the decision to design and conduct large trials with clinically meaningful outcomes. In phase III trials the primary endpoint should be the true clinically relevant outcome [1353,1354]. Clinically relevant endpoints for patients include (1) development of clinically manifest diabetic polyneuropathy, (2) progression of an already existing neuropathy, mirrored by the incidence of diabetic foot ulcers and amputations, (3) development of insensitive or painful feet, (4) reduction of pain or other debilitating symptoms, and (5), possibly, the gain in quality-adjusted life years, because quality of life is reduced in diabetic patients with polyneuropathy. With the exception of studies for the treatment of pain, such studies will require large numbers of patients and very long treatment or observation periods. In other areas of internal medicine, studies of an analogous design were performed with true outcome measures, e. g., thrombolysis in myocardial infarction, cholesterol-lowering therapy for prevention of myocardial infarction, angiotensin-converting enzyme inhibitor treatment of diabetic nephropathy, and digitalis trials. Exceptions may be acceptable if the validity of a surrogate variable has already been rigorously established. According to a model of the consequences of disease developed by the WHO in 1980, the aforementioned variables for diagnosing and staging diabetic neuropathy, which are also frequently used for quantitating therapeutic effects, are classified as measures of impairment (organ dysfunction or abnormalities of body structure). Much more important are measures of disability (the patient's functional performance) and of handicap (social disadvantages induced by impairment and disability) [1365]. The latter two categories have only rarely been included in pharmacologic studies of diabetic neuropathy.

Clinical Measures

The NIS-LL (Neuropathy Impairment Score in the Lower Limbs)—a modification of the NDS, the Neuropathy Disability Score, originally introduced by Dyck [1366] —quantitates neurologic function and is recommended for use in pharmaceutical trials [1367]. It represents deficits in polyneuropathies of the lower limbs, the maximum score being 88; it is weighted towards muscle examination, which contributes with 75% to the total score. Its advantage is that it only uses methods (touch pressure, pinprick, vibration, reflex, and joint position) that form part of a routine neurologic examination. Since neither autonomic disturbances nor erectile dysfunction nor acute and chronic painful symptoms are included, it can be used only as a part of the whole armamentarium to quantitate diabetic neuropathy. The score has not yet been shown to predict ultimate clinical outcomes.

Electrodiagnostic Measures

The Peripheral Nerve Society (PNS) [1368] has recently reassessed the suitability and appropriateness of putative endpoints to be employed in clinical trials. Neuropathic symptoms reducing quality of life are classified as being relevant; however, changes should be accompanied by at least the smallest changes of the NIS that physicians can detect, i.e., two points. This change of the NIS corresponds to a change in peroneal motor nerve conduction velocity (NCV) of 2.2 m/s, median sensory NCV of 1.9 m/s, and sural sensory amplitude of 3.8 μV. From these correlations it is deduced that if electrodiagnostic measures change by a certain magnitude, this change will be meaningful [1369]. The advantages of using electrodiagnostic measures are obvious: they are objective, sensitive, specific, reproducible, and widely available. However, they represent only the function of a small part of the peripheral nerve, their specificity for detecting *diabetic* neuropathy is relatively low, and the intraindividual variation of certain variables (amplitudes) is high. Electrodiagnostic measures may be influenced by external and internal factors such as electrode location, limb temperature, electrolyte concentration, or glucose concentration [1370].

Quantitative Sensory Testing

To characterize and quantitate cutaneous sensation, the PNS [1371] has proposed measuring thresholds of touch, pressure, vibration, coolness, warmth, and pain induced by various stimuli (heat, cold, mechanical). Methods used for quantitation include the method of limits, threshold tracking, titration, and the two-alternative forced-choice method. Quantitative sensory testing (QST) measurements are highly sensitive, simple, noninvasive, and nonaversive; they allow precise control of stimulus intensity and testing procedures; unlike electrodiagnostic measures they may help differentiate between deficits of small and large fibers, and they are appropriate for screening of large samples of patients for epidemiologic purposes or for inclusion into studies. On the other hand, important drawbacks are that they are influenced by alertness, mood, concentration, ambient noise, their relatively high intraindividual variability, a lack of standardization, and the long time needed to perform a complete assessment [1346].

Morphologic Analysis

Symptoms, signs, and neurophysiologic findings correlate with the degree of morphologic changes in peripheral nerves [1372]. Some parameters determined from sural nerve biopsy, like myelinated fiber density and the histogram of diameters, are accurate and reproducible. However, this technique is invasive, and there is little information as to whether neuropathologic measures predict the severity and course of diabetic polyneuropathy [1368]. Moreover, the rate of residual symptoms following nerve biopsy is not negligible [1373], at least not in patients with peripheral neuropathy, so it may be difficult to obtain approval from the institutional review boards.

Autonomic Function Tests

Measures of cardiovascular autonomic function tests (AFTs) based on changes in heart rate variability (HRV) may be used as markers of vagal and sympathetic dysfunction. Impairment of tests that are part of the classical test battery is associated with increased mortality in diabetic patients [1349]. Independent of the underlying disease, impairment of cardiovascular autonomic function is associated with increased mortality, e. g., in patients with alcoholic or nonalcoholic liver cirrhosis [1349,1374] or after myocardial infarction [1375, 1376]. This does not imply that a short-term improvement of cardiovascular reflex tests in diabetic patients treated with, e. g., α-lipoic acid, ACE inhibitors, or aldose reductase inhibitors will improve the prognosis, which must be proven using ultimate endpoints in long-term trials. Regrettably, neither of the two large scale long-term trials (DCCT [1358] and UKPDS [1377]) has evaluated clinical outcomes concomitantly with the aforementioned surrogate endpoints, leaving unanswered the question of whether influencing the surrogate is associated with improvement of neuropathic symptoms, deficits, or ultimate clinical outcomes, e. g., foot ulcers, amputations, and death.

Symptomatic Pain Treatment

Investigation of symptomatic treatment requires clear definitions of complaints and validated, accepted, and widely used instruments of pain assessment [1378, 1379]. Changes in pain expressed as the percentage of the maximum possible treatment effect, not absolute pain quantities, should be used as outcome measure. What should be regarded as real treatment success is a matter of definition: a 50% reduction in pain intensity has been proposed as a clinically relevant change [1380]. This variable cannot be substituted by other surrogate markers. Several clinical studies show that: (1) the course of pain over six months did not correlate with electrophysiologic results (e. g., NCV or motor and sensory nerve amplitudes) [1381]; (2) the function of small unmyelinated fibers as reflected by both pain and thermal thresholds, which deteriorated over time, did not correlate with the disappearance or persistence of pain [1382]; (3) morphologic changes of myelinated fiber density in the sural nerve correlated only with the changes in both motor and sensory NCV and amplitudes but not with any QST measure [1383]; (4) neurophysiologic measurements of the sural nerve did not allow any conclusion on sensory deficits [1384]; and (5), although the clinical neurologic examination correlated with a score derived from sensory symptoms, the combination of neurologic and neurophysiologic variables correlated only weakly with sensory symptoms such as tingling and numbness, but not with pain [1385].

Natural History

Due to the possibility that treatment within a clinical trial may only delay the progression of, but not improve preselected endpoints, the difference to be evaluated after the close of the study may depend on the natural course of these endpoints in the placebo-treated group. For this reason, knowledge of the natural course of symptoms, signs, psychophysical tests, and electrophysiologic measurements is crucial to determine, first, the number of patients needed for a therapeutic trial, and second, the time needed to achieve a therapeutic effect that is both statistically significant and clinically relevant.

Clinical polyneuropathy: The development of nerve damage is strongly related to metabolic control [1386–1396]. In population-based studies the overall incidence of distal symmetric polyneuropathy was 6.1 per 100 person-years in type 2 and 2.8 per 100 person-years in type 1 diabetic patients, derived from a six-year incidence of 15% with a relative risk of 2.6 in poorly controlled patients compared to those who were fairly well controlled [1389].

Painful symptoms: Changes in pain over time depend on the acuity of their appearance. Chronic pain does not change over years, while extreme pain of acute onset will subside within one or two years [1351,1397]. Pain due to acute, painful neuropathy, which is distinguished from other forms of neuropathy, disappears along with mental depression, weight loss, and impotence within 10 months [1398,1399]. Pain in painful mononeuropathy or radiculopathy will decrease over time [1400,1401]. By contrast, symptoms of chronic painful peripheral symmetric polyneuropathy may not change over the course of years [1381,1402–1404]. This seems to be at variance with the study of Benbow et al. [1382] who after 3.6 years observed a significant decrease in a pain index for 33 of 50 patients who could be followed up. However, only patients with a short duration of symptoms at the outset recovered completely.

QST: In type 2 diabetic patients vibration as well as pressure, warm, and cold thresholds deteriorated significantly by 7–36% after two years. The warm perception threshold increased by 0.9 °C and the cold perception threshold by 0.8 °C. Twenty-three out of 77 patients reached the risk stage for development of diabetic foot syndrome [1405]. MacLeod estimated the annual rate of deterioration for VPT on the great toe to be 0.4 V in healthy subjects and 2.5 V in those with diabetic neuropathy.

Electrodiagnostic measures: In diabetic patients NCV decreases usually by less than 1 m/s per year (Table 5.**32**) [1386,1391], sometimes not reaching a level of clinically meaningful change [1406]. It seems prudent not to include in studies patients with greatly reduced NCV, e. g., less than 30 m/s in the lower limbs, in order to exclude patients with far advanced forms of neuropathy in whom improvement is improbable.

Cardiovascular autonomic function tests (AFTs): In type 1 diabetic patients who had normal measurements at baseline, heart rate differences during deep breathing decreased by 1.02 ± 0.47 per year in a study over a decade [1407]. In general the heart rate difference during deep breathing decreases by 0–1.9/min per year [1408–1414] (Table 5.**33**), and the Valsalva ratio declines by 0.014–0.060 per year [1406,1408, 1410, 1413, 1414] (Table 5.**34**). These relatively slowly developing changes underline the need for long-term

Table 5.32 Changes in motor and sensory nerve conduction velocities (MNCV, SNCV) after five years in conventionally treated type 1 diabetic patients in the DCCT [1386]

	Primary prevention group	Secondary intervention group
Median MNCV (m/s)	−1.05 (−4.60 to +1.10)	−1.00 (−3.85 to +2.05)
Median SNCV (m/s)	−2.10 (−6.90 to +2.85)	−2.20 (−7.00 to +2.30)
Peroneal MNCV (m/s)	−2.70 (−4.90 to +0.30)	−0.70 (−3.50 to +2.00)
Sural SNCV (m/s)	−2.80 (−7.60 to +1.50)	−1.35 (−5.30 to +3.20)

Table 5.33 Natural decline per year of heart rate variation (inspiration/expiration difference) during deep breathing in diabetic patients

Change	Author
−1.9	Jacobsen et al. [1408]
−1.0	Sampson et al. [1407]
−1.2	Jermendy et al. [1409]
−1.0	Reichard et al. [1410]
−0.4	Quadri et al. [1411]
±0	Vanninen et al. [1412]
−0.7	Levitt et al. [1413]
−1.5	DCCT [1414]

Table 5.34 Natural course of the lying-to-standing ratio and the Valsalva ratio in diabetic patients (decline per year). The max/min (30/15) ratio was calculated using the longest and the shortest R-R intervals after standing up (around the 15th and the 30th heart beat) [1411]

Variable	Change	Author
Max/min 30:15 ratio	No significant change in 5 years	Quadri et al. [1411]
Valsalva ratio	−0.055	Jakobsen et al. [1408]
	−0.020	Reichard et al. [1410]
	−0.014	Levitt et al. [1413]
	−0.015	DCCT [1414]
	−0.060	Laudadio & Sima [1406]

trials using techniques with high precision and reproducibility to allow significant differences between treatment groups to be demonstrated.

Sample Size and Duration of Trials

The number of patients needed in pharmacologic studies to reach meaningful and significant results at the completion of a study depends on (1) the success rates in both the active drug and placebo-treated groups, (2) the absolute difference in success rates between the two groups, and (3) the statistical power specified at the outset, i. e., the probability of detecting a difference between the two arms of the study at a certain prespecified level of significance.

The absolute difference in success rates depends on the duration of treatment, the severity of neuropathy that defines inclusion in the trial, the natural course of endpoints, and the rate of improvement possible at all; e. g., morphologic changes may need a very long time to show any difference between placebo and active treatment arms. Prospective studies with intensified insulin therapy in type 1 diabetic patients [1358, 1395,1396,1415] as well as trials evaluating the effects of combined pancreas-kidney transplantation [1416–1418] suggest that the longer the diabetes duration and the more advanced the neuropathy, the longer will be the treatment time needed to identify any significant difference between groups. It is possible that stages of predominantly structural destruction may not be reversible at all. For this reason, Pfeifer and Schumer [1342] recommended that only patients with mild to moderate degrees of neuropathy should be included, and that these patients should be observed over three to five years to find clinically relevant changes.

Regarding statistical significance, negative results from a large number of small trials by no means prove inefficacy of the treatment under study, because the number of patients investigated was so small that the power of the statistical tests used was too low to detect small, but nonetheless real treatment effects [1419]. A meta-analysis of randomized parallel-group, placebo-controlled clinical trials with negative results showed that only 16% of the studies had a sufficient statistical power of more than 80% to detect a relative difference of 25% between the placebo arm and the actively treated patients, and only 36% of all studies had sufficient power to detect a difference of 50% between the two groups [1420]. For this reason, it is absolutely mandatory to precalculate the sample size needed to detect significant differences. Formulas and examples have been published by Campbell et al. [1421].

One requirement in calculating the number of patients needed in such studies is knowledge of the effect size that may be clinically meaningful. This implies that the clinical impact of the measured variable is known, which is not the case when surrogate variables are used. Cavaliere and coworkers [1341] showed that the median number of patients in studies to treat diabetic neuropathy is 30 (range 9–259), which is too small to demonstrate significant effects. Dyck and coworkers [1422] have calculated the sample size needed based on the follow-up results of the Rochester Diabetic Neuropathy Study using a composite score as the measure of treatment effects. This score includes electrophysiologic variables, VPT and HRV, and, assuming that a treatment effect of two points would be clinically meaningful, one would need 68 patients in each group to find a significant difference (two-tailed test, $P < 0.05$) with a probability of 90%. If treatment may only halt the progression of neuropathy without improving it, the study period must be lengthened to 3.7 years.

Using the annual incidence of diabetic foot ulcers as a real endpoint, Nicolucci et al. [1423] have calculated that 3000 patients have to be treated for five years to demonstrate efficacy of an aldose reductase inhibitor in reducing the incidence by 50%. This number was based on the following assumptions: (1) the annual incidence of foot ulcers in diabetic patients is 0.8% [1424], (2) an aldose reductase inhibitor may reduce the incidence by 50%, and (3) $\alpha = 0.05$ and $1-\beta = 0.80$.

With regard to the sample size needed in trials focusing on neuropathic pain, Moore et al. [1425] argued that group sizes in the range of 30–60 are required to have a 90% probability of obtaining a statistically significant effect, but nearly 500 patients per group are needed to achieve clinical relevance. These authors conclude that credible estimates of clinical efficacy are only likely to result from large trials or from pooling multiple trials of conventional (small) size.

Reproducibility

Numerous studies have reported the day-to-day reproducibility of electrophysiologic measures, QST, and AFTs. In large-scale multicenter studies the coefficients of variation were lowest for electrophysiologic measurements, slightly higher for VPT, and highest for AFTs (ranging from about 5% to 25%). Thus, while the intraindividual variability may be reasonably low, the intercenter variability may be quite high [1426–1430] (Tables 5.**35**, 5.**36**). This in turn leads to an additional increase in the number of patients needed to obtain significant treatment effects. Given equal probability and statistical power in a clinical trial, the number of patients to be included must increase if either the expected treatment difference will be small or the variability of the measurement is high. Hence, at a given probability of $\alpha = 0.05$ and a power of $1-\beta = 0.90$, the numbers in each group of patients must be 42 to detect a difference in NCV of 2.5 m/s, 175 patients are needed to detect a significant difference between amplitudes, and 550 patients are necessary to detect significant differences in VPT [1427]. With regard to the magnitude of the treatment effect, it is obvious that the number of patients in each group needed to detect a difference in NCV must be higher if the difference is smaller; e. g., the numbers required to detect a difference of 2 m/s or 3 m/s have been calculated at 262 and 116, respectively [1341]. Regrettably, the respective numbers of trials fulfilling these criteria were 2 (5%) and zero [1342].

To calculate the number of patients required it is therefore mandatory to know exactly the reproducibility of measurements used. Maser and colleagues [1431] showed that interobserver agreement varied depending on what was being investigated, e.g., sensory symptoms, sensation, or reflexes. Accordingly,

Table 5.**35** Coefficients of variation (combining intraindividual, interindividual, and intercenter variability) of various surrogate variables used in trials for treatment of diabetic neuropathy

Variables	Sundkvist et al. [1429]	Santiago et al. [1428]	Valensi et al. [1426]	Bril et al. [1427]
VPT	8.7–29.7	14.8–22.2	41.0	–
Median SNCV	1.6–12.7	5.4–9.1	19.6	3–4[a]
Median MNCV	2.9–9.5	3.9–7.2	11.7	3–4[a]
Sural SNAP	8.9–42.8	28.3–35.6	106.6	11–17[a]
Peroneal MA	13.4–80.4	19.6–32.8	87.9	9–15[a]

VPT, vibration perception threshold; M/SNCV, motor/sensory nerve conduction velocity; SNAP, sensory nerve action potential; MA, motor amplitude
[a] Triplicate measurements

Table 5.**36** Coefficients of variation (%) for autonomic function tests in diabetic patients

Variable	CV (%)	Author
30:15 ratio	1.5–18.1	Sundkvist et al. [1429]
Expiration/inspiration ratio	2.4–7.2	Sundkvist et al. [1429]
Valsalva ratio	3.8–24.4	Sundkvist et al. [1429]
Change in SBP to standing up	7±2	Ward and Kenny [1430]

SBP: systolic blood pressure

the reproducibility of the NSS is lower than that of the NDS, with an intraclass correlation coefficient of > 0.95 for the NDS but only of > 0.75 for the NSS [1432]. These results are corroborated by an Italian group: the coefficient of variation for symptom assessment with a questionnaire was 8–32 %, that for the neurologic examination 0–6.5 %, while for VPT at the great toe it was 4.4–28 % [1433]. If a tuning fork (Rydel-Seiffer, 128 Hz) was used by the same investigator, the intra-individual coefficient of variation in diabetic patients was 8.4 % [1434] in one study and 24 % in another [1435]. Therefore, clinical and psychophysical tests should be performed always at the same site on the patient's body and by the same investigator. The difference between the two great toes was more than 30 % in 24 % of all diabetic patients studied [1436]. Generally, intraindividual variabilities, either cross-sectionally between contralateral sites or longitudinally, are more pronounced in diabetic patients than in normal subjects. In diabetic patients the coefficients of variation of AFTs may also be higher, but this was not observed in all published studies [1437]. The large variability in psychophysical testing can be partially explained by changes in attention and ability to cooperate, but very large intraindividual variances may be an indication of feigned results [1438].

Factors influencing variation between centers may be differences in patient characteristics, the equipment used for measurement, the ability to use the equipment, varying skills and experience of technicians involved in measuring, changing the operators during a study, and differences between evaluation procedures used in different centers. Ideally, the bias due to all these factors can be reduced by rigid adherence to centralized training, identical equipment, a ban on changing operators, and centralized evaluation of test results. When interpreting individual values over time, measurement imprecision, which is inversely related to the absolute number of readings (i. e.; it is greater, the fewer readings there are) must be taken into account. Two values consecutively measured in the same patient can be judged with reasonable certainty to be biologically different only if the difference is larger than the coefficient of variation of this method in the given range of measurements multiplied by 2.6 [1439]; e. g., if NCV is 37 m/s at the first measurement and 43 m/s at the second measurement, the difference of 6 m/s can be interpreted as being a real change because it exceeds the product of the coefficient of variation 0.05×37 m/s $\times 2.6$, which is 4.8 m/s.

Whether the absolute difference in mean conduction velocities in groups of patients over time represents a relevant change is still under discussion. The formula given above does not seem to be appropriate to solving this problem. Dyck and O'Brien argue that the mean differences between treated and untreated groups of patients do not need to be larger than the reproducibility of the measurement, assuming that the variability in parallel group trials is identical in both groups [1369].

Factors Confounding Treatment Effects

A variety of confounding factors, known or unknown, during or after the completion of a study, may be superimposed on the true pharmacologic effects [1440]. Randomization in randomized, controlled trials (RCTs) is believed to distribute these factors evenly to the placebo and active treatment arms so that the difference observed between drug and placebo treatments can be ascribed to the true pharmacologic effect of the agent under study. For this reason, distinguishing true from perceived placebo effects in placebo-controlled clinical trials is not mandatory as long as the placebo effects are identical in both groups. However, this may not always be the case [1440].

The most impressive placebo effects are observed during treatment of pain [1441] where more than the often cited one-third of all placebo-treated patients may report pain relief [1442]. This was corroborated by a survey of 38 placebo-controlled studies for the treatment of painful diabetic neuropathy, which revealed that in 45 % (median, range 20–90 %) of all patients treated with placebo, pain was unspecifically reduced. The intensity of this placebo response may vary between different studies [1443] but shows positive correlation with pain intensity and inversely related to the duration of treatment [1444]. The apparent magnitude of the specific effect in RCTs may be modified either positively (e. g., by negative suggestion) or negatively (by positive suggestion) [1445].

The absolute amount and the direction of the placebo (nocebo) effect is determined by complex interactions between the patient, the placebo (drugs, applications, procedures), and the physician [1440, 1446]. In a given patient, unspecific effects may be augmented by pain intensity, positive expectation, the patient's attitudes towards his health, the disease, and the treating doctor, the way he is kept informed by the treating physician, the nurses, his family, what his treatment means to him, his conditioning by earlier treatment effects, positive suggestion, treatment experiences, and his degree of anxiety. Consequently, large unspecific and hence small treatment effects are observed if (1) the real drug is well known or assumed to be very potent [1445], (2) "active" placebos are used which may imitate effects or side effects of the study drug, (3) the patient is conditioned by earlier experience, or (4) he is positively influenced by the treating physician.

Attributes of the placebo drug which may increase unspecific effects include the way the drug is given, its assumed mechanism of action, its color, its impressiveness (i. e., its power to evoke awe), its obvious plausibility and credibility, and its costs [1442].

Physicians may induce higher unspecific effects if they have the appropriate clothing, habits, gestures, knowledge, positive attitudes towards the substance investigated and the patient treated, and their image of being well-known experts in the field.

Sometimes study design is compromised because it is impossible to conduct truly double-masked studies owing to typical effects that occur in many patients treated with the active drug, e. g., using tricyclic antidepressants, capsaicin, nerve growth factor, acupuncture, or transcutaneous electrical nerve stimulation. Sometimes the design of an "active" placebo may help to minimize this problem [1447].

The continuing use of placebo in studies for the treatment of various diseases may no longer be acceptable, since the declaration of Helsinki (1964) recommends that "every patient—including those of a control group —should be assured of the best proven diagnostic and therapeutic method," which, if already present, may preclude the use of placebo in some situations. Due to the differing interests of pharmaceutical companies, doctors, consumers, and health regulatory authorities, this is a matter of heated debate [1448–1450]. In trials of diabetic neuropathy, consequently, all patients included in studies should have their metabolic control improved, since this is the only generally accepted long-term approach to prevention, retardation, and, possibly, regression of diabetic micro-angiopathy and neuropathy. This requirement will become more important in the future than in the past because studies will last for years, not just for months, and for these long periods it may not be justifiable to neglect improvement of metabolic control. In pain treatment studies better metabolic control may reduce painful symptoms of diabetic neuropathy [1451] or change the perception of pain [1452], although this is still the subject of controversy [1453,1454]. Nevertheless, the requirement for improvement in glycemic control in all patients receiving active or placebo treatment may increase the need for larger numbers of patients to be included in such studies. Moreover, in future, treating symptoms such as pain may require control groups to be treated with drugs known from large RCTs or meta-analyses to be effective, rather than with placebo. In this situation, the aim of a study may sometimes be to show less severe or less frequent unexpected adverse events rather than superior efficacy.

Besides placebo effects and improvement in metabolic control, other time-dependent changes may occur in both groups: the investigator's experience in the use of the technical equipment will increase, the technique of interviewing patients may change, and the patients' familiarity with the psychophysical methods used may influence the results. Lifestyle changes, induced by increasing awareness of health problems during a study, e. g., improving metabolic control, abstaining from nicotine or alcohol misuse and the use of potentially neurotoxic drugs, taking additional vitamins, and changing both the quality and the quantity of fat consumption, may be more pronounced in patients with higher compliance to drug treatment.

Sometimes patient recruitment is by advertisements in local newspapers, specialized clinics or university hospitals, or, increasingly, via the Internet. This may presumably lead to entering patients into a study at the time when their complaints are at their worst. This effect may be exaggerated by choosing inclusion criteria that require quite high scores for pain. Subsequent pain scores are therefore lower due to biological variability, measurement errors, the natural course, and chance, since it is more likely that symptoms change from the 98% percentile to the 97% than to the 99% percentile. This tendency of extreme symptoms or findings to turn toward the individual's more typical state is known as the regression to the mean. The impact of this regression towards the mean can be minimized by using a relatively long run-in period without any therapeutic intervention but with multiple testing [1455], which may cause ethical problems.

Measures of Relevant Treatment Effects

Problems arising from the definition of treatment effects are divided into at least two distinct areas: the definition of treatment effects, and the appropriateness of presentation, which allows results to be translated to patients treated outside of studies.

Definitions of Clinically Relevant Treatment Effects

Clinically relevant success of drug treatment in studies of diabetic neuropathy is difficult to define and is therefore the subject of some controversy. The most frequently used technique, which is to investigate surrogate endpoints, is understandable but problematic [1354]. A meaningful change in NCV is defined as one which correlates with the minimum unequivocally detectable and relevant change of neuropathic symptoms and deficits. A change in motor NCV in the ulnar nerve by 4.6 m/s, median nerve by 2.5 m/s, and peroneal nerve by 2.2 m/s, on average by 2.9 m/s, was equivalent to a change in the NDS by two points. In a group of type 1 diabetic patients these changes were smaller: a change in peroneal motor NCV by 2.0 m/s and an average of 2.3 m/s, combining the ulnar, median, and peroneal nerves, equaled a change in the NDS by two points. Similar equations can be formulated for the changes in the NSS [1456]. NCV measurements, however, may fluctuate and reflect only the function of the remaining or, hopefully, regenerating large, myelinated fibers.

Internal consistency is an important criterion to check for plausibility of treatment-related changes; changes observed in different nerves do not need to show exactly the same magnitude, but the direction should be concordant. It is unclear how to interpret discordant changes of electrophysiologic measurements,

e. g., if NCV in one out of four nerves increases, two remain stable, and one decreases. To draw reliable conclusions about treatment effects, different studies using the same drug may be examined by looking for the patterns of changes, which should be similar. Two studies with the aldose reductase inhibitor tolrestat showed discordant results regarding the development of pain and paresthesias: in both studies pain decreased in both the placebo- and the drug-treated groups, whereas paresthesias improved during drug treatment in one study and during placebo treatment in the other [1457,1458]. A meta-analysis of aldose reductase inhibitor studies [1423] revealed a large variability between study results with regard to the composition of improved nerves and the magnitude of improvement in the same nerve. Internal consistency was lacking in 50% of all studies. A large variability of treatment effects within the same nerve in different studies may indicate that different populations of patients were studied, e. g., in different stages of neuropathy with different chances of any improvement. The variability of improvement between nerves in the same study may be due not only to measurement errors and changes by chance in small groups of patients, but also to different stages of neuropathy in different regions of the body, e. g., nerves in the upper part may well improve during therapy, whereas those in the lower part may not.

Presentation of Treatment Effects

The relative benefit of an active treatment over a control treatment is commonly expressed as the *relative risk reduction (RRR)* or the *odds* ratio:

	Improved (*n*)	Not improved (*n*)
Active treatment (*n*)	30	50
Placebo treatment (*n*)	5	45

Proportion of persisting disease in active treatment group: 50/80 = 0.625
Proportion of persisting disease in placebo group: 45/50 = 0.900
Relative risk (ratio of risks in treated to untreated patients): 0.625/0.900 = 0.694
Relative reduction of risk of persisting disease (RRR) (1–relative risk in treated patients/ relative risk in untreated patients):
1–(0.625/0.900) = 1–0.694 = 0.31 (31%)
Odds ratio for successful treatment in actively treated patients:
30/50 : 5/45 = 5.4
(i. e., the chance of being effectively treated is 5.4 times that of placebo-treated patients).

In this example and hence in all clinical trials when the prevalence of a certain disease, dysfunction or symptom is 100% in both the active treatment group and the placebo arm (defined by the inclusion criteria), the RRR reflects adequately the efficacy of an investigated drug in this group. Large RRRs, however, do not necessarily imply that a certain treatment may be justified for use in the population where the prevalence of a certain disease is less than 100%. Since RRRs may not mirror the real importance of a therapeutic intervention and odds ratios are not easy to understand for practicing physicians, it would be advantageous to have a number that demonstrates how effective a certain treatment will be. The calculation of the absolute risks and the absolute risk reduction (ARR) takes into account the prevalence of the risk, and by computing the number of patients needed to be treated (NNT) to obtain one successfully treated patient provides a figure which is easy to apply in clinical practice. It is defined as the difference between the absolute risk in treated patients and the absolute risk in untreated patients, i. e., ARR = abs. $risk_{untreated}$ – abs. $risk_{treated}$; using the numbers from the example above, it is 0.900–0.625 = 0.275. NNT is the reciprocal of this number, i.e., 1/0.275 = 3.64 [1459,1460]. A nomogram to facilitate the computation of this very important figure has been published [1461].

Some drawbacks must be mentioned which compromise the usefulness of this number to compare or combine treatment effects of different studies:

1. The mean NNT of a sample of studies is not the average of all weighted NNTs of these studies but is derived as the reciprocal of the arithmetic mean of the weighted absolute risk reductions.
2. In most instances differing periods of time and different endpoints or surrogate variables used do not allow direct comparison of studies. It is not possible to extrapolate NNTs beyond the time point investigated and to "normalize" NNTs from different studies to one common duration of treatment.
3. In all cases the 95% confidence interval for the NNT should be given, because in studies with small numbers of patients NNT is a rather crude estimate of the efficacy of the drug used. However, the formula for the calculation of the confidence interval given by Sackett et al. [1462] may not be appropriate for cross-over studies.
4. The absolute number of NNT does not answer the question whether a treatment of proven efficacy will be justified in clinical practice. This can only be decided if prevalence, severity, prognosis, efficacy, side effects, cultural influences on therapy, and the cost of treatment are taken into account.
5. NNTs may be overestimated if placebo and drug effects change in the same direction. To use NNTs correctly it is important to look for the appropriate comparator. In most cases this will not be a placebo treatment but another drug less effective than the new one. Thus, it has to be computed how many

patients must be transferred from the old to the new treatment and what effect can be expected from this change [1463].

To judge whether treatment results may justify the transfer to daily practice, it may be necessary to estimate the degree of heterogeneity between studies, which should not exceed the degree expected by chance alone [1464]. Groups of patients treated in different studies may in fact be suspected to be heterogeneous if the RRR differs by more than 20% (e. g., in the first study it may be 40%, in the second study less than 20%), or if the difference between the confidence intervals lying furthest apart is larger than 5% (e. g., the lowest risk reduction in study 1 may be 30% and the highest risk reduction in study 2 less than 25%). The confidence intervals can be computed according to Morris and Gardner [1465]. If there is heterogeneity between studies, it will be more difficult to generalize results from meta-analyses. Thompson and Pocock have proposed methods to reduce this problem of heterogeneity [1466].

Sometimes clinical studies that evaluated identical or different drugs can be compared using the "effect size," thus excluding the influence of varying placebo effects [1467]. It is defined as: $(M_{placebo} - M_{active})/SD_{placebo}$, $M_{placebo}$ representing for example the mean value of pain scores in the placebo group, M_{active} the mean value in the drug-treated group, and $SD_{placebo}$ the standard deviation of the placebo-treated group. Confidence intervals should be given and may be computed as proposed by Gardner and Altman [1468]. If mean values and standard errors are not available the effect size can be calculated as $t \times \sqrt{(1/N_{placebo} + 1/N_{active})}$ when N is the number of observations and t is the value of the t-statistics. To be relevant, the effect size should exceed 2, i. e., the difference between the placebo effect and the active drug effect should be more than two standard deviations. Improvements have been proposed by Sharp et al. [1469].

If multiple statistical tests are performed in the same sample of patients, which is the case in almost all studies, the null hypothesis will be rejected too often, leading to an inflated number of type 1 errors (the erroneous assumption of a "significant" difference between the two groups compared). If 100 tests are performed with a nominal probability of a type 1 error of $\alpha = 0.01$, then the global probability of getting at least one falsely significant result is 63% ($1 - 0.99^{100} = 63\%$); with $\alpha = 0.05$ the probability increases to > 99% [1470]. The Bonferroni method (nominal probability of a single test = global probability divided by the number of tests performed) will effectively reduce the erroneously high number of significant results. This method is, however, very conservative and may in itself lead to false adherence to the null hypothesis when differences really exist. The Bonferroni-Holm modification will reduce this problem [1471].

These rules of thumb may help as a first orientation but are no longer considered to be adequate methods to deal with the problem of multiple testing [1472], e. g., multiple analyses of variances may help circumvent these problems. This problem will often arise if, either at the end of a study or during the trial period, multiple symptoms or measurements between drug-treated and placebo-treated groups are compared.

Statistical Evaluation of RCTs

Adequate evaluation of treatment effects needs only comparisons between contrasting groups at the start and at the end of a study. Testing changes within each group and then comparing *P* values between groups may lead to incorrect conclusions.

The effects may be assessed "as intended" ("as randomized"), "per protocol," and "as treated" ("as received") [1473]. The main difference lies in the way in which these methods deal with the results of noncomplying patients. The term "noncompliance" in this context includes anything which may disturb the treatment to which a patient was randomly assigned, e. g., nonadherence, mistakes, perturbations, intercurrent illness, deviation from treatment design by the patients, protocol violations, withdrawal due to side effects, missing measurements due to any cause, unexpectedly large variability of centers, forgotten tablets, etc.

The "intention-to-treat" analysis, which is recommended as the primary approach to evaluation but is nevertheless used in less than one-half of all trials even in the 1990s [1474], compares the results of two groups of patients as they were randomized according to the study design. It provides information about the size of treatment effects in the typical study patient who was said to follow a certain treatment schedule because he was allocated to this treatment. Therefore, the comparison deals with the allocation to a certain treatment but not with the treatment itself. It reveals whether a drug works under the conditions of use as they are present in this particular study, which may be similar to those in the general patient population where nearly all causes for noncompliance will also exist. It is "use effectiveness," not "method effectiveness" that is analyzed. Method effectiveness (i. e., a certain substance is effective in killing certain bacteria) has to be proven in preceding studies. From the analyses of these foregoing studies, however, it may not be clear whether the use of a certain treatment has the same effect in general practice, since patients in controlled clinical trials may be—and in most cases are—selected, e. g., they differ with regard to compliance from the patients in the whole population.

The "per protocol" analysis compares the results only of those patients who apparently adhered to the protocol, i.e., patients who were identified as having violated the study design are excluded from further analysis and their results are ignored. The question answered is: How large is the difference between the mean result of patients who decided to take the drug and those patients who were to take the control medication. Neither the "as intended" analysis nor the "per protocol" analysis is suitable for providing information on the method effectiveness. The "as intended" analysis may diminish the apparent treatment effect, because noncompliers not taking the effective drug will remain within the group to which they were allocated but do not have any beneficial treatment effect. On the other hand, this may also reduce the apparent incidence of unexpected and severe adverse events. The "per protocol" analysis may augment the treatment effect, because noncompliers are excluded from the analysis whereby a certain subgroup with unknown but unique characteristics may be eliminated, e. g., patients with severe illness. Moreover, the number and severity of unexpected adverse events will apparently decrease, since patients given the active drug who experience severe side effects are more prone to stop taking study medication. They may not reach the end of the study and in this case their results will be discarded. If the patients excluded from the analysis are excluded not by chance but on the basis of a distinct characteristic, then the analysis no longer compares two groups derived from one common source, which is the real background of RCTs, but two distinct groups with different, albeit generally unknown personal traits. If the decision not to take the medication correlates with other features which themselves may influence the course of the disease, e. g., compliance, which may correlate with healthier lifestyle, etc., it may be very difficult to draw any conclusions from such analyses. In most cases it is not possible to ascertain whether the homogeneity of the population has been affected by the exclusion of patients, since the one variable which now may differ between the two groups was not evaluated at the outset. Only if no inhomogeneity is generated, which in fact cannot be guaranteed, will the "per protocol" analysis answer the questions in the same way as the "intent-to-treat" analysis (Table 5.**37**). The statistical power will, however, be reduced because of the smaller number of patients evaluated.

The "as treated" analysis compares the results of groups of patients as they were actually treated, i. e., noncompliers in the drug-treated group are added to the control group not taking active drug. The drawbacks described for the "per protocol" analysis also apply to the "as treated" analysis. Comparisons are made between patients who were allocated to medication and turned out to be compliant and patients who were allocated to placebo medication plus patients of the active-drug-treated group who were noncompliant and therefore excluded from the treatment group. This may confound results in an unforeseeable manner since patients do not change the groups by chance but due to certain characteristic yet unknown features. Patients in the actively treated group are no longer defined by the initial randomization but by other criteria, e. g., severity of disease, compliance, etc., which may correlate to the outcome independently of the allocation to treatment group [1475].

All these methods to evaluate study results can be used in modern RCTs and are valuable tools for analysis so long as their different meanings are appreciated. This may also be true for data evaluated retrospectively in the search for unexpected associations, as long as the problems with retrospective analysis and multiple comparisons are carefully addressed [1476].

Reporting of RCTs

In general, the effectiveness of a new agent should be proven in at least two studies performed independently in two different institutions—so-called pivotal studies—according to the principle that "science must be reproducible" [1477]. Evidence-based medicine [1462], which so far as possible should rule drug treatment, requires an overview over all randomized clinical trials ever performed with the drug in question. Increasingly, it has become clear that reporting of RCTs in the past has been far from perfect. For this reason, the Standards of Reporting Trials (SORT) and the Asilomar Working Group on Recommendations for Reporting of Clinical Trials in the Biomedical Literature have formulated a consensus statement known as the Consolidated Standards of Reporting Trials (CONSORT) statement [1478]. This statement includes a checklist and a flow diagram. The checklist contains various items all of which should be included in a report, and the flow chart is mandatory to describe the patients' further fate after recruitment for a study. These guidelines will, it is hoped, improve not only the reporting but also the planning and conducting of clinical trials [1479–1481].

Table 5.**37** Differences in the statistical evaluation of the results of RCTs with regard to noncompliers

Analysis	Noncompliers in the active drug-treated group	Apparent treatment effect
"Intent-to-treat"(as randomized)	Are evaluated in the group they were randomized to	Smaller
"Per protocol"	Are excluded from the evaluation	Probably changed
"As treated"(as received)	Are transferred to the placebo-treated group	Probably changed

Problems of Meta-analysis of Trials for the Treatment of Diabetic Neuropathy

Meta-analyses of RCTs add important information but are not the only determinants in the decision making for a given patient's treatment, since tradition, cultural influences, or opinion leaders may also influence the choice of a certain treatment [1482]. Because the retrieval of all relevant studies is of utmost importance, the search for relevant studies must include more than one literature retrieval system and has to use varying search strategies. Neither the sensitivity (the proportion of relevant studies found from among all known randomized controlled studies) nor the precision (the proportion of truly randomized clinical trials found under this label) will be 100%. Although not derived from studies in diabetic neuropathy, the following results may illustrate some of the difficulties: the search in Medline identified 17–82% of all relevant articles (mean 51%) and 32–91% (mean 77%) if only journals represented in Medline were included [1483]. Bias may be introduced in multiple ways [1484]. Evaluation only of published studies and only of those published in English may be misleading [1485]. Studies with negative results are published less frequently than studies yielding positive results [1486]. Presumably 25–50% of all clinical studies ever initiated, in most cases with negative results, are never published [1487]. Financial support from outside the university institutions and multicentric design correlate positively with later publication [1488]. However, corporate funding may not only accelerate the publication of results but also delay dissemination of new results for economical reasons [1489]. This may be more frequent than expected: about 20% of faculty members reported delaying the publication of studies due to corporate interests [1490,1491]. Only 51% (CI 45–57%, range 32–66%) of all published abstracts concerning randomized clinical trials are published at full length, in most cases within the following two years. There was only a weak correlation between "significant" study results and the number of patients included in a study [1492]. To reduce this publication bias the Cochrane Collaboration and other institutions were founded in order to collect both retrospectively and prospectively all randomized clinical trials, published or not [1493,1494]. Apart from negative unpublished results, the multiple publication of positive results and the publication of results in subgroups of patients who are also included in multicenter studies may lead to an erroneously positive picture, e. g., in a meta-analysis of capsaicin studies for the treatment of pain in diabetic neuropathy [1495–1499]. Tests which have not been generally accepted were proposed to test for bias in meta-analyses [1484,1500].

Moreover, studies sometimes lack appropriate design, performance, evaluation, and presentation, which precludes their inclusion in a meta-analytic evaluation. Even in 1990, an overview of 90 reports of randomized studies showed that in 30% it was unclear whether any randomization had been performed. In 41% of all studies statistical evaluation was inappropriate [1501]. For these reasons, criteria have been formulated which may allow the evaluation of study quality [1478,1502], requiring information on randomization, the method used, double-masked investigation, the manner of blinding, and frequency and causes of exclusion from a study [1380,1478]. Thus, not only the conduction, presentation, and evaluation of studies, but also meta-analysis itself has become the focus of scientific interest [1503,1504].

Some caveats should be borne in mind: meta-analytic techniques using randomized clinical studies do not necessarily provide information on the most effective and cheapest treatment for the individual patient with that patient's unique features of disease, which include severity, course, comorbidity, and clinical nuances [1505,1506]. Analogously to the CONSORT statement for the description of RCTs, the QUOROM statement may help improve the quality of meta-analyses [1507].

Cavaliere et al. have demonstrated specific problems of meta-analyses in studies for the treatment of diabetic neuropathy [1341]. A meta-analysis [1423] of aldose reductase inhibitor treatment showed that the number of studies suitable for meta-analysis was rather small: eight out of 25 studies had to be withdrawn (NCV not measured or not reported in 4 studies, no placebo group included in 1 study, inclusion of a subgroup from a previously published multicenter trial in 1 study, number of patients investigated unclear in 1 study, method of allocation to active or placebo treatment not reported in 1 study), and four more studies were excluded because they had used ponalrestat, an apparently ineffective aldose reductase inhibitor, thus leaving 13 studies for the final evaluation. Such a reduction of studies appropriate for meta-analysis is by no means infrequent. Whether the qualitatively best studies remain to be analyzed further or whether the formally best studies are evaluated is only rarely investigated during the meta-analytic process, since this requires frequent contacts with the authors.

The most important problems identified in meta-analyses [1341] of studies for the treatment of diabetic neuropathy are:(1) method of randomization not reported, (2) exclusion of more than 15% of the originally included patients from the evaluation, (3) failure to estimate the number of patients needed to answer a certain question or (vice versa) (4) failure to compute the statistical power needed to detect a given difference, and (5) no clinically relevant outcome measure. Items 3 and 4, however, can only be calculated if it is known what degree of improvement of a surrogate variable represents a true, clinically relevant advantage for the patient.

Placebo-controlled studies do not provide any information about whether a new therapy is superior to established ones since nonspecific effects may vary between studies. The proportion of patients with more than 50% reduction of pain varies from 7% to 37% in placebo-treated groups and from 5% to 63% in drug-treated groups [1380,1443,1444]. Trials comparing new drugs with established drugs in the treatment of pain in diabetic neuropathy have only rarely been performed, e. g., capsaicin versus amitriptyline [1508], gabapentin versus amitriptyline [1509], and carbamazepine versus the combination of nortriptyline/fluphenazine [1510]. However, these trials were too small to draw any definitive conclusions on the superiority of one particular agent over another in reducing pain.

External Validity of RCT Results

The applicability of study results is generally restricted, since for security reasons all patients with concurrent or earlier disorders or comedications are excluded. In one study for the treatment of diabetic neuropathy, out of 214 patients who were originally thought to be eligible, only 50 patients remained as qualified to participate after application of inclusion/exclusion criteria [1511]. Another rarely mentioned example is given by the DCCT. During the DCCT feasibility study, 1037 patients were selected as candidates, 656 (63%) of whom reached the phase of informed consent; eventually, 278 were admitted to the trial, i. e., only 27% of the originally selected candidates [1512,1513]. This highly selected population most probably is no longer representative of the whole population. Moreover, despite the explicit exclusion criterion of neuropathy requiring treatment, 39% of the 278 patients were diagnosed as having clinical neuropathy [1514].

The high exclusion rate is understandable since the aim of a study is to obtain an effect size large enough to reach clinical significance. This may be possible only if patients with a defined high or low grade of illness are included. Whether these patients should be extremely or only slightly ill depends on the effect under investigation. Whether the treatment effect and the spectrum of side effects, and the ratio of these two, observed during controlled studies will apply to the general population of patients, who often take comedications, suffer from concurrent illnesses, make mistakes in taking their drugs, and have unknown drug-drug interactions, is not clear when drugs are newly introduced. Moreover, the risk/benefit ratio may perhaps vary depending on the severity of symptoms or impairment. Thus, use of a certain drug and toleration of higher risks of unexpected adverse events may be justified if the severity is high, but this may change completely if the severity of disease is low before the start of treatment. To obtain unequivocal effects with a novel pain treatment in diabetic neuropathy, it may be advantageous to include only patients with a very high intensity of pain, e. g., more than 5–6 cm on the horizontal visual analogue scale, to have "space" for a significant reduction, e. g., from 6 cm to less than 3 cm. Such patients, however, are only rarely found: the overwhelming number of patients to be treated may suffer from pain with an intensity of "only" 3 cm. The treatment effect may reduce the pain intensity to 1.5 cm. Whether this reduction within a range of bearable pain may justify the use of a new drug with infrequent but dangerous side effects remains open. In addition, this smaller effect, namely the reduction of pain from "not very severe" to "a bit less severe" will be accompanied by a constant chance of side effects which does not change over the whole range of severity of disease, thus compromising the risk/benefit ratio.

In what way the recruitment of patients (through newspaper advertisements, from a specialized or a general out-patient clinic, or from an unselected population-based group) may influence generalizability is not clear. Presumably groups of study patients are more compliant than the "general," patient which leads Haynes and Dantes to conclude that "it is clearly not reasonable to generalize the results of a study among compliant volunteers to all people with similar disorders since the majority of people will be noncompliant under usual conditions," [1515] which implies that study results are generally better than what might be possible in general practice.

Even if a clinical outcome is adequately investigated methodologically and found to be beneficially influenced, the decision still has to be made what size of effect is needed for an agent to be used in general practice. This threshold, above which treatment will be both indicated and beneficial and below which it should not be used, can be constructed at least from an economic point of view by the formulation of two relevant endpoints: (1) the clinical outcome to be prevented by the treatment, and (2) the unwanted side effects that may occur during treatment. It may then be possible to calculate and compare the costs that are either spared by preventing clinical outcomes or required to treat unwanted side effects. This approach, however, ignores the fact that the quality of treatment effect and side effects cannot be counted only in terms of economic cost.

If the drugs being tested in studies for the treatment of diabetic neuropathy are thought to act via a hypothetical metabolic pathway which may be disturbed in diabetic neuropathy, a dilemma sometimes emerges because the treatment is aimed not at symptomatic improvement but at structural improvement, which may take years to become detectable. On the one hand, these agents would act best in diabetic patients with the least structural defects, i. e., in the very early stages of diabetic neuropathy, stage 0 or stage 1, in which the probability of developing symptomatic neuropathy may be about 30–40%. On the other hand, however, the fact that the spectrum, frequency, and severity of side effects are insufficiently known may preclude the use of a new drug in asymptomatic patients who will not inevitably become ill over time. New drugs may therefore be investigated only in patients already suffering from diabetic neuropathy, which in itself may prevent a meaningful treatment effect due to its advanced stage. This would increase the duration of the study, the number of patients needed to find smaller but nonetheless relevant effects, and the study costs. Although it would be better to test new drugs in the patients who would benefit most, it should be kept in mind that compounds which have been tested during the last years have shown unwanted, and sometimes disastrous, adverse reactions [1516–1520], while the beneficial effects were of only minor significance (Table 5.**38**).

Conclusions

Problems in one or more of the twelve areas described above may explain the relative scarcity of information on effective treatment of diabetic neuropathies. The most important appear to be the inhomogeneity of patients studied (in respect of both the form of neuropathy and the degree of metabolic control), differences in pathogenetic pathways (the relative importance of which may vary between individuals), advanced stages of neuropathy (which may preclude any significant improvement), the use of endpoints with rather large variability between individuals and between centers, the unknown relevance of endpoints used, study durations too short to allow for significant structural improvement, and, potentially, reliance upon pathogenetic hypotheses derived from animal studies [1521], the significance of which for the development of human diabetic neuropathy remain a matter of debate [1522–1525].

Table 5.**38** Serious adverse events in diabetic patients treated with investigational drugs against diabetic polyneuropathy

Agent	Serious adverse events
Sorbinil [1516]	Liver damage, skin hypersensitivity
Tolrestat [1517]	Liver damage
Zenarestat	Renal toxicity
Gangliosides [1518]	Guillain–Barré syndrome
Aminoguanidine [1519]	Liver damage, lupus-like and flu-like syndromes, vasculitis
Nerve growth factor [1520]	Hyperalgesia, myalgia

References

[1] Dyck PJ, Karnes JL, O'Brien PC, et al. Reassessment of tests and criteria for diagnosis and staged severity. Neurology 1992; 42: 1164–70.
[2] Dyck PJ, Davies JL, Litchy WJ, et al. Longitudinal assessment of diabetic polyneuropathy using a composite score in the Rochester Diabetic Neuropathy Study cohort. Neurology 1997; 49: 229–39.
[3] Dyck PJ, Kratz KM, Karnes JL, et al. The prevalence by staged severity of various types of diabetic neuropathy, retinopathy, and nephropathy in a population-based cohort: The Rochester Diabetic Neuropathy Study. Neurology 1993; 43: 817–24.
[4] Pirart J. Diabetes mellitus and its degenerative complications: A prospective study of 4,400 patients observed between 1947 and 1973. Part 1. Diabetes Care 1978; 1: 168–88.
[5] Pirart J. Diabetes mellitus and its degenerative complications: A prospective study of 4,400 patients observed between 1947 and 1973. Part 2. Diabetes Care 1978; 1: 252–63.
[6] Ziegler D, Hanefeld M, Ruhnau KJ, et al. Treatment of symptomatic diabetic peripheral neuropathy with the anti-oxidant alpha-lipoic acid. A 3-week multicenter randomized controlled trial (ALADIN Study). Diabetologia 1995; 38: 1425–33.
[7] Dyck PJ, Sherman WR, Hallcher LM, et al. Human diabetic endoneurial sorbital, fructose, and myo-inositol related to sural nerve morphometry. Ann Neurol 1980; 8: 590–6.
[8] Dyck PJ, Turner DW, Davies JL, et al. Electronic case-report forms of symptoms and impairements of peripheral neuropathy. Can J Neurol Sci 2002; 29: 258–66.
[9] Feldman EL, Stevens MJ, Thomas PK, et al. A practical two-step quantitative clinical and electrophysiological assessment for the diagnosis and staging of diabetic neuropathy. Diabetes Care 1994; 17: 1281–9.
[10] O'Brien PC, Dyck PJ. Procedures for setting normal values. Neurology 1995; 45: 17–23.
[11] Dyck PJ, Litchy WJ, Lehman KA, et al. Variables influencing neuropathic endpoints: the Rochester Diabetic Neuropathy Study of healthy subjects (RDNS-HS). Neurology 1995; 45: 1115–21.
[12] Dyck PJB, Dyck PJ. Diabetic polyneuropathy. Section III. In: Dyck PJ, Thomas PK, editors. Diabetic neuropathy. 2nd ed. Philadelphia, Pa: W.B. Saunders, 1999: 255–78.
[13] Thomas PK. Metabolic neuropathy. J R Coll Phys Lond 1973; 7: 154–60.
[14] Jordan WR. Neuritic manifestation in diabetes mellitus. Arch Int Med 1936; 57: 308–66.
[15] Watkins PJ, Thomas PK. Diabetes mellitus and the nervous system. J Neurol Neurosurg Psychiatry 1998; 65: 620–32.
[16] Newrick PG, Wilson AJ, Jakubowski J, et al. Sural nerve oxygen tension in man. London: BMJ Publishing, 1986.
[17] Schneider U, Quasthoff S, Mitrovic N, et al. Hyperglycaemia hypoxia alters after potential and fast K+ conductance of rat axons by cytoplasmic acidification. J Physiol Lond 1993; 465: 679–97.
[18] Gregersen G. Diabetic neuropathy: influence of age, sex, metabolic control, and duration of diabetes on motor conduction velocity. Neurology 1967; 17: 972–80.
[19] Ward JD, Barnes CG, Fisher DJ, et al. Improvement in nerve conduction following treatment in newly-diagnosed diabetics. Lancet 1971; 1: 428–30.
[20] Steiness IB. Vibratory perception in diabetics during arrested blood flow to the limb. Acta Med Scand 1959; 163: 195–205.
[21] Schneider U, Niedermeier W, Grafe P. The paradox between resistance to hypoxia and liability to hypoxic damage in hyperglycemic peripheral nerves. Evidence for glycolysis involvement. Diabetes 1993; 42: 981–7.

[22] Fraser DM, Campbell IW, Ewing DJ, et al. Peripheral and autonomic nerve function in newly diagnosed diabetes. Diabetes 1977; 26: 546–50.
[23] Pfeifer MA, Weinberg CF, Cook DC, et al. Autonomic neural dysfunction in recently diagnosed diabetic subjects. Diabetes Care 1984; 7: 447–53.
[24] Watkins PJ. The natural history of the diabetic neuropathies. Q J Med 1990; 77: 1209–18.
[25] Ozker RR, Richard NG, Schumaker OP. Acute polyneuritis following diabetic acidosis. Ohio State Med J 1959; 1521–2.
[26] Zochodne DW, Bolton CF, Wells GA, et al. Critical illness neuropathy: a complication of sepsis and multiple organ failure. Brain 1987; 110: 819–41.
[27] Cornblath DR, Drachman DB, Griffin JW. Demyelinating motor neuropathy in patients with diabetic polyneuropathy. Ann Neurol 1987; 22: 126–32.
[28] Stewart JD, McKelvey R, Durcan, et al. Chronic demyelinating polyneuropathy (CIDP) in diabetes. J Neurol Sci 1996; 142: 59–64.
[29] Dyck PJ, Swanson CJ, Low PA, et al. Prednisone responsive hereditary motor and sensory neuropathy. Mayo Clin Proc 1982; 57: 239–46.
[30] Danta G. Hypoglycemic peripheral neuropathy. Arch Neurol 1969; 21: 121–32.
[31] Harrison MJE. Muscle wasting after prolonged hypoglycaemic coma: case report with electrophysiological data. J Neurol Neurosurg Psychiatry 1976; 39: 465–70.
[32] Westfall SG, Felten DL, Mandelbaum JA, et al. Degenerative neuropathy in insulin-treated diabetic rats. J Neurol Sci 1983; 61: 93–107.
[33] Bril V. Role of electrophysiological studies in diabetic neuropathy. Can J Neurol Sci 1994; 21: S8–12.
[34] Daube JR. Electrophysiologic testing in diabetic neuropathy. In: Dyck PJ, Thomas PK, editors. Diabetic neuropathy. 2nd ed. Philadelphia: W.B. Saunders, 1999: 222–38.
[35] Dyck PJ. Evaluative procedures to detect, characterize, and assess the severity of diabetic neuropathy. Diabet Med 1991; 8: S48–51.
[36] Dyck PJ, Karnes JL, O'Brien PC, et al. The Rochester Diabetic Neuropathy Study: reassessment of tests and criteria for diagnosis and staged severity. Neurology 1992; 42: 1164–70.
[37] Arezzo JC. The use of electrophysiology for the assessment of diabetic neuropathy. Neurosci Res Commun 1997; 21: 13–23.
[38] Kimura J. Electrodiagnosis in diseases of nerve and muscle: principles and practice. 2nd ed. Philadelphia, Pa: Davis, 1989: 709.
[39] Daube JR. Clinical neurophysiology. Philadelphia, Pa: Davis, 1996: 533.
[40] Lamontagne A, Buchthal F. Electrophysiological studies in diabetic neuropathy. J Neurol Neurosurg Psychiatry 1970; 33: 442–52.
[41] Buchthal F. An introduction to electromyography. Copenhagen: Scandinavian University Books, 1957.
[42] Buchthal F, Rosenfalck A, Trojaborg W. Electrophysiological findings in entrapment of the median nerve at wrist and elbow. J Neurol Neurosurg Psychiatry 1974; 37: 340–60.
[43] Kimura J. Principles and pitfalls of nerve conduction studies. Ann Neurol 1984; 16: 415–29.
[44] Kimura J. Facts, fallacies and fancies of nerve conduction studies: 21st Annual Edward H Lambert Lecture. Muscle Nerve 1997; 20: 777–87.
[45] Kimura J. Electrically elicited blink reflex in diagnosis of multiple sclerosis: review of 260 patients over a seven-year period. Brain 1975; 98: 413–26.
[46] Hallet M, Chadwick D, Marsden CD. Cortical reflex myoclonus. Neurology 1979; 29: 1107–25.
[47] Deuschl G, Heinen F, Kleedorfer B. Clinical and polymyographic investigation of spasmodic torticollis. J Neurol 1992; 239: 9–15.
[48] Albers JW, Kelly JJ. Acquired inflammatory demyelinating polyneuropathies: clinical and electrodiagnostic features. Muscle Nerve 1989; 12: 435–51.
[49] Ashworth NL, Zochodne DW, Hahn AF, et al. Impact of plasma exchange on indices of demyelination in chronic inflammatory demyelinating polyradiculoneuropathy. Muscle Nerve 2000; 23: 206–10.
[50] Barohn RJ, Kissel JT, Warmolts JR, et al. Chronic inflammatory demyelinating polyradiculoneuropathy. Clinical characteristics, course, and recommendations for diagnostic criteria. Arch Neurol 1989; 46: 878–84.
[51] Dyck PJ, Daube J, O'Brien P, et al. Plasma exchange in chronic inflammatory demyelinating polyradiculoneuropathy. N Engl J Med 1986; 314: 461–5.
[52] Dyck PJ, Litchy WJ, Kratz KM, et al. A plasma exchange versus immune globulin infusion trial in chronic inflammatory demyelinating polyradiculoneuropathy. Ann Neurol 1994; 36: 838–45.
[53] Dyck PJ, O'Brien PC, Oviatt KF, et al. Prednisone improves chronic inflammatory demyelinating polyradiculoneuropathy more than no treatment. Ann Neurol 1982; 11: 136–41.
[54] Mendell JR, Barohn RJ, Freimer ML, et al. Randomized controlled trial of IVIG in untreated chronic inflammatory demyelinating polyradiculoneuropathy. Neurology 2001; 56: 445–9.
[55] Cornblath DR, Mellitts ED, Griffin JW, et al. Motor conduction studies in Guillain-Barré syndrome: description and prognostic value. Ann Neurol 1988; 23: 354–9.
[56] Albers JW, Kelly JJ. Sequential electrodiagnostic abnormalities in acute inflammatory demyelinating polyradiculoneuropathy. Muscle Nerve 1985; 8: 528–39.
[57] Miller GM, Peterson GW, Daube JR, et al. Prognostic value of electrodiagnosis in Guillain-Barré syndrome. Muscle Nerve 1988; 11: 769–74.
[58] Plasma Exchange/Sandoglobulin Guillain–Barré Syndrome Trial Group. Randomised trial of plasma exchange, intravenous immunoglobulin, and combined treatments in Guillain-Barré syndrome. Lancet 1997; 349: 225–30.
[59] Hahn AF, Bolton CF, Pillay N, et al. Plasma-exchange therapy in chronic inflammatory demyelinating polyneuropathy. A double-blind, sham-controlled, cross-over study. Brain 1996; 119: 1055–66.
[60] Greene D, Arezzo J, Brown M. Zenarestat Study Group. Effect of aldose reductase inhibition on nerve conduction and morphometry in diabetic neuropathy. Neurology 1999; 53: 580–91.
[61] Reichard P, Berglund B, Britz A, et al. Intensified conventional insulin treatment retards the microvascular complications of insulin-dependent diabetes mellitus (IDDM): the Stockholm Diabetes Intervention Study (SDIS) after 5 years. J Intern Med 1991; 230: 101–8.
[62] Reichard P, Nilsson B, Rosenqvist U. The effect of long-term intensified insulin treatment on the development of microvascular complications of diabetes mellitus. N Engl J Med 1993; 329: 304–9.
[63] Diabetes and Complications Trial (DCCT) Research Group. Effect of intensive diabetes treatment on nerve conduction in the diabetes control and complications trial. Ann Neurol 1995; 38: 869–80.
[64] Bril V, Ellison R, Ngo M, et al. Electrophysiological monitoring in clinical trials. Roche Neuropathy Study Group. Muscle Nerve 1998; 21: 1368–73.
[65] Casey EB, Jelliffe AM, Le Quesne PM, et al. Vincristine neuropathy – clinical and electrophysiological observations. Brain 1973; 96: 69–86.
[66] Guiheneuc P, Ginet J, Groleau JY, et al. Early phase of vincristine neuropathy in man. Electrophysiological evidence for a dying-back phenomenon, with transitory enhancement of spinal transmission of the monosynaptic reflex. J Neurol Sci 1980; 45: 355–66.
[67] Dolman CL. The pathology and pathogenesis of diabetic neuropathy. Bull N Y Acad Med 1967; 43: 773–83.
[68] Dyck PJ, Giannini C. Pathologic alterations in the diabetic neuropathies of humans: a review. J Neuropathol Exp Neurol 1996; 55: 1181–93.
[69] Dyck PJ, Lais A, Karnes JL, et al. Fiber loss is primary and multifocal in sural nerves in diabetic polyneuropathy. Ann Neurol 1986; 19: 425–39.
[70] Bischoff A. Diabetische Neuropathie. [Diabetic neuropathy. Pathologic anatomy, pathophysiology and pathogenesis on the basis of electron microscopic studies]. Dtsch Med Wochenschr 1968; 93: 237–41.
[71] Giannini C, Dyck PJ. Pathologic alterations in human diabetic polyneuropathy. In: Dyck PJ, Thomas PK, editors. Diabetic neuropathy. 2nd ed. Philadelphia, Pa: W.B. Saunders, 1999: 279–95.

[72] Kito S, Yamamura Y. [Diabetic neuropathy: a review of pathological studies]. Nippon Rinsho 1991; 49: 152–8.
[73] Reske-Nielsen E, Lundbaek K. Pathological changes in the central and peripheral nervous system of young long-term diabetics. II. The spinal cord and peripheral nerves. Diabetologia 1968; 4: 34–43.
[74] Brown MJ, Martin JR, Asbury AK. Painful diabetic neuropathy. A morphometric study. Arch Neurol 1976; 33: 164–71.
[75] Brown MJ, Asbury AK. Diabetic neuropathy. Ann Neurol 1984; 15: 2–12.
[76] Gwynne J, McMillan D. Advances and pathophysiology of vascular complications of diabetes. Introduction. Diabetes Care 1991; 14: 148–52.
[77] Perkins BA, Olaleye D, Zinman B, et al. Simple screening tests for peripheral neuropathy in the diabetes clinic. Diabetes Care 2001; 24: 250–6.
[78] McCombe PA, Pollard JD, McLeod JG. Chronic inflammatory demyelinating polyradiculoneuropathy. A clinical and electrophysiological study of 92 cases. Brain 1987; 110: 1617–30.
[79] Gorson K, Ropper A, Adelman L, et al. Influence of diabetes mellitus on chronic inflammatory demyelinating polyneuropathy. Muscle Nerve 2000; 23: 37–43.
[80] Kimura J, Yamada T, Stevland N. Distal slowing of motor nerve conduction velocity in diabetic polyneuropathy. J Neurol Sci 1979; 42: 291–302.
[81] Perkins BA, Olaleye D, Bril V. Carpal tunnel syndrome in patients with diabetic polyneuropathy. Diabetes Care 2001;25: 565–9.
[82] Thomas P. Diabetic neuropathy: models, mechanisms and mayhem. Can J Neurol Sci 1992; 19: 1–7.
[83] Said G, Slama G, Selva J. Progressive centripetal degeneration of axons in small fibre diabetic polyneuropathy. Brain 1983; 106: 791–807.
[84] Reeves M, Seigler D, Ayyar D, et al. Medial plantar sensory response. Sensitive indicator of peripheral nerve dysfunction in patients with diabetes mellitus. Am J Med 1984; 76: 842–6.
[85] Chroni E, Taub N, Panayiotopoulos CP. The importance of sample size for the estimation of F wave latency parameters in the peroneal nerve. Electroencephalogr Clin Neurophysiol 1996; 101: 375–8.
[86] Kohara N, Kimura J, Kaji R, et al. F-wave latency serves as the most reproducible measure in nerve conduction studies of diabetic poyneuropathy: multicentre analysis in healthy subjects and patients with diabetic polyneuropathy. Diabetologia 2000; 43: 915–21.
[87] Nobrega JAM, Manzano GM, Monteagudo PT. A comparison between different parameters in F-wave studies. Clin Neurophysiol 2001; 112: 866–8.
[88] Tuzun E, Oge AE, Ertas M, et al. F wave parameters and F tacheodispersion in mild diabetic neuropathy. Electromyogr Clin Neurophysiol 2001; 41: 273–9.
[89] Fagerberg S, Petersen I, Steg G, et al. Motor disturbances in diabetes mellitus: a clinical study using electromyography and conduction velocity determination. Acta Med Scand 1963; 174: 711–6.
[90] Perkins BA, Ngo M, Bril V. Symmetry of nerve conduction studies in different stages of diabetic neuropathy. Muscle Nerve 2002; 25: 212–7.
[91] Ponsford S. Sensory conduction in medial and lateral plantar nerves. J Neurol Neurosurg Psychiatry 1988; 51: 188–91.
[92] Pastore C, Izura V, Geijo-Barrientos E, et al. A comparison of electrophysiological tests for the early diagnosis of diabetic neuropathy. Muscle Nerve 1999; 22: 1667–73.
[93] Shin JB, Seong YJ, Lee HJ, et al. The usefulness of minimal F-wave latency and sural/radial amplitude ratio in diabetic polyneuropathy. Yonsei Med J 2000; 41: 393–7.
[94] Ozaki I, Baba M, Matsunaga M, et al. Deleterious effect of the carpal tunnel on nerve conduction in diabetic polyneuropathy. Electromyogr Clin Neurophysiol 1988; 28: 301–6.
[95] Rosenbaum R, Ochoa J. Carpal tunnel syndrome and other disorders of the median nerve. Boston: Butterworth-Heinemann, 1993.
[96] Wilbourn A. Diabetic entrapment and compression neuropathies. In: Dyck P, Thomas P, editors. Diabetic neuropathy. 2nd ed. Philadelphia, Pa: W.B. Saunders, 1999: 481–508.
[97] Kimura J, Ayyar D. The carpal tunnel syndrome: electrophysiological aspects of 639 symptomatic extremities. Electromyogr Clin Neurophysiol 1985; 25: 151–64.
[98] Bril V, Werb MR, Greene DA, et al. Single-fiber electromyography in diabetic peripheral polyneuropathy. Muscle Nerve 1996; 19: 2–9.
[99] Tkac I, Bril V. Glycemic control is related to the electrophysiologic severity of diabetic peripheral sensorimotor polyneuropathy. Diabetes Care 1998; 21: 1749–52.
[100] Feki I, Lefaucheur J. Correlation between nerve conduction studies and clinical scores in diabetic neuropathy. Muscle Nerve 2001; 24: 555–8.
[101] Perkins BA, Greene DA, Bril V. Glycemic control is related to the morphological severity of diabetic peripheral sensorimotor polyneuropathy. Diabetes Care 2001; 24: 748–52.
[102] Gregersen G. Variations in motor conduction velocity produced by acute changes of the metabolic state in diabetic patients. Diabetologia 1968; 4: 273–7.
[103] Ward JD, Barnes CG, Fisher DJ, et al. Improvement in nerve conduction following treatment in newly diagnosed diabetics. Lancet 1971; 1: 428–30.
[104] Young RJ, Ewing DJ, Clarke BF. Nerve function and metabolic control in teenage diabetics. Diabetes 1983; 32: 142–7.
[105] Pietri A, Ehle AL, Raskin P. Changes in nerve conduction velocity after six weeks of glucoregulation with portable insulin infusion pumps. Diabetes 1980; 29: 668–71.
[106] Dyke PJ. Detection, characterization, and staging of polyneuropathy: assessed in diabetics. Muscle Nerve 1988; 11: 21–32.
[107] Arezzo JC. New developments in the diagnosis of diabetic neuropathy. Am J Med 1999; 107: 9S-16S.
[108] Bril V, Nyunt M, Ngo M. Limits of the sympathetic skin response in patients with diabetic polyneuropathy. Muscle Nerve 2000; 23: 1427–30.
[109] Niakan E, Harati Y. Sympathetic skin response in diabetic peripheral neuropathy. Muscle Nerve 1988; 11: 261–4.
[110] Low PA. Clinical evaluation of autonomic function. In: Low P, editor. Clinical autonomic disorders: evaluation and management. Boston: Little, Brown, 1993: 157–67.
[111] Low PA, Pfeifer MA. Standardization of clinical tests for practice and clinical trials. In: Low PA, editor. Clinical autonomic disorders: evaluation and management. Boston: Little, Brown, 1993: 287–96.
[112] Low PA. Pitfalls in autonomic testing. In: Low PA, editor. Clinical autonomic disorders: evaluation and management. Boston: Little, Brown, 1993: 355–65.
[113] Consensus Statement: Proceedings of a Consensus Development Conference on Standardized Measures in Diabetic Neuropathy. Neurology 1992; 42: 1823–5.
[114] Risk MR, Bril V, Broadbridge C, et al. Heart rate variability measurement in diabetic neuropathy: review of methods. Diabetes Technol Ther 2001; 3: 63–76.
[115] Dyck PJ, Karnes J, O'Brien PC, et al. Detection thresholds of cutaneous sensation in humans. In: Griffin JW, Low PA, Poduslo JF, editors. Peripheral neuropathy. Philadelphia, Pa: W.B. Saunders, 1993: 706–28.
[116] Dyck PJ, Zimmerman I, Gillen DA, et al. Cool warm and heat-pain detection of receptors: testing methods and inferences about anatomic distribution of receptors. Neurol 1993; 43: 1500–08.
[117] Valk GD, de Sonnaville JJ, van Houtum W, et al. The assessment of diabetic polyneuropathy in daily clinical practice: reproducibility and validity of Semmes Weinstein monofilaments examination and clinical neurological examination. Muscle Nerve 1997; 20: 116–18.
[118] Dyck PJ, Dyck PJB, Velosa JA, et al. Patterns of quantitative sensation testing of hypoesthesia and hyperalgesia are predictive of diabetic polyneuropathy. A study of three cohorts. The Nerve Growth Factors Study Group. Diabetes Care 2000; 23: 510–17.
[119] Abbott CA, Vileikyte L, Williamson S, et al. Multicenter study of the incidence of and predictive risk factors for diabetic neuropathic foot ulceration. Diabetes Care 1998; 7: 1071–5.
[120] Dyck PJ, Davies JL, Litchy WJ, et al. Longitudinal assessment of diabetic polyneuropathy using a composite score in the Rochester Diabetic Neuropathy Study cohort. Neurol 1997; 49: 229–39.

[121] Young MJ, Breddy JL, Veves A, et al. The prediction of diabetic foot ulceration using vibration perception thresholds: a prospective study. Diabetes Care 1994; 17: 557–60.
[122] Apfel S, Schwartz S, Adornato BT, et al. For the rhNGF Clinical Investigators Group. Efficacy and safety of recombinant human nerve growth factor in patients with diabetic polyneuropathy. A randomized controlled trial. JAMA 2000; 284: 2215.
[123] Dyck PJ, Zimmerman IR, O'Brien PC, et al. Introduction of automated systems to evaluate touch-pressure, vibration, and thermal cutaneous sensation in man. Ann Neurol 1978; 4: 502–10.
[124] Bove F, Litwak MS, Arezzo JC, Baker EL. Quantitative sensory testing in occupational medicine. In: Baker E, editors. Seminars in occupational medicine. Stuttgart, Germany: Thieme Verlag, 1986: 185–90.
[125] Arezzo JC. Quantitative sensory testing for diabetic peripheral neuropathy. Wilmington, Del. Center for Advanced Study of Diabetes, 1988: 2; 3.
[126] Masson EA, Veves A, Fernando D, et al. Current perception thresholds: a new, quick, and reproducible method for the assessment of peripheral neuropathy in diabetes mellitus. Diabetologia 1989; 32: 724–28.
[127] Gruener G, Dyck PJ. Quantitative sensory testing: methodology, applications, and future directions. J Clin Neurophysiol 1994; 11: 568–83.
[128] Vinik AI, Suwanwalailom S, Stansberry KB, et al. Quantitative measurement of cutaneous perception in diabetic neuropathy. Muscle Nerve 1995; 18: 574–84.
[129] Yamitsky D, Fowler CJ. Quantitative sensory testing. In: Osselton JW, editor. Clinical neurophysiology: EMG, nerve conduction and evoked potentials. London: Butterworth-Heinemann, 1995: 253–70.
[130] Zaslansky R, Yarnitsky D. Clinical applications of quantitative sensory testing (QST). J Neurol Sci 1998; 153: 215–38.
[131] Dyck PJ, O'Brien PC. Quantitative sensation testing in epidemiological and therapeutic studies of peripheral neuropathy. Muscle Nerve 1999; 22: 659–62.
[132] American Diabetes Association and American Academy of Neurology. Report and recommendation of the San Antonio conference on diabetic neuropathy. Diabetes 1988; 37: 1000–4.
[133] Proceedings of a consensus development conference on standardized measures in diabetic neuropathy. Neurology 1992; 42: 1823–39.
[134] Dyck PJ. Quantitative sensory testing: a consensus report from the peripheral neuropathy association. Neurol 1993; 43: 1050–52.
[135] Cameron NE, Cotter MA. The relationship of vascular changes to metabolic factors in diabetes mellitus and their role in the development of peripheral nerve complications. Diabetes Metab Rev 1994; 10: 189–224.
[136] Brownlee M. Advanced products of nonenzymatic glycosylation and the pathogenesis of diabetic complications. In: Rifkin H, Porte D, editors. Diabetes mellitus: theory and practice. New York, NY: Elsevier Science, 1990: 279–91.
[137] Jamal GA. Pathogenesis of diabetic neuropathy: the role of the n-6 essential fatty acids and their eicosanoid derivations. Diabet Med 1990; 7: 574–9.
[138] Greene DA, Lattimer SA, Sima AA. Sorbitol, phosphoinositides, and sodium-potassium-ATPase in the pathogenesis of diabetic complications. N Engl J Med 1987; 316: 599–606.
[139] Giannini C, Dyck PJ. Basement membrane reduplication and pericyte degeneration precede development of diabetic polyneuropathy and are associated with its severity. Ann Neurol 1995; 37: 498–504.
[140] Tomlinson DR, Ferryhough P, Diemel LT. Neurotrophins and peripheral neuropathy. Philos Trans R Soc Lond B Biol Sci 1996; 351: 455–62.
[141] Nishikawa T, Edelstein D, Du XL, et al. Normalizing mitochondrial superoxide production blocks three pathways of hyperglycaemic damage. Nature 2000; 404: 787–90.
[142] Schaumburg HA, Berger AR, Thomas PK. Anatomical classification of peripheral nervous system disorders. In: Schaumburg HH, Berger AR, Thomas PK, editors. Disorders of peripheral nerves. 2nd ed. Philadelphia, Pa: Davis, 1992: 10–24.
[143] Schaumburg HH, Wisniewski H, Spencer PS. Ultrastructural studies of the dying-back process. I. Peripheral nerve terminal and axon degeneration in systemic acrylamide intoxication. J Neuropathol Exper Neurol 1974; 33: 260.
[144] Spencer PS, Schaumburg HH. Ultrastructural studies of the dying-back process. IV. Differential vulnerability of PNS and CNS fibers in experimental central peripheral distal axonopathies. J Neuropath Exper Neurol 1977; 36: 300.
[145] Wallengren J, Badendick K, Sundler F, et al. Innervation of the skin of the forearm in diabetic patients: relation to nerve function. Acta Derm Venereol 1995; 75: 37–42.
[146] Greene DM, Swets JA. Signal detection theory and psychophysics. New York, NY: John Wiley, 1996.
[147] Arezzo JC. The use of electrophysiology for the assessment of diabetic neuropathy. Neurosci Res Commun 1997; 21: 13–23.
[148] Thomas PK, Brown MJ. Diabetic polyneuropathy. In: Dyck PJ, Asbury AK, Winegard AI, et al, editors. Diabetic neuropathy. Philadelphia, Pa: W.B. Saunders, 1987: 56–65.
[149] Llewelyn JG, Thomas PK, Gilbey SG, et al. Pattern of myelinated fibre loss in the sural nerve in neuropathy related to type 1 (insulin-dependent) diabetes. Diabetologia 1988; 31: 162–67.
[150] Corso JF. The experiment psychology of sensory behavior. New York, NY: Holt, Rinehart & Winston, 1967.
[151] Dyck PJ, Karnes JL, Gillen DA, et al. Comparison of algorithms of testing for use in automated evaluation of sensation. Neurology 1990; 40: 1607.
[152] Dyck PJ, O'Brian PC, Kosanke JL, et al. A 4, 2, and 1 stepping algorithm for quick and accurate estimation of cutaneous sensation threshold. Neurology 1993; 43: 1508–12.
[153] Hilz MJ, Glorius SE, Beric A. Thermal perception thresholds: influence of determination paradigm and reference temperature. J Neurol Sci 1995; 129: 135–40.
[154] Yarnitsky D, Sprecher E. Thermal testing: normative data and repeatability for various test algorithms. J Neurol Sci 1994; 125: 39–45.
[155] Bertelsmann FW, Heimans JJ, Weber EJM, et al. Thermal discrimination thresholds in normal subjects and in patients with diabetic neuropathy. J Neurol Neurosurg Psychiatry 1985; 48: 686–90.
[156] Jamal GA, Hansen S, Weir AI, et al. An improved automated method for the measurement of thermal thresholds. 1. Normal subjects. J Neurol Neurosurg Psychiatry 1985; 48: 354–60.
[157] Gelber DA, Pfeifer MA, Broadstone VL, et al. Components of variance for vibratory and thermal thresholds testing in normal and diabetic subjects. J Diabetes Complications 1995; 9: 170–76.
[158] Gerr F, Letz R. Covariates of human peripheral function: vibrotactile and thermal thresholds II. Neurotoxicol Teratol 1994; 16: 105–12.
[159] Williams RT. The vibrating sensation in affections of the nervous system and in diabetes. Lancet 1905; i: 855–6.
[160] Guy RJ, Clark CA, Malcolm PN. Evaluation of thermal and vibration sensation in diabetic neuropathy. Diabetologia 1985; 28: 131–7.
[161] Boulton AJM, Kubrusly DB, Bowker JH, et al. Impaired vibratory perception and diabetic foot ulceration. Diabet Med 1986; 3: 335–37.
[162] Ziegler D, Mayer P, Wiefels K, et al. Assessment of small and large fiber function in long-term type 1 (insulin-dependent) diabetic patients with and without painful neuropathy. Pain 1988; 34: 1-10.
[163] Ziegler D, Mayer P, Wiefels K, et al. Evaluation of thermal, pain, and vibration sensation thresholds in newly diagnosed type 1 diabetic patients. J Neurol Neurosurg Psychiatry 1988; 11: 1420–4.
[164] Lavery LA, Armstrong DG, Vela SA, et al. Practical criteria for screening patients at high risk for diabetic foot ulcerations. Arch Intern Med 1998; 158: 157–62.
[165] Davis EA, Walsh P, Jones TW, et al. The use of biosthesiometry to detect neuropathy in children and adolescents with IDDM. Diabetes Care 1997; 20: 1448–53.
[166] Young MJ, Breddy JL, Veves A, et al. The prediction of diabetic foot ulceration thresholds: a prospective study. Diabetes Care 1994; 17: 557–60.

[167] Coppini DV, Young P, Wang C, et al. Risk factors associated with the development of end stage peripheral neuropathy: a 10-13 year follow up study. Diabet Med 1996; 13(Suppl 3): 85.
[168] Iggo A. Cutaneous thermoreceptors. In: von Euler C, Franzén O, Lindblom U, et al, editors. Somatosensory mechanisms. New York, London: Plenum Press, 1984: 261–72.
[169] Arezzo JC, Schaumburg HH, Laudadio C. Thermal sensitivity tester: device for quantitative assessment of thermal sense in diabetic neuropathy. Diabetes 1986; 35: 590–92.
[170] Sosenko JM, Kato M, Soto RA, et al. Specific assessments of warm and cool sensitivities in adult diabetic patients. Diabetes Care 1988; 11: 481.
[171] Sosenko JM, Kato M, Soto R, et al. Comparison of quantitative sensory-threshold measures for their association with foot ulceration in diabetic patients. Diabetes Care 1990; 13: 1057–61.
[172] Navarro X, Kennedy WR. Evaluation of thermal and pain sensitivity in type 1 diabetic patients. J Neurol Neurosurg Psychiat 1991; 54: 60–4.
[173] Kennedy WR, Wendelschafer-Crabb G, Johnson T. Quantitation of epidermal nerves in diabetic neuropathy. Neurology 1996; 47: 1042–48.
[174] Stocks EA, McArthur JC, Griffen JW, et al. An unbiased method of estimation of total epidermal nerve fibre length. J Neurocytol 1996; 25: 637–44.
[175] McCarthy BG, Hsieh ST, Stock A, et al. Cutaneous innervation in sensory neuropathies: evaluation by skin biopsy. Neurology 1995; 45: 1848–55.
[176] Dyck PJ, Zimmerman IR, Johnson DM, et al. A standard test of heat-pain responses using CASE IV. J Neurol Sci 1996; 136: 54–63.
[177] Hotta N, Sugimura K, Tsuchida I, et al. Use of the C64 quantitative tuning fork and the effect of niccritrol in diabetic neuropathy. Clin Ther 1994; 16: 1007.
[178] Vileikyte L, Hutchings G, Hollis S, et al. The tactile circumferential discriminator: a new simple screening device to identify diabetic patients at risk of foot ulceration. Diabetes Care 1997; 20: 623–26.
[179] Arezzo JC. New developments in the diagnosis of diabetic neuropathy. Am J Med 1999; 107: 9S-16S.
[180] Service FJ, Rizza RA, Daube JR, et al. Near normoglycaemia improved nerve conduction and vibration sensation in diabetic neuropathy. Diabetologia 1985; 28: 722–27.
[181] Apfel SC, Kessler JA, Adornato BT, et al. NGF Study Group. Recombinant human nerve growth factor in the treatment of diabetic polyneuropathy. Neurol 1998; 51: 695–702.
[182] Laudadio C, Sima AAF, The Ponalrestat Study Group. Progression rates of diabetic neuropathy in placebo patients in an 18-month clinical trial. J Diabetes Complications 1998; 12: 121–27.
[183] Yarnitsky D, Sprecher E, Tamir A, et al. Variance of sensory threshold measurements: discrimination of feigners from trustworthy performers. J Neurol Sci 1994; 125: 189–96.
[184] Dyck PJ, Kennedy WR, Kesserwani H, et al. Limitations of quantitative sensory testing when patients are biased toward a bad outcome. Neurol 1998; 50: 1213.
[185] Jordan WR. Neuritic manifestations in diabetes mellitus. Arch Intern Med 1936; 57: 307–66.
[186] Kahn R, Asbury AK, Porte DJ, et al. Report and recommendations of the San Antonio Conference on Diabetic Neuropathy. Neurology 1988; 38: 1161–5.
[187] Gadeberg P, Andersen H, Jakobsen J. Volume of ankle dorsiflexors and plantar flexors determined with stereological techniques. J Appl Physiol 1999; 86: 1670–5.
[188] Dyck PJ. Detection, characterization, and staging of polyneuropathy: assessed in diabetics. Muscle Nerve 1988; 11: 21–32.
[189] Bourque PR, Dyck PJ. Selective calf weakness suggests intraspinal pathology, not peripheral neuropathy. Arch Neurol 1990; 47: 79–80.
[190] Andersen H, Gadeberg PC, Brock B, et al. Muscular atrophy in diabetic neuropathy: a stereological magnetic resonance imaging study. Diabetologia 1997; 40: 1062–9.
[191] Dyck PJ, Kratz KM, Karnes JL, et al. The prevalence by staged severity of various types of diabetic neuropathy, retinopathy, and nephropathy in a population-based cohort: the Rochester Diabetic Neuropathy Study. Neurology 1993; 43: 817–24.
[192] Medical Research Council. Aids to the examination of the peripheral nervous system. Memorandum No. 45. London: Her Majesty's Stationary Office, 1976.
[193] Dyck PJ. Quantitating severity of neuropathy. In: Dyck PJ, Thomas PK, Griffin JW, et al, editors. Peripheral neuropathy. Philadelphia, Pa: W.B. Saunders, 1993: 686–97.
[194] Feldman EL, Stevens MJ, Thomas PK, et al. A practical two-step quantitative clinical and electrophysiological assessment for the diagnosis and staging of diabetic neuropathy. Diabetes Care 1994; 17: 1281–9.
[195] Fedele D, Comi G, Coscelli C, et al. A multicenter study on the prevalence of diabetic neuropathy in Italy. Italian Diabetic Neuropathy Committee. Diabetes Care 1997; 20: 836–43.
[196] Windebank AJ. Clinical evaluation of motor function. In: Dyck PJ, Thomas PK, Asbury AK, et al, editors. Diabetic neuropathy. Philadelphia, Pa: W.B. Saunders, 1987: 100–6.
[197] Andersen H, Jakobsen J. A comparative study of isokinetic dynamometry and manual muscle testing of ankle dorsal and plantar flexors and knee extensors and flexors. Eur Neurol 1997; 37: 239–42.
[198] Aitkens S, Lord J, Bernauer E, et al. Relationship of manual muscle testing to objective strength measurements. Muscle Nerve 1989; 12: 173–7.
[199] Delitto A. Isokinetic dynamometry. Muscle Nerve 1990; 13(Suppl): S53-S57.
[200] Hislop HJ, Perrine JJ. The isokinetic concept of exercise. Phys Ther 1967; 47: 114–7.
[201] Knutsson E, Martensson A. Isokinetic measurements of muscle strength in hysterical paresis. Electroencephalogr Clin Neurophysiol 1985; 61: 370–4.
[202] Robinson ME, O'Connor PD, Shirley FR, et al. Variability of isometric and isotonic leg exercise. Utility for detection of submaximal efforts. J Occup Rehabil 1994; 4: 163–9.
[203] Lin PC, Robinson ME, Carlos J, et al. Detection of submaximal effort in isometric and isokinetic knee extension tests. J Orthop Sports Phys Ther 1996; 24: 19–24.
[204] Simonsen JC. Coefficient of variation as a measure of subject effort. Arch Phys Med Rehabil 1995; 76: 516–20.
[205] Dvir Z, David G. Suboptimal muscular performance: measuring isokinetic strength of knee extensors with new testing protocol. Arch Phys Med Rehabil 1996; 77: 578–81.
[206] Norregaard J, Lykkegaard JJ, Bulow PM, et al. The twitch interpolation technique for the estimation of true quadriceps muscle strength. Clin Physiol 1997; 17: 523–32.
[207] Bland JM, Altman DG. A note on the use of the intraclass correlation coefficient in the evaluation of agreement between two methods of measurement. Comput Biol Med 1990; 20: 337–40.
[208] Holmback AM, Porter MM, Downham D, et al. Reliability of isokinetic ankle dorsiflexor strength measurements in healthy young men and women. Scand J Rehabil Med 1999; 31: 229–39.
[209] Wennerberg D. Reliability of an isokinetic dorsiflexion and plantar flexion apparatus. Am J Sports Med 1991; 19: 519–22.
[210] Pincivero DM, Lephart SM, Karunakara RA. Reliability and precision of isokinetic strength and muscular endurance for the quadriceps and hamstrings. Int J Sports Med 1997; 18: 113–7.
[211] Andersen H. Reliability of isokinetic measurements of ankle dorsal and plantar flexors in normal subjects and in patients with peripheral neuropathy. Arch Phys Med Rehabil 1996; 77: 265–8.
[212] Farrell M, Richards JG. Analysis of the reliability and validity of the kinetic communicator exercise device. Med Sci Sports Exerc 1986; 18: 44–9.
[213] Patterson LA, Spivey WE. Validity and reliability of the Lido Active Isokinetic System. J Orthop Sports Phys Ther 1992; 15: 32–6.
[214] Bemben MG, Grump KJ, Massey BH. Assessment of technical accuracy of the Cybex II isokinetic dynamometer and analog recording system. J Orthop Sports Phys Ther 1988; 10: 12–7.
[215] The National Isometric Muscle Strength. (NIMS) Database Consortium. Muscular weakness assessment: use of normal isometric strength data. Arch Phys Med Rehabil 1996; 77: 1251–5.

[216] Perusse L, Lortie G, Leblanc C, et al. Genetic and environmental sources of variation in physical fitness. Ann Hum Biol 1987; 14: 425–34.
[217] Gibbons LE, Videman T, Battie MC. Determinants of isokinetic and psychophysical lifting strength and static back muscle endurance: a study of male monozygotic twins. Spine 1997; 22: 2983–90.
[218] Vandervoort AA, McComas AJ. Contractile changes in opposing muscles of the human ankle joint with aging. J Appl Physiol 1986; 61: 361–7.
[219] Phillips SK, Rook KM, Siddle NC, et al. Muscle weakness in women occurs at an earlier age than in men, but strength is preserved by hormone replacement therapy. Clin Sci Colch 1993; 84: 95–8.
[220] Jubrias SA, Odderson IR, Esselman PC, et al. Decline in isokinetic force with age: muscle cross-sectional area and specific force. Pflugers Arch 1997; 434: 246–53.
[221] Borges O, Essen, Gustavsson B. Enzyme activities in type I and II muscle fibres of human skeletal muscle in relation to age and torque development. Acta Physiol Scand 1989; 136: 29–36.
[222] Doherty TJ, Vandervoort AA, Taylor AW, et al. Effects of motor unit losses on strength in older men and women. J Appl Physiol 1993; 74: 868–74.
[223] Hakkinen K, Pakarinen A. Muscle strength and serum testosterone, cortisol and SHBG concentrations in middle-aged and elderly men and women. Acta Physiol Scand 1993; 148: 199–207.
[224] Phillips W, Hazeldene R. Strength and muscle mass changes in elderly men following maximal isokinetic training. Gerontology 1996; 42: 114–20.
[225] Cartee GD. Aging skeletal muscle: response to exercise. Exerc Sport Sci Rev 1994; 22: 91–120.
[226] Grimby G, Aniansson A, Hedberg M, et al. Training can improve muscle strength and endurance in 78- to 84-yr-old men. J Appl Physiol 1992; 73: 2517–23.
[227] Milner Brown HS. Muscle strengthening in a post-polio subject through a high-resistance weight-training program. Arch Phys Med Rehabil 1993; 74: 1165–7.
[228] Era P, Lyyra AL, Viitasalo JT, et al. Determinants of isometric muscle strength in men of different ages. Eur J Appl Physiol 1992; 64: 84–91.
[229] Fugl-Meyer AR, Gustafsson L, Burstedt Y. Isokinetic and static plantar flexion characteristics. Eur J Appl Physiol 1980; 45: 221–34.
[230] DiBrezzo R, Fort IL, Brown B. Relationships among strength, endurance, weight and body fat during three phases of the menstrual cycle. J Sports Med Phys Fitness 1991; 31: 89–94.
[231] Kaiser P. Physical performance and muscle metabolism during beta-adrenergic blokkade in man. Acta Physiol Scand Suppl 1984; 536: 1–53.
[232] Carre F, Handschuh R, Beillot J, et al. Effects of captopril chronic intake on the aerobic performance and muscle strength of normotensive trained subjects. Int J Sports Med 1992; 13: 308–12.
[233] Rantanen T, Guralnik JM, Sakari-Rantala R, et al. Disability, physical activity, and muscle strength in older women: the Women's Health and Aging Study. Arch Phys Med Rehabil 1999; 80: 130–5.
[234] Booth FW, Weeden SH, Tseng BS. Effect of aging on human skeletal muscle and motor function. Med Sci Sports Exerc 1994; 26: 556–60.
[235] Rantanen T, Guralnik JM, Foley D, et al. Midlife hand grip strength as a predictor of old age disability. JAMA 1999; 281: 558–60.
[236] Whipple RH, Wolfson LI, Amerman PM. The relationship of knee and ankle weakness to falls in nursing home residents: an isokinetic study. J Am Geriatr Soc 1987; 35: 13–20.
[237] Agre JC, Rodriquez AA, Franke TM. Strength, endurance, and work capacity after muscle strengthening exercise in postpolio subjects. Arch Phys Med Rehabil 1997; 78: 681–6.
[238] Larsson L, Karlsson J. Isometric and dynamic endurance as a function of age and skeletal muscle characteristics. Acta Physiol Scand 1978; 104: 129–36.
[239] Milner Brown HS, Miller RG. Increased muscular fatigue in patients with neurogenic muscle weakness: quantification and pathophysiology. Arch Phys Med Rehabil 1989; 70: 361–6.
[240] Hulten B, Thorstensson A, Sjodin B, et al. Relationship between isometric endurance and fibre types in human leg muscles. Acta Physiol Scand 1975; 93: 135–8.
[241] Thorstensson A, Karlsson J. Fatiguability and fibre composition of human skeletal muscle. Acta Physiol Scand 1976; 98: 318–22.
[242] Backman E, Johansson V, Hager B, et al. Isometric muscle strength and muscular endurance in normal persons aged between 17 and 70 years. Scand J Rehabil Med 1995; 27: 109–17.
[243] Petrofsky JS, Lind AR. Aging, isometric strength and endurance, and cardiovascular responses to static effort. J Appl Physiol 1975; 38: 91–5.
[244] Hainaut K, Duchateau J. Muscle fatigue, effects of training and disuse. Muscle Nerve 1989; 12: 660–9.
[245] De Visser M, Reimers CD. Muscle imaging. In: Engel AG, Franzini-Armstrong C, editors. Myology. New York: McGraw-Hill Inc., 1994: 795–806.
[246] Sartoris DJ. Cross-sectional imaging of the diabetic foot. J Foot Ankle Surg 1994; 33: 531–45.
[247] Barohn RJ, Bazan C, Timmons JH, et al. Bilateral diabetic thigh muscle infarction. J Neuroimaging 1994; 4: 43–4.
[248] Fleckenstein JL, Watumull D, Conner KE, et al. Denervated human skeletal muscle: MR imaging evaluation. Radiology 1993; 187: 213–8.
[249] Gundersen HJ, Bendtsen TF, Korbo L, et al. Some new, simple and efficient stereological methods and their use in pathological research and diagnosis. Acta Pathologica Microbiologica et Immunologica Scandinavica 1988; 96: 379–94.
[250] Roberts N, Cruz-Orive LM, Reid NMK, et al. Unbiased estimation of human body composition by the Cavalieri method using magnetic resonance imaging. J Microsc 1993; 171: 239–53.
[251] Gundersen HJ, Jensen EB. The efficiency of systematic sampling in stereology and its prediction. J Microsc 1987; 147: 229–63.
[252] Said GG, Slama G, Selva J. Progressive centripetal degeneration of axons in small fibre diabetic polyneuropathy. Brain 1983; 106: 791–807.
[253] Dyck PJ, Winkelmann RK, Bolton CF. Quantitation of Meissner's corpuscles in hereditary neurologic disorders. Charcot-Marie-Tooth disease, Roussy-Levy syndrome, Dejerine-Sottas disease, hereditary sensory neuropathy, spinocerebellar degenerations, and hereditary spastic paraplegia. Neurology 1966; 16: 10–7.
[254] Bloom SR, Polak JM. Regulatory peptides and the skin. Clin Exp Dermatol 1983; 8: 3–18.
[255] Thompson RJ, Day INM. Protein gene product 9.5: a new neuronal and neuroendocrine marker. In: Marangos PJ, Campbell, Cohen RM, editors. Neuronal and glial proteins: structure, function and clinical application. Neurobiological research. Vol 2. Millbrae, CA, USA: California Academic Press Inc, 1988: 209–328.
[256] Dalsgaard CJ, Rydh M, Haegerstrand A. Cutaneous innervation in man visualized with protein gene product 9.5 (PGP 9.5) antibodies. Histochemistry 1989; 92: 385–90.
[257] Karanth SS, Springall DR, Kuhn DM, et al. An immunocytochemical study of cutaneous innervation and the distribution of neuropeptides and protein gene product 9.5 in man and commonly employed laboratory animals. Am J Anat 1991; 191: 369–83.
[258] Arthur RP, Shelley WB. The innervation of human epidermis. J Invest Derm 1959; 32: 397–411.
[259] Lauria G. Innervation of the human epidermis. A historical review. Ital J Neurol Sci 1999; 20: 63–70.
[260] Wang L, Hilliges M, Jernberg T, et al. Protein gene product 9.5-immunoreactive nerve fibres and cells in human skin. Cell Tissue Res 1990; 261: 25–33.
[261] Kennedy WR, Wendelschafer-Crabb G. The innervation of human epidermis. J Neurol Sci 1993; 115: 184–200.
[262] Hilliges M, Wang L, Johansson O. Ultrastructural evidence for nerve fibers within all vital layers of the human epidermis. J Invest Derm 1995; 104: 134–7.
[263] Kennedy WR, Wendelschafer-Crabb G, Walk D. Utility of skin biopsy and skin blister in neurological practice. J Clin Neuromusc Dis 2000; 1: 196–203.
[264] Scott LJC, Griffin JW, Luciano C, et al. Quantitative analysis of epidermal innervation in Fabry disease. Neurology 1999; 52: 1249–54.

[265] Holland NR, Stocks A, Hauer P, et al. Intraepidermal nerve fiber density in patients with painful sensory neuropathy. Neurology 1997; 48: 708–11.
[266] Holland NR, Crawford TO, Hauer P, et al. Small-fiber sensory neuropathies: clinical course and neuropathology of idiopathic cases. Ann Neurol 1998; 44: 47–59.
[267] Periquet MI, Novak V, Collins MP, et al. Painful sensory neuropathy. Neurology. 1999; 53: 1641–7.
[268] Selim M, Wendelschafer-Crabb G, Kennedy WR, et al. Neuropathological diagnosis of enteric diabetic autonomic neuropathy. Clin Auton Res 2001; 11: 186.
[269] Kennedy WR, Wendelschafer-Crabb G, Johnson T, et al. A skin blister method to study epidermal nerves in peripheral nerve disease. Muscle Nerve 1999; 22: 360–71.
[270] Wendelschafer-Crabb G, Kennedy WR, Nolan M, et al. Regeneration of nerves during reepithelialization of human skin. Cambridge, England: Peripheral Nerve Society, 1997.
[271] Levy DM, Terenghi G, Gu X-H, et al. Immunohistochemical measurements of nerves and neuropeptides in diabetic skin: relationship to tests of neurological function. Diabetologia 1992; 35: 889–97.
[272] McCarthy BG, Hsieh S-T, Stocks A, et al. Cutaneous innervation in sensory neuropathies. Neurology 1995; 45: 1848–55.
[273] Kennedy WR, Wendelschafer-Crabb G, Johnson T. Quantitation of epidermal nerves in diabetic neuropathy. Neurology 1996; 47: 1042–8.
[274] Lauria G, McArthur JC, Hauer PE, et al. Neuropathological alterations in diabetic truncal neuropathy: evaluation by skin biopsy. J Neurol Neurosurg Psychiatry 1998; 65: 762–6.
[275] Herrmann DN, Griffin JW, Hauer P, et al. Epidermal nerve fibers density and sural nerve morphometry in peripheral neuropathies. Neurology 1999; 53: 1634–40.
[276] McArthur JC, Stocks EA, Hauer P, et al. Epidermal nerve fiber density. AMA Arch Neurol 1998; 55: 1513–20.
[277] Hilliges M, Johansson O. Comparative analysis of numerical estimation methods of epithelial nerve fibers using tissue sections. J Periph Nerv Syst 1999; 4: 53–7
[278] Johansson O, Wang L, Hilliges M, et al. Intraepidermal nerves in human skin: PGP 9.5 immunohistochemistry with special reference to the nerve density in skin from different body regions. J Periph Nerv Syst 1999; 4: 43–52.
[279] Wendelschafer-Crabb G, Kennedy WR, Hazen E, et al. Distribution of epidermal nerves in control and diabetic subjects. Distribution of epidermal nerves in control and diabetic subjects. J Periph Nerv Syst 1999; 4: 201.
[280] Lauria G, Nolland N, Hauer P, et al. Epidermal innervation: changes with aging, topographic location and in sensory neuropathy. J Neurol Sci 1999; 164: 172–8.
[281] Simone DA, Nolano M, Wendelschafer-Crabb G, et al. Intradermal injection of capsaicin in humans: diminished pain sensation associated with rapid degeneration of intracutaneous nerve fibers. J Neurosci 1998; 18: 8947–59.
[282] Nolano M, Simone DA, Wendelschafer-Crabb G, et al. Topical capsaicin in humans: parallel loss of epidermal nerve fibers and pain sensation. Pain 1999; 81: 135–45.
[283] Kennedy WR, Khalili N, Wendelschafer-Crabb G, et al. Probe size influences detection of pain sensation after topical capsaicin induced epidermal denervation. Am Acad Neurol 2000; 54(Suppl 3): A179.
[284] Boulton AJM, Gries FA, Jervell JA. Guidelines for the diagnosis and outpatient management of diabetic peripheral neuropathy. Diabetic Med 1998; 15: 508–14.
[285] Dyck JB, Dyck PJ. Diabetic polyneuropathy. In: Dyck PJ, Thomas PK, editors. Diabetic neuropathy. Philadelphia, Pa: W.B. Saunders, 1999: 255–78.
[286] Vinik AI, Holland MT, Le Beau JM. Diabetic neuropathies. Diabetes Care 1992; 15: 1926–75.
[287] Neundörfer B. Die diabetische Polyneuropathie aus neurologischer Sicht. Internist 1984; 25: 613–9.
[288] Neundörfer B, editor. Polyneuritiden und Polyneuropathien. Weinheim, Deerfield Beach/Florida: VCH, 1987.
[289] Thomas PK, Brown M. Diabetic polyneuropathy. In: Dyck PJ, Thomas PK, Asbury AK, et al, editors. Diabetic neuropathy. Philadelphia, Pa: W.B. Saunders, 1987: 56–65.
[290] Dyck PJ, Kratz KM, Karnes JL, et al. The prevalence by staged severity of various types of diabetic neuropathy, retinopathy, and nephropathy in a population-based cohort: The Rochester Diabetic Neuropathy Study. Neurology 1993; 43: 817–24.
[291] Dyck PJ, Karnes JL, Daube J, et al. Clinical and neuropathological criteria for the diagnosis and staging of diabetic polyneuropathy. Brain 1985; 108: 861–80.
[292] Harris M, Eastman R, Cowie C. Symptoms of sensory neuropathy in adults with NIDDM in the U.S. population. Diabetes Care 1993; 16: 1446–52.
[293] Dyck PJ, Litchy WJ, Lehman KA, et al. Variables influencing neuropathic endpoints: The Rochester Diabetic Neuropathy Study of Healthy Subjects (RDNS-HS). Neurology 1995; 45: 1115–21.
[294] O'Brien PC, Dyck PJ. Procedures for setting normal values. Neurology 1995; 45: 17–23.
[295] Neundörfer B. Polyneuropathien: Standards. Nervenheilk 1995; 14: 164–74.
[296] Dyck PJ. Detection, characterization, and staging of polyneuropathy: assessed in diabetics. Muscle Nerve 1988; 11: 21–32.
[297] Dyck PJ, Sherman WR, Hallcher LM, et al. human diabetic endoneurial sorbital, fructose and myo-inositol related to sural nerve morphometry. Ann Neurol 1980; 8: 590–6.
[298] Feudell P. Neuropathia diabetica. Die Erkrankungen peripherer Nerven bei Diabetes Mellitus. Berlin: VEB Verlag Volk und Gesundheit, 1963.
[299] Gibbels, Schliep G. Diabetische Polyneuropathie: Probleme der Diagnostik und Nosologie. Fortschr Neurol Psychiat 1970; 38: 369–436.
[300] Bischoff A. Die diabetische Neuropathie. Stuttgart, Germany: Thieme Verlag, 1963.
[301] Neundörfer B. Differentialtypologie der Polyneuritiden und Polyneuropathien. Schriftenreihe Neurologie. Vol 11. Berlin, Heidelberg, New York: Springer, 1973.
[302] Bonkalo A. Relation between neuritis and the clinical background in diabetes mellitus. Arch Intern Med 1950; 85: 944–54.
[303] Daeppen J. Les Neuropathies diabétiques. Praxis 1960; 49: 902–15.
[304] Gomensoro JB, Temesio P, Ferrari A. Neuropatia diabetica. Rev Clin Esp 1961; 80: 1–15.
[305] Mayne N. Neuropathy in the diabetic and non-diabetic populations. Lancet 1965; II: 1313–6.
[306] Neundörfer B. Ein Beitrag zur Differentialdiagnose fehlender oder abgeschwächter Achillessehnenreflexe. Dtsch Med Wochenschr 1970; 95: 2474–7.
[307] Said G. Diabetic neuropathy: an update. J Neurol 1996; 243: 431–40.
[308] Hirson C, Feinmann EL, Wade JH. Diabetic neuropathy. BMJ 1953; I: 1408–13.
[309] Collens WS, Zilinsky JD, Boas LC. Quantitative estimation of vibratory sense as a guide for treatment of peripheral neuritis in diabetes. Proc Am Diabet Assoc 1947; 6: 457–68.
[310] Sabin TD, Geschwind N, Waxman SG. Patterns of clinical deficits in peripheral nerve disease. In: Waxman SG, editors. Physiology and pathobiology of axons. New York, NY: Raven Press, 1978: 431–8.
[311] Said G, Goulon-Goeau C, Slama G, et al. Severe early-onset polyneuropathy in insulin-dependent diabetes mellitus: a clinical and pathological study. N Engl J Med 1992; 326: 1257–63.
[312] Said G, Slama G, Selva J. Progressive centripetal degeneration of axons in small fibre type diabetic polyneuropathy. A clinical and pathological study. Brain 1983; 106: 791–807.
[313] Low PA. McLeod JG. Autonomic neuropathies. In: Low PA, editors. Clinical autonomic disorders. 2nd ed. Philadelphia, Pa: Lippincott-Raven, 1997: 463–86.
[314] Fagius J. Microneurographic findings in diabetic polyneuropathy with special reference to sympathetic nerve activity. Diabetologia 1982; 23: 415–20.
[315] Tackmann W, Kaeser HE, Berger W, et al. Autonomic disturbances in relation to sensorimotor peripheral neuropathy in diabetes mellitus. J Neurol 1981; 224: 273–81.
[316] Canal N, Comi G, Saibene V, et al. The relationship between peripheral and autonomic neuropathy in insulin dependent diabetes: a clinical and instrumental evaluation. In: Canal N, Pozza G, editors. Peripheral neuropathies. Amsterdam:

Elsevier Science, North Holland Biomedical Press, 1978: 247–55.
[317] Fraser DM, Campbell IW, Ewing DJ, et al. Peripheral and autonomic nerve function in newly diagnosed diabetes. Diabetes 1977; 26: 546–50.
[318] Kennedy WR, Sakuta M, Sutherland D, et al. Quantitaton of the sweating deficiency in diabetes. Ann Neurol 1984; 15: 482–8.
[319] Pfeifer MA, Cook D, Brodsky J, et al. Quantitative evaluation of cardiac parasympathetic activity in normal and diabetic man. Diabetes 1982; 31: 339–45.
[320] Nicholson GA, Dawkins JL, Blair IP, et al. The gene for hereditary sensory neuropathy type I (HSN-I) maps to chromosome 9q22.1-q22.3. Nat Genet 1996; 13: 101–4.
[321] Dyck PJ, Benstead TJ, Conn DL, et al. Nonsystemic vasculitic neuropathy. Brain 1987; 110: 843–53.
[322] Stewart JD, McKelvey R, Duncan L, et al. Chronic inflammatory demyelinating polyneuropathy (CIDP) in diabetes. J Neurol Sci 1996; 142: 59–64.
[323] Pirart J. Diabetic neuropathy: a metabolic or a vascular disease? Diabetes 1965; 14: 1–9.
[324] Ellenberg M. Diabetic neuropathy cachexia. Diabetes 1974; 23: 418–23.
[325] Greenbaum D. Observations on the homogenous nature and pathogenesis of diabetic neuropathy. Brain 1964; 87: 215–32.
[326] Rucker CW. The causes of paralysis of the third, fourth and sixth cranial nerves. Am J Ophthalmol 1966; 61: 1293–8.
[327] Rush JA, Younge BR. Paralysis of cranial nerves III, IV, and VI: cause and prognosis in 1000 cases. Arch Ophthalmol 1981; 99: 76–9.
[328] Richards BW, Jones FR, Younge BR. Causes and prognosis in 4,278 cases of paralysis of the oculomotor, trochlear, and abducens nerves. Am J Ophthalmol 1992; 113: 489–96.
[329] Goldstein JE, Cogan DG. Diabetic ophthalmoplegia with special reference to the pupil. Arch Ophthalmol 1960; 64: 592–600.
[330] Zorilla E, Kozak EP. Ophthalmoplegia in diabetes mellitus. Ann Intern Med 1967; 67: 968–83.
[331] Teuscher AU, Meienberg O. Ischaemic oculomotor nerve palsy. Clinical features and vascular risk factors in 23 patients. J Neurol 1988; 232: 144–9.
[332] Watanabe K, Hagura R, Akunama Y, et al. Characteristic of cranial nerve palsies in diabetic patients. Diabetes Res Clin Pract 1990; 10: 19–27.
[333] Jackson WPU. Ocular nerve palsy with severe headache in diabetics. Br Med J 1955; 2: 408–9.
[334] Ross AT. Recurrent cranial nerve palsies in diabetes. Neurology 1962; 12: 180–5.
[335] Raff MC, Sangalang V, Asbury AK. Ischemic mononeuropathy multiplex associated with diabetes mellitus. Arch Neurol 1968; 18: 487–99.
[336] Said G, Lacroix C, Fujimura H, Blas C, Faux N. The peripheral neuropathy of necrotizing arteritis: a clinicopathologic study. Ann Neurol 1988; 23: 461–5.
[337] Nukada H, McMorran PO. Perivascular demyelination and intramyelinic oedema in reperfusion nerve injury. J Anat 1994; 185: 259–66.
[338] Hopf HC, Gutmann L. Diabetic third nerve palsy: evidence for a mesencephalic lesion. Neurology 1990; 40: 1041–5.
[339] Sunderland S, Hughes ESR. Pupilloconstriction pathway and the nerves to the ocular muscles in man. Brain 1946; 69: 301–9.
[340] Kerr FWL, Hollowell OW. Location of pupillomotor and accommodation fibres in the oculomotor nerve: experimental studies on paralytic mydriasis. J Neurol Neurosurg Psychiatry 1964; 27: 473–81.
[341] Korczyn AD. Prevalence of diabetes mellitus in Bell's palsy. Lancet 1971; 2: 489.
[342] Aminoff MJ, Miller AL. The prevalence of diabetes mellitus in patients with Bell's palsy. Acta Neurol Scand 1972; 48: 381–4.
[343] Adour KK, Bell DN, Wingerd J. Bell palsy. Dilemma of diabetes mellitus. Arch Otolaryngol 1974; 99: 114–7.
[344] Pecket P, Schattner A. Concurrent Bell's palsy and diabetes mellitus: a diabetic mononeuropathy? J Neurol Neurosurg Psychiatry 1982; 45: 652–5.
[345] Abraham-Inpijn L, Devries PP, Hart AA. Predisposing factors in Bell's palsy: a clinical study with reference to diabets mellitus, hypertension, clotting mechanism and lipid disturbance. Clin Otolaryngol 1982; 7: 99–105.
[346] Takahashi A, Sobue I. Concurrence of facial paralysis and diabetes mellitus: prevalence, clinical features and prednisolone treatment. In: Goto Y, Horinchi A, Kogure K, editors. Diabetic neuropathy. Amsterdam: Excerpta Med, 1982: 173–8.
[347] Stewart JD. Diabetic truncal neuropathy: topography of the sensory deficit. Ann Neurol 1989; 25: 233–8.
[348] Chaudhuri KR, Wren DR, Werring D, et al. Unilateral abdominal muscle herniation with pain: a distinctive variant of diabetic radiculopathy. Diabet Med 1997; 14: 803–7.
[349] Schulz A. Diabetische Radiculopathie der unteren Thorakalsegmente mit Bauchdekkenparesen. Verh Dtsch Ges Inn Med 1966; 72: 1171–5.
[350] Wessely P, Schnaberth G. Kasuistischer Beitrag zu einer seltenen Lokalisation diabetischer Neuropathie. Wien Klin Wochenschr 1973; 85: 710–2.
[351] Ellenberg M. Diabetic truncal mononeuropathy-a new clinical syndrome. Diabetes Care 1978; 1: 10–3.
[352] Sun SF, Streib EW. Diabetic thoracoabdominal neuropathy: clinical and electrodiagnostic features. Ann Neurol 1981; 9: 75–9.
[353] Schulz A. Brennende Schmerzen an Rumpp und Oberschenkel mit Bandeckenparesen. Dtsch Med Wochenschr 1972; 97: 1568–9.
[354] Longstreth GF, Newcomer AD. Abdominal pain caused by diabetic radiculopathy. Ann Intern Med 1977; 86: 166–8.
[355] Child DL, Yates DAH. Radicular pain in diabetes. Rheumatol Rehabil 1978; 17: 195–6.
[356] Boulton AJM, Angus E, Ayyar DR, et al. Diabetic thoracic polyradiculopathy presenting as an abdominal swelling. Br Med J 1984; 289: 798–9.
[357] Parry GJ, Floberg J. Diabetic truncal neuropathy presenting as abdominal hernia. Neurology 1989; 39: 1488–90.
[358] Weeks RA, Thomas PK, Gale AN. Abdominal pseudohernia caused by diabetic truncal radiculoneuropathy. J Neurol Neurosurg Psychiatry 1999; 66: 405.
[359] Garland H. Diabetic amyotrophy. Br Med J 1955; 2: 1287–90.
[360] Bastron JA, Thomas JE. Diabetic polyradiculopathy: clinical and electromyographic findings in 105 patients. Mayo Clin Proc 1981; 56: 725–32.
[361] Kitka DG, Breuer AC, Wilbourne AJ. Thoracic root pain in diabetes: the spectrum of clinical electromyographic findings. Ann Neurol 1982; 11: 80–5.
[362] Bruns L. Über neuritische Lähmungen beim Diabetes Mellitus. Berl Klin Wochenschr 1890; 27: 509–15.
[363] Garland H, Taverner D. Diabetic myelopathy. Br Med J 1953; 1: 1405–8.
[364] Calverley JR, Mulder DW. Femoral neuropathy. Neurology 1960; 10: 963–7.
[365] Williams IR, Mayer RF. Subacute proximal diabetic neuropathy. Neurology 1976; 26: 108–16.
[366] Coppack SW, Watkins PJ. The natural history of diabetic femoral neuropathy. Q J Med 1991; 79: 307–13.
[367] Casey EB, Harrison MJE. Diabetic amyotrophy: a follow-up study. Br Med J 1972; 1: 656–9.
[368] Asbury AK. Renaut bodies: a forgotten endoneurial structure. J Neuropathol Exp Neurol 1973; 32: 334–43.
[369] Said G, Goulou-Goeau C, Lacroix C, et al. Nerve biopsy findings in different pattern of proximal diabetic neuropathy. Ann Neurol 1994; 35: 559–69.
[370] Llewelyn JG, Thomas PK, King RHM. Epineurial microvasculitis in proximal diabetic neuropathy. J Neurol 1998; 245: 159–65.
[371] Said G, Elgrably F, Lacroix C, et al. Painful proximal diabetic neuropathy inflammatory nerve lesions and spontaneous favourable outcome. Ann Neurol 1997; 41: 762–70.
[372] Bradley WG, Chad D, Verghese JP, et al. Painful lumbosacral plexopathy with elevated erythrocyte sedimentation rate: a treatable inflammatory syndrome. Ann Neurol 1984; 15: 457–64.
[373] Wilbourne AJ. Diabetic entrapment and compression neuropathies. In: Dyck PJ, Thomas PK, editors. Diabetic neuropathy. 2nd ed. Philadelphia, Pa: W.B. Saunders, 1999: 481–508.

[374] Mulder DW, Lambert EH, Bastron JA, et al. The neuropathies associated with diabetes mellitus. Neurology 1961; 11: 275–84.
[375] Fry IK, Hardwick C, Scott CW. Diabetic neuropathy: a survey and follow-up in 66 cases. Guy's Hosp Rep 1962; 111: 113–29.
[376] Fraser DM, Campbell IW, Ewing DJ, et al. Mononeuropathy in diabetes mellitus. Diabetes 1979; 28: 96–101.
[377] Thomas PK. Painful neuropathies. In: Bonica JJ, Liebeskind JC, Albe-Fessaed DG, editors. Advances in pain research and therapy. New York, NY: Raven Press, 1979: 103–101.
[378] Gilliatt RW, Willison RG. Peripheral nerve conduction in diabetic neuropathy. J Neurol Neurosurg Psychiatry 1962; 25: 11–8.
[379] Ochoa J, Fowler TJ, Gilliatt RW. Anatomical changes in peripheral nerves compressed by pneumatic tourniquet. J Anat 1972; 113: 433–55.
[380] King RHM, Llewelyn JG, Thomas PK, et al. Diabetic neuropathy: abnormalities of Schwann cell and perineurial basal lamina. Implications for diabetic neuropathy. Neuropathol Appl Neurobiol 1989; 5: 339–55.
[381] Krendel DA, Costigan DA, Hopkins LC. Successful treatment of neuropathies in patients with diabetes mellitus. Arch Neurol 1995; 52: 1053–61.
[382] Bell DS. Stroke in the diabetic patient. Diabetes Care 1994; 17: 213–9.
[383] Cryer PE, Fisher JN, Shamoon H. Hypoglycemia. Diabetes Care 1994; 17: 734–55.
[384] Miles WR, Root HF. Psychologic tests applied in diabetic patients. Arch Intern Med 1922; 30: 767–77.
[385] Ryan CM. Neurobehavioral complications of type I diabetes. Examination of possible risk factors. Diabetes Care 1988; 11: 86–93.
[386] Gold AE, Deary IJ, Jones RW, et al. Severe deterioration in cognitive function and personality in five patients with long-standing diabetes: a complication of diabetes or a consequence of treatment? Diabet Med 1994; 11: 499–505.
[387] Ryan CM, Williams TM, Finegold DN, et al. Cognitive dysfunction in adults with type 1 (insulin-dependent) diabetes mellitus of long duration; effects of recurrent hypoglycaemia and other chronic complications. Diabetologia 1993; 36: 329–34.
[388] Deary IJ, Crawford JR, Hepburn DA, et al. Severe hypoglycemia and intelligence in adult patients with insulin-treated diabetes. Diabetes 1993; 42: 341–4.
[389] Ryan CM, Williams TM. Effects of insulin-dependent diabetes on learning and memory efficiency in adults. J Clin Exp Neuropsychol 1993; 15: 685–700.
[390] The DCCT Research Group. Effects of intensive diabetes therapy on neuropsychological function in adults in the Diabetes Control and Complications Trial. Ann Intern Med 1996; 124: 379–88.
[391] Wredling R, Levander S, Adamson U, et al. Permanent neuropsychological impairment after recurrent episodes of severe hypoglycaemia in man. Diabetologia 1990; 33: 152–7.
[392] Lincoln NB, Faleiro RM, Kelly C, et al. Effect of long-term glycemic control on cognitive function. Diabetes Care 1996; 19: 656–8.
[393] Reichard P, Berglund A, Britz A, et al. Hypoglycaemic episodes during intensified insulin treatment: increased frequency but no effect on cognitive function. J Intern Med 1991; 229: 9–16.
[394] Kramer L, Fasching P, Madl C, et al. Previous episodes of hypoglycemic coma are not associated with permanent cognitive brain dysfunction in IDDM patients on intensive insulin treatment. Diabetes 1998; 47: 1909–14.
[395] Biessels GJ. Cerebral complications of diabetes: clinical findings and pathogenetic mechanisms. Neth J Med 1999; 54: 35–45.
[396] Tun PA, Nathan DM, Perlmuter LC. Cognitive and affective disorders in elderly diabetics. Clin Geriatr Med 1990; 6: 731–46.
[397] Strachan MWJ, Deary IJ, Ewing FME, et al. Is type II diabetes associated with an increased risk of cognitive dysfunction? A critical review of published studies. Diabetes Care 1997; 20: 438–45.
[398] Stewart R, Liolitsa D. Type 2 diabetes mellitus, cognitive impairment and dementia. Diabet Med 1999; 16: 93–112.
[399] Croxson SCM, Jagger C. Diabetes and cognitive impairment: a community based study of elderly subjects. Age Ageing 1995; 24: 421–4.
[400] Kalmijn S, Feskens EJM, Launer LJ, et al. Glucose intolerance, hyperinsulinaemia and cognitive function in a general population of elderly men. Diabetologia 1995; 38: 1096–102.
[401] Vanhanen M, Koivisto K, Karjalainen L, et al. Risk for non-insulin-dependent diabetes in the normoglycaemic elderly is associated with impaired cognitive function. Neuroreport 1997; 8: 1527–30.
[402] Ott A, Stolk RP, Hofman A, et al. Association of diabetes mellitus and dementia: The Rotterdam Study. Diabetologia 1996; 39: 1392–7.
[403] Leibson CL, Rocca WA, Hanson VA, et al. Risk of dementia among persons with diabetes mellitus: a population-based cohort study. Am J Epidemiol 1997; 145: 301–8.
[404] Ott A, Stolk RP, Van Harskamp F, et al. Diabetes mellitus and the risk of dementia: The Rotterdam Study. Neurology 1999; 53: 1937–42.
[405] Curb JD, Rodriguez BL, Abbott RD, et al. Longitudinal association of vascular and Alzheimer's dementias, diabetes, and glucose tolerance. Neurology 1999; 52: 971–5.
[406] Peyrot M, Rubin RR. Levels and risks of depression and anxiety symptomatology among diabetic adults. Diabetes Care 1997; 20: 585–90.
[407] Lustman PJ, Griffith LS, Gavard JA, et al. Depression in adults with diabetes. Diabetes Care 1992; 15: 1631–9.
[408] Di Mario U, Morano S, Valle E, et al. Electrophysiological alterations of the central nervous system in diabetes mellitus. Diabetes Metab Rev 1995; 11: 259–78.
[409] Stockard JJ, Pope-Stockard JE, Sharbrough FW. Brainstem auditory evoked potentials in neurology: methodology, interpretation and clinical application. In: Aminoff MJ, editors. Electrodiagnosis in clinical neurology. New York: Churchill Livingstone, 1992: 503–36.
[410] Donald MW, Williams Erdahl DL, Surridge DHC, et al. Functional correlates of reduced central conduction velocity in diabetic subjects. Diabetes 1984; 33: 627–33.
[411] Khardori R, Soler NG, Good DC, et al. Brainstem auditory and visual evoked potentials in type 1 (insulin-dependent) diabetic patients. Diabetologia 1986; 29: 362–5.
[412] Parisi V, Uccioli L. Visual electrophysiological responses in persons with type 1 diabetes. Diabetes Metab Res Rev 2001; 17: 12–8.
[413] Moreo G, Mariani E, Pizzamiglio G, et al. Visual evoked potentials in NIDDM: a longitudinal study. Diabetologia 1995; 38: 573–6.
[414] Ziegler O, Guerci B, Algan M, et al. Improved visual evoked potential latencies in poorly controlled diabetic patients after short-term strict metabolic control. Diabetes Care 1994; 17: 1141–7.
[415] Nakamura R, Noritake M, Hosoda Y, et al. Somatosensory conduction delay in central and peripheral nervous system of diabetic patients. Diabetes Care 1992; 15: 532–5.
[416] Gupta PR, Dorfman LJ. Spinal somatosensory conduction in diabetes. Neurology 1981; 31: 841–5.
[417] Bax G, Lelli S, Grandis U, et al. Early involvement of central nervous system type I diabetic patients. Diabetes Care 1995; 18: 559–62.
[418] Picton TW. The P300 wave of the human event-related potential. J Clin Neurophysiol 1992; 9: 456–79.
[419] Mooradian AD, Perryman K, Fitten J, et al. Cortical function in elderly non-insulin dependent diabetic patients. Behavioral and electrophysiologic studies. Arch Intern Med 1988; 148: 2369–72.
[420] Pozzessere G, Valle E, de-Crignis S, et al. Abnormalities of cognitive functions in IDDM revealed by P300 event-related potential analysis. Comparison with short-latency evoked potentials and psychometric tests. Diabetes 1991; 40: 952–8.
[421] Reske-Nielsen E, Lundbaek K, Rafaelsen OJ. Pathological changes in the central and peripheral nervous system of young long-term diabetics. Diabetologia 1965; 1: 233–41.
[422] Peress NS, Kane WC, Aronson SM. Central nervous system findings in a tenth decade autopsy population. Progr Brain Res 1973; 40: 473–83.
[423] Soininen H, Puranen M, Helkala EL, et al. Diabetes mellitus and brain atrophy: a computed tomography study in an elderly population. Neurobiol Aging 1992; 13: 717–21.

[424] Araki Y, Nomura M, Tanaka H, et al. MRI of the brain in diabetes mellitus. Neuroradiology 1994; 36: 101–3.
[425] Lunetta M, Damanti AR, Fabbri G, et al. Evidence by magnetic resonance imaging of cerebral alterations of atrophy type in young insulin-dependent diabetic patients. J Endocrinol Invest 1994; 17: 241–5.
[426] Ylikoski A, Erkinjuntti T, Raininko R, et al. White matter hyperintensities on MRI in the neurologically nondiseased elderly. Analysis of cohorts of consecutive subjects aged 55 to 85 years living at home. Stroke 1995; 26: 1171–7.
[427] Sredy J, Sawicki DR, Notvest RR. Polyol pathway activity in nervous tissues of diabetic and galactose-fed rats: effect of dietary galactose withdrawal or tolrestat intervention therapy. J Diabetes Complications 1991; 5: 42–7.
[428] Knudsen GM, Jakobsen J, Barry DI, et al. Myo-inositol normalizes decreased sodium permeability of the blood-brain barrier in streptozotocin diabetes. Neuroscience 1989; 29: 773–7.
[429] Ryle C, Leow CK, Donaghy M. Nonenzymatic glycation of peripheral and central nervous system proteins in experimental diabetes mellitus. Muscle Nerve 1997; 20: 577–84.
[430] Mooradian AD. The antioxidative potential of cerebral microvessels in experimental diabetes mellitus. Brain Res 1995; 671: 164–9.
[431] Kumar JS, Menon VP. Effect of diabetes on levels of lipid peroxides and glycolipids in rat brain. Metabolism 1993; 42: 1435–9.
[432] Makar TK, Rimpel-Lamhaouar K, Abraham DG, et al. Antioxidant defense systems in the brains of type II diabetic mice. J Neurochem 1995; 65: 287–91.
[433] Mankovsky BN, Metzger BE, Molitch ME, et al. Cerebrovascular disorders in patients with diabetes mellitus. J Diabetes Complications 1997; 10: 228–42.
[434] Smith MA, Sayre LM, Monnier VM, et al. Radical ageing in Alzheimer's disease. Trends Neurosci 1995; 18: 172–6.
[435] Gispen WH, Biessels GJ. Cognition and synaptic plasticity in diabetes mellitus. Trends Neurosci 2000; 23: 542–9.
[436] Hoyer S. Is sporadic Alzheimer disease the brain type of non-insulin dependent diabetes mellitus? A challenging hypothesis. J Neural Transm 1998; 105: 415–22.
[437] Frolich L, Blum-Degen D, Bernstein HG, et al. Brain insulin and insulin receptors in aging and sporadic Alzheimer's disease. J Neural Transm 1998; 105: 423–38.
[438] Biller J, Love BB. Diabetes and stroke. Med Clin North Am 1993; 77: 95–110.
[439] Kilander L, Nyman H, Boberg M, et al. Hypertension is related to cognitive impairment: a 20-year follow-up of 999 men. Hypertension 1998; 31: 780–6.
[440] Kuusisto J, Koivisto K, Mykkänen L, et al. Essential hypertension and cognitive function: the role of hyperinsulinemia. Hypertension 1993; 22: 771–9.
[441] Geldmacher DS, Whitehouse PJ. Evaluation of dementia. N Engl J Med 1996; 335: 330–6.
[442] Meneilly GS, Cheung E, Tessier D, et al. The effect of improved glycemic control on cognitive functions in the elderly patient with diabetes. J Gerontol 1993; 48: M117-M121.
[443] Gradman TJ, Laws A, Thompson LW, et al. Verbal learning and/or memory improves with glycemic control in older subjects with non-insulin-dependent diabetes mellitus. J Am Geriatr Soc 1993; 41: 1305–12.
[444] Zorilla E, Kozak GP. Ophthalmoplegia in diabetes mellitus. Ann Intern Med 1967; 67: 968–76.
[445] Thomas PK, Olsson Y. Microscopic anatomy and function of the connective tissue components of peripheral nerve. In: Dyck PJ, Thomas PK, Lambert EH, et al, editors. Peripheral neuropathy. Philadelphia, Pa: W.B. Saunders, 1984: 97–120.
[446] Asbury AK, Aldredge H, Hershberg R, et al. Oculomotor palsy in diabetes mellitus: a clinical-pathological study. Brain 1970; 93: 555–66.
[447] Bortolami R, Veggetti A, Callegari E, et al. Afferent fibers and sensory ganglion cells within the oculomotor nerve in some mammals and man. I Anatomical investigations. Arch Ital Biol 1977; 115: 355–85.
[448] Bortolami R, Calza L, Lucchi ML, et al. Peripheral territory and neuropeptides of the trigeminal ganglion neurons centrally projecting through the oculomotor nerve demonstrating by fluorescent retrograde double-labeling compared with immunocytochemistry. Brain Res 1991; 547: 82–8.
[449] Bortolami R, D'Alessandro R, Manni E. The origin of pain in ischemic-diabetic third-nerve palsy. Arch Neurol 1993; 50: 795.
[450] Manni E, Bortolami R, Pettorossi VE, et al. Trigeminal afferent fibers in the trunk of the oculomotor nerve of lambs. Exp Neurol 1976; 50: 465–76.
[451] Thomas PK. Painful neuropathies. In: Bonica JJ, Liebeskind JC, Albe-Fessard DG, editors. Advances in pain research and therapy. New York, NY: Raven Press, 1979: 103–10.
[452] Torebjörk HE, La Motte RH , Robinson CJ. Peripheral neural correlates of magnitude of cutaneous pain and hyperalgesia: simultaneous recordings in humans of sensory judgements of pain and evoked responses in nociceptors with C fibers. J Neurophysiol 1984; 51: 325–39.
[453] Cline MA, Ochoa JL, Torebjörk E. Chronic hyperalgesia and skin warming caused by sensitized C nociceptors. Brain 1989; 112: 621–47.
[454] Ochoa JL. Positive sensory symptoms in neuropathy: mechanisms and aspects of treatment. In: Asbury AK, Thomas PK, editors. Peripheral nerve disorders. Oxford: Butterworth Heinemann, 1995: 44–58.
[455] Thomas PK. The anatomical substratum of pain: evidence derived from morphometric studies of peripheral nerve. Can J Neurol Sci 1974; 1: 92–7.
[456] Campbell JN, Raja SN, Meyer RA, et al. Myelinated afferents signal the hyperalgesia associated with nerve injury. Pain 1988; 32: 89–94.
[457] Dyck PJ, Lambert H, O'Brien PC. Pain in peripheral neuropathy related to rate and kind of fiber degeneration. Neurology 1976; 26: 466–71.
[458] Llewelyn JG, Gilbey SG, Thomas PK, et al. Sural nerve morphometry in diabetic autonomic and painful sensory neuropathy: a clinicopathological study. Brain 1991; 114: 867–92.
[459] Castellanos F, Mascias J, Zabala JA, et al. Acute painful diabetic neuropathy following severe weight loss. Muscle Nerve 1996; 19: 463–7.
[460] Britland ST, Young RJ, Sharma AK, et al. Acute remitting painful diabetic polyneuropathy: a comparison of peripheral nerve fibre pathology. Pain 1992; 48: 361–70.
[461] Brown MJ, Martin JR, Asbury AK. Painful diabetic neuropathy: a morphometric study. Arch Neurol 1976; 33: 164–71.
[462] Asbury AK, Fields HL. Pain due to peripheral nerve damage: an hypothesis. Neurology 1984; 34: 1587–90.
[463] Wall PD, Gutnick M. Ongoing activity in peripheral nerves: the physiology and pharmacology of impulses originating in a neuroma. Exp Neurol 1974; 43: 580–93.
[464] Scadding JW. Development of ongoing activity, mechanosensitivity and adrenaline sensitivity in severed peripheral nerve axons. Exp Neurol 1981; 73: 345–64.
[465] Llewelyn JG, Thomas PK, Fonseca V, et al. Acute painful diabetic neuropathy precipitated by strict glycaemic control. Acta Neuropathol 1986; 72: 157–63.
[466] Thomas PK, Scadding JW. Treatment of pain in diabetic neuropathy. In: Dyck PJ, Thomas PK, Asbury AK, et al, editors. Diabetic neuropathy. Philadelphia: W.B. Saunders, 1987: 216–22.
[467] Britland ST, Young RJ, Sharma AK, et al. Association of painful and painless diabetic neuropathy with different patterns of nerve fibre degeneration and regeneration. Diabetes 1990; 39: 898–908.
[468] Aitken JT, Thomas PK. Retrograde changes in fibre size following nerve section. J Anat 1962; 96: 121–9.
[469] Dyck PJ, Lais AC, Karnes JL, et al. Permanent axotomy, a model of axonal atrophy and secondary demyelination and regeneration. Ann Neurol 1981; 9: 575–83.
[470] Cragg BG, Thomas PK. Changes in conduction velocity and fibre size proximal to peripheral nerve lesions. J Physiol (London) 1961; 157: 315–27.
[471] Devor M, Govrin-Lippmann R. Maturation of axonal sprouts after nerve crush. Exp Neurol 1979; 64: 260–70.
[472] Sugimura K, Dyck PJ. Sural nerve myelin thickness and axis cylinder caliber in human diabetes. Neurology 1981; 31: 1087–91.
[473] Doupe J, Cullen CH, Chance CQ. Post-traumatic pain and the causalgic syndrome. J Neurol Neurosurg Psychiatry 1944; 7: 33–48.
[474] Granit R, Leksell L, Skoglund CR. Fibre interaction in injured or compressed region of nerve. Brain 1944; 67: 125–40.

[475] Seltzer Z, Devor M. Ephaptic transmission in chronically damaged peripheral nerves. Neurology 1979; 29: 1061–4.
[476] Nielsen VK. Pathophysiology of hemifacial spasm I: Ephaptic transmission and ectopic excitation. Neurology 1984; 34: 418–26.
[477] Sanders DB. Ephaptic transmission in hemifacial spasm: a single fiber EMG study. Muscle Nerve 1989; 12: 690–4.
[478] Wall PD, Devor M. Sensory afferent impulses originate from dorsal root ganglia as well as from the periphery in normal and injured rat nerves. Pain 1983; 17: 321–39.
[479] Said G, Slama G, Selva J. Progressive centripetal degeneration of axons in small fibre type diabetic polyneuropathy. A clinical and pathological study. Brain 1983; 106: 791–807.
[480] Archer AG, Roberts VC, Watkins PJ. Blood flow patterns in painful diabetic neuropathy. Diabetologia 1984; 27: 563–7.
[481] Morley GK, Mooradian AD, Levine AS et al. Mechanism of pain in diabetic neuropathy. Effect of glucose on pain perception in humans. Am I Med 1984; 77: 79–82.
[482] Boulton AJM, Drury J, Clarke B, Ward JD. Continuous subacute insulin infusion in the management of painful diabetic neuropathy. Diabetes Care 1982; 5: 386–90.
[483] Simon GS, Dewey WL. Narcotics and diabetes I. The effects of streptozotocin-induced diabetes on the antinociceptive potency of morphine. J Pharmacol Exp Ther 1981; 218: 318–23.
[484] Tuck RR, Schmelzer JD, Low PA. Endoneurial blood flow and oxygen tension in the sciatic nerves of rats with experimental diabetic neuropathy. Brain 1984; 107: 935–50.
[485] Schneider U, Quasthoff S, Mitrovic N, et al. Hyperglycaemic hypoxia alters after potential and fast K^+ conductance of rat axons by cytoplasmic acidification. J Physiol 1993; 465: 679–97.
[486] Hillman P, Wall PD. Inhibitory and excitatory factors influencing the receptive fields of lamina 5 spinal cord cells. Exp Brain Res 1969; 9: 284–306.
[487] Archer AG, Watkins PJ, Thomas PK, et al. The natural history of acute painful diabetic neuropathy. J Neurol Neurosurg Psychiatry 1983; 46: 491–9.
[488] Wall PD. Future trends in pain research. Philos Trans R Soc Lond B Biol Sci 1985; 308: 393–405.
[489] Melzack R, Wall PD. Pain mechanisms: a new theory. Science 1965; 150: 971–9.
[490] Bowsher D. Neurogenic pain syndromes and their management. Br Med Bull 1991; 47: 644–66.
[491] Crook J, Rideout E, Browne G. The prevalence of pain complaints in a general population. Pain 1984; 18: 299–314.
[492] Merskey H. Classification of chronic pain. Pain 1986; 3: 215–7.
[493] Chan AW, MacFarlane IA, Bowsher DR, et al. Chronic pain in patients with diabetes mellitus: comparison with non-diabetic population. Pain Clin 1990; 3: 147–59.
[494] Ziegler D. Diagnosis, staging and epidemiology of diabetic peripheral neuropathy. Diabetes Nutr Metab 1994; 7: 342–8.
[495] Dyck PJ, Kratz KM, Karnes JL, et al. The prevalence by staged severity of various types of diabetic neuropathy, retinopathy, and nephropathy in a population-based cohort: The Rochester Diabetic Neuropathy Study. Neurology 1993; 43: 817–24.
[496] Galer BS, Gianas A, Jensen MP. Painful diabetic neuropathy: epidemiology, pain description, and quality of life. Diabetes Res Clin Pract 2000; 47: 123–8.
[497] Asbury AK, Fields HL. Pain due to peripheral nerve damage: a hypothesis. Neurology 1984; 34: 1587–90.
[498] Pfeifer MA, Ross DR, Schrager JP, et al. A highly successful and novel model for treatment of chronic painful diabetic peripheral neuropathy. Diabetes Care 1993; 16: 1103–15.
[499] Rajbhandari SM, Jarratt JA, Griffiths PD, Ward JD. Diabetic neuropathic pain in a leg amputated 44 years previously. Pain 1999; 83: 627–9.
[500] Thomas PK, Scadding JW. Treatment of pain in diabetic neuropathy. In: Dyck PJ, Thomas PK, Asbury AK, et al, editors. Diabetic neuropathy. Philadelphia, Pa: W.B. Saunders, 1987: 216–22.
[501] Thomas PK. Painful diabetic neuropathy: mechanisms and treatment. Diabetes Nutr Metab 1994; 7: 359–68.
[502] Watkins PJ. The natural history of the diabetic neuropathies. Q J Med 1990; 77: 1209–18.
[503] Boulton AJM, Scarpello JHB, Armstrong WD, Ward JD. The natural history of painful diabetic neuropathy—a 4-year study. Postgrad Med J 1983; 59: 556–9.
[504] Young RJ, Ewing DJ, Clarke BF. Chronic and remitting painful diabetic neuropathy. Diabetes Care 1988; 11: 34–40.
[505] Benbow SJ, Chan AW, Bowsher D, et al. A prospective study of painful symptoms, small-fibre function and peripheral vascular disease in chronic painful diabetic neuropathy. Diabetic Med 1993; 11: 17–21.
[506] Archer AG, Watkins PJ, Thomas PK, et al. The natural history of acute painful neuropathy in diabetes mellitus. J Neurol Neurosurg Psychiatry 1983; 46: 491–9.
[507] Ellenberg M. Diabetic neuropathic cachexia. Diabetes 1974; 23: 418–23.
[508] Steele JM, Young RJ, Lloyd GG, Clarke BF. Clinically apparent eating disorders in young diabetic women: associations with painful neuropathy and other complications. Br Med J 1987; 294: 859–66.
[509] Caravati CM. Insulin neuritis: a case report. Va Med Mon 1933; 59: 745–6.
[510] Llewelyn JG, Thomas PK, Fonseca V, et al. Acute painful diabetic neuropathy precipitated by strict glycaemic control. Acta Neuropathol 1986; 72: 157–63.
[511] Tesfaye S, Malik R, Harris N, et al. Arterio-venous shunting and proliferating new vessels in acute painful neuropathy of rapid glycaemic control (insulin neuritis). Diabetologia 1996; 39: 329–35.
[512] Chan AW, MacFarlane IA, Bowsher D. Short term fluctuations in blood glucose concentrations do not alter pain perception in diabetic patients with and without painful peripheral neuropathy. Diabetes Res 1990; 14: 15–9.
[513] Asbury AK. Focal and multifocal neuropathies of diabetes. In: Dyck PJ, Thomas PK, Asbury AK, et al, editors. Diabetic neuropathy. Philadelphia, Pa: W B Saunders, 1987. 45–55.
[514] Zorilla E, Kozak GP. Ophthalmoplegia in diabetes mellitus. Ann Intern Med 1967; 67: 968–74.
[515] Chaudhuri KR, Wren DR, Werring D, Watkins PJ. Unilateral abdominal muscle herniation with pain: a distinctive variant of diabetic radiculopathy. Diabetic Med 1997; 14: 803–7.
[516] Melzack R. Measurement of the dimensions of pain experience. In: Bromm B, editors. Pain measurement in man. Amsterdam: Elsevier Science, 1984: 327–48.
[517] Conno F De, Caraceni A, Gamba A, et al. Pain measurement in cancer patients: a comparison of six methods. Pain 1994; 57: 161-166.
[518] Williams RC. Toward a set of reliable and valid measures for chronic pain assessment and outcome research. Pain 1988; 35: 239–51.
[519] Scott J, Huskisson EC. Graphic representation of pain. Pain 1976; 2: 175–84.
[520] Collins SL, Moore RA, McQuay HJ. The visual analogue pain intensity scale: what is moderate pain in millimetres? Pain 1997; 72: 95–7.
[521] Melzack R. The McGill Pain Questionnaire: major properties and scoring methods. Pain 1975; 1: 277–99.
[522] Masson EA, Hunt L, Gem JM, Boulton AJM. A novel approach to the diagnosis and assessment of symptomatic diabetic neuropathy. Pain 1989; 38: 25–8.
[523] Galer BS, Jensen MP. Development and preliminary validation of a pain measure specific to neuropathic pain: the Neuropathic Pain Scale. Neurology 1997; 48: 332–8.
[524] Chan AW, MacFarlane IA. The impact of chronic pain on quality of life in diabetes. Pract Diabetes 1989; 6: 249–53.
[525] Vileikyte L, Bundy C, Shaw J, et al. Neuroqol: The first specific quality of life scale for diabetic neuropathy. Diabetologia 1998; 41(Suppl 1): A274.
[526] Young RJ, Clarke BF. Pain relief in diabetic neuropathy: the effectiveness of imipramine and related drugs. Diabet Med 1985; 2: 363–6.
[527] Vinik AI, Milicevic Z. Recent advances in the diagnosis and treatment of diabetic neuropathy. Endocrinologist 1996; 6: 443–61.
[528] Benbow SJ, Cossins L, MacFarlane IA. Painful diabetic neuropathy. Diabet Med 1999; 16: 632–44.

[529] Ziegler D. Pharmacological treatment of painful diabetic neuropathy. In: Veves A, editors. Contemporary endocrinology: clinical management of diabetic neuropathy. Totowa, NJ: Humana Press, 1998: 147–69.
[530] Amthor K-F, Dahl-Jorgensen K, Berg TJ, et al. The effect of 8 years of strict glycaemic control on peripheral nerve function in IDDM patients: the Oslo Study. Diabetologia 1994; 37: 579–84.
[531] The Diabetes Control and Complications Trial Research Group. The effect of intensive diabetes therapy on the development and progression of neuropathy. Ann Intern Med 1995; 122: 561–8.
[532] Reichard P, Pihl M, Rosenqvist U, Sule J. Complications in IDDM are caused by elevated blood glucose level: The Stockholm Diabetes Intervention Study (SDIS) at 10-year follow up. Diabetologia 1996; 39: 1483–8.
[533] Ohkubo Y, Kishikawa H, Araki E, et al. Intensive insulin therapy prevents the progression of diabetic microvascular complications in Japanese patients with non-insulin-dependent diabetes mellitus: a randomized prospective 6-year study. Diabetes Res Clin Pract 1995; 28: 103–17.
[534] Prospective Diabetes Study UK (UKPDS) Group. Intensive blood glucose control with sulphonylureas or insulin compared with conventional treatment and risk of complications in patients with type 2 diabetes. Lancet 1998; 352: 837–53.
[535] Gæde P. Vede P, Parving H-H, Pederson O. Intensified multifactorial intervention in patients with type 2 diabetes mellitus and microalbuminuria: the Steno type 2 randomised study. Lancet 1999; 353: 617–22.
[536] Ziegler D, Dannehl K, Wiefels K, Gries FA. Differential effects of near-normoglycaemia for 4 years on somatic nerve dysfunction and heart rate variation in type 1 diabetic patients. Diabet Med 1992; 9: 622–9.
[537] Ziegler D, Piolot R. Prevention of diabetic neuropathy by near-normoglycemia. A 12-year prospective study from the diagnosis of IDDM. Diabetes 1998; 47 (Suppl 1): A63.
[538] Ziegler D. Electrophysiologic assessment: relationship to glycaemic control. In: Hotta N, Greene DA, Ward JD, et al, editors. Diabetic neuropathy: new concepts and insights. Amsterdam: Elsevier Science, 1995: 59–69.
[539] Tattersall R. Is pancreas transplantation for insulin-dependent diabetics worthwhile? N Engl J Med 1989; 321: 112–4.
[540] Kennedy WR, Navarro X, Goetz FC, et al. Effects of pancreatic transplantation on diabetic neuropathy. N Engl J Med 1990; 322: 1031–7.
[541] Solders G, Tydén G, Persson A, Groth C-G. Improvement of nerve conduction in diabetic neuropathy. A follow-up study 4 yr after combined pancreatic and renal transplantation. Diabetes 1992; 41: 946–51.
[542] Martinenghi S, Comi G, Galardi G, et al. Amelioration of nerve conduction velocity following simultaneous kidney/pancreas transplantation is due to the glycaemic control provided by the pancreas. Diabetologia 1997; 40: 1110–2.
[543] Müller-Felber W, Landgraf R, Scheuer R, et al. Diabetic neuropathy 3 years after successful pancreas and kidney transplantation. Diabetes 1993; 42: 1482–6.
[544] Allen RDM, Al-Habri IS, Morris JGL, et al. Diabetic neuropathy after pancreas transplantation: determinants of recovery. Transplantation 1997; 63: 830–8.
[545] Cameron NE, Cotter MA. The relationship of vascular changes to metabolic factors in diabetes mellitus and their role in the development of peripheral nerve complications. Diabetes /Metab Rev 1994; 10: 189–224.
[546] Nicolucci A, Carinci F, Cavaliere D, et al. A meta-analysis of trials on aldose reductase inhibitors in diabetic peripheral neuropathy. Diabet Med 1996; 13: 1017–26.
[547] Nicolucci A, Carinci F, Graepel JG, et al. The efficacy of tolrestat in the treatment of diabetic peripheral neuropathy. A meta-analysis of individual patient data. Diabetes Care 1996; 19: 1091–6.
[548] Masson EA, Boulton AJM. Aldose reductase inhibitors in the treatment of diabetic neuropathy. A review of the rationale and clinical evidence. Drugs 1990; 39: 190–202.
[549] The γ-Linolenic Acid Multicenter Trial Group. Treatment of diabetic neuropathy with γ-linolenic acid. Diabetes Care 1993; 16: 8–15.
[550] Horrobin DF. Essential fatty acids in the management of impaired nerve function in diabetes. Diabetes 1997; 46(Suppl 2): S90-S93.
[551] Ziegler D, Reljanovic M, Mehnert H. Gries FA. α-Lipoic acid in the treatment of diabetic polyneuropathy in Germany: current evidence from clinical trials. Exp Clin Endocrinol Diabetes 1999; 107: 421–30.
[552] Shindo H, Tawata M, Aida K, Onaya T. Clinical efficacy of a stable prostacyclin analog, iloprost, in diabetic neuropathy. Prostaglandins 1991; 41: 85–96.
[553] Younger DS, Rosoklija G, Hays AP, et al. Diabetic peripheral neuropathy: a clinicopathologic and immunohistochemical analysis of sural nerve biopsies. Muscle Nerve 1996; 19: 722–7.
[554] Said G, Elgrably F, Lacroix C, et al. Painful proximal diabetic neuropathy: inflammatory nerve lesions and spontaneous favorable outcome. Ann Neurol 1997; 41: 762–70.
[555] Krendel DA, Costigan DA, Hopkins LC. Successful treatment of neuropathies in patients with diabetes mellitus. Arch Neurol 1995; 52: 1053–61.
[556] Gregersen G. Myo-Inositol supplementation. In: Dyck PJ, Thomas PK, Asbury AK, et al, editors. Diabetic neuropathy. Philadelphia, Pa: W.B. Saunders, 1987: 188–9.
[557] Yuen EC, Mobley WC. Therapeutic potential of neurotrophic factors for neurological disorders. Ann Neurol 1996; 40: 346–54.
[558] Riaz SS, Tomlinson DR. Neurotrophic factors in peripheral neuropathies: pharmacological strategies. Prog Neurobiol 1996; 49: 125–43.
[559] Yagihashi S, Kamijo S, Baba M, et al. Effect of aminoguanidine on functional and structural abnormalities in peripheral nerve of STZ-induced diabetic rats. Diabetes 1992; 41: 47–52.
[560] Dyck PJ, O'Brien PC. Meaningful degrees of prevention or improvement of nerve conduction in controlled clinical trials of diabetic neuropathy. Diabetes Care 1989; 9: 649–52.
[561] Boulton AJM, Levin S, Comstock J. A multicentre trial of the aldose-reductase inhibitor, tolrestat, in patients with symptomatic diabetic neuropathy. Diabetologia 1990; 33: 431–7.
[562] Sorbinil Retinopathy Trial Research Group. The Sorbinil Retinopathy Trial: neuropathy results. Neurology 1993; 43: 1141–9.
[563] Greene DA, Arezzo JC, Brown MB, Zenarestat Study Group. Effect of aldose reductase inhibition on nerve conduction and morphometry in diabetic neuropathy. Neurology 1999; 53: 580–91.
[564] Goto Y, Hotta N, Shigeta Y, et al. Effects of an aldose reductase inhibitor, epalrestat, on diabetic neuropathy. Clinical benefit and indication for the drug assessed from the results of a placebo-controlled double-blind study. Biomed Pharmacother 1995; 49: 269–77.
[565] Ziegler D, Mühlen H, Rathmann W, Gries FA. Effects of one year's treatment with gamma-linolenic acid (EF4) on diabetic neuropathy. Diabetes 1993; 42(Suppl 1): 99A.
[566] Nagamatsu M, Nickander KK, Schmelzer JD, et al. Lipoic acid improves nerve blood flow, reduces oxidative stress and improves distal nerve conduction in experimental diabetic neuropathy. Diabetes Care 1995; 18: 1160–7.
[567] Ziegler D, Hanefeld M, Ruhnau KJ, et al. The ALADIN Study Group. Treatment of symptomatic diabetic peripheral neuropathy with the antioxidant α-lipoic acid. A 3-week multicentre randomized controlled trial (ALADIN Study). Diabetologia 1995; 38: 1425–33.
[568] Ruhnau K-J, Meissner HP, Finn J-R, et al. Effects of 3-week oral treatment with the antioxidant thioctic acid (α-lipoic acid) in symptomatic diabetic polyneuropathy. Diabet Med 1999; 16: 1040–3.
[569] Ziegler D, Hanefeld M, Ruhnau K-J, et al. ALADIN III Study group. Treatment of symptomatic diabetic polyneuropathy with the antioxidant α-lipoic acid. A 7-month multicenter randomized controlled trial (ALADIN III Study). Diabetes Care 1999; 22: 1296–301.
[570] Ziegler D, Schatz H, Conrad F, et al, DEKAN Study Group. Effects of treatment with the antioxidant α-lipoic acid on cardiac autonomic neuropathy in NIDDM patients. A 4-month randomized controlled multicenter trial (DEKAN study). Diabetes Care 1997; 20: 369–73.

[571] Reljanovic M, Reichel C, Rett K, et al. The ALADIN II Study group. Treatment of diabetic peripheral neuropathy with the antioxidant thioctic acid (α-lipoic acid). A two-year multicenter randomized double blind placebo controlled trial (ALADIN II). Free Radic Res 1999; 31: 171–9.
[572] Rathmann W, Haastert B, Delling B, et al. Postmarketing surveillance of adverse drug reactions: a correlation study approach using multiple data sources. Pharmacoepidemiol Drug Saf 1998; 7: 51–7.
[573] Ziegler D. The design of clinical trials for treatment of diabetic neuropathy. Neurosci Res Commun 1997; 21: 83–91.
[574] Tütüncü NB, Bayraktar M, Varli K. Reversal of defective nerve conduction with vitamin E supplementation in type 2 diabetes. Diabetes Care 1998; 21: 1915–8.
[575] Malik RA, Williamson S, Abbott C, et al. Effect of angiotensin-converting-enzyme (ACE) inhibitor trandolapril on human diabetic neuropathy: randomised double blind placebo controlled trial. Lancet 1998; 352: 1978–81.
[576] Suzuki S, Okuda Y, Asano M, et al. Effects of beraprost sodium on diabetic peripheral neuropathy in type 2 diabetic patients. Diabetes Res 1999; 34: 29–35.
[577] Shindo H, Tawata M, Inoue M, et al. The effect of prostaglandin E1.αCD on vibratory threshold determined with the SMV-5 vibrometer in patients with diabetic neuropathy. Diabetes Res Clin Pract 1994; 24: 173–80.
[578] Toyota T, Hirata Y, Ikeda Y, et al. Lipo-PGE1, a new lipid-encapsulated preparation of prostaglandin E1: placebo- and prostaglandin E1-controlled multicenter trials in patients with diabetic neuropathy and leg ulcers. Prostaglandins 1993; 46: 453–68.
[579] Walk D. Immunotherapy of neuropathies in patients with diabetes mellitus requires closer scrutiny. Arch Neurol 1996; 53: 590–1.
[580] Krendel DA. Immunotherapy of neuropathies in patients with diabetes mellitus requires closer scrutiny (in reply). Arch Neurol 1996; 53: 591–2.
[581] Stevens MJ, Lattimer SA, Feldman EL, et al. Acetyl-L-carnitine deficiency as a cause of altered nerve myo-inositol content, Na,K-ATPase activity, and motor conduction velocity in the streptozotocin-diabetic rat. Metabolism 1996; 45: 865–72.
[582] Quatraro A, Roca P, Donzella C, et al. Acetyl-l-carnitine for symptomatic diabetic neuropathy. Diabetologia 1995; 38: 123.
[583] Bril V, Ellison R, Ngo M, et al. Electrophysiological monitoring in clinical trials. Muscle Nerve 1998; 21: 1368–73.
[584] Levi-Montalcini R. The nerve growth factor 35 years later. London: Science, 1987.
[585] Apfel SC, Kessler JA, Adornato BT, et al. Recombinant human nerve growth factor in the treatment of diabetic polyneuropathy. Neurology 1998; 51: 695–702.
[586] Bravenboer B, Hendrikse PH, Oey LP, et al. Randomized double-blind placebo-controlled trial to evaluate the effect of the ACTH4-9 analogue ORG 2766 in IDDM patients with neuropathy. Diabetologia 1994; 37: 408–13.
[587] Valk GD, Kappelle AC, Tjon-A-Tsien AML, et al. Treatment of diabetic polyneuropathy with the neurotrophic peptide ORG 2766. J Neurol 1996; 243: 257–63.
[588] Cohen KL, Lucibello FE, Chomiak MA. Lack of effect of clonidine and pentoxifylline in short-term therapy of diabetic peripheral neuropathy. Diabetes Care 1990; 13: 1074–7.
[589] Cohen SM, Mathews T. Pentoxifylline in the treatment of distal diabetic neuropathy. Angiology 1991; 42: 741–6.
[590] De Leeuw IH, Roy P Van, Moeremans M, Driessens M. Clinical experience with cyclandelate in insulin-dependent diabetic patients with neuropathy. Drugs 1987; 33(Suppl 2): 125–30.
[591] Heimans JJ, Drukarch B, Matthaei I, et al. Cyclandelate in diabetic neuropathy. A double-blind, placebo-controlled, randomized, cross-over study. Acta Neurol Scand 1991; 84: 483–6.
[592] Janka HU, Schuh D, Nuber A, Mehnert H. Der Einfluß von Ginkgo biloba Spezialextrakt EGb 761 auf die diabetische Neuropathie. Geriatr Forsch 1992; 2: 173–9.
[593] Hendriksen PH, Oey PL, Wieneke GH, et al. Antihypoxic treatment at an early stage of diabetic neuropathy: an electrophysiological study with sabeluzole. Acta Neurol Scand 1992; 86: 506–11.
[594] Laupacis A, Sackett DL, Roberts RS. An assessment of clinically useful measures of the consequences of treatment. N Engl J Med 1988; 318: 1728–33.
[595] Cook RJ, Sackett DL. The number needed to treat: a clinically useful measure of treatment effect. Br Med J 1995; 310: 452–4.
[596] McQuay HJ, Moore RA. Using numerical results from systematic reviews in clinical practice. Ann Intern Med 1997; 126: 712–20.
[597] Philipp M, Fickinger M. Psychotropic drugs in the management of chronic pain syndromes. Pharmacopsychiatry 1993; 26: 221–34.
[598] Onghena P, van Houdenhove B. Antidepressant-induced analgesia in chronic non-malignant pain: a meta-analysis of 39 placebo-controlled studies. Pain 1992; 49: 205–19.
[599] McQuay HJ, Tramer M, Nye BA, et al. A systematic review of antidepressants in neuropathic pain. Pain 1996; 68: 217–27.
[600] Sindrup SH. Antidepressants in the treatment of diabetic neuropathy symptoms. Pharmacodynamic,—kinetic, and genetic aspects. Dan Med Bull 1994; 41: 66–78.
[601] Kingery WS. A critical review of controlled clinical trials for peripheral neuropathic pain and complex regional pain syndromes. Pain 1997; 73: 123–39.
[602] Low PA, Dotson RM. Symptomatic treatment of painful neuropathy. JAMA 1998; 280: 1863–4.
[603] Sindrup SH, Jensen TS. Efficacy of pharmacological treatments of neuropathic pain: an update and effect related to mechanism of drug action. Pain 1999; 83: 389–400.
[604] McQuay HJ, Moore RA. Antidepressants and chronic pain. Br Med J 1997; 314: 763–4.
[605] Max MB, Kishore-Kumar R, Schafer SC, et al. Efficacy of desipramine in painful diabetic neuropathy: a placebo controlled trial. Pain 1991; 45: 3–9.
[606] Max MB, Lynch SA, Muir J, et al. Effects of desipramine, amitriptyline, and fluoxetine on pain in diabetic neuropathy. N Engl J Med 1992; 326: 1250–6.
[607] Max MB, Culnane M, Schafer SC, et al. Amitriptyline relieves diabetic neuropathy pain in patients with normal or depressed mood. Neurology 1987; 37: 589–96.
[608] McQuay HJ, Carroll D, Glynn CJ. Dose-response for analgesic effect of amitriptyline in chronic pain. Anaesthesia 1993; 48: 281–5.
[609] Gomez-Perez FJ, Rull JA, Dies H, et al. Nortriptyline and fluphenazine in the symptomatic treatment of diabetic neuropathy. A double-blind cross-over study. Pain 1985; 23: 395–400.
[610] Gomez-Perez FJ, Choza R, Rios JM, et al. Nortriptyline-fluphenazine vs. carbamazepine in the symptomatic treatment of diabetic neuropathy. Arch Med Res 1996; 27: 525–9.
[611] Sindrup SH, Gram LF, Brosen K, Eshoj O, Mogensen EF. The selective serotonin reuptake inhibitor paroxetine is effective in the treatment of diabetic neuropathy symptoms. Pain 1990; 42: 135–44.
[612] Sindrup SH, Bjerre U, Dejgaard A, et al. The selective serotonin reuptake inhibitor citalopram relieves the symptoms of diabetic neuropathy. Clin Pharmacol Ther 1992; 52: 547–52.
[613] Henry JA, Alexander CA, Sener EK. Relative mortality from overdose of antidepressants. Br Med J 1995; 310: 221–4.
[614] Abajo FJ, Rodriguez LAG, Montero D. Association between selective serotonin reuptake inhibitors and upper gastrointestinal bleeding: population based case-control study. Br Med J 1999; 319: 1106–9.
[615] Rull JA, Quibrera R, Gonzalez-Millan H, Castaneda LO. Symptomatic treatment of peripheral diabetic neuropathy with carbamazepine (Tegretol): double blind crossover trial. Diabetologia 1969; 5: 215–8.
[616] Ocaranza Ochoa J, Cervantes Amezcua A, Macias Torres V, Casilas Ochoa O, Pere Becerra JL. La carbamazepina en el tratamiento de la neuropatia diabetica: informe preliminar. Prensa Med Mex 1968; 33: 132–5.
[617] Wilton TD. Tegretol in the treatment of diabetic neuropathy. S Afr Med J 1974; 48: 869–72.
[618] McQuay H, Carroll D, Jadad AR, et al. Anticonvulsant drugs for management of pain: a systematic review. Br Med J 1995; 311: 1047–52.

[619] Backonja M, Beydoun A, Edwards KR, et al. Gabapentin for the symptomatic treatment of painful neuropathy in patients with diabetes mellitus. JAMA 1998; 280: 1831–6.
[620] Morello CM, Leckband SG, Stoner CP, et al. Randomized double-blind study comparing the efficacy of gabapentin with amitriptyline on diabetic peripheral neuropathy pain. Arch Intern Med 1999; 159: 1931–7.
[621] Dejgaard A, Petersen P, Kastrup J. Mexiletine for treatment of chronic painful diabetic neuropathy. Lancet 1988; 2: 9–11.
[622] Wright JM, Oki JC, Graves L. Mexiletine in the symptomatic treatment of diabetic peripheral neuropathy. Ann Pharmacother 1997; 31: 29–33.
[623] Stracke H, Meyer UE, Schumacher HE, Federlin K. Mexiletine in the treatment of diabetic neuropathy. Diabetes Care 1992; 15: 1550–5.
[624] Oskarsson P, Ljunggren J-G, Lins P-E. The Mexiletine Study Group. Efficacy and safety of mexiletine in the treatment of painful diabetic neuropathy. Diabetes Care 1997; 20: 1594–7.
[625] Jarvis B, Coukell AJ. Mexiletine. A review of its therapeutic use in painful diabetic neuropathy. Drugs 1998; 56: 691–707.
[626] Kastrup J, Petersen P, Dejgard A, et al. Intravenous lidocaine infusion—a new treatment of chronic painful diabetic neuropathy? Pain 1987; 28: 69–75.
[627] Bach FW, Jensen TS, Kastrup J, et al. The effect of intravenous lidocaine on nociceptive processing in diabetic neuropathy. Pain 1990; 40: 29–34.
[628] Wallace MS, Laitin S, Licht D, Yaksh TL. Concentration – effect relations for intravenous lidocaine infusions in human volunteers. Anesthesiology 1997; 86: 1262–72.
[629] Ferrante FM, Paggioli J, Cherukuri S, Arthur GR. The analgesic response to intravenous lidocaine in the treatment of neuropathic pain. Anesth Analg 1995; 82: 91–7.
[630] Saudek CD, Werns S, Reidenberg MM. Phenytoin in the treatment of diabetic symmetrical neuropathy. Clin Pharmacol Ther 1977; 22: 196–9.
[631] Chadda VS, Mathur MS. Double blind study of the effects of diphenylhydantoin sodium on diabetic neuropathy. J Assoc Phys Ind 1978; 26: 403–6.
[632] Zeigler D, Lynch SA, Muir J, et al. Transdermal clonidine versus placebo in painful diabetic neuropathy. Pain 1992; 48: 403–8.
[633] Byas-Smith MG, Max MB, Muir J, Kingman A. Transdermal clonidine compared to placebo in painful diabetic neuropathy using a two-stage. Pain 1995; 60: 267–74.
[634] McQuay HJ. Opioid use in chronic pain. Acta Anaesthesiol Scand 1997; 41: 175–83.
[635] Arner S, Meyerson BA. Lack of analgesic effect of opioids on neuropathic and idiopathic forms of pain. Pain 1988; 33: 11–23.
[636] Jadad AR, Carroll D, Glynn CJ, et al. Morphine responsiveness of chronic pain: double-blind randomised crossover study with patient-controlled analgesia. Lancet 1992; 339: 1367–71.
[637] Dellemijn PL, Vanneste JAL. Randomised double-blind active-placebo-controlled crossover trial of intravenous fentanyl in neuropathic pain. Lancet 1997; 349: 753–8.
[638] Moulin DE, Iezzi A, Amireh R, et al. Randomised trial of oral morphine for chronic non-cancer pain. Lancet 1996; 347: 143–7.
[639] Dellemijn P. Are opioids effective in relieving neuropathic pain? Pain 1999; 80: 453–62.
[640] Harati Y, Gooch C, Swenson M, et al. Double-blind randomized trial of tramadol for the treatment of the pain of diabetic neuropathy. Neurology 1998; 50: 1842–6.
[641] Sindrup SH, Andersen G, Madsen C, et al. Tramadol relieves pain and allodynia in polyneuropathy: a randomized, double-blind, controlled trial. Pain 1999; 83: 85–90.
[642] Low PA, Opfer-Gehrking TL, Dyck PJ, et al. Double-blind, placebo-controlled study of the application of capsaicin cream in chronic distal painful polyneuropathy. Pain 1995; 62: 163–8.
[643] Chad DA, Aronin N, Lundstrom R, et al. Does capsaicin relieve the pain of diabetic neuropathy? Pain 1990; 42: 387–8.
[644] Scheffler NM, Sheitel PL, Lipton MN. Treatment of painful diabetic neuropathy with capsaicin 0.075%. J Am Podiatr Med Assoc 1991; 81: 288–93.
[645] Basha KM, Whitehouse FW. Capsaicin: a therapeutic option for painful diabetic neuropathy. Henry Ford Hosp Med J 1991; 39: 138–40.
[646] The Capsaicin Study Group. Treatment of painful diabetic neuropathy with topical capsaicin. Arch Intern Med 1991; 151: 2225–9.
[647] The Capsaicin Study Group. Effect of treatment with capsaicin on daily activities of patients with painful diabetic neuropathy. Diabetes Care 1992; 15: 159–65.
[648] Tandan R, Lewis GA, Badger GB, Fries TJ. Topical capsaicin in painful diabetic neuropathy. Diabetes Care 1992; 15: 15–8.
[649] Biesbroeck R, Bril V, Hollander P, et al. A double-blind comparison of topical capsaicin and oral amitriptyline in painful diabetic neuropathy. Adv Ther 1995; 12: 111–20.
[650] Zhang WY, Li Wan Po A. The effectiveness of topically applied capsaicin. A meta-analysis. Eur J Clin Pharmacol 1994; 46: 517–22.
[651] Nolano M, Simone DA, Wendelschafer-Crabb G, et al. Topical capsaicin in humans: parallel loss of epidermal nerve fibers and pain sensation. Pain 1999; 81: 135–45.
[652] Nelson KA, Park KM, Robinovitz E, et al. High-dose oral dextromethorphan versus placebo in painful diabetic neuropathy and postherpetic neuralgia. Neurology 1997; 48: 1212–8.
[653] Ertas M, Sagduyu A, Arac N, et al. Use of levodopa to relieve pain from painful symmetrical diabetic polyneuropathy. Pain 1998; 75: 257–9.
[654] Weber W, Walter-Sack I. Klinische Bedeutung von Vitamin B1, B6, B12 in der Schmerztherapie. Klin Wochenschr 1988; 66: 274–6.
[655] Straub RH, Rokitzki L, Schumacher T, et al. No evidence of deficiency of vitamins A, E, β-carotene, B1, B2, B6, B12 and folate in neuropathic type II diabetic women. Int J Vitam Nutr Res 1993; 63: 239–40.
[656] Levin ER, Hanscom TA, Fisher M, et al. The influence of pyridoxine in diabetic peripheral neuropathy. Diabetes Care 1981; 4: 606–9.
[657] McCann VJ, Davis RE. Pyridoxine and diabetic neuropathy: a double-blind controlled study. Diabetes Care 1983; 6: 102–3.
[658] Schaumburg H, Kaplan J, Windebank A, et al. Sensory neuropathy from pyridoxine abuse: a new megavitamin syndrome. N Engl J Med 1983; 309: 445–8.
[659] Janka HU, Rietzel S, Mehnert H. Der Einfluß von Neurobion auf die Temperatursensibilität bei Patienten mit diabetischer Neuropathie. In: Rietbrock N, editors. Pharmakologie und klinische Anwendung hochdosierter B-Vitamine. Darmstadt, Germany: Steinkopff, 1991: 87–97.
[660] Stracke H, Lindemann A, Federlin K. A benfotiamine-vitamin B combination in treatment of diabetic polyneuropathy. Exp Clin Endocrinol Diabetes 1996; 104: 311–6.
[661] Haupt E, Ledermann H, Köpcke W. Benfotiamine in treatment of diabetic polyneuropathy. J Peripher Nerv Syst 1997; 2: 270.
[662] Quatraro A, Minei A, De Rosa N, Giugliano D. Calcitonin in painful diabetic neuropathy. Lancet 1992; 339: 746–7.
[663] Gallai V, Mazzotta G, Montesi S, et al. Effect of uridine in the treatment of diabetic neuropathy: an electrophysiological study. Acta Neurol Scand 1992; 86: 3–7.
[664] Biesenbach G, Grafinger P, Eichbauer-Sturm G, Zazgornik J. Cerebrolysin in der Behandlung der schmerzhaften diabetischen Neuropathie. Wien Med Wochenschr 1997; 147: 63–6.
[665] Cohen KL, Harris S. Efficacy and safety of nonsteroidal antiinflammatory drugs in the therapy of diabetic neuropathy. Arch Intern Med 1987; 147: 1442–4.
[666] Foster AVM, Eaton C, McConville DO, Edmonds ME. Application of OpSite film: a new and effective treatment of painful diabetic neuropathy. Diabetic Med 1994; 11: 768–72.
[667] Tawata M, Kurihara A, Nitta K, et al. The effects of goshajinkigan, a herbal medicine, on subjective symptoms and vibratory threshold in patients with diabetic neuropathy. Diabetes Res Clin Pract 1994; 26: 121–8.
[668] Tesfaye S. Painful diabetic neuropathy. Aetiology and nonpharmacological treatment. In: Veves A, editor. Clinical

management of diabetic neuropathy. Totowa, NJ: Humana Press, 1998: 133–46.
[669] Abuaisha BB, Costanzi, Boulton AJM. Acupuncture for the treatment of chronic painful peripheral diabetic neuropathy: a long-term study. Diabetes Res Clin Pract 1998; 39: 115–21.
[670] Kumar D, Marshall HJ. Diabetic peripheral neuropathy: amelioration of pain with transcutaneous electrostimulation. Diabetes Care 1997; 20: 1702–5.
[671] Kumar D, Alvaro MS, Julka IS, Marshall HJ. Diabetic peripheral neuropathy. Effectiveness of electrotherapy and amitriptyline for symptomatic relief. Diabetes Care 1998; 21: 1322–5.
[672] Lundeberg T. Electrical stimulation techniques. Lancet 1996; 348: 1672–3.
[673] Tesfaye S, Watt J, Benbow SJ, et al. Electrical spinal-cord stimulation for painful diabetic peripheral neuropathy. Lancet 1996; 348: 1696–701.
[674] Davies HTO, Crombie IK, Lonsdale M, Macrae WA. Consensus and contention in the treatment of chronic nerve-damage pain. Pain 1991; 47: 191–6.
[675] Virani A, Mailis A, Shapiro LE, Shear NH. Drug interactions in human neuropathic pain pharmacotherapy. Pain 1997; 73: 3–13.
[676] American Diabetes Association and American Academy of Neurology. Consensus Statement: Report and recommendations of the San Antonio Conference on Diabetic Neuropathy. Diabetes Care 1988; 11: 592–7.
[677] Kahn R. Proceedings of a consensus development conference on standardized measures in diabetic neuropathy. Diabetes Care 1992; 15: 1081–103.
[678] Neil HAW. Epidemiology of diabetic autonomic neuropathy. In: Bannister R, Mathias CJ, editors. Autonomic failure. 3rd edition. Oxford: Oxford Medical Publications, 1992: 683–97.
[679] Broadstone VL, Roy T, Self M, Pfeifer MA. Cardiovascular autonomic dysfunction: diagnosis and prognosis. Diabet Med 1991; 8: S88–93.
[680] Ewing DJ. Analysis of heart rate variability and other noninvasive tests with special reference to diabetes mellitus. In: Bannister R, Mathias CJ, editors. Autonomic failure. 3rd edition. Oxford: Oxford Medical Publications, 1992: 312–33.
[681] Kahn JE, Zola B, Juni JE, Vinik AI. Decreased exercise heart rate and blood pressure response in diabetic subjects with cardiac autonomic neuropathy. Diabetes Care 1986; 9: 389–94.
[682] Roy TM, Peterson HR, Snider HL, et al. Autonomic influence on cardiovascular performance in diabetic subjects. Am J Med 1989; 87: 382–8.
[683] Bottini P, Tantucci Scionti L, Dottorini ML, et al. Cardiovascular response to exercise in diabetic patients: influence of autonomic neuropathy of different severity. Diabetologia 1995; 38: 244–50.
[684] Zola B, Khan JK, Juni JE, Vinik AI. Abnormal cardiac function in diabetic patients with autonomic neuropathy in the absence of ischemic heart disease. J Clin Endocrinol Metab 1986; 63: 208–14.
[685] Kahn JE, Zola B, Juni JE, Vinik AI. Radionuclide assessment of left ventricular diastolic filling in diabetes mellitus with and without cardiac autonomic neuropathy. J Am Coll Cardiol 1986; 7: 1303–9.
[686] Mustonen J, Uusitupa M, Lansimies E, et al. Autonomic nervous function and its relationship to cardiac performance in middle-aged diabetic patients without clinically evident cardiovascular disease. J Intern Med 1992; 232: 65–72.
[687] Young LH, Ramahi TM, McNulty PH. Heart disease in diabetes mellitus: a clinical and metabolic perspective. Diabetes Nutr Metab 1994; 7: 233–49.
[688] Faerman I, Faccio E, Milei J, et al. Autonomic neuropathy and painless myocardial infarction in diabetic patients: histologic evidence of their relationship. Diabetes 1977; 12: 1147–58.
[689] Niakan E, Harati Y, Rolak LA, et al. Silent myocardial infarction and diabetic cardiovascular autonomic neuropathy. Arch Intern Med 1986; 146: 2229–30.
[690] Nesto RW, Phillips RT, Kett KG, et al. Angina and exertional myocardial ischemia in diabetic and nondiabetic patients: assessment by exercise thallium scintigraphy. Ann Intern Med 1988; 108: 170–5.
[691] Koistinen MJ. Prevalence of asymptomatic myocardial ischaemia in diabetic subjects. Br Med J 1990; 301: 92–5.
[692] Milan Study on Atherosclerosis and Diabetes (MiSAD) Group. Prevalence of unrecognized silent myocardial ischemia and its association with atherosclerosis risk factors in non insulin-dependent diabetes mellitus. Am J Cardiol 1997; 79: 134–9.
[693] Chiariello M, Indolfi C. Silent myocardial ischemia in patients with diabetes mellitus. Circulation 1996; 93: 2089–91.
[694] Nesto RW. Screening for asymptomatic coronary artery disease in diabetes. Diabetes Care 1999; 22: 1393–5.
[695] Hume L, Oakley GD, Boulton AJM, et al. Asymptomatic myocardial ischemia in diabetes and its relationship to diabetic neuropathy: an excercise electrocardiography study in middle-aged diabetic men. Diabetes Care 1986; 9: 384–8.
[696] Murray DP, O'Brien T, Mulrooney R, O'Sullivan DJ. Autonomic dysfunction and silent myocardial ischaemia on exercise testing in diabetes mellitus. Diabet Med 1990; 7: 580–4.
[697] Ambepitiya G, Kopelman PG, Ingram D, et al. Exertional myocardial ischemia in diabetes: a quantitative analysis of anginal perceptual threshold and the influence of autonomic function. J Am Coll Cardiol 1990; 15: 72–7.
[698] Langer A, Freeman MR, Josse RG, et al. Detection of silent myocardial ischemia in diabetes mellitus. Am J Cardiol 1991; 67: 1073–8.
[699] Marchant B, Umachandran V, Stevenson R, et al. Silent myocardial ischemia: role of subclinical neuropathy in patients with and without diabetes. J Am Coll Cardiol 1993; 22: 1433–7.
[700] Hikita H, Kurita A, Takase B, et al. Usefulness of plasma beta-endorphin level, pain threshold and autonomic function in assessing silent myocardial ischemia in patients with and without diabetes mellitus. Am J Cardiol 1993; 72: 140–3.
[701] Langer A, Freeman MR, Josse RG, Armstrong PW. Metaiodobenzylguanidine imaging in diabetes mellitus: assessment of cardiac sympathetic denervation and its relation to autonomic dysfunction and silent myocardial ischemia. J Am Coll Cardiol 1995; 25: 610–8.
[702] Koistinen MJ, Airaksinen KEJ, Huikuri HV, et al. No difference in cardiac innervation of diabetic patients with painful and asymptomatic coronary artery disease. Diabetes Care 1996; 19: 231–5.
[703] Weiner DA, Ryan TJ, Parsons L, et al. Significance of silent myocardial ischemia during exercise testing in patients with diabetes mellitus: a report from the coronary artery surgery study (CASS) registry. Am J Cardiol 1991; 68: 729–34.
[704] Neil HAW, Thompson AV, John S, et al. Diabetic autonomic neuropathy: the prevalence of impaired heart rate variability in a geographically defined population. Diabet Med 1989; 6: 20–4.
[705] Stephenson J, Fuller JH. EURODIAB IDDM Complications Study Group. Microvascular and acute complications in IDDM patients: the EURODIAB IDDM Complications Study. Diabetologia 1994; 37: 278–85.
[706] Masaki KH, Schatz IJ, Burchfield CM, et al. Orthostatic hypotension predicts mortality in elderly men. Honolulu Heart Program. Circulation 1998; 98: 2290–5.
[707] Luukinen H, Koski K, Laippala P, Kivelä S-L. Prognosis of diastolic and systolic orthostatic hypotension in older persons. Arch Intern Med 1999; 159: 273–80.
[708] Bannister R, Mathias C. Management of postural hypotension. In: Mathias CJ, Bannister R, editors. Autonomic failure. 4th edition. Oxford: Oxford University Press, 1999: 342–56.
[709] Sampson MJ, Wilson S, Karagiannis P, et al. Progression of diabetic autonomic neuropathy over a decade in insulin-dependent diabetics. Q J Med 1990; 75: 635–46.
[710] Watkins PJ, Edmonds ME. Diabetic autonomic failure. In: Mathias CJ, Bannister R, editors. Autonomic failure. 4th edition. Oxford: Oxford University Press, 1999: 378–86.
[711] Hoeldtke RD, Davis KM, Joseph J, et al. Hemodynamic effects of octreotide in patients with autonomic neuropathy. Circulation 1991; 84: 168–76.
[712] DiBona GF, Wilcox CS. The kidney and the sympathetic nervous system. In: Mathias CJ, Bannister R, editors. Auto-

nomic failure. 4th edition. Oxford: Oxford University Press, 1999: 143–50.
[713] Reid W, Ewing DJ, Lightman SL, et al. Vasopressin secretion in diabetic subjects with and without autonomic neuropathy: responses to osmotic and postural stimulation. Clin Sci 1989; 77: 589–97.
[714] Ogi M, Kojima S, Kuramochi M. Effect of postural change on urine volume and urinary sodium excretion in diabetic nephropathy. Am J Kidney Dis 1998; 31: 41–8.
[715] Hoeldtke RD, Streeten DHP. Treatment of orthostatic hypotension with erythropoietin. N Engl J Med 1993; 329: 611–5.
[716] Biaggioni I, Robertson D, Krantz S, et al. The anemia of primary autonomic failure and its reversal with recombinant erythropoietin. Ann Intern Med 1994; 121: 181–6.
[717] Winkler AS, Marsden J, Chaudhurit KR, et al. Erythopoietin depletion and anemia in diabetes mellitus. Diabet Med 1999; 16: 813–9.
[718] Cotroneo P, Ricerca BM, Todaro L, et al. Blunted erythopoietin response to anaemia in patients with type 1 diabets. Diabetes Metab Res Rev 2000; 16: 172–6.
[719] Spallone V, Cicconetti E, Maiello MR, et al. Role of autonomic neuropathy in erythropoietin regulation in non proteinuric type 1 and type 2 diabetic patients. Diabetologia 2000; 43(Suppl 1): A250.
[720] Yun YS, Lee HC, Yoo NC, et al. Reduced erythopoietin responsiveness to anaemia in diabetic patients before advanced diabetic nephropathy. Diabetes Res Clin Pract 1999; 46: 223–9.
[721] Yki-Järvinen H, Utrianen T. Insulin-induced vasodilatation: physiology or pharmacology? Diabetologia 1998; 41: 369–79.
[722] Porcellati F, Fanelli C, Bottini P, et al. Mechanisms of arterial hypotension after therapeutic dose of subcutaneous insulin in diabetic autonomic neuropathy. Diabetes 1993; 42: 1055–64.
[723] Mathias CJ, Bannister R. Postprandial hypotension in autonomic disorders. In: Mathias CJ, Bannister R, editors. Autonomic failure. 4th edition. Oxford: Oxford University Press, 1999: 283–95.
[724] Wieling W, van Lieshout JJ, van Leeuwen AM. Physical manoeuvres that reduce postural hypotension in autonomic failure. Clin Auton Res 1993; 3: 57–65.
[725] Ten Harkel AD, Van Lieshout JJ, Wieling W. Treatment of orthostatic hypotension with sleeping in the head-up tilt position, alone and in comination with fludrocortisone. J Intern Med 1992; 232: 139–45.
[726] Low PA, Gilden JL, Freeman R, et al. Efficacy of midodrine vs placebo in neurogenic orthostatic hypotension. A randomized, double-blind multicenter study. Midodrine Study Group. JAMA 1997; 227: 1046–51.
[727] Hoeldtke RD, D'Dorisio TM, Boden G. Treatment of autonomic neuropathy with a somatostatin analogue, SMS 201-995. Lancet 1986; ii: 602–5.
[728] Lipsitz LA, Jansen RWMM, Connely CM, et al. Haemodynamic and neurohumoral effects of caffeine in elderly patients with symptomatic postprandial hypotension: a double-blind, randomized, placebo-controlled study. Clin Sci 1994; 87: 259–67.
[729] Ziegler D. Diabetic cardiovascular autonomic neuropathy: prognosis, diagnosis and treatment. Diabetes Metab Rev 1994; 10: 339–82.
[730] Ziegler D, Laux G, Dannehl K, et al. Assessment of cardiovascular autonomic function: age-related normal ranges and reproducibility of spectral analysis, vector analysis, and standard tests of heart rate variation and blood pressure responses. Diabet Med 1992; 9: 166–75.
[731] Lawrence GP, Home PD, Murray A. Repeatability of measurements and sources of variability in tests of cardiovascular autonomic function. Br Heart J 1992; 68: 205–11.
[732] Wieling W, Karemaker JM. Measurement of heart rate and blood pressure to evaluate disturbances in neurocardiovascular control. In: Mathias CJ, Bannister R, editors. Autonomic failure. 4th edition. Oxford: Oxford University Press, 1999: 196–210.
[733] Mathias CJ, Bannister R. Investigation of autonomic disorders. In: Mathias CJ, Bannister R, editors. Autonomic failure. 4th edition. Oxford: Oxford University Press, 1999: 169–95.
[734] Ricordi L, Rossi M, Marti G, et al. Hypertension in diabetes: an additional factor determining autonomic neuropathy. Diabetes Nutr Metab 1989; 2: 269–75.
[735] Airaksinen KEJ, Koistinen MJ, Ikäheimo MJ, et al. Effect of coronary artery disease on parasympathetic cardiovascular reflexes in NIDDM patients. Diabetes Care 1990; 13: 83–6.
[736] Kronert K, Holder K, Kuschmierz G, et al. Influence of cardiovascular diseases upon the results of the cardiovascular reflex tests in diabetic and nondiabetic subjects. Acta Diabetol Lat 1990; 27: 1–0.
[737] Flapan AD, Nolan J, Neilson JMM, Ewing DJ. Effect of captopril on cardiac parasympathetic activity in chronic cardiac failure secondary to coronary artery disease. Am J Cardiol 1992; 69: 532–5.
[738] Kaufman ES, Bosner MS, Bigger JT, et al. Effects of digoxin and enalapril on heart period variability and response to head-up tilt in normal subjects. Am J Cardiol 1993; 72: 95–9.
[739] Kleiger RE, Miller JP, Bigger JT, Moss AJ, and the Multicenter Post-Infarction Research Group. Decreased heart rate variability and its association with increased mortality after acute myocardial infarction. Am J Cardiol 1987; 59: 256–62.
[740] Ewing DJ, Campbell IM, Clarke BF. The natural history of diabetic autonomic neuropathy. Q J Med 49 1980; 49: 95–108.
[741] Stubbs TA, Macdonald IA. Systematic and regional haemodynamic effects of caffeine and alcohol in fasting subjects. Clin Auton Res 1995; 5: 123–7.
[742] Hayano J, Yamada M, Sakakibara Y, et al. Short- and long-term effects of cigarette smoking on heart rate variability. Am J Cardiol 1990; 65: 84–8.
[743] Maser RE, Pfeifer MA, Dorman JS, et al. Diabetic autonomic neuropathy and cardiovascular risk. Arch Intern Med 1990; 150: 1218–22.
[744] Spallone V, Maiello MR, Cicconetti E, Menzinger G. Autonomic neuropathy and cardiovascular risk factors in insulin-dependent and non insulin-dependent diabetes. Diabetes Res Clin Pract 1997; 34: 169–79.
[745] Peterson HR, Rothschild M, Weinberg CR, et al. Body fat and the activity of the autonomic nervous system. N Engl J Med 1988; 318: 1077–83.
[746] Rossi M, Marti G, Ricordi L, et al. Cardiac autonomic dysfunction in obese subjects. Clin Sci 1989; 76: 567–72.
[747] Straub RH, Thum M, Hollerbach C, et al. Impact of obesity on neuropathic late complications in NIDDM. Diabetes Care 1994; 17: 1290–4.
[748] Veglio M, Carpano-Maglioli P, Tonda L, et al. Autonomic neuropathy in non-insulin-dependent diabetic patients: correlation with age, sex, duration and metabolic control of diabetes. Diabete Metab 1990; 16: 200–6.
[749] Bellavere F, Cardone C, Ferri M, et al. Standing to lying heart rate variation. A new simple test in the diagnosis of diabetic autonomic neuropathy. Diabet Med 1987; 4: 41–3.
[750] Marfella R, Giugliano D, Di Maro G, et al. The squatting test. A useful tool to assess both parasympathetic and sympathetic involvement of the cardiovascular autonomic neuropathy in diabetes. Diabetes 1994; 43: 607–12.
[751] Bernardi L. Clinical evaluation of arterial baroreflex activity in diabetes. Diabetes Nutr Metab 2000; 13: 331–40.
[752] Imholtz BP, Wieling W, van Montfrans GA, Wesseling KH. Fifteen years experience with finger arterial pressure monitoring: assessment of the technology. Cardiovasc Res 1998; 38: 605–16.
[753] Eckberg DL, Convertino VA, Fritsch JM, Doerr DF. Reproducibility of human vagal carotid baroreceptor-cardiac reflex responses. Am J Physiol 1992; 263(1): R215–20.
[754] Parati G, Di Rienzo M, Omboni S, Mancia G. Computer analysis of blood pressure and heart rate variability in subjects with normal and abnormal autonomic cardiovascular control. In: Mathias CJ, Bannister R, editors. Autonomic failure. 4th edition. Oxford: Oxford University Press, 1999: 211–23.
[755] Mortara A, La Rovere T, Pinna GD, et al. Arterial baroreflex modulation of heart rate on chronic heart failure: clinical and hemodynamic correlates and prognostic implications. Circulation 1997; 96: 3450–8.
[756] La Rovere MT, Bigger JT, Marcus FI, Mortara A, Schwartz PJ, for the ATRAMI Investigators. Baroreflex sensitivity and

heart-rate variability in prediction of total cardiac mortality after myocardial infarction. Lancet 1998; 351: 478–84.
[757] Bennett T, Hosking DJ, Hampton JR. Baroreflex sensitivity and responses to the Valsalva manoeuvre in subjects with diabetes mellitus. J Neurol Neurosurg Psychiatry 1976; 39: 178–83.
[758] Olshan AR, O'Connor DT, Cohen IM, et al. Baroreflex dysfunction in patients with adult-onset diabetes and hypertension. Am J Med 1983; 74: 233–42.
[759] Weston PJ, James MA, Panerai R, et al. Abnormal baroreceptor-cardiac reflex sensitivity is not detected by conventional tests of autonomic function in patients with insulin-dependent diabetes mellitus. Clin Sci 1996; 91: 59–64.
[760] Weston PJ, Panerai RB, McCullogh A, et al. Assessment of baroreceptor-cardiac reflex sensitivity using time domain analysis in patients with IDDM and the relation to left ventricular mass index. Diabetologia 1996; 39: 1385–91.
[761] Frattola A, Parati G, Gamba P, et al. Time and frequency domain estimates of spontaneous baroreflex sensitivity provide early detection of autonomic dysfunction in diabetes mellitus. Diabetologia 1997; 40: 1470–75.
[762] Lefrandt JD, Hoogenberg K, van Roon AM, et al. Baroreflex sensitivity is depressed in microalbuminuric type 1 diabetic patients at rest and during sympathetic manoeuvres. Diabetologia 1999; 42: 1345–9.
[763] McDowell TS, Hajduczok G, Abboud FM, Chapleau MW. Baroreflex dysfunction in diabetes mellitus. II. Site of baroreflex impairment in diabetic rabbits. Am J Physiol 1994; 266: H244–9.
[764] Lawrence IG, Weston PJ, Bennett MA, et al. Is impaired baroreflex sensitivity a predictor or cause of sudden death in insulin-dependent diabetes mellitus? Diabet Med 1997; 14: 82–5.
[765] Kahn JK, Sisson JC, Vinik AI. QT interval prolongation and sudden cardiac death in diabetic autonomic neuropathy. J Clin Endocrinol Metab 1987; 64: 751–4.
[766] Bellavere F, Ferri G, Guarini L, et al. Prolonged QT period in diabetic autonomic neuropathy: a possible role in sudden cardiac death? Br Heart J 1988; 59. 379–83.
[767] Ewing DJ, Boland O, Neilson JMM, et al. Autonomic neuropathy, QT interval lengthening, and unexpected deaths in male diabetic patients. Diabetologia 1991; 34: 182–5.
[768] Lo SSS, St. John Sutton M, Leslie RDG. Information on type 1 diabetes mellitus and QT interval from identical twins. Am J Cardiol 1993; 72: 305–9.
[769] Sivieri R, Veglio M, Chinaglia A, et al. Prevalence of QT prolongation in a type 1 diabetic population and its association with autonomic neuropathy. The Neuropathy Study Group of the Italian Society for the Study of Diabetes. Diabet Med 1993; 10: 920–4.
[770] Veglio M, Borra M, Stevens LK, et al. EURODIAB IDDM Complications Study Group. The relation between QTc interval prolongation and diabetic complications. The EURODIAB IDDM Complications Study Group. Diabetologia 1999; 42: 68–75.
[771] Dekker JM, Feskens EJ, Schouten EG, et al. QT duration is associated with levels of insulin and glucose tolerance. Zutphen Elderly Study. Diabetes 1996; 45: 376–80.
[772] Gastaldelli A, Emdin M, Conforti F, et al. Insulin prolongs the QTc interval in humans. Am J Physiol Regul Integre Comp Physiol 2000; 279: R2022–2025.
[773] Marfella R, Nappo F, De Angelis L, et al. The effect of acute hyperglycaemia on QTc duration in healthy man. Diabetologia 2000; 43: 571–5.
[774] Whitsel EA, Boyko EJ, Siscovick DS. Reassessing the role of QTc in the diagnosis of autonomic failure among patients with diabetes. Diabetes Care 2000; 23: 241–7.
[775] Sawicki PT, Dähne R, Bender R, Berger M. Prolonged QT interval as a predictor of mortality in diabetic nephropathy. Diabetologia 1996; 39: 77–81.
[776] Veglio M, Sivieri R, Chinaglia A, Scaglione L, Cavallo-Perin P. QT interval prolongation and mortality in type 1 diabetic patients. A 5-year cohort prospective study. Diabetes Care 2000; 23: 1381–3.
[777] Sawicki PT, Kiwitt S, Bender R, Berger M. The value of QT interval dispersion for identification of total mortality risk in non-insulin-dependent diabetes mellitus. J Intern Med 1998; 243: 49–56.
[778] Veglio M, Chinaglia A, Cavallo Perin P. The clinical utility of QT interval assessment in diabetes. Diabetes Nutr Metab 2000; 13: 356–65.
[779] Mølgaard H, Hermansen K. Evaluation of cardiac autonomic neuropathy by heart rate variability. In: Mogensen CE, Standl E, editors. Research methodologies in human diabetes. Part 1. Berlin: Walter de Gruyter, 1995: 219–40.
[780] van Ravenswaaij-Arts CMA, Kollée LAA, Hopman JCW, et al. Heart rate variability. Ann Intern Med 1993; 118: 436–47.
[781] Spallone V, Menzinger G. Diagnosis of cardiovascular autonomic neuropathy in diabetes. Diabetes 1997; 46(Suppl 2): S67–76.
[782] Pagani M, Montano N, Porta A, et al. Relationship between spectral components of cardiovascular variabilities and direct measures of muscle sympathetic nerve activity in humans. Circulation 1997; 95: 1441–8.
[783] Malliani A, Pagani M, Lombardi F, Cerutti S. Cardiovascular neural regulation explored in the frequency domain. Circulation 1991; 84: 482–92.
[784] Bernardi L, Ricordi L, Lazzari P, et al. Impaired circadian modulation of sympatho-vagal activity in diabetes: a possible explanation for altered temporal onset of cardiovascular disease. Circulation 1992; 96: 1443–52.
[785] Bellavere F, Balzani I, De Masi G, et al. Power spectral analysis of heart-rate variations improves assessment of diabetic cardiac autonomic neuropathy. Diabetes 1992; 41: 633–40.
[786] Rossi M, Ricordi L, Mevio E, et al. Autonomic nervous system and microcirculation in diabetes. J Auton Nerv Syst 1990; 30: S133–6.
[787] Bernardi L, Ricordi L, Ferrari MR, et al. Application of chaos theory (approximate entropy) to detect cardiac autonomic dysfunction in diabetes (Abstract). Diabetologia 1995; 38(Suppl 1): A241.
[788] Ziegler D, Piolot R, Straßburger K, et al. Normal ranges and reproducibility of statistical, geometric, frequency domain, and non-linear measures of 24-hour heart rate variability. Horm Metab Res 1999; 31. 672–9.
[789] Verdecchia P, Schillaci G, Guerrieri M, et al. Circadian blood pressure changes and left ventricular hyperthrophy in essential hypertension. Circulation 1990; 81: 528–36.
[790] O'Brien E, Sheridan J, O'Malley K. Dippers and non-dippers. Lancet 1988; ii: 397.
[791] Spallone V, Bernardi L, Ricordi L, et al. Relationship between the circadian rhythms of blood pressure and sympathovagal balance in diabetic autonomic neuropathy. Diabetes 1993; 42: 1745–52.
[792] Poulsen PL, Ebbehøj E, Hansen KW, Mogensen KW. 24-h blood pressure and autonomic function is related to albumin excretion within the normoalbuminuric range in IDDM patients. Diabetologia 1997; 40: 718–25.
[793] Hansen HP, Rossing P, Tarnow L, et al. Circadian rhythm of arterial blood pressure and albuminuria in diabetic nephropathy. Kidney Int 1996; 50: 579–85.
[794] Nielsen FS, Hansen HP, Jacobsen P, et al. Increased sympathetic activity during sleep and nocturnal hypertension in type 2 diabetic patients with diabetic nephropathy. Diabet Med 1999; 16: 555–62.
[795] Roman MJ, Pickering TG, Schwartz JE, et al. Is the absence of a normal nocturnal fall in blood pressure (nondipping) associated with cardiovascular target organ damage? J Hypertens 1997; 15: 969–78.
[796] Gambardella S, Frontoni S, Spallone V, et al. Increased left ventricular mass in normotensive diabetic patients with autonomic neuropathy. Am J Hypertens 1993; 6: 97–102.
[797] Liniger C, Favre L, Assal J-P. Twenty-four hour blood pressure and heart rate profiles of diabetic patients with abnormal cardiovascular reflexes. Diabet Med 1991; 8: 420–7.
[798] Verdecchia P, Porcellati C, Schillaci G, et al. Ambulatory blood pressure and risk of cardiovascular disease in type II diabetes mellitus. Diabetes Nutr Metab 1994; 7: 223–31.
[799] Nakano S, Fukuda M, Hotta F, et al. Reversed circadian blood-pressure rhythm is associated with occurrences of both fatal and nonfatal vascular events in NIDDM subjects. Diabetes 1998; 47: 1501–6.
[800] Nakano S, Ogihara M, Tamura C, et al. Reversed circadian blood-pressure rhythm independently predicts endstage renal failure in non-insulin-dependent diabetes mellitus subjects. J Diabetes Complications 1999; 13: 224-31.

[801] Furlan R, Guzzetti S, Crivellaro W, et al. Continuous 24-hour assessment of the neural regulation of systemic arterial pressure and R-R variabilities in ambulant subjects. Circulation 1990; 81: 537–47.
[802] Quyyumi AA. Circadian rhythms in cardiovascular disease. Am Heart J 1990; 120: 726–33.
[803] Hjalmarson Å, Gilpin EA, Nicod P, et al. Differing circadian patterns of symptom onset in subgroups of patients with acute myocardial infarction. Circulation 1989; 80: 267–75.
[804] Spallone V, Bernardi L, Maiello MR, et al. Twenty-four-hour pattern of blood pressure and spectral analysis of heart rate variability in diabetic patients with various degrees of autonomic neuropathy. Comparison to standard cardiovascular tests. Clin Sci 1996; 91(Suppl): 105–7.
[805] Ziegler D, Piolot R. Evaluation of 24-hour Holter ECG compared with autonomic function tests in detecting diabetic cardiovascular autonomic neuropathy. Diabetologia 1999; 42(Suppl 1): A294.
[806] Task Force of the European Society of Cardiology and the North American Society of Pacing and Electrophysiology. Heart rate variability. Standards of measurement, physiological interpretation, and clinical use. Circulation 1996; 93: 1043–65.
[807] Ewing DJ, Martyn CN, Young RJ, Clarke BF. The value of cardiovascular autonomic function tests: 10 years experience in diabetes. Diabetes Care 1985; 8: 491–8.
[808] Melon P, Schwaiger M. Imaging of metabolism and autonomic innervation of the heart by positron emission tomography. Eur J Nucl Med 1992; 19: 453–64.
[809] Münch G, Nguyen N, Wieland D, Schwaiger M. Assessment of sympathetic cardiac innervation by scintigraphic techniques. In: van der Wall EE, et al, editors. Cardiac positron emission tomography. Dordrecht, Netherlands: Kluwer Academic Publishers, 1995: 183–99.
[810] Dae MW, Botvinick EH. Imaging of the heart using metaiodobenzylguanidine. J Thorac Imaging 1990; 5: 31–6.
[811] Glowniak JV. Cardiac studies with metaiodobenzylguanidine: a critique of methods and interpretation of results. J Nucl Med 1995; 36: 2133–7.
[812] Langen K-J, Ziegler D, Weise F, et al. Evaluation of QT interval length, QT dispersion and myocardial m-iodobenzylguanidine uptake in insulin-dependent diabetic patients with and without autonomic neuropathy. Clin Sci 1997; 92: 325–33.
[813] Standl E, Schnell O. A new look at the heart in diabetes mellitus: from ailing to failing. Diabetologia 2000; 43: 1455–69.
[814] Ziegler D. Cardiovascular autonomic neuropathy: clinical manifestations and measurement. Diabetes Rev 1999; 7: 342–57.
[815] Matsuo S, Takahashi M, Nakamura Y, Kinoshita M. Evaluation of cardiac sympathetic innervation with iodine-123-metaiodobenzylguanidine imaging in silent myocardial ischemia. J Nucl Med 1996; 37: 712–7.
[816] Tsuchimochi S, Tamaki N, Tadamura E, et al. Age and gender differences in normal myocardial adrenergic neuronal function evaluated by iodine-123-MIBG imaging. J Nucl Med 1995; 36: 969–74.
[817] Morozumi T, Kusuoka H, Fukuchi K, et al. Myocardial iodine-123-metaiodobenzylguanidine images and autonomic nerve activity in normal subjects. J Nucl Med 1997; 38: 49–52.
[818] Mitrani RD, Klein LS, Miles WM, et al. Regional cardiac sympathetic denervation in patients with ventricular tachycardia in the absence of coronary artery disease. J Am Coll Cardiol 1993; 22: 1344–53.
[819] Stevens MJ, Dayanikli F, Raffel DM, et al. Scintigraphic assessment of regionalized defects in myocardial sympathetic innervation and blood flow regulation in diabetic autonomic neuropathy. J Am Coll Cardiol 1998; 31: 1575–84.
[820] Stevens MJ, Raffel DM, Allman KC, et al. Cardiac sympathetic dysinnervation in diabetes. Implications for cardiovascular risk. Circulation 1998; 98: 961–8.
[821] Di Carli MF, Bianco-Battles D, Landa ME, et al. Effects of autonomic neuropathy on coronary blood flow in patients with diabetes mellitus. Circulation 1999; 100: 813–9.
[822] Schnell O, Muhr D, Weiss M, et al. Reduced myocardial ^{123}I-metaiodobenzylguanidine uptake in newly diagnosed IDDM patients. Diabetes 1996; 45: 801–5.
[823] Ziegler D, Weise F, Langen K-J, et al. Effect of glycaemic control on myocardial sympathetic innervation assessed by [^{123}I]metaiodobenzylguanidine scintigraphy: a 4-year prospective study in IDDM patients. Diabetologia 1998; 41: 443–51.
[824] Stevens MJ, Raffel DM, Allman KC, et al. Regression and progression of cardiac sympathetic dysinnervation complicating diabetes; an assessment by C-11 hydroxyephedrine and positron emission tomography. Metabolism 1999; 48: 92–101.
[825] The Diabetes Control and Complications Trial Research Group. The effect of intensive diabetes therapy on the development and progression of neuropathy. Ann Intern Med 1995; 122: 561–8.
[826] Schnell O, Muhr D, Weiss M, et al. Three-year follow-up on scintigraphically assessed cardiac sympathetic denervation in patients with long-term type 1 diabetes. J Diab Comp 1997; 11: 307–13.
[827] Schnell O, Muhr D, Dresel S, et al. Partial restoration of scintigraphically assessed cardiac sympathetic denervation in newly diagnosed patients with insulin-dependent (type 1) diabetes mellitus at one-year follow-up. Diabet Med 1997; 14: 57–62.
[828] Sundkvist G, Lilja B. Autonomic neuropathy predicts deterioration in glomerular filtration rate in patients with IDDM. Diabetes Care 1993; 16: 773–9.
[829] Spallone V, Gambardella S, Maiello MR, et al. Relationship between autonomic neuropathy, 24-h blood pressure profile and nephropathy in normotensive IDDM patients. Diabetes Care 1994; 17: 578–84.
[830] Bikkina M, Alpert MA, Mukerji R, et al. Diminished short-term heart rate variability predicts inducible ventricular tachycardia. Chest 1998; 113: 312–6.
[831] Töyry JP, Niskanen LK, Lansimies EA, Partanen KP, Uusitupa MI. Autonomic neuropathy predicts the development of stroke in patients with non-insulin-dependent diabetes mellitus. Stroke 1996; 27: 1316–8.
[832] Cencetti S, Lagi A, Cipriani M, et al. Autonomic control of the cerebral circulation during normal and impaired peripheral circulatory control. Heart 1999; 82: 365–72.
[833] Linsted U, Jaeger H, Petry A. The neuropathy of the autonomic nervous system. An additional anesthetic risk in diabetes mellitus. Anaesthesist 1993; 42: 521–7.
[834] Schuyler MR, Niewoehner DE, Inkley SR, Kohn R. Abnormal lung elasticity in juvenile diabetes mellitus. Am Rev Respir Dis 1976; 113: 37–41.
[835] Schernthaner G, Haber P, Krummer R, Ludwig H. Lung elasticity in juvenile onset diabetes mellitus. Am Rev Respir Dis 1977; 116: 544–6.
[836] Schnapf BM, Banks RA, Silverstein JH, et al. Pulmonary function in insulin-dependent diabetes mellitus with limited joint mobility. Am Rev Respir Dis 1984; 130: 930–2.
[837] Primhak RA, Whincup G, Tsanakas JN, Milner RD. Reduced vital capacity in insulin-dependent diabetes. Diabetes 1987; 36: 324–6.
[838] Sandler M, Bunn AE, Stewart RI. Cross-section study of pulmonary function in patients with insulin-dependent diabetes mellitus. Am Rev Respir Dis 1987; 135: 223–9.
[839] Bell D, Collier A, Matthews DM, et al. Are reduced lung volumes in IDDM due to defect in connective tissue? Diabetes 1988; 37: 829–31.
[840] Sandler M. Is the lung a "target organ" in diabetes mellitus? Arch Intern Med 1990; 150: 1385–8.
[841] Ramirez LC, Dal Nogare A, Hsia C, et al. Relationship between diabetes control and pulmonary function in insulin-dependent diabetes mellitus. Am J Med 1991; 91: 371–6.
[842] Wanke T, Formanek D, Auinger M, et al. Inspiratory muscle performance and pulmonary function changes in insulin-dependent diabetes mellitus. Am Rev Respir Dis 1991; 143: 97–100.
[843] Strojek K, Ziora D, Sroczynski, Oklek K. Pulmonary complications of type 1 (insulin-dependent) diabetic patients. Diabetologia 1992; 35: 1173–6.
[844] Douglas NJ, Campbell IW, Ewing DJ, et al. Reduced airway vagal tone in diabetic patients with autonomic neuropathy. Clin Sci 1981; 61: 581–4.
[845] Bruni B, Dottorini ML, Peccini F, et al. Volumi polmonari e tono bronchiale nel diabete insulino-dipendente con neuropatia autonomica. Med Torac 1990; 12: 421–7.

[846] Santos e Fonseca CMC, Manço JC, Gallo L, et al. Cholinergic bronchomotor tone and airway caliber in insulin-dependent diabetes mellitus. Chest 1992; 101: 1038–43.
[847] Heaton RW, Guy RJC, Gray BJ, et al. Diminished bronchial reactivity to cold air in diabetic patients with autonomic neuropathy. Br Med J 1984; 289: 149–51.
[848] Tantucci C, Scionti L, Bruni B, et al. Bronchial reactivity and control of breathing in diabetic autonomic neuropathy. Diabetes Nutr Metab 1988; 1: 315–22.
[849] Bertherat J, Lubetzki J, Lockhart A, Regnard J. Decreased bronchial response to methacholine in IDDM patients with autonomic neuropathy. Diabetes 1991; 40: 1100–6.
[850] Vianna LG, Gilbet SG, Barnes NC, et al. Cough threshold to citric acid in diabetic patients with and without autonomic neuropathy. Thorax 1988; 43: 569–71.
[851] Rhind GB, Gould GA, Ewing DJ, Clarke BF, Douglas NJ. Increased bronchial reactivity to histamine in diabetic autonomic neuropathy. Clin Sci 1987; 73: 401–5.
[852] Hansen LA, Prakash UBS, Colby TV. Pulmonary complications in diabetes mellitus. Mayo Clin Proc 1989; 64: 791–9.
[853] Estenne M, Primo G, Yernault JC. Cardiorespiratory response to dynamic exercise after human heart-lung transplantation. Thorax 1987; 42: 629–30.
[854] Banner NR, Lloyd MH, Hamilton RD, et al. Cardiopulmonary response to dynamic exercise after heart and combined heart-lung transplantation. Br Heart J 1989; 61: 215–23.
[855] Kimoff RJ, Cheong TH, Cosio MG, et al. Pulmonary denervation in humans. Effects on dyspnea and ventilatory pattern during exercise. Am Rev Respir Dis 1990; 142: 1034–40.
[856] Tantucci C, Bottini P, Dottorini ML, et al. Ventilatory response to exercise in diabetic subjects with autonomic neuropathy. J Appl Physiol 1996; 81: 1978–86.
[857] Wanke T, Formanek D, Auinger M, et al. Mechanical load on the inspiratory muscles during exercise hyperpnea in patients with type 1 (insulin-dependent) diabetes mellitus. Diabetologia 1992; 35: 425–8.
[858] Soler NG, Eagleton LE. Autonomic neuropathy and the ventilatory responses of diabetics to progressive hypoxemia and hypercarbia. Diabetes 1982, 31: 609–14.
[859] Williams JG, Morris AI, Hayter RC, Ogilvie CM. Respiratory responses of diabetics to hypoxia, hypercapnia, and exercise. Thorax 1984; 39: 529–34.
[860] Montserrat JM, Cochrane GM, Wolf C, et al. Ventilatory control in diabetes mellitus. Eur J Respir Dis 1985; 67: 112–7.
[861] Sobotka PA, Liss HP, Vinik AI. Impaired hypoxic ventilatory drive in diabetic patients with autonomic neuropathy. J Clin Endocrinol Metab 1986; 62: 658–63.
[862] Nishimura M, Miyamoto K, Suzuki A, et al. Ventilatory and heart rate responses to hypoxia and hypercapnia in patients with diabetes mellitus. Thorax 1989; 44: 251–7.
[863] Wanke T, Abrahamian H, Lahrmann H, et al. No effect of naloxone on ventilatory response to progressive hypercapnia in IDDM patients. Diabetes 1993; 42: 282–7.
[864] Homma I, Kageyama S, Nagai T, et al. Chemosensitivity in patients with diabetic neuropathy. Clin Sci 1981; 61: 599–603.
[865] Tantucci C, Scionti L, Bottini P, et al. Influence of autonomic neuropathy of different severity on the hypercapnic drive to breathing in diabetic patients. Chest 1997; 112: 145–53.
[866] Kostreva DR, Hopp FA, Zupercu EJ, et al. Respiratory inhibition with sympathetic afferent stimulation in the canine and primate. J Appl Physiol 1978; 44: 718–24.
[867] Champagnat J, Denavit-Saubie M, Henry JL, Leviel V. Catecholaminergic depressant effect on bulbar respiratory mechanisms. Brain Res 1979; 160: 57–68.
[868] Bolm P, Fuxe K. Pharmacological studies on a possible role of central noradrenaline neurons in respiratory control. J Pharm Pharmacol 1973; 25: 351–2.
[869] Gross PM, Heistad DD, Strait MR, et al. Cerebral vascular responses to physiological stimulation of sympathetic pathways in cats. Circ Res 1979; 44: 288–94.
[870] Heistad DD, Marcus ML, Gross PM. Effects of sympathetic nerves on cerebral vessels in dog, cat and monkeys. Am J Physiol 1978; 235: 544–52.
[871] Tantucci C, Bottini P, Fiorani C, et al. Influence of diabetic autonomic neuropathy on cerebral vascular reactivity to hypercapnia. Diabetologia 1998; 41 (Suppl): A305.
[872] Grunstein RR, Ho KY, Berthon-Jones M, et al. Central sleep apnea is associated with increased ventilatory response to carbon dioxide and hypersecretion of growth hormone in patients with acromegaly. Am J Respir Crit Care Med 1994; 150: 496–502.
[873] Chapman KR, Bruce EN, Gothe B. Possible mechanisms of periodic breathing during sleep. J Appl Physiol 1988; 64: 1000–8.
[874] Xie A, Rutherford R, Rankin F, et al. Hypocapnia and increased ventilatory responsiveness in patients with idiopathic central sleep apnea. Am J Respir Crit Care Med 1995; 152: 1950–5.
[875] Wilcox I, Grunstein RR, Collins FL, et al. The role of central chemosensitivity in central apnea of heart failure. Sleep 1993; 16: S37–8.
[876] Keyl C, Lemberge P, Rodig G, et al. Changes in cardiac autonomic control during nocturnal repetitive oxygen desaturation episodes in patients with coronary artery disease. J Cardiovasc Risk 1996; 3: 221–7.
[877] Page MM, Watkins PJ. Cardiorespiratory arrest and diabetic autonomic neuropathy. Lancet 1978; i: 14–6.
[878] Ewing DJ, Campbell IW, Clarke BF. Mortality in diabetic autonomic neuropathy. Lancet 1978; i: 601–3.
[879] Srinivasan G, Sanders G. Cardiorespiratory arrest and diabetes. Lancet 1978; i: 935–6.
[880] Guilleminault C, Briskin JG, Greenfield MS, Silvestri R. The impact of the autonomic nervous system dysfunction on breathing during sleep. Sleep 1981; 4: 263–78.
[881] Rees PJ, Prior JG, Cochrane GM, Clark TJ. Sleep apnea in diabetic patients with autonomic neuropathy. J R Soc Med 1981; 74: 192–5.
[882] Mondini S, Guilleminault C. Abnormal breathing patterns during sleep in diabetes. Ann Neurol 1985; 17: 391–5.
[883] Catterall JR, Calverley PMA, Ewing DJ, et al. Breathing, sleep and diabetic autonomic neuropathy. Diabetes 1984; 33: 1025–7.
[884] Ficker JH, Dertinger SH, Siegfried W, et al. Obstructive sleep apnea and diabetes mellitus: the role of cardiovascular autonomic neuropathy. Eur Respir J 1998; 11: 14–9.
[885] Bottini P, Cordoni MC, Dottorini ML, et al. Diabetic autonomic neuropathy promotes obstructive sleep apnea while central sleep apnea is prevented by decreased CO_2 peripheral chemosensitivity. Diabetes 2000; 49(Suppl 1): A162.
[886] Neumann C, Martinez D, Schmid H. Nocturnal oxygen desaturation in diabetic patients with severe autonomic neuropathy. Diabetes Res Clin Pract 1995; 28: 97–102.
[887] Remmers JE, De Groot WJ, Sauerland EK, Anch AM. Pathogenesis of upper airway occlusion during sleep. J Appl Physiol 1978; 44: 931–8.
[888] Wheatley JR, Mezzanotte WS, Tangel DJ, White DP. Influence of sleep on genioglossal muscle activation by negative pressure in normal men. Am Rev Respir Dis 1993; 148: 597–605.
[889] Weiner D, Mitra J, Salamone J, Cherniack NS. Effects of chemical stimuli on nerves supplying upper airway muscle. J Appl Physiol 1982; 52: 530–6.
[890] DeWeese EL, Sullivan TY. Effects of upper airway anesthesia on pharyngeal patency during sleep. J Appl Physiol 1988; 64: 1346–53.
[891] Villa MP, Multari G, Montesano M, et al. Sleep apnoea in children with diabetes mellitus: effect of glycaemic control. Diabetologia 2000; 43: 696–702.
[892] Huizinga JD. Pathophysiology of GI motility related to interstitial cells of Cajal. Am J Physiol 1998; 275: G381–386.
[893] Gonella J, Bouvier M, Blanquet F. Extrinsic nervous control of motility of the small intestine and related sphincters. Physiol Rev 1987; 67: 902–1053.
[894] Rundles RW. Diabetic neuropathy: General review with report of 125 cases. Medicine 1945; 24: 111–60.
[895] Horowitz M. Gastric and oesophageal emptying in insulin-dependent diabetes mellitus. J Gastroenterol Hepatol 1986; 1: 97–113.
[896] Wegener M. Gastrointestinal transit disorders in patients with insulin-treated diabetes mellitus. Dig Dis Sci 1990; 8: 23–36.
[897] Horowitz M. Relationships between oesophageal transit and solid and liquid gastric emptying in diabetes mellitus. Eur J Nucl Med 1991; 18: 229–34.
[898] Keshavarzian A, Iber FL, Vaeth J. Gastric emptying in patients with insulin-requiring diabetes mellitus. Am J Gastroenterol 1987; 82: 29–35.

[899] Lucas PD, Sardar AM. Effects of diabetes on cholinergic transmission in two rat gut preparations. Gastroenterology 1991; 100: 123–8.
[900] Takahashi T, Nakamura K, Itoh H. Impaired expression of nitric oxide synthase in the gastric myenteric plexus of spontaneously diabetic rats. Gastroenterology 1997; 113: 1535–44.
[901] Watkins CC, Sawa A, Jaffrey S, et al. Insulin restores neuronal nitric oxide synthase expression and function that is lost in diabetic gastropathy. J Clin Invest 2000; 106: 373–84.
[902] Konturek JW, Fischer H, Gromotka PM, Dommschke W. Endogenous nitric oxide in the regulation of gastric secretory and motor activity in humans. Aliment Pharmacol Ther 1999; 13: 1683–91.
[903] Yoshida MM, Schuffler MD, Sumi MS. There are no morphological abnormalities of the gastric wall or abdominal vagus in patients with gastroparesis. Gastroenterology 1988; 94: 907–14.
[904] Ejskjaer NT, et al. Novel surgical treatment and gastric pathology in diabetic gastroparesis. Diabet Med 1999; 16: 488–95.
[905] Fraser R, Horowitz M, Maddox AP, et al. Hyperglycaemia slows gastric emptying in type 1 diabetes mellitus. Diabetologia 1990; 33: 675–80.
[906] Horowitz M, Harding PE, Maddox AP, et al. Gastric and oesophageal emptying in patients with type 2 (non-insulin-dependent) diabetes mellitus. Diabetologia 1989; 32: 151–9.
[907] Schvarcz E, Palmer M, Aman J, et al. Hypoglycaemia increases the gastric emptying rate in patients with type 1 diabetes mellitus. Diabet Med 1993; 10: 660–3.
[908] Barnett JL, Owyang C. Serum glucose concentration as a modulator of interdigestive gastric motility. Gastroenterology 1988; 94: 739–44.
[909] Fraser R, Horowitz M, Dent J. Hyperglycaemia stimulates pyloric motility in normal subjects. Gut 1991; 32: 475–8.
[910] Hasler WL, Soudah HC, Dulai G, Owyang C. Mediation of hyperglycaemia-evoked gastric slow-wave dysrhythmias by endogenous prostaglandins. Gastroenterology 1995; 108: 1096–104.
[911] Jebbink RJA, Samsom M, Bruijs PP, et al. Hyperglycaemia induces abnormalities of gastric myoelectrical activity in patients with type 1 diabetes mellitus. Gastroenterology 1994; 107: 1390–7.
[912] Bjornsson E, Urbanavicius V, Eliasson B, et al. Effects of hyperglycaemia on interdigestive gastrointestinal motility in humans. Scand J Gastroenterol 1994; 20: 1096–104.
[913] Russo A, Fraser R, Horowitz M. The effect of acute hyperglycaemia on small intestinal motility in normal subjects. Diabetologia 1996; 39: 984–9.
[914a] de Boer SY, Masclee AA, Lam WF, et al. Hyperglycaemia modulates gallbladder motility and small intestinal transit time in man. Dig Dis Sci 1993; 38: 2228–35.
[914b] de Boer SY, Masclee AA, Lam WF, Lamers CB. Effect of acute hyperglycemia on oesophageal motility and lower oesophageal sphincter pressure in humans. Gastroenterology 1992; 103: 775–80.
[915] Sims MA, Hasler WL, Chey WD, et al. Hyperglycaemia inhibits mechanoreceptor-mediated gastrocolonic responses and colonic peristaltic reflexes in healthy humans. Gastroenterology 1995; 108: 350–9.
[916] Maleki D, Camilleri M, Zinsmeister AR, Rizza RA. Effect of acute hyperglycaemia on colorectal motor and sensory function in humans. Am J Physiol 1997; 273: G859–864.
[917] Russo A, Sun WM, Sattawatthamrong Y, et al. Acute hyperglycaemia affects anorectal motor and sensory function in normal subjects. Gut 1997; 41: 494–9.
[918] Avsar E, Ersoz O, Karisik E, et al. Hyperglycaemia-induced attenuation of rectal perception depends upon pattern of rectal balloon inflation. Dig Dis Sci 1997; 42: 2206–12.
[919] Lam WF, Masclee AA, de Boer SY, Lamers CB. Hyperglycaemia reduces gastric secretory and plasma pancreatic polypeptide to modified sham feeding in humans. Digestion 1993; 54: 48–53.
[920] Yeap B, Russo A, Fraser R, et al. Hyperglycaemia affects cardiovascular autonomic nerve function in normal subjects. Diabetes Care 1996; 19: 880–2.
[921] Kong M-F, King P, Macdonald I, et al. Euglycaemic hyperinsulinaemia does not affect gastric emptying in type 1 and type 2 diabetes mellitus. Diabetologia 1999; 42: 365–72.
[922] Horowitz M, Edelbroek M, Wishart J, Straathof J. Relationship between oral glucose tolerance and gastric emptying in normal healthy subjects. Diabetologia 1993; 36: 857–62.
[923] Bytzer P, Talley NJ, Leemon M, et al. Prevalence of gastrointestinal symptoms associated with diabetes mellitus: a population-based survey of 15,000 adults. Arch Intern Med 2001; 161:1989–96.
[924] Feldman M, Schiller LR. Disorders of gastrointestinal motility associated with diabetes mellitus. Ann Intern Med 1983; 98: 378–84.
[925] Clouse RE, Lustman PJ. Gastrointestinal symptoms in diabetic patients: lack of association with neuropathy. Am J Gastroenterol 1989; 84: 868.
[926] Schvarcz E, Palmer M, Ingberg CM, et al. Increased prevalence of upper gastrointestinal symptoms in long-term type 1 diabetes mellitus. Diabet Med 1996; 13: 478–81.
[927] Maleki D, Locke R, Camilleri M, et al. Gastrointestinal tract symptoms among persons with diabetes mellitus in the community. Arch Intern Med 2000; 160: 2808–16.
[928] Ricci JA, et al. Upper gastrointestinal symptoms in a U.S. national sample of adults with diabetes. Scand J Gastroenterol 2000; 35: 152–9.
[929] Spangeus A, et al. Prevalence of gastrointestinal symptoms in young and middle-aged diabetic patients. Scand J Gastroenterol 1999; 34: 1196–202.
[930] Talley NJ, Young L, Bytzer P, et al. Impact of chronic gastrointestinal symptoms in diabetes mellitus on health-related quality of life. Am J Gastroenterol 2001; 96: 71–6.
[931] Oldenburg B, Diepersloot RJA, Hoekstra JBL. High seroprevalence of Helicobacter pylori in diabetes mellitus. Dig Dis Sci 1996; 41: 458.
[932] Samsom M, Salet GAM, Roelofs JMM, et al. Compliance of the proximal stomach and dyspeptic symptoms in patients with type 1 diabetes mellitus. Dig Dis Sci 1995; 40: 2037.
[933] Hebbard GS, Sun WM, Dent J, Horowitz M. Hyperglycaemia affects proximal gastric motor and sensory function in normal subjects. Eur J Gastroenterol Hepatol 1996; 8: 211–7.
[934] Jones KL, Horowitz M, Berry M, et al. The blood glucose concentration influences postprandial fullness in insulin-dependent diabetes mellitus. Diabetes Care 1997; 20: 1141–6.
[935] Rayner CK, Samsom M, Jones KL, Horowitz M. Relationships between upper gastrointestinal motor and sensory function with glycaemic control (review). Diabetes Care 2001; 24: 371–81.
[936] Talley NJ, Bytzer P, Hammer J, et al. Psychological distress is linked to gastrointestinal symptoms in diabetes mellitus. Am J Gastroenterol 2001; 96: 1033–8.
[937] Horowitz M, Maddoz AF, Wishart J, et al. Relationships between oesophageal transit and solid and liquid gastric emptying in diabetes mellitus. Eur J Nucl Med 1991; 18: 229–34.
[938] Keshavarzian A, Iber FL, Nasrallah S. Radionuclide oesphageal emptying and manometric studies in diabetes mellitus. Am J Gastroenterol 1987; 82: 625–31.
[939] Murray PE, Lombart MG, Ache J, et al. Esophageal function in diabetes mellitus with special reference to acid studies and relationship to peripheral neuropathy. Am J Gastroenterol 1987; 82: 840–3.
[940] Borgstrom PS, Olsson R, Sundkvist G, et al. Pharyngeal and oesphageal transit and solid and liquid gastric emptying in diabetes mellitus. Br J Radiol 1988; 61: 817–21.
[941] Russell COH, Gannan R, Coatsworth J, et al. Relationship among oesophageal dysfunction, diabetic gastroenteropathy, and peripheral neuropathy. Dig Dis Sci 1983; 28: 289–93.
[942] Stewart IM, Hosking DJ, Preston BJ, et al. Oesophageal motor changes in diabetes mellitus. Thorax 1976; 31: 278–83.
[943] Westin L, Lilja B, Sundkvist G. Oesophagus scintigraphy in patients with diabetes mellitus. Scand J Gastroenterol 1986; 21: 1200–4.
[944] Lluch I, et al. Gastroesophageal reflux in diabetes mellitus. Am J Gastroenterol 1999; 94: 919–24.
[945] Maddern GJ, Horowitz M, Jamieson GG. The effect of domperidone on oesophageal emptying in diabetic autonomic neuropathy. Br J Clin Pharmacol 1985; 19: 441–4.

[946] Horowitz M, Maddox A, Harding PE, et al. Effect of cisapride on gastric emptying in insulin-dependent diabetes mellitus. Gastroenterology 1987; 92: 1899–907.

[947] Kao CH, Wang SJ, Pang DY. Effects of oral erythromycin on upper gastrointestinal motility in patients with non-insulin-dependent diabetes mellitus. Nucl Med Commun 1995; 16: 790–3.

[948] Jorgensen F, Bosen F, Andersen B, et al. Oesophageal transit in patients with autonomic dysfunction. The effect of treatment with fluodrocortisone. Clin Phys 1991; 11: 83–92.

[949] Jones KL, Wishart J, Berry M, et al. Effects of fedotozine on gastric emptying and upper gastrointestinal symptoms in diabetic gastroparesis. Aliment Pharmacol Ther 2000; 14: 937–43.

[950] Sun WM, Hebbard GS, Malbert C-H, et al. Spatial patterns of fasting and fed antropyloric pressure waves in humans. J Physiol (Lond) 1997; 503: 455–62.

[951] Malbert C-H, Mathis CJ. Antropyloric modulation of transpyloric flow of liquids in pigs. Gastroenterology 1994; 107: 37–46.

[952] Hausken T, Odegaard S, Matre K, Berstad A. Antroduodenal motility and movements of luminal contents studied by duplex sonography. Gastroenterology 1992; 102: 1583–90.

[953] Horowitz M, Dent J, Fraser R, et al. Role and integration of mechanisms controlling gastric emptying. Dig Dis Sci 1994; 39: S7–13.

[954] Apiroz F, Malagelada JR. Gastric tone measured by an electronic barostat in health and postsurgical gastroparesis. Gastroenterology 1987; 92: 934–43.

[955] Hebbard GS. Physiology and pathophysiology of gastric emptying. Gastroenterol Int 1998; 11: 150–60.

[956] Horowitz M, Dent J. Disordered gastric emptying; mechanical basis, assessment and treatment. Bailliere's Clin Gastroenterol 1991; 5: 371–407.

[957] Lee JS, Camilleri M, Zinsmeister AR, et al. Towards office-based measurement of gastric emptying in symptomatic diabetics using C13 octanoic acid breath test. Am J Gastroenterol 2000; 95: 2251–61.

[958] Jones KL, Horowitz M, Wishart JM, et al. Relationships between gastric emptying, intragastric meal distribution and blood glucose concentrations in diabetes mellitus. J Nucl Med 1995; 36: 2220–8.

[959] Weytjens C, Keymeulen B, van Haleweyn C, et al. Rapid gastric emptying of a liquid meal in long-term type 2 diabetes mellitus. Diabet Med 1998; 15: 1022–7.

[960] Camilleri M, Hasler WL, Parkman HP, et al. Measurement of gastrointestinal motility in the GI laboratory. Gastroenterology 1998; 115: 747–62.

[961] Stacher G, Shernthaner G, Francesconi M, et al. Cisapride versus placebo for 8 weeks on glycaemic control and gastric emptying in insulin-dependent diabetes: a double-blind cross-over trial. J Clin Endocrinol Metab 1999; 84: 2357–62.

[962] Ziegler D, Schadewaldt P, Pour Mirza A, et al. C13 octanoic breath test for non-invasive assessment of gastric emptying in diabetic patients; validation and relationship to gastric symptoms and cardiovascular autonomic function. Diabetologia 1996; 39: 823–30.

[963] Dutta U, Padhy AK, Ahuja V, Sharma MP. Double-blind controlled trial of cisapride on gastric emptying in diabetics. Trop Gastroenterol 1999; 20: 116–9.

[964] Urbain JL, Vekemans M, Bouillon R, et al. Characterisation of gastric antral motility disturbances in diabetes using scintigraphic technique. J Nucl Med 1993; 34: 576–81.

[965] Nowak TV, Johnson CP, Kalbfleisch JH, et al. Highly variable gastric emptying in patients with insulin dependent diabetes mellitus. Gut 1995; 37: 23–9.

[966] Phillips WT, Schwartz JG, McMahon CA. Rapid gastric emptying of an oral glucose solution in type 2 diabetic patients. J Nucl Med 1992; 33: 1496–500.

[967] Schwartz JG, Green GM, Guan GM, et al. Rapid emptying of a solid pancake meal in type II diabetic patients. Diabetes Care 1996; 19: 468–71.

[968] Samsom M, Jebbink RJA, Akkermans LMA, et al. Abnormalities of antroduodenal motility in type 1 diabetes. Diabetes Care 1996; 19: 21–7.

[969] Fraser R, Horowitz M, Maddox A, Dent J. Postprandial antropyloroduodenal motility and gastric emptying in gastroparesis—effects of cisapride. Gut 1994; 35: 172–8.

[970] Nguyen HN, Silny J, Wuller S, et al. Abnormal postprandial duodenal chyme transport in patients with longstanding insulin dependent diabetes mellitus. Gut 1997; 41: 624–31.

[971] Kawagishi T, Nishizawa Y, Emoto M, et al. Gastric myoelectrical activity in patients with diabetes: role of glucose control and autonomic nerve function. Diabetes Care 1997; 20: 848–54.

[972] Jones KL, Tonkin A, Horowitz M, et al. The rate of gastric emptying is a determinant of postprandial hypotension in non-insulin diabetes mellitus. Clin Sci 1998; 94: 65–70.

[973] Iber FL, Parveen S, Vandrunen M, et al. Relation of symptoms to impaired stomach, small bowel, and colonic motility in long-standing diabetes. Dig Dis Sci 1993; 38: 45–50.

[974] Chandalia M, Garg A, Lutjohann D, et al. Beneficial effects of high dietary fibre intake in patients with type 2 diabetes mellitus. N Engl J Med 2000; 342: 1392–8.

[975] Cunningham KM, Read NW. The effect of incorporating fat into different components of a meal on gastric emptying and postprandial blood glucose and insulin responses. Br J Nutr 1989; 61: 285–90.

[976] Trinick TR, Laker MF, Johnston DG, et al. Effect of guar gum on second-meal glucose tolerance in normal man. Clin Sci 1986; 71: 49–55.

[977] Melga P, Mansi C, Ciuchi E, et al. Chronic administration of levosulpiride and glycaemic control in IDDM patients with gastroparesis. Diabetes Care 1997; 20: 55–8.

[978] Thompson RG, Pearson L, Schoenfeld SL, Kolterman OG. Pramlintide, a synthetic analog of human amylin, improves the metabolic profile of patients with type 2 diabetes using insulin. The Pramlintide in Type 2 Diabetes Group. Diabetes Care 1998; 21: 987–93.

[979] Buse J, Fineman M, Gottlieb A, et al. Effects of five-day dosing of synthetic exendin-4 (AC2993) in people with type 2 diabetes. Diabetes 2000; 49(Suppl): A100.

[980] Kong M-F, Horowitz M, Jones KL, et al. Natural history of gastroparesis. Diabetes Care 1999; 22: 503–7.

[981] Holzapfel A, Festa A, Stacher-Janotta G, et al. Gastric emptying in type II (non-insulin dependent) diabetes mellitus before and after therapy readjustment: no influence of actual blood glucose concentration. Diabetologia 1999; 42: 1410–2.

[982] Samsom M, Smout AJPM, Goozen HG. Medical and surgical treatment of gastroparesis. Gastroenterol Int 1998; 11: 169–76.

[983] Janssens J, Peeters TL, Vantrappen G, et al. Erythromycin improves delayed gastric emptying in diabetic gastroparesis. N Engl J Med 1990; 322: 1028–31.

[984] Horowitz M, Harding PE, Chatterton BE, et al. Acute and chronic effect of domperidone on gastric emptying in diabetic autonomic neuropathy. Dig Dis Sci 1985; 30: 1–9.

[985] Soykan I, Sarosiek I, MacCallum RW. The effect of chronic oral domperidone therapy on gastrointestinal symptoms, gastric emptying, and quality of life in patients with gastroparesis. Am J Gastroenterol 1997; 92: 979–80.

[986] Silvers D, Kipnes M, Broadstone V, et al. Domperidone in the management of diabetic gastroparesis: efficacy, tolerability and quality of life outcomes in a multicentre controlled trial. Clin Ther 1998; 20: 438–53.

[987] Schade RR, Dugas MC, Lhotsky DM, et al. Effect of metoclopramide on gastric liquid emptying in patients with diabetic gastroparesis. Dig Dis Sci 1985; 30: 10–5.

[988] Richards RD, Davenport KS, MacCallum RW. The treatment of idiopathic and diabetic gastroparesis with acute intravenous and chronic oral erythromycin. Am J Gastroenterol 1993; 88: 203–7.

[989] Coulie B, Tack J, Peeters TL, Janssens J. Involvement of two different pathways in the motor effects of erythromycin on the gastric antrum in humans. Gut 1998; 43: 395–400.

[990] Di Baise JK, Quigley EMM. Efficacy of long-term intravenous erythromycin in the management of severe gastroparesis: one center's experience. J Clin Gastroenterol 1999; 28: 131–4.

[991] Jones KL, Berry M, Kong M-F, et al. Hyperglycaemia attenuates the gastrokinetic effect of erythromycin and effects the perception of postprandial hunger in normal subjects. Diabetes Care 1999; 22: 339–44.

[992] Petrakis IE, Vrachassotakis N, Sciacca V, et al. Hyperglycaemia attenuates erythromycin-induced acceleration of solid-phase gastric emptying in idiopathic and diabetic gastroparesis. Scand J Gastroenterol 1999; 34: 396–403.

[993] Camilleri M, Malagelada JR, Abell TL, et al. Effect of six weeks of treatment with cisapride in gastroparesis and intestinal pseudoobstruction. Gastroenterology 1989; 96: 704–12.
[994] De Caestecker JS, Ewing DJ, Tothill P, et al. Evaluation of oral cisapride and metoclopramide in diabetic autonomic neuropathy: an eight week double-blind cross-over study. Aliment Pharmacol Ther 1989; 3: 69–81.
[995] Havelund T, Oster-Jorgensen E, Eshoj O, et al. Effects of cisapride on gastroparesis in patients with insulin-dependent diabetes mellitus. A double-blind controlled trial. Acta Med Scand 1987; 222: 339–43.
[996] Tonini M, De Ponti F, Di Nucci A, Crema F. Review article: cardiac adverse effects of gastrointestinal prokinetics. Aliment Pharmacol Ther 1999; 13: 1585–91.
[997] Ganzini L, Casey DE, Hoffman WF, McCall AI. The prevalence of metoclopramide-induced tardive dyskinesia and acute extra-pyramidal movements. Arch Intern Med 1993; 153: 1469–75.
[998] Farup CE, Leidy NK, Murray M, et al. Effect of domperidone on the health-related quality of life of patients with symptoms of diabetic gastroparesis. Diabetes Care 1998; 21: 1699–706.
[999] Gaber AO, Oxley D, Karas J, et al. Changes in gastric emptying in recipients of combined pancreas-kidney transplants. Dig Dis 1991; 9: 437–43.
[1000] Camilleri M. Tegaserod. Aliment Pharmacol Ther 2001; 15: 277–89.
[1001] Talley NJ, Verlinden M, MacCallum RW, et al. Efficacy of a motilin receptor agonist (ABT-229) for relief of dyspepsia in type 1 diabetes mellitus: a randomised double-blind placebo controlled trial. Gut 2001; 49: 359–401.
[1002] Camilleri M, Malagelada JR. Abnormal intestinal motility in diabetics with gastroparesis syndrome. Eur J Clin Invest 1984; 14: 420–7.
[1003] Dooley CP, Newihi HM, Zeidler A, et al. Abnormalities of the migrating motor complex in diabetics with autonomic neuropathy and diarrhoea. Scand J Gastroenterol 1988; 23: 217–23.
[1004] Chang EB, Bergenstal RM, Field M. Diarrhea in streptozotocin treated rats. J Clin Invest 1985; 75: 1666–70.
[1005] Fedorak R, Field M, Chang E. Treatment of diabetic diarrhoea with clonidine. Ann Intern Med 1985; 102: 197–9.
[1006] Tsai ST, Vinik AL, Brunner JF. Diabetic diarrhoea and somatostatin. Ann Intern Med 1986; 105: 139.
[1007] Grodzki M, Mazurkewicz-Rozynska E, Czyzk A. Diabetic cholecystopathy. Diabetologia 1968; 4: 345–8.
[1008] Read NW. The relationship between colonic motility and secretion. Scand J Gastroenterol 1984; 19(Suppl 84): 45–63.
[1009] Baker WNW, Mann CV. The rectosigmoid junction zone: another sphincter. In: Thomas PA, Mann CV, editors. Alimentary sphincters and their disorders. London: Macmillan Press, 1981: 210–1.
[1010] Kawagishi T, Nishizawa Y, Okuno Y, et al. Segmental gut transit in diabetes mellitus: effect of cisapride. Diabetes Res Clin Pract 1992; 17: 137–44.
[1011] Battle WM, Snape WJ, Alavi A, et al. Colonic dysfunction in diabetes mellitus. Gastroenterology 1980; 79: 1217–21.
[1012] Yanni G, Snape WJ. Effect of erythromycin on colonic motility in patients with constipation. Gastroenterology 1992; 103: A1384.
[1013] Jameson JS, Rogers J, Misiewicz JJ, et al. Oral or intravenous erythromycin has no effect on human distal colonic motility. Aliment Pharmacol Ther 1992; 6: 589–95.
[1014] Martin M. Diabetic neuropathy: a clinical study of 150 cases. Brain 1958; 76: 594–624.
[1015] Sun WM, Katsinelos P, Horowitz M, Read NW. Disturbances in anorectal function in patients with diabetes mellitus and faecal incontinence. Eur J Gastroenterol Hepatol 1996; 8: 1007–12.
[1016] Hackett GI. Impotence—the most neglected complication of diabetes. Diabetes Res 1995; 28: 75–83.
[1017] NIH consensus development panel on impotence. Impotence. JAMA 270: 83–90, 1993.
[1018] Wagner G, Saenz de Tejada I. Update on male erectile dysfunction. Br Med J 1998; 316: 678–82.
[1019] Feldman HA, Goldstein I, Hatzichristou DG, Krane RJ, McKinlay JB. Impotence and its medical and psychosocial correlates: results of the Massachusetts male ageing study. J Urol 1994; 151: 54–61.
[1020] Johannes CB, Araujo AB, Feldman HA, Derby CA, Kleinman KP, McKinlay JB. Incidence of erectile dysfunction in men 40 to 69 years old: longitudinal results from the Massachusetts male aging study. J Urol 2000; 163: 460–3.
[1021] Klein R, Klein BE, Lee KE, Moss SE, Cruickshanks KJ. Prevalence of self-reported erectile dysfunction in people with long-term IDDM. Diabetes Care 1996; 19:135–41.
[1022] Fedele D, Coscelli C, Santeusanio F, Bortolotti A, Chatenoud L, Colli E, Landoni M, Parazzini F. Erectile dysfunction in diabetic subjects in Italy. Diabetes Care 1998; 21: 1973–7.
[1023] Parazzini F, Menchini FF, Bortolotti A, Calabro A, Chatenoud L, Colli E, Landoni M, Lavezzari M, Turchi P, Sessa A, Mirone V. Frequency and determinants of erectile dysfunction in Italy. Eur Urol 2000; 37: 43–9.
[1024] Lustman PJ, Clouse RE. Relationship of psychiatric illness to impotence in men with diabetes. Diabetes Care 1990; 13: 893–5.
[1025] Lue TF, Takamura T, Schmidt RA, Tanagho EA. Hemodynamics of erection in the monkey. J Urol 1983; 130: 1237–41
[1026] Lue TF, Tanagho EA. Physiology of erection and pharmacological management of impotence. J Urol 1987; 137: 829–35.
[1027] Andersson KE, Wagner G. Physiology of penile erection. Physiol Rev 1995; 75: 191–236.
[1028] Mandrek K. Electrophysiological methods in smooth muscle physiology. Corpus cavernosum in vitro. World J Urol 1994; 12: 262–5.
[1029] Mersdorf A, Goldsmith P, Diederichs W, Padula C, Lue T F, Fishman I, Tanagho EA.: Ultrastructural changes in impotent penile tissue. J Urol 1991; 145: 749–56.
[1030] Andersson KE, Holmquist F. Regulation of tone in penile cavernous smooth muscle. World J Urol 1994; 12: 249–61.
[1031] Andersson KE, Stief CG. Neurotransmission and the contraction and relaxation of penile erectile tissues. World J Urol 1997; 15: 14–20.
[1032] Ignarro JL, Bush PA, Buga GM, Wood KS, Fukoto JM, Raifer J. Nitric oxide and cyclic GMP formation upon electrical field stimulation cause relaxation of corpus cavernosum smooth muscle. Biochem Biophys Res Commun 1990; 170: 843–6.
[1033] Holmquist F, Hedlund H, Andersson KE. L-N-nitro arginine inhibits non-adrenergic, non cholinergic relaxation of human isolated corpus cavernosum. Acta Physiol Scand 1991; 141: 383–90.
[1034] Lue TF. Erectile dysfunction. N Engl J Med 2000; 342: 1802–13.
[1035] Saenz de Tejada I, Goldstein I. Diabetic penile neuropathy. Urol Clin North Am 1988; 15: 17–22.
[1036] Seftel AD, Vaziri ND, Ni Z, Razmjouei K, Fogarty J, Hampel N, Polak J, Wang RZ, Ferguson K, Block C, Haas C. Advanced glycation end products in human penis: elevation in diabetic tissue, site of deposition, and possible effect through iNOS or eNOS. Urology 1997; 50: 1016–26.
[1037] Hirata K, Kuroda R, Sakoda T, Katayama M, Inoue N, Suematsu M, Kawashima S, Yokoyama M. Inhibition of endothelial nitric oxide synthase activity by protein kinase C. Hypertension 1995; 25: 180–5.
[1038] Saenz de Tejada I, Goldstein I, Azadzoi K, Krane RJ, Cohen RA. Impaired neurogenic and endothelium-mediated relaxation of penile smooth muscle from diabetic men with impotence. N Engl J Med 1989; 320: 1025–30.
[1039] Keegan A, Cotter MA, Cameron NE. Effects of diabetes and treatment with the antioxidant α-lipoic acid on endothelial and neurogenic responses of corpus cavernosum in rats. Diabetologia 1999; 42: 343–50.
[1040] Elabbady AA, Gagnon C, Hassouna MM, Begin LR, Elhilali MM. Diabetes mellitus increases nitric oxide synthase in penises but not in major pelvic ganglia of rats. Br J Urol 1996; 76: 196–202.
[1041] Vernet D, Cai L, Garban H, Babbitt ML, Murray FT, Rajfer J, Gonzalez-Cadavid NF: Reduction of penile nitric oxide

synthase in diabetic BB/WORdp (type I) and BBZ/WORdp (type II) rats with erectile dysfunction. Endocrinology 1995; 136:5709–17.
[1042] Sato K. The physiology, pharmacology, and biochemistry of the eccrine sweat gland. Rev Physiol Biochem Pharm 1977; 79: 51–131.
[1043] Kuno Y. Human perspiration. Springfield, Ill.: Charles C. Thomas, 1956.
[1044] Ogawa T, Low PA. Autonomic regulation of temperature and sweating. In: Low PA, editor. Clinical autonomic disorders: evaluation and management. Boston: Little, Brown and Company, 1993: 79–91.
[1045] Baker MA, Doris PA. Effect of dehydration on hypothalamic control of evaporation in the cat. J Physiol 1982; 322: 457–68.
[1046] Nakashima T, Hori T, Kiyohara T, Shibata M. Osmosensitivity of preoptic thermosensitive neurons in hypothalamic slices in vitro. Pflugers Arch 1985; 405: 112–7.
[1047] Fortney SM, Nadel ER, Wenger CB, Bove JR. Effect of blood volume on sweating rate and body fluids in exercising humans. J Appl Physiol 1981; 51: 1594–600.
[1048] Kasting NW, Veale WL, Cooper KE. Vasopressin: a homeostatic effector in the febrile process. Neurosci Biobehav Rev 1982; 6: 215–22.
[1049] Clark WG, Lipton JM. Brain and pituitary peptides in thermoregulation. [Review]. Pharmacol Ther 1983; 22: 249–97.
[1050] Sugenoya J, Kihara M, Ogawa T, et al. Effects of thyrotropin releasing hormone on human sudomotor and cutaneous vasomotor activities. Eur J Appl Physiol 1988; 57: 632–8.
[1051] Tache Y, Pittman Q, Brown M. Bombesin-induced poikilothermy in rats. Brain Res 1980; 188: 525–30.
[1052] Hori T, Yamasaki M, Kiyohara T, Shibata M. Responses of preoptic thermosensitive neurons to poikilothermia-inducing peptides—bombesin and neurotensin. Pflugers Arch 1986; 407: 558–60.
[1053] Clark WG, Lipton JM, Said SI. Hyperthermic responses to vasoactive intestinal polypeptide (VIP) injected into the third cerebral ventricle of cats. Neuropharmacology 1978; 17: 883–5.
[1054] Ogawa T, Low PA. Autonomic regulation of temperature and sweating. In: Low PA, editor. Clinical autonomic disorders: evaluation and management. 2nd edition. Philadelphia, Pa.: Lippincott-Raven, 1997: 83–96.
[1055] Low PA. Laboratory evaluation of autonomic function. In: Low PA, editor. Clinical autonomic disorders: evaluation and management. 2nd edition. Philadelphia, Pa.: Lippincott-Raven, 1997: 179–208.
[1056] List CF, Peet MM. Sweat secretion in man. I. Sweating responses in normal persons. Arch Neurol Psychiatry 1938; 39: 1228–37.
[1057] Kennedy WR, Sakuta M, Sutherland D, Goetz FC. Quantitation of the sweating deficit in diabetes mellitus. Ann Neurol 1984; 15: 482–8.
[1058] Guttmann L. The management of the quinizarin sweat test (QST). Postgrad Med J 1947; 23: 353–66.
[1059] Silverman JJ, Powell VE. Simple technique for outlining sweat pattern. War Med 1945; 7: 178–80.
[1060] Randall WC. Quantitation and regional distribution of sweat glands in man. J Clin Invest 1946; 25: 761–7.
[1061] Macmillan AL, Spalding JM. Human sweating response to electrophoresed acetylcholine: a test of postganglionic sympathetic function. J Neurol Neurosurg Psychiatry 1969; 32: 155–60.
[1062] Herrmann F, Prose PH, Sulzberger MB. Studies on sweating. IV. A new quantitative method of assaying sweat-delivery to circumscribed areas of the skin surface. J Invest Dermatol 1951; 17: 241–9.
[1063] Richter CP. Instructions for using the cutaneous resistance recorder, or dermometeron peripheral nerve injuries, sympathectomies, and paravertebral blocks. J Neurosurg 1946; 3: 181–91.
[1064] Shahani BT, Halperin JJ, Boulu P, Cohen J. Sympathetic skin response: a method of assessing unmyelinated axon dysfunction in peripheral neuropathies. J Neurol Neurosurg Psychiatry 1984; 47: 536–42.
[1065] Netsky MG. Studies on secretion in man. I. Innervation of the sweat glands of the upper extremity; newer methods of studying sweating. Arch Neurol Psychiatry 1948; 60: 279–87.
[1066] Darrow CW. Sensory, secretory and electrical changes in the skin following bodily excitation. J Exp Psychol 1927; 10: 197–226.
[1067] Ogawa T, Asayama M, Miyagawa T. Effects of sweat gland training by repeated local heating. Jpn J Physiol 1982; 32: 971–81.
[1068] Lang E, Foerster A, Pfannmuller D, Handwerker HO. Quantitative assessment of sudomotor activity by capacitance hygrometry. Clin Auton Res 1993; 3: 107–15.
[1069] Low PA, Caskey PE, Tuck RR, et al. Quantitative sudomotor axon reflex test in normal and neuropathic subjects. Ann Neurol 1983; 14: 573–80.
[1070] Adams T, Steinmetz MA, Manner DB, et al. An improved method for water vapor detection. Ann Biomed Eng 1983; 11: 117–29.
[1071] Low PA, Walsh JC, Huang CY, McLeod JG. The sympathetic nervous system in diabetic neuropathy. A clinical and pathological study. Brain 1975; 98: 341–56.
[1072] Fealey RD. The thermoregulatory sweat test. In: Low PA, editor. Clinical autonomic disorders: evaluation and management. Boston: Little, Brown and Company, 1993: 217–29.
[1073] Fealey RD, Low PA, Thomas JE. Thermoregulatory sweating abnormalities in diabetes mellitus. Mayo Clin Proc 1989; 64: 617–28.
[1074] Low PA. Sudomotor function and dysfunction. In: Asbury AK, McKhann GM, McDonald WI, editors. Diseases of the nervous system. Philadelphia: WB Saunders; 1986: 596–605.
[1075] Lang E, Spitzer A, Claus D, et al. Stimulation of sudomotor axon reflex mechanism by carbachol in healthy subjects and patients suffering from diabetic polyneuropathy. Acta Neurol Scand 1995; 91: 251–4.
[1076] Low PA, Zimmerman BR, Dyck PJ. Comparison of distal sympathetic with vagal function in diabetic neuropathy. Muscle Nerve 1986; 9: 592–6.
[1077] Schondorf R. The role of sympathetic skin responses in the assessment of autonomic function. In: Low PA, editor. Clinical autonomic disorders: evaluation and management. Boston: Little, Brown and Company, 1993: 231–41.
[1078] Davison MA, Koss MC. Brainstem loci for activation of electrodermal response in the cat. Am J Physiol 1975; 229: 930–4.
[1079] Sato A, Schmidt RF. Somatosympathetic reflexes: afferent fibers, central pathways, discharge characteristics. Physiol Rev 1973; 53: 916–47.
[1080] Knezevic W, Bajada S. Peripheral autonomic surface potential. A quantitative technique for recording sympathetic conduction in man. J Neurol Sci 1985; 67: 239–51.
[1081] Yokota T, Matsunaga T, Okiyama R, et al. Sympathetic skin response in patients with multiple sclerosis compared with patients with spinal cord transection and normal controls. Brain 1991; 114: 1381–94.
[1082] Soliven B, Maselli R, Jaspan J, et al. Sympathetic skin response in diabetic neuropathy. Muscle Nerve 1987; 10: 711–6.
[1083] Niakan E, Harati Y. Sympathetic skin response in diabetic peripheral neuropathy. Muscle Nerve 1988; 11: 261–4.
[1084] Maselli RA, Jaspan JB, Soliven BC, et al. Comparison of sympathetic skin response with quantitative sudomotor axon reflex test in diabetic neuropathy. Muscle Nerve 1989; 12: 420–3.
[1085] Schondorf R, Gendron D. Evaluation of sudomotor function in patients with peripheral neuropathy [abstract]. Neurology 1990; 40(Suppl 1): 386.
[1086] Shahani BT, Day TJ, Cros D, et al. RR interval variation and the sympathetic skin response in the assessment of autonomic function in peripheral neuropathy. Arch Neurol 1990; 47: 659–64.
[1087] Ravits JM, Baker M, Hallett M, et al. A comparative study of electrophysiologic tests of autonomic function in patients with primary autonomic failure [abstract]. Muscle Nerve 1986; 9: 657.
[1088] Gutrecht JA, Suarez GA, Denny BE. Sympathetic skin response in multiple sclerosis. J Neurol Sci 1993; 118: 88–91.

[1089] Smith SE, Smith SA, Brown PM, et al. Pupillary signs in diabetic autonomic neuropathy. Br Med J 1978; 2: 924–7.
[1090] Hreidarsson AB. Acute, reversible autonomic nervous system abnormalities in juvenile insulin-dependent diabetes. A pupillographic study. Diabetologia 1981; 20: 475–81.
[1091] Pfeifer MA, Weinberg CR, Cook DL, et al. Autonomic neural dysfunction in recently diagnosed diabetic subjects. Diabetes Care 1984; 7: 447–53.
[1092] Alexandridis E, Hain G. Frequency of flicker stimulus-dependent pupillary oscillation in diabetics. Fortschr Ophthalmol 1985; 82: 187–8.
[1093] Kuroda N, Taniguchi H, Baba S, Yamamoto M. The pupillary light reflex in borderline diabetics. J Int Med Res 1989; 17: 205–11.
[1094] Straub RH, Jeron A, Kerp L. The pupillary light reflex. 2. Prevalence of pupillary autonomic neuropathy in diabetics using age-dependent and age-independent pupillary parameters. Ophthalmologica 1992; 204: 143–8.
[1095] Schwingshandl J, Simpson JM, Donaghue K, et al. Pupillary abnormalities in type I diabetes occurring during adolescence. Comparisons with cardiovascular reflexes. Diabetes Care 1993; 16: 630–3.
[1096] Löwenstein O, Loewenfeld IE. The pupil. In: Davson H, editors. The eye. New York, N.Y.: Academic Press, 1970: 255–337.
[1097] Sigsbee B, Torkelson R, Kadis G, et al. Parasympathetic denervation of the iris in diabtes mellitus. J Neurol Neurosurg Psychiatry 1974; 37: 1031–5.
[1098] Alexandridis E. The pupil. New York, N.Y.: Springer, 1985.
[1099] Neil HAW, Smith SA. A simple clinical test of pupillary autonomic function. Correlation with cardiac autonomic function tests in diabetes. Neuroophthalmol 1989; 9: 237–42.
[1100] Cüppers C. Eine neue Methode zur stetigen Registrierung der konsensuellen Pupillenlichtreaktion. Klin Mon Augenheilkd 1951; 119: 411–7.
[1101] Ishikawa S, Naito M, Inaba K. A new videopupillography. Ophthalmologica 1970; 160: 248–59.
[1102] Straub RH, Arnolds BJ, Kerp L. Biometry with a video-genlock interface and a computer-based image-analyzing system: use as a TV-videopupillometer. Biomed Instrum Technol 1993; 27: 43–8.
[1103] Pfeifer MA, Cook D, Brodsky J, et al. Quantitative evaluation of sympathetic and parasympathetic control of iris function. Diabetes Care 1982; 5: 518–28.
[1104] Straub RH, Thies U, Kerp L. The pupillary light reflex. 1. Age-dependent and age-independent parameters in normal subjects. Ophthalmologica 1992; 204: 134–42.
[1105] Straub RH, Thies U, Jeron A, et al. Valid parameters for investigation of the pupillary light reflex in normal and diabetic subjects shown by factor analysis and partial correlation. Diabetologia 1994; 37: 414–9.
[1106] Hreidarsson AB. Pupil size in insulin-dependent diabetes. Relationship to duration, metabolic control, and log-term manifestations. Diabetes 1982; 31: 442–8.
[1107] Straub RH, Thies U, Jeron A, et al. Valid parameters for investigation of the pupillary light reflex in normal and diabetic subjects shown by factor analysis and partial correlation. Diabetologia 1994; 37: 414–9.
[1108] Straub RH, Zietz B, Palitzsch KD, Schölmerich J. Impact of disease duration on cardiovascular and pupillary autonomic nervous function in IDDM and NIDDM patients. Diabetes Care 1996; 19: 960–7.
[1109] Straub RH, Andus T, Lock G, et al. Cardiovascular and pupillary autonomic and somatosensory neuropathy in chronic diseases with autoimmune phenomena. A comparative study of patients with Crohn disease, ulcerative colitis, systemic lupus erythematosus, progressive systemic sclerosis and type I diabetes mellitus. Med Clin 1997; 92: 647–53.
[1110] Straub RH, Gluck T, Zeuner M, et al. Association of pupillary parasympathetic hyperreflexia and systemic inflammation in patients with systemic lupus erythematosus. Br J Rheumatol 1998; 37: 665–70.
[1111] Straub RH, Antoniou E, Zeuner M, et al. Association of autonomic nervous hyperreflexia and systemic inflammation in patients with Crohn's disease and ulcerative colitis. J Neuroimmunol 1997; 80: 149–57.
[1112] The St. Thomas's Diabetic Study Group. Failure of improved glycaemic control to reverse diabetic autonomic neuropathy. Diabet Med 1986; 4: 330–4.
[1113] Ziegler D, Cicmir I, Mayer P, et al. The natural course of peripheral and autonomic neural function during the first two years after diagnosis of type 1 diabetes. Klin Wochenschr 1988; 66: 1085–92.
[1114] Karachaliou F, Karavanaki K, Greenwood R, Baum JD. Consistency of pupillary abnormality in children and adolescents with diabetes. Diabet Med 1997; 14: 849–53.
[1115] Pena MM, Donaghue KC, Fung AT, et al. The prospective assessment of autonomic nerve function by pupillometry in adolescents with type 1 diabetes mellitus. Diabet Med 1995; 12: 868–73.
[1116] Namba K, Utsumi T, Kitazawa A. Diabetes mellitus and pupil (a preliminary report). Nippon Ganka Gakkai Zasshi 1980; 84: 398–405.
[1117] Smith SA, Smith SE. Reduced pupillary light reflexes in diabetic autonomic neuropathy. Diabetologia 1983; 24: 330–2.
[1118] Clark CV. Ocular autonomic nerve function in proliferative diabetic retinopathy. Eye 1988; 2: 96–101.
[1119] Vos A de, Marcus JT, Reulen JP, et al. The pupillary light reflex in diabetes mellitus: evaluation of a newly developed infrared light reflection method. Diabetes Res 1989; 10: 191–5.
[1120] Hilsted J, Galbo H, Christensen NJ. Impaired cardiovascular responses to graded exercise in diabetic autonomic neuropathy. Diabetes 1979; 28: 313–9.
[1121] Kahn JK, Zola B, Juni JE, Vinik AI. Decreased exercise heart rate and blood pressure responses in diabetic subjects with cardiac autonomic neuropathy. Diabetes Care 1986; 9: 389–94.
[1122] Bottini P, Tantucci C, Scionti L, et al. Cardiovascular response to exercise in diabetic patients: influence of autonomic neuropathy of different severity. Diabetologia 1995; 38: 244–50.
[1123] Bergström B, Manhem P, Bramnert M, et al. Impaired responses of plasma catecholamines to exercise in diabetic patients with abnormal heart rate reactions to tilt. Clin Phys 1989; 9: 259–67.
[1124] Nugent AM, Steele IC, Al-Modaris F, et al. Exercise responses in patients with IDDM. Diabetes Care 1997; 20: 1814–21.
[1125] Kremser CB, Levitt NS, Borow KM, et al. Oxygen uptake kinetics during exercise in diabetic neuropathy. J Appl Physiol 1988; 65: 2665–71.
[1126] Tantucci C, Bottini P, Dottorini ML, et al. Ventilatory response to exercise in diabetic subjects with autonomic neuropathy. J Appl Physiol 1996; 81: 1978–86.
[1127] Estacio RO, Regensteiner JG, Wolfel EE, et al. The association between diabetic complications and exercise capacity in NIDDM patients. Diabetes Care 1998; 21: 291–5.
[1128] Radice M, Rocca A, Bedon E, et al. Abnormal response to exercise in middle-aged NIDDM patients with and without autonomic neuropathy. Diabet Med 1996; 13(3): 259–65.
[1129] Hilsted J, Galbo H, Christensen NJ, et al. Haemodynamic changes during graded exercise in patients with diabetic autonomic neuropathy. Diabetologia 1982; 22: 318–23.
[1130] Donckier JE, De Coster PM, Buysschaert M, et al. Exercise and posture-related changes of atrial natriuretic factor and cardiac function in diabetes. Diabetes Care 1989; 12: 475–80.
[1131] Hilsted J, Low PA. Diabetic autonomic neuropathy. In: Low PA, editor. Clinical autonomic disorders. 2nd edition. Philadelphia, Pa.: Lippincott-Raven, 1997: 487–509.
[1132] Low PA, Walsh JC, Huang CY, McLeod JC. The sympathetic nervous system in diabetic neuropathy. Brain 1975; 98: 341–56.
[1133] Scognamiglio R, Fasoli G, Ferri M, et al. Myocardial dysfunction and abnormal left ventricular exercise response in autonomic diabetic patients. Clin Cardiol 1995; 18: 276–82.
[1134] Raev DC. Left ventricular function and specific diabetic complications in other target organs in young insulin-dependent diabetics: an echocardiographic study. Heart Vessels 1994; 9: 121–8.

[1135] Rowell LB, Detry J-MR, Blackmon Jr, Wyss C. Importance of the splanchnic vascular bed in human blood pressure regulation. J Appl Physiol 1972; 32: 213–20.

[1136] Galbo H. Hormonal and metabolic adaptation to exercise. Stuttgart, Germany: Thieme Verlag, 1983.

[1137] Hilsted J, Galbo H, Christensen NJ. Impaired responses of catecholamines, growth hormone and cortisol to graded exercise in diabetic autonomic neuropathy. Diabetes 1980; 29: 257–62.

[1138] Bottini P, Boschetti E, Pampanelli S, et al. Contribution of autonomic neuropathy to reduced plasma adrenaline responses to hypoglycemia in IDDM: evidence for a nonselective defect. Diabetes 1997; 46(5): 814–23.

[1139] Smith GD, Watson LP, Mathias CJ. Differing haemodynamic and catecholamine responses to exercise in three groups with peripheral autonomic dysfunction: insulin-dependent diabetes mellitus, familial amyloid polyneuropathy and pure autonomic failure. J Auton Nerv Syst 1998; 10: 125–34.

[1140] Endo A, Kinugawa T, Ogino K, et al. Cardiac and plasma catecholamine responses to exercise in patients with type 2 diabetes: prognostic implications for cardiac-cerebrovascular events. Am J Med Sci 2000; 320: 24–30.

[1141] Veves A, Saouaf R, Donaghue VM, et al. Aerobic exercise capacity remains normal despite impaired endothelial function in the micro- and macrocirculation of physically active IDDM patients. Diabetes 1997; 46: 1846–52.

[1142] Smit AAJ, Halliwill JR, Low PA, Wieling W. Topical review. Pathophysiological basis of orthostatic hypotension in autonomic failure. Physiol 1999; 519: 1–10.

[1143] Cryer PE, Silverberg AB, Santiago JV, Shah SD. Plasma catecholamines in diabetes: the syndromes of hypoadrenergic and hyperadrenergic postural hypotension. Am J Med 1978; 64: 407–16.

[1144] Hilsted J, Parving H-H, Christensen NJ, et al. Hemodynamics in diabetic orthostatic hypotension. J Clin Invest 1981; 68: 1427–34.

[1145] Laederach-Hofmann K, Weidmann P, Ferrari P. Hypovolemia contributes to the pathogenesis of orthostatic hypotension in patients with diabetes mellitus. Am J Med 1999; 106: 50–8.

[1146] Nakano S, Ishii T, Kitazawa M, et al. Effects of posture on the plasma hormonal and renal water-electrolyte excretory responses to acute water loading in diabetic subjects with hypoadrenergic orthostatic hypotension. J Diabetes Complications 1996; 10: 274–9.

[1147] Banner NR, Meuring William TDM, Patel N, et al. Altered cardiovascular and neurohumoral responses to head-up tilt after heart-lung transplantation. Circulation 1990; 82: 863–71.

[1148] Low PA, Opfer-Gehrking TL, Textor SC, et al. Comparison of the postural tachycardia syndrome (POTS) with orthostatic hypotension due to autonomic failure. J Auton Nerv Syst 1994; 50: 181–8.

[1149] Purewal TS, Goss DE, Zanone MM, et al. The splanchnic circulation and postural hypotension in diabetic autonomic neuropathy. Diabetic Med 1995; 12: 513–22.

[1150] Dejgaard A, Hilsted J, Christensen NJ. Noradrenaline and isoproterenol kinetics in diabetic patients with and without autonomic neuropathy. Diabetologia 1986; 29: 773–7.

[1151] Dejgaard A. Pathophysiology and treatment of diabetic neuropathy. Diabetic Med 1998; 15: 97–112.

[1152] The effect of intensive diabetes therapy on measures of autonomic nervous system function in the Diabetes Control and Complications Trial. (DCCT). Diabetologia 1998; 41: 416–23.

[1153] Kennedy FP, Bolli GB, Go VL, et al. The significance of impaired pancreatic polypeptide and epinephrine responses to hypoglycemia in patients with insulin-dependent diabetes mellitus. J Clin Endocrinol Metab 1987; 64: 602–8.

[1154] Maher TD, Tanenberg RJ, Greenberg BZ, et al. Lack of glucagon response to hypoglycemia in diabetic autonomic neuropathy. Diabetes 1977; 26: 196–200.

[1155] Taborsky GJ Jr, Ahren B, Havel PJ. Autonomic mediation of glucagon secretion during hypoglycemia: implications for impaired alpha-cell responses in type 1 diabetes. Diabetes 1998; 47: 995–1005.

[1156] Cryer PE. Iatrogenic hypoglycemia as a cause of hypoglycemia-associated autonomic failure in IDDM. A vicious circle. Diabetes 1992; 41: 255–60.

[1157] Fanelli CG, Epifano L, Rambotti AM, et al. Meticulous prevention of hypoglycemia normalizes the glycemic thresholds and magnitude of most of neuroendocrine responses to, symptoms of, and cognitive function during hypoglycemia in intensively treated patients with short-term IDDM. Diabetes 1993; 42: 1683–9.

[1158] Amiel S, Archibald H, Chusney G, et al. Ketone infusion lowers hormonal responses to hypoglycaemia: evidence for acute cerebral utilization of a non-glucose fuel. Clin Sci 1991; 81: 189–94.

[1159] Veneman T, Mitrakou A, Mokan M, et al. Effects of hyperketonemia and hyperlactacidemia on symptoms, cognitive dysfunction and counterregulatory hormone responses during hypoglycemia in normal humans. Diabetes 1994; 43: 1311–7.

[1160] Maran A, Cranston I, Lomas J, et al. Protection by lactate of cerebral function during hypoglycaemia. Lancet 1994; 343: 16–20.

[1161] Fanelli C, Di Vincenzo A, Modarelli F, et al. Post-hypoglycaemic hyperketonaemia does not contribute to brain metabolism during insulin-induced neuroglycopenia in humans. Diabetologia 1993; 36: 1191–7.

[1162] Fanelli CG, Pampanelli S, Porcellati F, et al. Effects of rate of fall of blood glucose on responses of counterregulatory hormones, symptoms and cognitive functions to hypoglycemia in type 1 diabetes mellitus in the postprandial state. Diabetologia 2002 in press.

[1163] Maran A, Crepaldi C, Trupiani S, et al. Brain function rescue effect of lactate following hypoglycaemia is not an adaptation process in both normal and type I diabetic subjects. Diabetologia 2000; 43: 733–41.

[1164] Bolli GB, Fanelli C. Physiology of glucose counterregulation to hypoglycemia. In: Service FJ, editor. Hypoglycemic disorders. Philadelphia, Pa.: W.B. Saunders, 1999: 467–93.

[1165] Gerich J, Mokan M, Veneman T, et al. Hypoglycemia unawareness. Endocr Rev 1991; 12: 356–71.

[1166] Mitrakou A, Ryan C, Veneman T, et al. Hierarchy of glycemic thresholds for counterregulatory hormone secretion, symptoms, and cerebral dysfunction. Am J Physiol 1991; 260: E67–74.

[1167] Bolli GB, Dimitriadis GD, Pehling GB, et al. Abnormal glucose counterregulation after subcutaneous insulin in insulin-dependent diabetes mellitus. N Engl J Med 1984; 310: 1706–11.

[1168] Bolli GB, De Feo P, Compagnucci P, et al. Abnormal glucose counterregulation in insulin-dependent diabetes mellitus. Interaction of anti-insulin antibodies and impaired glucagon and epinephrine secretion. Diabetes 1983; 32: 134–41.

[1169] Bolli GB. From physiology of glucose counterregulation to prevention of hypoglycaemia in type 1 diabetes mellitus. Diabetes Nutr Metab 1990; 3: 333–49.

[1170] Gerich J, Davis J, Lorenzi M, et al. Hormonal mechanisms of recovery from insulin-induced hypoglycemia in man. Am J Physiol 1979; 236: E380–85.

[1171] Fanelli C, Pampanelli S, Lalli C, et al. Long-term intensive therapy of IDDM patients with clinically overt autonomic neuropathy: effects on hypoglycemia unwareness and counterregulation. Diabetes 1997; 46: 1172–81.

[1172] Mitrakou A, Fanelli C, Veneman T, et al. Reversibility of unawareness of hypoglycemia in patients with insulinoma. N Engl J Med 1993; 329: 834–39.

[1173] Amiel S, Sherwin R, Simonson D, Tamborlane W. Effect of intensive insulin therapy on glycemic thresholds for counterregulatory hormone release. Diabetes 1988; 37: 901–07.

[1174] Schwartz NS, Clutter WE, Shah SD, Cryer PE. Glycemic thresholds for activation of glucose counterregulatory systems are higher than the threshold for symptoms. J Clin Invest 1987; 79: 777–81.

[1175] Fanelli C, Pampanelli S, Epifano L, et al. Long-term recovery from unawareness, deficient counterregulation and lack of cognitive dysfunction during hypoglycaemia following institution of a rational, intensive insulin therapy in IDDM. Diabetologia 1994; 37: 1265–76.

[1176] Fanelli CG, Pampanelli S, Porcellati F, Bolli GB. Shift of glycaemic thresholds for cognitive function in hypoglycaemia unawareness in humans. Diabetologia 1998; 41: 720–23.
[1177] Cranston I, Lomas J, Maran A, et al. Restoration of hypoglycaemia awareness in patients with long duration insulin-dependent diabetes. Lancet 1994; 344: 283–87.
[1178] Dagogo-Jack S, Rattarasarn C, Cryer PE. Reversal of hypoglycaemia unawareness, but not defective glucose counterregulation, in IDDM. Diabetes 1994; 43: 1426–14.
[1179] Heller S, Cryer P. Reduced neuroendocrine and symptomatic responses to subsequent hypoglycemia after one episode of hypoglycemia in nondiabetic humans. Diabetes 1991; 40: 223–26.
[1180] Veneman T, Mitrakou A, Mokan M, et al. Induction of hypoglycemia unawareness by asymptomatic nocturnal hypoglycemia. Diabetes 1993; 42: 1233–37.
[1181] Fanelli CG, Paramore DS, Hershey T, et al. Impact of nocturnal hypoglycemia on hypoglycemic cognitive dysfunction in type 1 diabetes. Diabetes 1998; 47: 1920–27.
[1182] Dagogo-Jack SE, Cryer PE. Hypoglycemia-associated autonomic failure in insulin-dependent diabetes mellitus. Recent antecedent hypoglycemia reduces autonomic responses to, symptoms of, and defenses against subsequent hypoglycemia. J Clin Invest 1993; 91: 819–28.
[1183] Ovalle F, Fanelli CG, Paramore DS, et al. Brief twice-weekly episodes of hypoglycemia reduce detection of clinical hypoglycemia in type 1 diabetes mellitus. Diabetes 1998; 47: 1472–79.
[1184] Bolli GB. How to ameliorate the problem of hypoglycemia in intensive as well as non-intensive treatment of type 1 diabetes mellitus. Diabetes Care 1999; 22(Suppl 2): B43–52.
[1185] McCall A, Fixman L, Fleming N, et al. Chronic hypoglycemia increases brain glucose transport. Am J Physiol 1986; 251: E442–47.
[1186] McCall AL, Millington WR, Wurtman RJ. Metabolic fuel and aminoacid transport into the brain in experimental diabetes mellitus. Proc Natl Acad Sci USA 1982; 79: 5406–10.
[1187] Boyle PJ, Nagy RJ, O'Connor AM, et al. Adaptation in brain glucose uptake following recurrent hypoglycemia. Proc Natl Acad Sci USA 1994; 91: 9352–56.
[1188] Boyle P, Kempers S, O'Connor AM, Nagy RJ. Brain glucose uptake and hypoglycemia unawareness in patients with insulin-dependent diabetes mellitus. N Engl J Med 1995; 333: 1726–31.
[1189] Fanelli CG, Dence CS, Markham J, et al. Blood-to-brain glucose transport and cerebral glucose metabolism are not reduced in poorly controlled type 1 diabetes. Diabetes 1998; 47: 1444–14.
[1190] Segel S, Fanelli C, Dence C, et al. Blood-to-brain glucose transport is not increased following hypoglycemia. Diabetes 2000; 49(Suppl 1): A65.
[1191] Davis SN, Shavers C, Costa F, Mosqueda-Garcia R. Role of cortisol in the pathogenesis of deficient counterregulation after antecedent hypoglycemia in normal humans. J Clin Invest 1996; 98: 680–91.
[1192] De Kloet E, Ratka A, Reul J, et al. Corticosteroid receptor types in brain regulation and putative function. Ann NY Acad Sci 1987; 512: 351–61.
[1193] Pampanelli S, Lalli C, Sindaco P Del, et al. Effect of recent, antecedent hypoglycaemia and response of cortisol per se, on responses to susequent hypoglycaemia in humans. Diabetologia 1997; 99: A27.
[1194] Bolli GB, Di Marchi RD, Park GD, Pramming S, Koivisto VA. Insulin analogues and their potential in the management of diabetes mellitus. Diabetologia 1999; 42: 1151–67.
[1195] Kendall DM, Rooney DP, Smets YFC, Salazar Bolding L, Robertson RP. Pancreas transplantation restores epinephrine response and symptom recognition during hypoglycemia in patients with long-standing type I diabetes and autonomic neuropathy. Diabetes 1997; 46: 249–57.
[1196] Fritsche A, Stumvoll M, Haring HU, Gerich JE. Reversal of hypoglycemia unawareness in a long-term type 1 diabetic patient by improvement of beta-adrenergic sensitivity after prevention of hypoglycemia. J Clin Endocrinol Metab 2000; 85(2): 523–25.
[1197] Porcellati F, Fanelli C, Bottini P, et al. Mechanisms of arterial hypotension after therapeutic dose of subcutaneous insulin in diabetic subjects with and without autonomic neuropathy. Diabetes 1993; 42: 1055–64.
[1198] Bottini P, Boschetti E, Pampanelli S, et al. Contribution of autonomic neuropathy to reduced plasma adrenaline responses to hypoglycemia in IDDM: evidence for a non-selective defect. Diabetes 1997; 46: 814–23.
[1199] Bolli GB, Owens DR. Insulin glargine. Lancet 2000; 356: 443–5.
[1200] Rattner R, Hirsch IB, Neifing JL, et al. For the USA Study group of Insulin glargine in type 1 diabetes: less hypoglycemia with insulin glargine in intensive treatment for type 1 diabetes. Diabetes Care 2000; 23: 639–43.
[1201] Pampanelli S, Fanelli C, Lalli C, et al. Long-term intensive insulin therapy in IDDM: effects of HbA1c, risk for severe and mild hypoglycaemia, status of counterregulation and awareness of hypoglycaemia. Diabetologia 1996; 39: 677–86.
[1202] Mayfield JA, Reiber GE, Sanders LJ, et al. Preventive foot care in people with diabetes. Diabetes Care 1998; 21: 2161–77.
[1203] Consensus Development on Diabetic Foot Wound Care. Diabetes Care 1999; 22: 1354–60.
[1204] Boulton AJM. Why bother educating the multidisciplinary team and the patient: the example of prevention of lower extremity amputation in diabetes. Patient Educ Couns 1995; 26: 183–8.
[1205] Ramsey SD, Newton K, Blough D, et al. Incidence, outcomes and cost of foot ulcers in patients with diabetes. Diabetes Care 1999; 22: 382–7.
[1206] Boyko EJ, Ahroni JH, Smith DG, Davignon D. Increased mortality associated with diabetic foot ulcer. Diabet Med 1996; 13: 967–72.
[1207] Shaw JE, Boulton AJM. Charcot foot. Foot 1995; 5: 65–70.
[1208] Connor H. Diabetic foot disease—where is the evidence? Diabet Med 1999; 16: 799–800.
[1209] Boulton AJM, Vileikyte L. Diabetic foot problems and their management around the world. In: Bowker JH, Pfeifer MA, editors. Levin and O'Neal's 'The diabetic foot.' 6th edition. St Louis: CV Mosby, 2001: 261–270.
[1210] Young MJ, Veves A, Breddy JL, Boulton AJM. The prediction of diabetic foot ulceration using vibration perception thresholds. Diabetes Care 1994; 17: 557–61.
[1211] Abbott CA, Vileikyte L, Williamson SH, et al. Multicenter study of the incidence and predictive factors for diabetic foot ulceration. Diabetes Care 1998; 21: 1071–5.
[1212] Holzer SE, Camerato A, Martens L, et al. Costs and duration of care for lower extremity ulcers in patients with diabetes. Clin Ther 1998; 20: 169–81.
[1213] Eneroth M, Apelqvist J, Troeng T, Persson BM. Operations, total hospital stay and costs of critical limb ischaemia: a population-based, longitudinal outcome study of 321 patients. Acta Orthop Scand 1996; 67: 459–65.
[1214] Jude EB, Boulton AJM. End-stage complications of diabetic neuropathy. Diabetes Rev 1999; 7: 395–410.
[1215] Vileikyte L. Psychological aspects of diabetic peripheral neuropathy. Diabetes Rev 1999; 7: 387–96.
[1216] Boulton AJM, Gries FA, Jervell J. Guidelines for the diagnosis and outpatient management of diabetic peripheral neuropathy. Diabet Med 1998; 15: 508–14.
[1217] Mason J, O'Keeffe C, McIntosh A, et al. A systematic review of foot ulcer prevention in patients with type 2 diabetes. 1: Prevention. Diabet Med 1999; 16: 801–12.
[1218] Litzelman DK, Marriott DJ, Vinicor F. Independent physiological predictors of foot lesion in patients with NIDDM. Diabetes Care 1997; 20: 1273–8.
[1219] Reiber GE, Vileikyte L, Boyko EJ, et al. Causal pathways for incident lower-extremity ulcers in patients with diabetes from two settings. Diabetes Care 1999; 22: 157–62.
[1220] Katoulis EC, Ebdon-Parry M, Hollis S, et al. Postural instability in diabetic neuropathic patients at risk of foot ulceration. Diabet Med 1997; 14: 296–300.
[1221] Murray HJ, Young MJ, Boulton AJM. The relationship between callus formation, high foot pressures and neuropathy in diabetic foot ulceration. Diabet Med 1996; 13: 979–82.

[1222] Frykberg RG, Lavery LA, Pham H, et al. Role of neuropathy and high foot pressures in diabetic foot ulceration. Diabetes Care 1998; 21: 1714–9.
[1222a] Boulton AJM. The pathway to ulceration: aetiopathogenesis. In: Boulton AJM, Connor H, Cavanagh PR, editors. The foot in diabetes. 3rd edition. Chichester: John Wiley & Sons, 2000: 19–31.
[1223] International working group on the Diabetic Foot. International Consensus on the Diabetic Foot. Amsterdam; 1999.
[1223a] Abbott CA, Carrington AL, Ashe H, et al. The North-West Diabetes Foot Care Study: incidence of, and risk factors for, new diabetic foot ulceration in a community-based patient cohort. Diabetic Med 2002; 19: 377–84.
[1224] Young MJ, Boulton AJM, MacLeod AF, et al. A multicentre study of the prevalence of diabetic peripheral neuropathy in the UK hospital clinic population. Diabetologia 1993; 36: 150–4.
[1225] McCabe CJ, Stevenson RC, Dolan AM. Evaluation of a diabetic foot screening and prevention programme. Diabet Med 1998; 15: 80–4.
[1226] Uccioli L, Faglia E, Montocine G, et al. Manufactured shoes in the prevention of diabetic foot ulcers. Diabetes Care 1995; 18: 1376–8.
[1227] Colagiuri S, Marsden LL, Naidu V, Taylor L. The use of orthotic devices to arrest plantar callus in people with diabetes. Diabetes Res Clin Pract 1995; 28: 29–36.
[1228] Van Schie CHM, Whalley A, Vileikyte L, et al. The use of injected liquid silicone in the diabetic neuropathic foot: a randomised controlled trial. Diabetes Care 2000; 23: 634–8.
[1229] Frykberg RG. Charcot Foot: an update on pathogenesis and management. In: Boulton AJM, Connor H, Cavanagh PR, editors. The foot in diabetes. 3rd ed. Chichester: John Wiley, 2000: 235-260.
[1230] Armstrong DG, Todd WF, Lavery LA, et al. The natural history of acute Charcot's arthropathy in a diabetic foot specialty clinic. Diabet Med 1997; 14: 357–63.
[1231] Young MJ. Classification of ulcers and its relevance to management. In: Boulton AJM, Connor H, Cavanagh PR, editors. The foot in diabetes. 3rd ed. Chichester: John Wiley, 2000: 61–72.
[1232] Armstrong DG, Lavery LA, Harkless LB. Validation of a diabetic wound classification system. Diabet Med 1998; 21: 855–9.
[1233] Witte MB, Barbul A. General principles of wound healing. Surg Clin North Amer 1997; 77: 509–27.
[1234] Hehenberger K, Heilbron JD, Brismar K, Hansson A. Inhibited proliferation of fibroblasts derived from chronic diabetic wounds and normal dermal fibroblasts treated with high glucose in associated with increased formation of 1-lactate. Wound Repair Regen 1998; 6: 135–41.
[1235] Blakytny R, Jude EB, Gibson JM, et al. Lack of insulin-like growth factor 1 in basal keratinocyte layer of diabetic skin and diabetic foot ulcers. J Pathol 2000; 190: 589–94.
[1236] Ferguson MWJ, Herrick SE, Spencer MJ, et al. The histology of diabetic foot ulcers. Diabet Med 1996; 13(Suppl 1): 530–5.
[1237] Mason J, O'Keeffe CO, Hutchinson A, et al. A systematic review of foot ulcers in patients with type 2 diabetes. II: Treatment. Diabet Med 1999; 16: 889–909.
[1238] Caputo GM. The rational use of antimicrobial agents in diabetic foot infections. In: Boulton AJM, Connor H, Cavanagh PR, editors. The foot in diabetes. 3rd ed. Chichester: John Wiley, 2000: 143–52.
[1239] Chantelau EA, Tanudjaja T, Altenhofer F, et al. Antibiotic treatment for uncomplicated neuropathic forefoot ulcers in diabetes: a controlled trial. Diabet Med 1996; 13: 156–9.
[1240] Lipsky BA. Evidence-based antibiotic therapy of diabetic foot infections. FEMS Immunol Med Microbiol 1999; 26: 267–76.
[1241] Tentolouris N, Jude EB, Smirnoff I, et al. Methicillin resistant Staphylococcus aureus: an increasing problem in a diabetic foot clinic. Diabet Med 1999; 16: 767–71.
[1242] Wieman TJ, Smiell JM, Yachin S. Efficacy and safety of a topical gel formulation of recombinant human platelet-derived growth factor-BB (Becaplermin) in patients with chronic neuropathic diabetic foot ulcers. Diabetes Care 1998; 21: 822–7.
[1243] Thomas S. Larval Therapy. In: Boulton AJM, Connor H, Cavanagh PR, editors. The Foot in Diabetes. 3rd ed. Chichester, UK: J Wiley, 2000: 185–92.
[1244] Gough A, Clapperton M, Rolando N, et al. Randomised placebo-controlled trial of granulocyte-colony stimulating factor in diabetic foot infection. Lancet 1997; 350: 855–9.
[1245] Pittet D, Wyssa B, Herter-Clavel C, et al. Outcome of diabetic foot infections treated conservatively: a retrospective cohort study with long-term follow-up. Arch Int Med 1999; 159: 851–6.
[1246] Adler A, Boyko EJ, Ahroni JH, Smith DG. Lower extremity amputation in diabetes: the independent effects of peripheral vascular disease, sensory neuropathy and foot ulcers. Diabetes Care 1999; 22: 1029–38.
[1247] Krasner DL, Sibbald RG. Nursing management of chronic wounds. Nurs Clin North Am 1999; 34: 933–53.
[1248] Cameron NE, Cotter MA. Metabolic and vascular factors in the pathogenesis of diabetic neuropathy. Diabetes 1997; 46: S31–37.
[1249] Yasaki S, Jakobsen J, Dyck PJ. Hypoglycaemic polyneuropathy. In: Dyck PJ, Thomas PK, editors. Diabetic neuropathy. Philadelphia: W.B. Saunders Co, 1999: 445–55.
[1250] Abood L. Neuronal metabolism. In: Vinken P, Bruyn G, editors. Handbook of clinical neurology. Amsterdam: North Holland Publishing Co, 1970: 1821.
[1251] Yasaki S, Dyck P. Duration and severity of hypoglycaemia needed to induce neuropathy. Brain Res 1991; 531: 8–15.
[1252] Sidenius P, Jakobsen J. Peripheral neuropathy in rats induced by insulin treatment. Diabetes 1983; 32: 383–6.
[1253] Sidenius P, Jakobsen J. Anterograde fast component of axonal transport during insulin induced hypoglycaemia in nondiabetic and diabetic rats. Diabetes 1987; 36: 853–8.
[1254] Mohseni S, Lillesaar C, Theodorsson E, Hildebrand C. Hypoglycaemic neuropathy: occurrence of axon terminals in plantar skin and plantar muscle of diabetic BB/Wor rats treated with insulin implants. Acta Neuropathol 2000; 99: 257–62.
[1255] Tomlinson DR, James P. Impaired orthograde axonal transport in acute hypoglycaemia, an effect mediated via hypothermia. Med Biol 1984; 64: 34–7.
[1256] Kedes L, Field J. Hypothermia: a clue to hypoglycaemia. N Engl J Med 1964; 271: 785.
[1257] Tesfaye S, Malik R, Ward JD. Vascular factors in diabetic neuropathy. Diabetologia 1994; 37: 847–54.
[1258] Ibrahim S, Harris N, Radatz M, et al. A new minimally invasive technique to show nerve ischaemia in diabetic neuropathy. Diabetologia 1999; 42: 737–42.
[1259] Nukada H, Dyck PJ. Microsphere embolization of nerve capillaries and fiber degeneration. Am J Pathol 1984; 115: 275–87.
[1260] McManis P, Low PA. Factors affecting the relative viability of centrifascicular and subperineurial axons in acute peripheral nerve ischaemia. Exp Neurol 1988; 99: 84–95.
[1261] Yasaki S, Dyck P. Spatial distribution of fiber degeneration in hypoglycaemic neuropathy in rats. J Neuropathol Exp Neurol 1991; 50: 681–92.
[1262] Giannini C, Dyck PJ. Pathologic alterations in human diabetic polyneuropathy. In: Dyck PJ, Thomas PK, editors. Diabetic neuropathy. Philadelphia: W.B. Saunders Co, 1999: 279–95.
[1263] Jaspan J, Wollman R, Bernstein L. Hypoglycaemia peripheral neuropathy in association with insulinoma: implication of glucopenia rather than hyperinsulinaemia. Medicine 1982; 61: 33.
[1264] Akanuma T. Effect of acute hypoglycaemia on peripheral nerve blood flow in rats. St Marianna Med 1993; 21: 623.
[1265] Hata A. Effect of nitric acid on sciatic nerve blood flow in acute hypoglycaemia. St Marianna Med 1996; 24: 370.
[1266] Zochodne DW, Low PA. Adrenergic control of nerve blood flow. Exp Neurol 1990; 109: 300–7.
[1267] Polderman K, Stehouwer C, Kamp G van, Gooran L. Effects of insulin infusion on endothelium-derived vasoactive substances. Diabetologia 1996; 39: 1284–92.
[1268] Kihara M, Zollman P, Smithson I, et al. Hypoxic effects of exogenous insulin on normal and diabetic peripheral nerve. Am J Physiol 1994; 266: E980–985.

[1269] Steinberg H, Brechtel G, Johnson A, et al. Insulin-mediated skeletal muscle vasodilation is nitric oxide dependent. A novel action of insulin to increase nitric oxide production. J Clin Invest 1994; 94: 1172–9.
[1270] Stevens E, Carrington AL, Tomlinson DR. Nerve ischaemia in diabetic rats: time-course of development, effects of insulin treatment plus comparison of streptozotocin and BB models. Diabetologia 1994; 37: 43–8.
[1271] Danta G. Hypoglycaemic peripheral neuropathy. Arch Neurol 1969; 21: 121–32.
[1272] Jayasinghe K, Nimalasuriya A, Dharmadasa K. A case of insulinoma with peripheral neuropathy. Postgrad Med J 1983; 59: 189–90.
[1273] Daggett P, Naberro J. Neurological aspects of insulinoma neuritis. Postgrad Med J 1984; 60: 577–81.
[1274] Conri C, Ducloux G, Lagueny A, et al. Polyneuropathy in type 1 multiple endocrine syndrome. Presse Med 1990; 19: 247–50.
[1275] Tintore M, Montalban J, Cervera C, et al. Peripheral neuropathy in association with insulinoma: clinical features and neuropathology of a new case [letter]. J Neurol Neurosurg Psychiatry 1994; 57: 1009–10.
[1276] Stern K, Dancey T, McNaughton F. Sensory disturbances following insulin treatment of psychoses. J Ment Nerv Dis 1942; 95: 183.
[1277] Ziegler D. Minor neurologic signs and symptoms following insulin coma therapy. J Ment Nerv Dis 1954; 120: 75.
[1278] Control D, Trial C. Effect of intensive diabetes treatment on nerve conduction in the Diabetes Control and Complications Trial. Ann Neurol 1995; 38: 869–80.
[1279] Lins P-E, Adamson U. Neurological manifestations of hypoglycaemia. In: Frier B, Fisher CM, editors. Hypoglycaemia and diabetes: clinical and physiological aspects. London: Edward Arnold, 1993: 347–54.
[1280] Caravati CM. Insulin neuritis: a case report. Va Med Mon 1933; 59: 745–6.
[1281] Jordan W. Neuritic manifestations in diabetic mellitus. Arch Intern Med 1936; 57: 307.
[1282] Rundles R. Diabetic neuropathy. General review with reports of 125 cases. Medicine 1945; 24: 111.
[1283] Rudy A, Epstein S. Review of 100 cases of "diabetic neuropathy" followed from 1 to 10 years. J Clin Endocrinol Metab 1945; 5: 92–8.
[1284] Martin M. Diabetic neuropathy: A clinical review of 150 cases. Brain 1953; 76: 594.
[1285] Ellenberg M. Diabetic neuropathy precipitating after institution of diabetic control. Am J Med Sci 1958; 236: 466–71.
[1286] Krentz A. Acute symptomatic diabetic neuropathy associated with normalisation of haemoglobin A1. J R Soc Med 1989; 82: 157–63.
[1287] Llewelyn JG, Thomas PK, Fonseta V, et al. Acute painful neuropathy precipitated by strict glycaemic control. Acta Neuropathol (Berl) 1986; 72: 157–63.
[1288] Tesfaye S, Malik R, Harris ND, et al. Arterio-venous shunting and proliferating new vessels in acute painful neuropathy of rapid glycaemic control (insulin neuritis). Diabetologia 1996; 39: 329–35.
[1289] Watkins PJ, Edmonds ME. Clinical features of diabetic neuropathy. In: Pickup J, Williams G, editors. Textbook of diabetes. Oxford: Blackwell, 1997: 50.1–50.20.
[1290] Boulton AJM, Armstrong WD, Scarpello JHB, Ward JD. The natural history of painful diabetic neuropathy: a four year study. Postgrad Med J 1983; 59: 556–9.
[1291] Ward JD, Barnes CG, Fisher DJ, Jessop JD. Improvement in nerve conduction following treatment in newly diagnosed diabetics. Lancet 1971; i: 428–31.
[1292] UKPDS Group. Intensive blood glucose control with sulphonylureas or insulin compared with conventional treatment and risk of complication in patients with type 2 diabetes (UKPDS 33). Lancet 1998; 352: 837–53.
[1293] Ellenberg M. Diabetic neuropathic cachexia. Diabetes 1974; 23: 418–23.
[1294] Archer AG, Watkins PJ, Thomas PK, et al. The natural history of acute painful neuropathy in diabetes mellitus. J Neurol Neurosurg Psychiatry 1983; 46: 491–9.
[1295] Boulton AJM. Current and emerging treatments for the diabetic neuropathies. Diabetes Rev 1999; 7: 379–86.
[1296] Tesfaye S, Harris ND, Jakubowski J, et al. Impaired blood flow and arterio-venous shunting in human diabetic neuropathy: a novel technique of nerve photography and fluorescein angiography. Diabetologia 1993; 36: 1266–74.
[1297] Eaton SEM, Ibrahim S, Harris ND, et al. Can differences in sural nerve haemodynamics explain the painful symptoms of neuropathy? Diabetes 2000; 49(1): A163.
[1298] Chantelau E, Kohner E. Why do some cases of retinopathy worsen when diabetic control improves. London: BMJ Publishing, 1997.
[1299] Paques M, Massin P, Gaudric A. Growth factors and diabetic retinopathy. Diabetes Metab 1997; 23: 125–30.
[1300] Antonetti D, Barber A, Hollinger L, et al. Vascular endothelial growth factor induces rapid phosphorylation of tight junction proteins occludin and zonula occluden 1. A potential mechanism for vascular permeability in diabetic retinopathy and tumors. J Biol Sci 1999; 274: 23463-7.
[1301] Hyer S, Sharp P, Burrin J, Kohner E. Progression of diabetic retinopathy and changes in serum insulin-like growth factor 1 (IGF-1) during continuous subcutaneous insulin infusion. Horm Metab Res 1989; 21: 18–22.
[1302] Scott RS, Brown LJ, Clifford P. Use of health services in diabetic persons. II Hospital admissions. Diabetes Care 1985; 8: 43–7.
[1303] Charalambous C, Schofield I, Malik RA. Acute diabetic emergencies and their management. Care Crit Ill 1999; 15: 132–5.
[1304] Paton RC. Haemostatic changes in diabetic coma. Diabetologia 1981; 21: 172–7.
[1305] Roe TF, Crawford TO, Huff KR, et al. Brain infarction in children with diabetic ketoacidosis. J Diabetes Complications 1996; 10: 100–8.
[1306] Ng CK, Sigmund CJ, Lagos LA, Chernin M. Hepatic infarctions and diabetic ketoacidosis. Gastroenterology 1977; 73: 804–7.
[1307] Faigel DO, Metz DC. Prevalence, etiology, and prognostic significance of upper gastrointestinal hemorrhage in diabetic ketoacidosis. Dig Dis Sci 1996; 41: 1–8.
[1308] Tesfaye S, Stevens LK, Stephenson JM, et al. Prevalence of diabetic peripheral neuropathy and its relation to glycaemic control and potential risk factors: the EURODIAB IDDM Complications Study. Diabetologia 1996; 39: 1377–84.
[1309] Johnson DD, Palumbo PJ, Chu CP. Diabetic ketoacidosis in a community-based population. Mayo Clin Proc 1980; 55(2): 83–8.
[1310] Krentz AJ, Singh BM, Wright AD, Nattrass M. Effects of autonomic neuropathy on glucose, fatty acid, and ketone body metabolism following insulin withdrawal in patients with insulin-dependent diabetes. J Diabetes Complications 1994; 8: 105–10.
[1311] Timperley WR, Preston FE, Ward-JD. Cerebral intravascular coagulation in diabetic ketoacidosis. Lancet 1974; 1: 952–6.
[1312] Andersen JM. Diabetic ketoacidosis presenting as neurosurgical emergencies. Br Med J 1974; 3: 22–3.
[1313] Preston FE, Timperley WR, Ward JD. Diabetic ketoacidosis presenting as neurosurgical emergencies. Br Med J 1974; 3: 341–2.
[1314] Ozrer RR, Richard NG, Schumaker OP. Acute polyneuritis following diabetic acidosis. Ohio State Med J 1959; 55: 1521.
[1315] Williams E, Timperley WR, Ward JD, Duckworth T. Electron microscopical studies of vessels in diabetic peripheral neuropathy. J Clin Pathol 1980; 33: 462–70.
[1316] Maccario M. Neurological dysfunction associated with nonketotic hyperglycemia. Arch Neurol 1968; 19: 525–34.
[1317] Davenport A, Ahmad R. Hyperosmolar non-ketotic hyperglycemia manifested as ascending polyneuropathy. South Med J 1990; 83: 250–2.
[1318] O'Mahony D, Ferriss JB, Perry I. Fulminant severe retinopathy in a newly diagnosed diabetic without risk factors. J Intern Med 1989; 226: 63–6.
[1319] Weintraub N, Plaut S, Shalev N, Sharan H. Severe neuropathy in a young diabetic. Harefuah 1994; 127: 305–9.
[1320] Bonfanti R, Bognetti E, Meschi F, et al. Disseminated intravascular coagulation and severe peripheral neuropathy complicating ketoacidosis in a newly diagnosed diabetic child. Acta Diabetol 1994; 31: 173–4.

[1321] Sullivan PA, Gonggrijp H, Crowley MJ, et al. Plasma angiotensin II concentrations in diabetic ketoacidosis and in hyperosmolar non-ketotic hyperglycemia. Acta Diabetol Lat 1981; 18: 139–46.
[1322] Christlieb AR. Renin-angiotensin-aldosterone system in diabetes mellitus. Diabetes 1976; 25: 820–5.
[1323] Kilby A. Diabetic ketosis with gross hyperlipoproteinaemia and followed by severe peripheral neuropathy. Proc R Soc Med 1972; 65: 786.
[1324] Walker D, Carrington A, Cannan SA, et al. Peripheral nerve structural abnormalities do not explain the reduction in nerve conduction velocity or nerve blood flow in the streptozotocin diabetic rat. J Anat 1999; 195: 419–27.
[1325] Wolff A. Neuropathy associated with transient diabetes mellitus in 2 cats. Mod Vet Pract 1984; 65: 726–8.
[1326] Pont A, Rubino JM, Bishop D, Peal R. Diabetes mellitus and neuropathy following Vacor ingestion in man. Arch Intern Med 1979; 139: 185–7.
[1327] LeWitt PA. The neurotoxicity of the rat poison Vacor. A clinical study of 12 cases. N Engl J Med 1980; 302: 73–7.
[1328] Lee TH, Doi K, Yoshida M, Baba S. Morphological study of nervous system in Vacor-induced diabetic rats. Diabetes Res Clin Pract 1988; 4: 275–9.
[1329] Mayatepek E, Hoffmann GF, Baumgartner R, et al. Atypical vitamin B12-unresponsive methylmalonic aciduria in sibship with severe progressive encephalomyelopathy: a new genetic disease? Eur J Pediatr 1996; 155: 398–403.
[1330] Danta G. Hypoglycemic peripheral neuropathy. Arch Neurol 1969; 21: 121–32.
[1331] Danta G. Clinical features of peripheral neuropathy associated with hypoglycemia. Adv Metab Disord 1973; 2(suppl): 465–79.
[1332] Kihara M, Zollman PJ, Smithson IL, et al. Hypoxic effect of exogenous insulin on normal and diabetic peripheral nerve. Am J Physiol 1994; 266: E980–985.
[1333] Conri C, Ducloux G, Lagueny A, et al. Polyneuropathy in type I multiple endocrine syndrome. Presse Med 1990; 19: 247–50.
[1334] Cornblath DR, Drachman DB, Griffin JW. Demyelinating motor neuropathy in patients with diabetic polyneuropathy. Ann Neurol 1987; 22: 126.
[1335] Timperley WR, Boulton AJ, Davies-Jones GA, et al. Small vessel disease in progressive diabetic neuropathy associated with good metabolic control. J Clin Pathol 1985; 38: 1030–8.
[1336] Stewart JD, McKelvey R, Durcan L, et al. Chronic inflammatory demyelinating polyneuropathy (CIDP) in diabetics. J Neurol Sci 1996; 142: 59–64.
[1337] Dyck PJB, Norell JE, Dyck PJ. Microvasculitis and ischemia in diabetic lumbosacral radiculoplexus neuropathy. Neurology 1999; 53: 2113–21.
[1338] Pascoe MK, Low PA, Windebank AJ, Litchy WJ. Subacute diabetic proximal neuropathy. Mayo Clin Proc 1997; 72: 1123–32.
[1339] Ellenberg M. Diabetic neuropathic cachexia. Diabetes 1974; 23: 418–23.
[1340] Poet JL, Le Pommelet C, Tonolli-Serabian I, et al. Abdominal neuropathy of motor expression of diabetic origin. Apropos of a case. Rev Med Interne 1994; 15: 329–31.
[1341] Cavaliere D, Scorpiglione N, Belfiglio M, et al. Quality assessment of randomised clinical trials on medical treatment of diabetic neuropathy. Diab Nutr Metab 1994; 7: 287–94.
[1342] Pfeifer MA, Schumer MP. Clinical trials of diabetic neuropathy: Past, present, and future. Diabetes 1995; 44: 1355–61.
[1343] Sima AAF, Laudadio C. Design of controlled clinical trials for diabetic neuropathy. Semin Neurol 1996; 16: 187–91.
[1344] Ziegler D. The design of clinical trials for treatment of diabetic neuropathy. Neurosci Res Comm 1997; 21: 83–91.
[1345] Luft D. Interpretation of clinical trials for the treatment of diabetic neuropathy. Drugs Today 1998; 34: 157–75.
[1346] Consensus statement. Standardized measures in diabetic neuropathy. Diabetes Care 1992; 15: 1080–107.
[1347] Thomas PK. Painful diabetic neuropathy: Mechanisms and treatment. Diab Nutr Metab 1994; 7: 359–68.
[1348] Ziegler D. Diagnosis, staging and epidemiology of diabetic peripheral neuropathy. Diab Nutr Metab 1994; 7: 342–8.
[1349] Ziegler D. Diabetic cardiovascular autonomic neuropathy: prognosis, diagnosis and treatment. Diab Metab Rev 1994; 10: 339–83.
[1350] Dyck PJ, Kratz KM, Karnes JL, et al. The prevalence by staged severity of various types of diabetic neuropathy, retinopathy, and nephropathy in a population-based cohort: The Rochester Diabetic Neuropathy Study. Neurology 1993; 43: 817–24.
[1351] Young RJ, Ewing DJ, Clarke BF. Chronic and remitting painful diabetic polyneuropathy. Correlations with clinical features and subsequent changes in neurophysiology. Diabetes Care 1988; 11: 34–40.
[1352] Temple RJ. A regulatory authority's opinion about surrogate endpoints. In: Nimmo WS, Tucker GT, editors. Clinical measurement in drug evaluation. New York: John Wiley, 1995: 57.
[1353] Fleming TR, DeMets DL. Surrogate end points in clinical trials: are we being misled? Ann Intern Med 1996; 125: 605–13.
[1354] Boissel JP, Collet JP, Moleur P, Haugh M. Surrogate endpoints: a basis for a rational approach. Eur J Clin Pharmacol 1992; 43: 235–44.
[1355] Dyck PJ, Litchy WJ, Lehman KA, et al. Variables influencing neuropathic endpoints: the Rochester Diabetic Neuropathy Study of Healthy Subjects. Neurology 1995; 45: 1115–21.
[1356] Young MJ, Breddy JL, Veves A, Boulton AJM. The prediction of diabetic neuropathic foot ulceration using vibration perception thresholds. Diabetes Care 1994; 17: 557–60.
[1357] Abbott CA, Vileikyte L, Williamson S, et al. Multicenter study of the incidence of and predictive risk factors for diabetic neuropathic foot ulceration. Diabetes Care 1998; 21: 1071–5.
[1358] The Diabetes Control and Complications Trial Research Group. The effect of intensive treatment of diabetes on the development and progression of long-term complications in insulin-dependent diabetes mellitus. N Engl J Med 1993; 329: 977–86.
[1359] Echt DS, Liebson PR, Mitchell LB, et al. Mortality and morbidity in patients receiving encainide, flecainide, or placebo: the Cardiac Arrhythmia Suppression Trial. N Engl J Med 1991; 324: 781–8.
[1360] Waldo AL, Camm AJ, de Ruyter H, et al. Effect of D-sotalol on mortality in patients with left ventricular dysfunction after recent and remote myocardial infarction. The SWORD Investigators. Survival with oral D-sotalol. Lancet 1996; 348: 7–12.
[1361] The Alpha-Tocopherol, Beta-Carotene Cancer Prevention Study Group. The effect of vitamin E and beta-carotene on the incidence of lung cancer and other cancers in male smokers. N Engl J Med 1994; 330: 1029–35.
[1362] Omenn GS, Goodman GE, Thornquist MD, et al. Effects of a combination of beta-carotene and vitamin A on lung cancer and cardiovascular disease. N Engl J Med 1996; 334: 1150–5.
[1363] Riggs BL, Hodgson SF, O'Fallon WM, et al. Effect of fluoride treatment on the fracture rate in postmenopausal women with osteoporosis. N Engl J Med 1990; 322: 802–9.
[1364] Sobel BE, Furberg CD. Surrogates, semantics, and sensible public policy. Circulation 1997; 95: 1661–3.
[1365] World Health Organization. International classification of impairment , disabilities, and handicaps. Geneva, Switzerland: WHO, 1980.
[1366] Dyck PJ. Detection, characterization, and staging of polyneuropathy: assessed in diabetics. Muscle Nerve 1988; 11: 21–32.
[1367] Bril V. NIS-LL: the primary measurement scale for clinical trial endpoints in diabetic peripheral neuropathy. Eur Neurol 1999; 41(suppl 1): 8–13.
[1368] Peripheral Nerve Society. Diabetic polyneuropathy in controlled clinical trials: consensus report of the Peripheral Nerve Society. Ann Neurol 1995; 38: 478–82.
[1369] Dyck PJ, O'Brien PC. Meaningful degrees of prevention or improvement of nerve conduction in controlled clinical trials of diabetic neuropathy. Diabetes Care 1989; 12: 649–52.

[1370] Orskov L, Worm M, Schmitz O, et al. Nerve conduction velocity in man: influence of glucose, somatostatin and electrolytes. Diabetologia 1994; 37: 1216–20.
[1371] Peripheral Neuropathy Association. Quantitative sensory testing: a consensus report from the Peripheral Neuropathy Association. Neurology 1993; 43: 1050–2.
[1372] Dyck PJ, Sherman WR, Hallcher LM, et al. Human diabetic endoneurial sorbitol, fructose, and myo-inositol related to sural nerve morphometry. Ann Neurol 1980; 8: 590–6.
[1373] Thomas PK. Nerve biopsy. Diabet Med 1997; 14: 345–6.
[1374] American Academy of Neurology. Assessment Clinical autonomic testing report of the Therapeutics and Technology Assessment Subcommittee of the American Academy of Neurology, 1996; 46: 873–80.
[1375] La Rovere MT, Bigger JT Jr, Marcus FI, et al. Baroreflex sensitivity and heart-rate variability in prediction of total cardiac mortality after myocardial infarction. ATRAMI (Autonomic Tone and Reflexes After Myocardial Infarction) Investigators. Lancet 1998; 351: 478–84.
[1376] Schwartz PJ, La Rovere MT. ATRAMI: a mark in the quest for the prognostic value of autonomic markers. Autonomic tone and reflexes after myocardial infarction. Eur Heart J 1998; 19: 1593–5.
[1377] UK Prospective Diabetes Study (UKPDS) Group. Intensive blood-glucose control with sulphonylureas or insulin compared with conventional treatment and risk of complications in patients with type 2 diabetes (UKPDS 33). Lancet 1998; 352: 837–53.
[1378] Boulton AJM, Ward JD. Diabetic neuropathies and pain. Clin Endocrinol Metab 1986; 15: 917–31.
[1379] Scott J, Huskisson EC. Graphic representation of pain. Pain 1976; 2: 175–84.
[1380] McQuay H, Carroll D, Moore A. Variation in the placebo effect in randomised controlled trials of analgesics: all is as blind as it seems. Pain 1995; 64: 331–5.
[1381] Greene DA, Brown MJ, Braunstein SN, et al. Comparison of clinical course and sequential electrophysiological tests in diabetics with symptomatic polyneuropathy and its implications for clinical trials. Diabetes 1981; 30: 139–47.
[1382] Benbow SJ, Chan AW, Bowsher D, et al. A prospective study of painful symptoms, small-fibre function and peripheral vascular disease in chronic painful diabetic neuropathy. Diabet Med 1994; 11: 17–21.
[1383] Veves A, Malik RA, Lye RH, et al. The relationship between sural nerve morphometric findings and measures of peripheral nerve function in mild diabetic neuropathy. Diabet Med 1991; 8: 917–21.
[1384] Valk GD, Nauta JJP, Strijers RLM, Bertelsmann FW. Clinical examination versus neurophysiological examination in the diagnosis of diabetic polyneuropathy. Diabet Med 1992; 9: 716–21.
[1385] Valk GD, Grootenhuis PA, Bouter LM, Bertelsmann FW. Complaints of neuropathy related to the clinical and neurophysiological assessment of nerve function in patients with diabetes mellitus. Diab Res Clin Pract 1994; 26: 29–34.
[1386] The Diabetes Control and Complications Trial Research Group. The effect of intensive diabetes therapy on the development and progression of neuropathy. Ann Intern Med 1995; 122: 561–8.
[1387] The Diabetes Control and Complications Trial Research Group. Effect of intensive diabetes treatment on nerve conduction in the Diabetes Control and Complications Trial. Ann Neurol 1995; 38: 869–80.
[1388] Lloyd CE, Becker D, Ellis D, Orchard TJ. Incidence of complications in insulin-dependent diabetes mellitus: a survival analysis. Am J Epidemiol 1996; 143: 431–41.
[1389] Forrest KY, Maser RE, Pambianco G, et al. Hypertension as a risk factor for diabetic neuropathy: a prospective study. Diabetes 1997; 46: 665–70.
[1390] Sands ML, Shetterly SM, Franklin GM, Hamman RF. Incidence of distal symmetric (sensory) neuropathy in NIDDM. San Luis Val Diabetes Study. Diabetes Care 1997; 20: 322–9.
[1391] Ziegler D, Piolot R, Gries FA. The natural history of diabetic neuropathy is governed by the degree of glycaemic control. A 10-year prospective study in IDDM. Diabetologia 1996; 39(suppl 1): A35.
[1392] Töyry JP, Niskanen LK, Mäntysaari-MJ, et al. Occurrence, predictors, and clinical significance of autonomic neuropathy in NIDDM. Ten-year follow-up from the diagnosis. Diabetes 1996; 45: 308–15.
[1393] Partanen J, Niskanen L, Lehtinen J, et al. Natural history of peripheral neuropathy in patients with non-insulin-dependent diabetes mellitus. N Engl J Med 1995; 333: 89–94.
[1394] Mustonen J, Uusitupa M, Mäntysaari M, et al. Changes in autonomic nervous function during the 4-year follow-up in middle-aged diabetic and nondiabetic subjects initially free of coronary heart disease. J Intern Med 1997; 241: 227–35.
[1395] Amthor K-F, Dahl-Jorgensen K, Berg TJ, et al. The effect of 8 years of strict glycaemic control on peripheral nerve function in IDDM patients: the Oslo study. Diabetologia 1994; 37: 579–84.
[1396] Reichard P, Pihl M, Rosenqvist U, Sule J. Complications in IDDM are caused by elevated blood glucose levels: the Stockholm Diabetes Intervention Study (SDIS) at 10-year follow-up. Diabetologia 1996; 39: 1483–8.
[1397] Watkins PJ. Natural history of the diabetic neuropathies. Q J Med 1990; 77: 1209–18.
[1398] Archer AG, Watkins PJ, Thomas PK, et al. The natural history of acute painful neuropathy in diabetes mellitus. J Neurol Neurosurg Psychiatry 1983; 46: 491–9.
[1399] D'Costa DF, Price DE, Burden AC. Diabetic neuropathic cachexia associated with malabsorption. Diabet Med 1992; 9: 203–5.
[1400] Coppack SW, Watkins PJ. The natural history of diabetic femoral neuropathy. Q J Med 1991; 79: 307–13.
[1401] Sühler K, Parhofer K, Richter WO, et al. Diabetische Radikulopathie. Dtsch Med Wochenschr 1990; 115: 1665–9.
[1402] Bischoff A. The natural course of diabetic neuropathy. A follow up. In: Gries FA, Freund HJ, Rabe F, Berger H, editors. Aspects of autonomic neuropathy in diabetes. Horm Metab Res (Suppl 9), 1980: 98–100.
[1403] Boulton AJM, Scarpello JH, Armstrong WD, Ward JD. The natural history of painful diabetic neuropathy—a 4-year study. Postgrad Med J 1983; 59: 556–9.
[1404] Mayne N. The short-term prognosis in diabetic neuropathy. Diabetes 1968; 17: 270–3.
[1405] Sosenko JM, Kato M, Soto R, Bild DE. A prospective study of sensory function in patients with type 2 diabetes. Diabet Med 1993; 10: 110–4.
[1406] Laudadio C, Sima AAF. Progression rates of diabetic neuropathy in placebo patients in an 18-month clinical trial. J Diabetes Compl 1998; 12: 121–7.
[1407] Sampson MJ, Wilson S, Karagiannis P, et al. Progression of diabetic autonomic neuropathy over a decade in insulin-dependent diabetics. Q J Med 1990; 75: 635–46.
[1408] Jakobsen J, Christiansen JS, Kristoffersen I, et al. Autonomic and somatosensory nerve function after 2 years of continuous subcutaneous insulin infusion in type I diabetes. Diabetes 1988; 37: 452–5.
[1409] Jermendy G, Toth L, Uvrös P, et al. Cardiac autonomic neuropathy and QT interval length. A follow-up study in diabtic patients. Acta Cardiol 1991; 46: 189–200.
[1410] Reichard P, Berglund B, Britz A, et al. Intensified conventional insulin treatment retards the microvascular complications of insulin-dependent diabetes mellitus (IDDM): the Stockholm Diabetes Intervention Study (SDIS) after 5 years. J Intern Med 1991; 230: 101–8.
[1411] Quadri R, Ponzani P, Zanone M, et al. Changes in autonomic nervous function over a 5-year period in non-insulin-dependent diabetic patients. Diabet Med 1993; 10: 916–9.
[1412] Vanninen E, Uusitupa M, Länsimies E, et al. Effect of metabolic control on autonomic function in obese patients with newly diagnosed type 2 diabetes. Diabet Med 1993; 10: 66–73.
[1413] Levitt NS, Stansberry KB, Wynchank S, Vinik AI. The natural progression of autonomic neuropathy and autonomic function tests in a cohort of people with IDDM. Diabetes Care 1996; 19: 751–4.
[1414] The Diabetes Control and Complications Trial Research Group. The effect of intensified diabetes therapy on measures of autonomic nervous system function in the Diabe-

tes Contol and Complication Trial (DCCT). Diabetologia 1998; 41: 416–23.
[1415] Reichard P, Nilsson B-Y, Rosenqvist U. The effect of long-term intensified insulin treatment on the development of microvascular complications of diabetes mellitus. N Engl J Med 1993; 329: 304–9.
[1416] Navarro X, Kennedy WR, Loewenson RB, Sutherland DER. Influence of pancreas transplantation on cardiorespiratory reflexes, nerve conduction, and mortality in diabetes mellitus. Diabetes 1990; 39: 802–6.
[1417] Solders G, Tydén G, Persson A, Groth C-G. Improvement of nerve conduction in diabetic neuropathy. A follow-up study 4 yr after combined pancreatic and renal transplantation. Diabetes 1992; 41: 946–51.
[1418] Müller-Felber W, Landgraf R, Scheuer R, et al. Diabetic neuropathy 3 years after successful pancreas and kidney transplantation. Diabetes 1993; 42: 1482–6.
[1419] Altman DG, Bland JM. Absence of evidence is not evidence of absence. Br Med J 1995; 311: 485.
[1420] Moher D, Dulberg CS, Wells GA. Statistical power, sample size, and their reporting in randomized controlled trials. JAMA 1994; 272: 122–4.
[1421] Campbell MJ, Julious SA, Altman DG. Estimating sample sizes for binary, ordered categorical, and continuous outcomes in two group comparisons. Br Med J 1995; 311: 1145–8.
[1422] Dyck PJ, Davies JL, Litchy WJ, O'Brien PC. Longitudinal assessment of diabetic polyneuropathy using a composite score in the Rochester Diabetic Neuropathy Study cohort. Neurology 1997; 49: 229–39.
[1423] Nicolucci A, Carinci F, Cavaliere D, et al. On behalf of the Italian study group for the implementation of the St. Vincent Declaration. A meta-analysis of trials on aldose reductase inhibitors in diabetic peripheral neuropathy. Diabet Med 1996; 13: 1017–26.
[1424] Young MJ, Breddy JL, Veves A, Boulton AJM. The prediction of diabetic neuropathic foot ulceration using vibration perception thresholds: a prospective study. Diabetes Care 1994; 17: 557–60.
[1425] Moore RA, Gavaghan D, Tramer MR, et al. Size is everything – large amounts of information are needed to overcome random effects in estimating direction and magnitude of treatment effects. Pain 1998; 78: 209–16.
[1426] Valensi P, Attali J-R, Gagant S, and the French Group for Research and Study of Diabetic Neuropathy. Reproducibility of parameters for assessment of diabetic neuropathy. Diabet Med 1993; 10: 933–9.
[1427] Bril V, Ellison R, Ngo M, et al. Roche Neuropathy Study Group. Electrophysiological monitoring in clinical trials. Muscle Nerve 1998; 21: 1368–73.
[1428] Santiago JV, Sönksen PH, Boulton AJM, et al. The Tolrestat Study Group. Withdrawal of the aldose reductase inhibitor tolrestat in patients with diabetic neuropathy: effect on nerve function. J Diabetes Complications 1993; 7: 170–8.
[1429] Sundkvist G, Armstrong FM, Bradbury JE, et al. The United Kingdom/Scandinavian Ponalrestat Trial. Peripheral and autonomic nerve function in 259 diabetic patients with peripheral neuropathy treated with ponalrestat (an aldose reductase inhibitor) or placebo for 18 months. J Diabetes Complications 1992; 6: 123–30.
[1430] Ward C, Kenny RA. Reproducibility of orthostatic hypotension in symptomatic elderly. Am J Med 1996; 100: 418–22.
[1431] Maser RE, Nielsen VK, Bass EB, et al. Measuring diabetic neuropathy. Assessment and comparison of clinical examination and quantitative sensory testing. Diabetes Care 1989; 12: 270–5.
[1432] Dyck PJ, Kratz KM, Lehman KA, et al. The Rochester diabetic neuropathy study: design, criteria for types of neuropathy, selection bias, and reproducibility of neuropathic tests. Neurology 1991; 41: 799–807.
[1433] Gentile S, Turco S, Corigliano G, Marmo R, the SIMSDN Group. Simplified diagnostic criteria for diabetic distal polyneuropathy. Acta Diabetol 1995; 32: 7–12.
[1434] Thivolet C, El Farkh J, Petiot A, et al. Measuring vibration sensations with graduated tuning fork. Simple and reliable means to detect diabetic patients at risk of neuropathic foot ulceration. Diabetes Care 1990; 13: 1077–80.
[1435] Liniger C, Albeanu A, Bloise D, Assal JPh. The tuning fork revisited. Diabet Med 1990; 7: 859–64.
[1436] Williams G, Gill JS, Aber V, Mather HM. Variability in vibration perception thresholds among sites: a potential source of error in biothesiometry. Br Med J 1988; 296: 233–5.
[1437] Krönert K, Luft D, Baumann B, et al. Reduced intraindividual variability of repeated cardio-vascular reflex tests: an additional marker of autonomic neuropathy in insulin-dependent (type I) diabetes mellitus? Acta Diabetol Lat 1986; 23: 279–89.
[1438] Yarnitsky D, Sprecher E, Tamir A, et al. Variance of sensory threshold measurements: discrimination of feigners from trustworthy performers. J Neurol Sci 1994; 125: 186–9.
[1439] Hänseler E, Keller H. Rationale Beurteilung von Labordaten. Probleme und Grenzen. Internist 1994; 35: 609–18.
[1440] Ernst E, Resch KL. Concept of true and perceived placebo effects. Br Med J 1995; 311: 551–3.
[1441] Richardson PH. Placebo effects in pain management. Pain Rev 1994; 1: 15–32.
[1442] Turner JA, Deyo RA, Loeser JD, et al. The importance of placebo effects in pain treatment and research. JAMA 1994; 271: 1609–14.
[1443] McQuay H, Carroll D, Jadad AR, et al. Anticonvulsant drugs for management of pain: a systematic review. Br Med J 1995; 311: 1047–52.
[1444] Hässler R, Chantelau E, Schopen M. Placebo-Wirkung bei der schmerzhaften diabetischen Polyneuropathie. Eine Literaturstudie. Z Allg Med 1995; 71: 333–8.
[1445] Kleijnen J, de Craen AJM, van Everdingen J, Krol L. Placebo effect in double-blind clinical trials: a review of interactions with medications. Lancet 1994; 344: 1347–9.
[1446] Pearce JMS. The placebo enigma. Q J Med 1995; 88: 215–20.
[1447] Max MB, Culnane M, Schafer SC, et al. Amitriptyline relieves diabetic neuropathy pain in patients with normal or depressed mood. Neurology 1987; 37: 589–96.
[1448] Rothman KJ, Michels KB. The continuing unethical use of placebo controls. N Engl J Med 1994; 331: 394–8.
[1449] Collier J. Confusion over use of placebos in clinical trials. Br Med J 1995; 311: 821–2.
[1450] Cleophas TJM, v d Meulen J, Kalmansohn RB. Clinical trials: specific problems associated with the use of a placebo control group. Br J Clin Pharmacol 1997; 43: 219–21.
[1451] Boulton AJM, Drury J, Clarke B, Ward JD. Continuous subcutaneous insulin infusion in the management of painful diabetic neuropathy. Diabetes Care 1982; 5: 386–90.
[1452] Morley GK, Mooradian AD, Levine AS, Morley JE. Mechanisms of pain in diabetic peripheral neuropathy. Effect of glucose on pain perception in humans. Am J Med 1984; 77: 79–82.
[1453] Chan AW, MacFarlane IA, Bowsher DR, Wells JCD. Does acute hyperglycaemia influence heat pain thresholds ? J Neurol Neurosurg Psychiatry 1988; 51: 688–90.
[1454] Luft D, Lay A, Benda N, et al. Pain intensity and blood pressure reactions during a cold pressor test in IDDM patients. Diabetes Care 1996; 19: 722–5.
[1455] Bland JM, Altman DG. Some examples of regression towards the mean. Br Med J 1994; 309: 780.
[1456] Dyck PJ, Bushek W, Spring EM, et al. Vibratory and cooling detection thresholds compared with other tests in diagnosing and staging diabetic neuropathy. Diabetes Care 1987; 10: 432–40.
[1457] MacLeod AF, Boulton AJM, Owens DR, et al, and the North European Tolrestat Study Group Belgium, Holland and UK. A multicentre trial of the aldose-reductase inhibitor tolrestat, in patients with symptomatic diabetic peripheral neuropathy. Diabete Metab 1992; 18: 14–20.
[1458] Boulton AJM, Levin S, Comstock J. A multicentre trial of the aldose-reductase inhibitor, tolrestat, in patients with symptomatic diabetic neuropathy. Diabetologia 1990; 33: 431–7.
[1459] Laupacis A, Sackett DL, Roberts RA. An assessment of clinically useful measures of the consequences of treatment. N Engl J Med 1988; 318: 1728–33.

[1460] Cook RJ, Sackett DL. The number needed to treat: a clinically useful measure of treatment effect. Br Med J 1995; 310: 452–4.
[1461] Chatellier G, Zapletal E, Lemaitre D, et al. The number needed to treat: a clinically useful nomogram in its proper context. Br Med J 1996; 312: 426–9.
[1462] Sackett D, Rosenberg W, Haynes B, Richardson S. Evidence-based medicine—how to practice and teach EBM. New York, Edinburgh, London, Melbourne, Tokyo: Churchill Livingstone International, 1996.
[1463] De Craen AJM, Vickers AJ, Tijssen JGP, Kleijnen J. Number-needed-to-treat and placebo-controlled trials. Lancet 1998; 351: 310.
[1464] L'Abbé KA, Detsky AS, O'Rourke K. Meta-analysis in clinical research. Ann Intern Med 1987; 107: 224–33.
[1465] Morris JA, Gardner MJ. Calculating confidence intervals for relative risks (odds ratios) and standardised ratios and rates. Br Med J 1988; 296: 1313-6.
[1466] Thompson SG, Pocock SJ. Can meta-analyses be trusted? Lancet 1991; 338: 1127–30.
[1467] Onghena P, van Houdenhove B. Antidepressant-induced analgesia in chronic non-malignant pain: a meta-analysis of 39 placebo-controlled studies. Pain 1992; 49: 205–19.
[1468] Gardner MJ, Altman DG. Confidence intervals rather than P values: estimation rather than hypothesis testing. Br Med J 1986; 292: 746–50.
[1469] Sharp SJ, Thompson SG, Altman DG. The relation between treatment benefit and underlying risk in meta-analysis. Br Med J 1996; 313: 735–8.
[1470] Bland JM, Altman DG. Multiple significance tests: the Bonferroni method. Br Med J 1995; 310: 170.
[1471] Ludbrook J. Multiple comparison procedures updated. Clin Exp Pharmacol Physiol 1998; 25: 1032–937.
[1472] Windeler J, Holle R. Beurteilung klinischer Studien. Hinweise zum kritischen Literaturstudium. Internist 1997; 38: 337–43.
[1473] Sheiner LB, Rubin DB. Intention-to-treat analysis and the goals of clinical trials. Clin Pharmacol Ther 1995; 57: 6–15.
[1474] Hollis S, Campbell F. What is meant by intention to treat analysis? Survey of published randomised controlled trials. Br Med J 1999; 319: 670–4.
[1475] Lee YJ, Ellenberg JH, Hirtz DG, Nelson KB. Analysis of clinical trials by treatment actually received: is it really an option? Stat Med 1991; 10: 1595–605.
[1476] Michels KB, Rosner BA. Data trawling: to fish or not to fish. Lancet 1996; 348: 1152–3.
[1477] Demol P, Weihrauch TR. Multinationale klinische Therapiestudien (MTS). Design, Management und Kosten. Med Klin 1997; 92: 117–23.
[1478] Begg C, Cho M, Eastwood S, et al. Improving the qualitiy of reporting of randomized controlled trials: the CONSORT statement. JAMA 1996; 276: 637–9.
[1479] Freemantle N, Mason JM, Haines A, Eccles MP. CONSORT: an important step toward evidence-based health care. Consolidated Standards of Reporting Trials. Ann Intern Med 1997; 126: 81–3.
[1480] Rennie D. How to report randomized controlled trials. The CONSORT statement. JAMA 1996; 276: 649.
[1481] Altman D. Better reporting of randomised contolled trials: the CONSORT statement. Br Med J 1996; 313: 570–1.
[1482] Mulrow CD, Cook DJ, Davidoff F. Systematic reviews: critical links in the great chain of evidence. Ann Intern Med 1997; 126: 389–91.
[1483] Dickersin K, Scherer R, Lefebvre C. Identifying relevant studies for systematic reviews. Br Med J 1994; 309: 1286–91.
[1484] Eggert M, Smith GD. Bias in location and selection of studies. Br Med J 1998; 316: 61–6.
[1485] Egger M, Zellweger-Zähner T, Schneider M, et al. Language bias in randomised controlled trials published in English and German. Lancet 1997; 350: 326–9.
[1486] Easterbrook PJ, Berlin JA, Gopalan R, Matthews DR. Publication bias in clinical research. Lancet 1991; 337: 867–72.
[1487] Dickersin K, Min YI. Publication bias: the problem that won't go away. Ann N Y Acad Sci 1993; 703: 135–48.
[1488] Dickersin K, Min Y-I, Meinert CL. Factors influencing publication of research results. Follow-up of applications submitted to two institutional review boards. JAMA 1992; 267: 374–8.
[1489] Dong BJ, Hauck WW, Gambertoglio JG, et al. Bioequivalence of generic and brand-name levothyroxine products in the treatment of hypothyroidism. JAMA 1997; 277: 1205–13.
[1490] Blumenthal D, Campbell EG, Anderson MS, et al. Withholding research results in academic life science: Evidence from a national survey of faculty. JAMA 1997; 277: 1224–8.
[1491] Deyo RA, Psaty BM, Simon GS, et al. The messenger under attack—intimidation of researchers by special-interest groups. N Engl J Med 1997; 336: 1176–80.
[1492] Scherer RW, Dickersin K, Langenberg P. Full publication of results initially presented as abstracts: a meta-analysis. JAMA 1994; 272: 158–62.
[1493] Editorial. Cochrane's legacy. Lancet 1992; 340: 1131–2.
[1494] Bero L. The Cochrane Collaboration. Preparing , maintaining, and disseminating systematic reviews of the effectiveness of health care. JAMA 1996; 274: 1935–8.
[1495] Zhang WY, Li Wan Po A. The effectiveness of topically applied capsaicin. Eur J Clin Pharmacol 1994; 46: 517–22.
[1496] Scheffler NM, Sheitel PL, Lipton MN. Treatment of painful diabetic neuropathy with capsaicin 0.075%. J Am Podiatr Med Assoc 1991; 81: 288–93.
[1497] Tandan R, Lewis GA, Krusinski PB, et al. Topical capsaicin in painful diabetic neuropathy. Controlled study with long-term follow-up. Diabetes Care 1992; 15: 8–14.
[1498] The Capsaicin Study Group. Treatment of painful diabetic neuropathy with topical capsaicin—a multicenter, double-blind, vehicle-controlled study. Arch Intern Med 1991; 151: 2225–9.
[1499] Chad DA, Aronin N, Lundstrom R, et al. Does capsaicin relieve the pain of diabetic neuropathy? Pain 1990; 42: 387–8.
[1500] Eggert M, Smith GD, Schneider M, Minder C. Bias in meta-analysis detected by a simple, graphical test. Br Med J 1997; 31: 629–34.
[1501] Eggert M, Smith GD. Bias in location and selection of studies. Br Med J 1998; 316: 61–6.
[1502] Altman DG, Doré CJ. Randomisation and baseline comparisons in clinical trials. Lancet 1990; 335: 149–53.
[1503] The Asilomar working group on recommendations for reporting of clinical trials in the biomedical literature. Checklist of information for inclusion in reports of clinical trials. Ann Intern Med 1996; 124: 741–3.
[1504] Sacks HS, Berrier J, Reitman D, et al. Meta-analyses of randomized controlled trials. N Engl J Med 1987; 316: 450–5.
[1505] Guyatt GH, Sackett DL, Sinclair JC, et al, for the Evidence-Based Medicine Working Group. Users' guides to the medical literature. IX. A method for grading health care recommendations. JAMA 1995; 274: 1800–4.
[1506] Feinstein AR, Horwitz RI. Problems in the "evidence" of "evidence based medicine". Am J Med 1997; 103: 529–35.
[1507] Moher D, Cook DJ, Eastwood S, et al. Improving the quality of reports of metaanalyses of randomised controlled trials: the QUOROM statement. Lancet 1999; 354: 1896–900.
[1508] Biesbroeck R, Bril V, Hollander P, et al. A double-blind comparison of topical capsaicin and oral amitriptyline in painful diabetic neuropathy. Adv Ther 1995; 12: 111–20.
[1509] Morello CM, Leckband SG, Moorhouse DF, Sahagian GA. Randomized double-blind study comparing the efficacy of gabapentin with amitriptyline on diabetic periperal neuropathy pain. Arch Intern Med 1999; 159: 1931–7.
[1510] Gomez-Perez FJ, Choza R, Rios JM, et al. Nortriptyline-fluphenazine vs. carbamazepine in the symptomatic treatment of diabetic neuropathy. Arch Med Res 1996; 27: 525–9.
[1511] Krentz AJ, Honigsberger L, Nattrass M. Selection of patients with symptomatic diabetic neuropathy for clinical trials. Diabete Metab 1989; 15: 416–9.
[1512] The DCCT Research Group. Diabetes control and complications trial (DCCT). Results of feasibility study. Diabetes Care 1987; 10: 1–9.
[1513] The DCCT Research Group. Diabetes control and complications trial (DCCT). Design and methodological considerations for the feasibility phase. Diabetes 1986; 35: 530–45.
[1514] The DCCT Research Group. Factors in development of diabetic neuropathy. Baseline analysis of neuropathy in fea-

sibility phase of diabetes control and complications trial (DCCT). Diabetes 1988; 37: 476–81.

[1515] Haynes RB, Dantes R. Patient compliance and the conduct and interpretation of therapeutic trials. Controlled Clin Trials 1987; 8: 12–9.

[1516] Spielberg SP, Shear NH, Cannon M, et al. In-vitro assessment of a hypersensitivity syndrome associated with sorbinil. Ann Intern Med 1991; 114: 720–4.

[1517] Nicolucci A, Carinci F, Graepel JG, et al. The efficacy of tolrestat in the treatment of diabetic peripheral neuropathy. A meta-analysis of individual patient data. Diabetes Care 1996; 19: 1091–6.

[1518] Raschetti R, Maggini M, Popoli P, et al. Gangliosides and Guillain-Barré syndrome. J Clin Epidemiol 1995; 48: 1399–405.

[1519] Freedman BI, Wuerth J-P, Cartwright K, et al. Design and baseline characteristics for the Aminoguanidine Clinical Trial in Overt Type 2 Diabetic Nephropathy (ACTION II). Controlled Clin Trials 1999; 20: 493–510.

[1520] Dyck PJ, Peroutka S, Rask C, et al. Intradermal recombinant human nerve growth factor induces pressure allodynia and lowered heat-pain thresholds in humans. Neurology 1997; 48: 501–5.

[1521] Cameron NE, Cotter MA. Potential therapeutic approaches to the treatment or prevention of diabetic neuropathy: evidence from experimental studies. Diabet Med 1993; 10: 593–605.

[1522] Thomas PK. Diabetic neuropathy. Human and experimental. Drugs 1986; 32(suppl 2): 36–42.

[1523] Tomlinson DR. Polyols and myo-inositol in diabetic neuropathy – of mice and men. Mayo Clin Proc 1989; 64: 1030–3.

[1524] Hounsom L, Tomlinson DR. Does neuropathy develop in animal models? Clin Neurosci 1997; 4: 380–9.

[1525] Malone JI, Lowitt S, Korthals JK, et al. The effect of hyperglycemia on nerve conduction and structure is age dependent. Diabetes 1996; 45: 209–15.

[1526] Alici B, Gumustas MK, Ozkara H, Akkus E, Demirel G, Yencilek F, Hattat H. Apoptosis in the erectile tissues of diabetic and healthy rats. Br J Urol Int 2000; 85:326–9.

[1527] Rosen RC, Riley A, Wagner G, Osterloh IH, Kirkpatrick J, Mishra A. The International Index of Erectile Function (IIEF): a multidimensional scale for assessment of erectile dysfunction. Urology 1997;49: 822–30.

[1528] Ewing DJ, Clarke BF. Diabetic autonomic neuropathy: present insights and future prospects. Diabetes Care 1986; 9: 648–65.

[1529] Jovanovic L. Sex and the woman with diabetes: desire versus dysfunction. IDF Bull 1998; 43: 23–8.

[1530] Azad N, Emanuele NV, Abraira C, Henderson WG, Colwell J, Levin SR, Nuttall FQ, Comstock JP, Sawin CT, Silbert C, Rubino FA, the VA CSDM Group. The effects of intensive glycemic control on neuropathy in the VA Cooperative Study on type II diabetes mellitus. J Diabetes Complications 2000; 13: 307–13.

[1531] Shabsigh R. The effects of testosterone on the cavernous tissue and erectile function. World J Urol 1997; 15: 21–26.

[1532] Hartmann U. Pyschological subtypes of erectile dysfunction. World J Urol 1997; 15: 256–64

[1533] Truss MC, Becker AJ, Schultheiss D, Jonas U. Intracavernous pharmacotherapy. World J Urol.1997; 15: 71–7.

[1534] Vogt HJ, Brandl P, Kockott G, Schmitz JR, Wiegand MH, Schadrack J, Gierend M. Double-blind, placebo-controlled safety and efficacy trial with yohimbine hydrochloride in the treatment of nonorganic erectile dysfunction. Int J Impot Res 1997; 9: 155–61.

[1535] Ernst E, Pittler MH. Yohimbine for erectile dysfunction: a systematic review and meta-analysis of randomized clinical trials. J Urol 1998; 159: 433–36.

[1536] Rampin O, Bernabe J, Guilano F. Spinal control of penile erection. World J Urol 1997; 15: 2–13.

[1537] Padma-Nathan H, Auerbach S, Lewis R, Lewand M, et al. Efficacy and safety of apomorphine vs. placebo for male erectile dysfunction. J Urol 1999; 161: 821.

[1538] Lewis R, Agre K, Rudd D. Efficacy of apomorphine vs. placebo for erectile dysfunction in patients with hypertension. J Urol 1999; 161: 822.

[1539] Reproductive Health Drugs Advisory Committee. Urology Subcomittee. FDA briefing package, April 10, 2000, pp 42–110.

[1540] Küthe A, Wiedentoth A, Stief C, Mägert H, Forssmann W, Jonas U. Identification of 13 PDE isoforms in human cavernous tissue. Eur Urol 1999; 35: 404.

[1541] Taher A, Stief CG, Raida M, Jonas U, Forssmann WG. Cyclic nucleotide phosphodiesterase activity in human cavernous smooth muscle and the effect of various selective inhibitors. Int J Impot Res 1992; 4(suppl 2): P11.

[1542] Rendell MS, Rajfer J, Wicker PA, Smith MD. Sildenafil for treatment of erectile dysfunction in men with diabetes: a randomized controlled trial. Sildenafil Diabetes Study Group. JAMA 1999; 281: 421–6.

[1543] Boulton AJM, Selam J-L, Sweeney M, Ziegler D. Sildenafil citrate for the treatment of erectile dysfunction in men with type II diabetes mellitus. Diabetologia 2001; 44: 1296–301.

[1544] Sellam R, Ziegler D, Boulton AJM. Sildenafil citrate is effective and well tolerated for the treatment of erectile dysfunction in men with type 1 or type 2 diabetes mellitus (abstract). Diabetologia 2000; 43(suppl 1): A253.

[1545] Mitka M. Some men who take Viagra die—why? JAMA 2000; 283: 590–3.

[1546] Shakir SAW, Wilton LV, Boshier A, Layton D, Heeley E. Cardiovascular events in users of sildenafil: results from first phase of prescription event monitoring in England. Br Med J 2001; 322: 651–2.

[1547] Herrmann HC, Chang G, Klugherz BD, Mahoney PD. Hemodynamic effects of sildenafil in men with severe coronary artery disease. N Engl J Med 2000; 342:1622–6.

[1548] De Angelis L, Marfella MA, Siniscalchi M, Marino L, Nappo F, Giugliano F, De Lucia D, Giugliano D. Erectile and endothelial dysfunction in type II diabetes: a possible link. Diabetologia 2001; 44: 1155–60.

[1549] Desouza C, Parulkar A, Lumpkin D, Akers D, Fonseca V. Acute and chronic effects of low dose sildenafil on endothelial function in type 2 diabetes. Diabetes 2001; 50 (suppl 2): 439.

[1550] Katz SD, Balidemaj K, Homma S, Wu H, Wang J, Maybaum S. Acute type 5 phosphodiesterase inhibition with sildenafil enhances flow mediated vasodilation in patients with chronic heart failure. J Am Coll Cardiol 2000; 36: 845–51.

[1551] Cheitlin MD, Hutter AM, Brindis RG, Ganz P, Kaul S, Russell RO, Zusman RM. Use of sildenafil (Viagra) in patients with cardiovascular disease. Circulation 1999; 99: 168–77.

[1552] Stolk EA, Busschbach JJ, Caffa M, Meuleman EJ, Rutten FF. Cost utility analysis of sildenafil compared with papaverine-phentolamine injections. Br Med J 2000; 320:1165–8.

[1553] Smith KJ, Roberts MS. The cost-effectiveness of sildenafil. Ann Intern Med 2000; 132: 933–7.

[1554] Saenz de Tejada I, Emmick J, Anglin G, Fredlund P, Segal S. The effect of as-needed tadalafil (IC351) treatment of erectile dysfunction in men with diabetes. Int J Impot Res 2001; 13(suppl 4): S46.

[1555] Goldstein I. Vardenafil demonstrates improved erectile function in diabetic men with erectile dysfunction. Fourth Congress of the European Society for Sexual and Impotence Research (ESSIR), Rome, Oct 1, 2001.

[1556] Becker AJ, Stief CG, Machtens S, Schultheiss D, Truss MC, Jonas U. Oral phentolamine as treatment for erectile dysfunction. J Urol 1998; 159: 1214–16.

[1557] Linet OI, Ogrinc FG. Efficacy and safety of intracavernosal alprostadil in men with erectile dysfunction. The Alprostadil Study Group. N Engl J Med 1996; 334: 873–7.

[1558] Shabsigh R, Padma-Nathan H, Gittleman M, McMurray J, Kaufman J, Goldstein I. Intracavernous alprostadil alfadex is more efficacious, better tolerated, and preferred over intraurethral alprostadil plus optional actis: a comparative, randomized, crossover, multicenter study. Urology 2000; 55:109–13.

[1559] Porst H, Buvat J, Meuleman EJH, Michal V, Wagner G. Final results of a prospective multi-center study with self-injection therapy with PGE_1 after 4 years of follow-up. Int J Impot Res 1996; 6: 151, D118.

[1560] Padma-Nathan H, Hellstrom WJ, Kaiser FE, Labasky RF, Lue TF, Nolten WE, Norwood PC, Peterson CA, Shabsigh R, Tam PY. Treatment of men with erectile dysfunction with transurethral alprostadil. Medicated Urethral System for Erection (MUSE) Study Group. N Engl J Med 1997; 336: 1–7.
[1561] Porst H. Transurethrale Alprostadilapplikation mit MUSE ("medicated urethral system for erection"). Urologe [A] 1998; 37: 410–16.
[1562] Spivack AP, Peterson CA, Cowley C, Hall M, Nemo KJ, Stephens D, Tam PY, Todd CK, Place VA, Gesundheit N, VIVUS-MUSE Study Group. Long-term safety profile of transurethral alprostadil for the treatment of erectile dysfunction (abstract). J Urol 1997; 157(suppl): 203.
[1563] Fulgham PF, Cochran JS, Denman JL, Feagins BA, Gross MB, Kadesky KT, Kadesky MC, Clark AR, Roehrborn CG. Disappointing initial results with transurethral alprostadil for erectile dysfunction in a urology practice setting. J Urol 1998; 160: 2041–6
[1564] Dutta TC, Eid JF. Vacuum constriction devices for erectile dysfunction: a long-term, prospective study of patients with mild, moderate, and severe dysfunction. Urology 1999; 54: 891–3.
[1565] Paro M, Prashar A, Prosdocimi M, Cherian PV, Fiori MG, Sima AAF. Urinary bladder dyfunction in the BB/W diabetic rat. J Urol 1994; 151: 781–6.
[1566] Ellenberg M. Development of urinary bladder dysfunction in diabetes mellitus. Ann Int Med 1980; 92: 321–3.
[1567] Kaplan SA, Te AE, Blavas JG. Urodynamic findings in patients with diabetic cystopathy. J Urol 1995; 153: 342–4.
[1568] Starer P, Libow L. Cystometric evaluation of bladder dysfunction in elderly diabetic patients. Arch Intern Med 1990; 150: 810–16.
[1569] Thon WF, Stief CG. Blasenfunktionsstörungen als urologische Diabetes-Komplikation. Kassenarzt 1996; 23: 40–8.
[1570] Thon WF, Grünewald V. Neurostimulation. Curr Opin Urol1993; 3: 295–302.
[1571] Grünewald V, Thon W F, Jonas U. Neuromodulation bei neurogener Blasenfunktionsstörung. In: Stöhrer M, Madersbacher H, Palmtag H, editors. Neurogene Blasenfunktionsstörungen. Berlin: Springer, 1996: 163–175.
[1572] Thon WF. Elektrostimulation der sakralen Spinalnerven bei Blasenfunktionsstörungen. Med Welt 1994; 45: 195–203.
[1573] Eri LM, Tveter KJ. Alpha blockade in the treatment of symptomatic benign prosatic hyperplasia. J Urol 1995; 154: 923–34.

6 Socioeconomic Aspects

W. Rathmann and J. Ward

Direct Costs of Diabetic Neuropathy

A substantial proportion of the economic burden of diabetes is attributable to its complications, in particular, cardiovascular disease. In the United States, direct medical costs attributable to diabetes in 1997 totaled $44.1 billion, including $11.8 billion (27%) for excess prevalence of diabetes-related chronic complications [1]. The major cost factors were cardiovascular disease (17.2%), followed by neurologic (3.4%) and renal (2.3%) complications.

Costs of Medical Care For Diabetic Neuropathy

There are few cost-of-illness studies assessing the economic impact of diabetic neuropathy. The American Diabetes Association estimated $1.5 billion total health care expenditures attributable to diabetes for treatment of neurologic diseases in the US in 1997 [1]. The most cost-intensive health care sector was inpatient care, accounting for about 70% ($1.0 billion), whereas outpatient treatment comprised only 8% ($119 million). Neurologic disorders included not only peripheral neuropathy, neuralgia, and neuritis, but also cerebrovascular disease, transient ischemic attacks, and stroke, which are major cost factors.

Based on the US 1987 National Hospital Discharge Survey, diabetic polyneuropathy, mononeuropathy, amyotrophy, and peripheral autonomic neuropathy alone contributed to about 36 000 hospital admissions with an average length of stay of 8.6 days and average costs per day of $596 [2]. Total inpatient costs for these disorders in the US were estimated to amount to $184 million in 1987. Costs for inpatient treatment of diabetic foot problems were not given separately in this analysis.

In an earlier study based on US national data from 1980, health care expenditures for treatment of neuropathy in type 2 diabetic patients comprised 2% ($240 millions) of total costs attributable to diabetes [3]. Hospital treatment was found to be the major factor, contributing to about 90% of costs. Expenditures for chronic skin ulcers, which are closely related to peripheral neuropathy, were estimated to amount to $145 million in the type 2 diabetic population.

Using data from a large health maintenance organization in the US, Selby et al. estimated excess costs of hospitalization for disorders of the peripheral nervous system in diabetic patients compared to an age- and sex-matched nondiabetic control group [4]. Diabetic patients were 1.5-fold more likely to be hospitalized for treatment of neuropathy, yielding annual excess costs of $137 000 among these 85 000 patients, which was a minor cost factor (< 0.01% of total excess costs) compared to other complications, in particular cardio-vascular and end-stage renal disease.

In the UK, Williams estimated that about 13% of total costs of care for diabetic patients could be attributed to peripheral neuropathy and vascular disease [5]. In another British study, nationwide direct health and social care costs in the type 1 diabetic population were estimated as US$157 million in 1992 [6]. Neurologic complications, which were not further specified, were reported to comprise 1.2% ($2.0 million), almost completely due to hospital treatment.

More recently, expenditures of inpatient care for diabetic neuropathy in the United Kingdom were estimated. From 1991 to 1995, routine hospital data from a large population of more than 400 000 people, whose demographic characteristics largely reflect those of the UK, were analyzed for admissions for mononeuritis and inflammatory and toxic neuropathy [7]. Diabetic patients comprised 7.8% of all subjects with one of these admission diagnoses, accounting for 12.2% ($151 346) of total hospital costs for these disorders over a study period of four years. There are no comparable comprehensive analyses of the costs of diabetic neuropathy in other health care systems.

In conclusion, cost-of-illness studies on diabetic neuropathy suggested that nerve disorders contribute directly to only a small proportion of total health care costs (about 2%) in the diabetic population, mostly due to hospital treatment. However, most of these analyses were based on the International Classification of Diseases (ICD) coding of principal diagnoses, and the attributable costs of neuropathy in diabetic foot complications were not included, which has probably led to an underestimation of the real economic impact of diabetic neuropathy.

Costs of Medication

Overall, prescription drug costs in people with diabetes have been found to be about three-fold higher than in nondiabetic patients [8]. The most important cost factors were cardiovascular drugs and antidiabetic agents. Compared to these drug groups, pharmacologic treatment of neuropathy was a minor cost factor. Nationwide prescription drug costs in German primary care practices attributable to diabetic neuropathy were estimated to amount to US$61 million in 1996, which was about 1.4% of total estimated annual drug costs in diabetic patients [9]. It is noteworthy that about one-third of these medication costs were due to drugs without proven effectiveness in symptomatic diabetic nerve disorders (e. g. vitamin B, vasodilator drugs). These results indicate the urgent need for cost-effective drug treatment guidelines for symptomatic diabetic neuropathy. Furthermore, economic studies assessing the cost-effectiveness or cost-utility of drug treatment of diabetic neuropathy are currently lacking.

Potential Cost Savings by Prevention of Diabetic Neuropathy

The effect of intensive diabetes therapy on the incidence of neuropathy in type 1 diabetes was estimated using a simulation model based on data from the Diabetes Control and Complications Trial (DCCT) [10]. The cumulative incidence of neuropathy was predicted to be 31% at age 70 years in people receiving intensive therapy, compared to 57% with conventional treatment (46% reduction). The predicted total lifetime costs per type 1 diabetic patient for intensive insulin therapy were $99 822, which was, on average $33 746 more than for conventional insulin therapy. The model estimated an overall average gain of 15.3 additional years of life free from any significant microvascular or neurologic complication and a 5.1-year increase in survival. When length of life was adjusted for quality of life using utilities for blindness, end-stage renal disease, and lower extremity amputation, the incremental cost per quality-adjusted life year (QALY) gained under intensive insulin therapy was $19 987, which was within the range of other accepted therapeutic interventions in chronic diseases.

A similar probabilistic model was used for type 2 diabetic subjects, assuming that the effects of intensive diabetes treatment observed in type 1 diabetes (hazard rate for complications) can be applied [11]. A lifetime incidence for symptomatic distal neuropathy of 10% under intensive care was estimated, compared to 31% under standard treatment (reduction: 68%). The cumulative incidence of lower extremity amputations also decreased from 15% to 5% (a drop of 67%). Therefore, under intensive care, the predicted average lifetime costs per type 2 diabetic person for neuropathy and lower extremity amputation were $1469 compared to $4381 under standard treatment (difference: $2912). A small randomized clinical trial in middle-aged type 2 diabetic patients in Japan (Kumamoto study) indicated a 60% risk reduction for clinical neuropathy over ten years in subjects receiving intensified versus conventional insulin treatment, yielding 2.2 additional years free of this disorder [12]. Total average direct costs for microvascular, neuropathic, and macrovascular complications combined in the trial patients (hospitalizations, drugs, ophthalmic treatment) were about 50% lower in the intense-treatment group (conventional: $15 565; intense: $7591). Thus, improved glycemic control carries a considerable cost-saving potential with respect to neurologic complications of diabetes.

Methodologic Considerations

There are no representative studies estimating the cost distribution of the various medical problems related to diabetic neuropathy, e. g., paresthesia and pain, neuropathic foot ulcer and amputation, or autonomic dysfunction. It has been stated that this may be a result of the disparate way in which diabetic patients with neuropathy and neuropathy-related complications use health services, e. g., episodes of lower limb complications spread over many different clinical specialties. This points to another methodologic problem in assessing neuropathy-related costs: different specialists will use different diagnostic terms for the same clinical problem, making valid comparisons or data aggregation difficult. Furthermore, in some cases the link between neuropathy and specific symptoms or disorders will be less evident (e. g., autonomic dysfunction of the gastrointestinal or genitourinary tract). Thus, previous studies most likely largely underestimated the economic impact of nerve disorders in diabetes.

■ Costs of Foot Ulcer and Lower-Extremity Amputation

Neuropathy is the major risk factor leading to foot ulceration and lower extremity amputation. Most previous cost-of-illness studies of diabetic foot ulcers and amputations have only estimated direct costs (hospitalizations, procedures, wound care, etc.). Only a few of these economic studies have been performed outside the US (e. g., Sweden, The Netherlands, UK). It is therefore important to note that economic estimates are not applicable to other health care systems and may even not be valid for the same geographic region at different periods (e. g., change in reimbursement, move from acute care to rehabilitation).

Cost-of-Illness Studies: Data Sources

A variety of study approaches have been used to estimate the health care costs of diabetic foot complications. The strengths and weaknesses of the various study designs need to be considered. Center-based studies (e. g., diabetic foot clinics) allow a comprehensive assessment of the total costs in a well-defined population; however, a referral bias towards more severe cases is likely. Large automated databases (health maintenance organizations, private insurance companies) facilitate detailed assessment of procedures in large patient populations. However, diagnoses usually have low specificity (e. g., ICD coding for foot ulcer) and are restricted to persons enrolled in these health insurance plans, who are often younger, healthier, and higher educated than the general population. National data on hospital admissions for diabetic foot complications or amputations are often incomplete and comprise only one cost component. Finally, economic models (decision analyses, Markov models), which have been used to predict long-term economic consequences, depend on the quality of the underlying epidemiologic data. Unfortunately, there are few prospective studies of long-term outcomes of diabetic foot complications. The main results of these studies are summarized in Tables 6.**1**–6.**3**.

Center-Based Studies

In Sweden, Apelquist et al. have found that in diabetic patients in whom primary healing of their foot ulcer could be achieved, outpatient costs were the major cost factor, comprising about two-thirds of total expenditures [13]. As expected, in patients requiring amputations, inpatient costs were more important (83% total costs), leading to about seven-fold higher total average costs than in primary healing. It is noteworthy that in both groups (healed ulcer and amputations) an enormous range and overlap of costs was observed, depending on the individual clinical course of the patients (Table 6.**1**). This should be kept in mind when average costs for treatment of foot complications are calculated, e. g., for reimbursement. Costs in patients with primary healing increased with the severity of the lesions in the Swedish study, e. g., average total costs in patients with deep ulcerations were roughly three-fold higher than those for treatment of superficial ulcers. Thus, from an economic perspective, too, early intervention in foot ulcerations is mandatory. Other risk factors for increased health care costs were a healing time of more than two months and the presence of impaired peripheral circulation.

In the group requiring primary amputation, total costs for patients with minor amputations (US$33 540) were only about two-third of the costs for subjects who underwent major amputations ($50 700), mainly because hospital stays were shorter. It is further noteworthy that average costs were substantially higher for minor amputations than for subjects with primary ulcer healing without amputation, which was due to the longer wound healing periods in this population.

In the same cohort of diabetic patients, the long-term costs over a period of three years were assessed (Table 6.**1**) [14]. Long-term costs for patients with initial primary healing were higher in subjects with critically impaired peripheral circulation, which was mainly due to a higher incidence of new ulcerations. In both patients with initial minor and major amputation, health care costs were substantially higher, which was explained by cost-intensive inpatient care especially during the first year of follow-up. In long-term care, home care and social services became the major cost factors. High expenditures also occurred because of recurrent ulcers and amputations in this high-risk population with a poor prognosis. Almost half of the patients died within the three-year follow-up period.

Maximum limb salvage in patients with severe diabetic foot complications (ischemia, sepsis) can be achieved by prolonged hospital treatment including surgical revascularization. In the United States, at the New England Deaconess Hospital in Boston, the incidence of amputations fell from 44% to 7% from 1984 to 1990 as the result of an intensive multidisciplinary approach [15]. Length of hospital stay, average bypass graft costs (1984: $19 470; 1990: $15 796), and average costs of amputations (1984: $20 248; 1990: $18 341) all decreased over this period. Although quality of care improved and the overall costs decreased, the Medicare reimbursement for foot complications was insufficient, resulting in an overall loss of about $7500 per admission.

Resource use over one year was assessed among 151 patients from a diabetic foot clinic in Belgium, representing the whole range of severity of foot problems [16]. Mean annual costs per ulcer was $5227. The most important cost contributor was inpatient treatment (72%), followed by drugs (11%). The 16 (11%) severe wounds requiring amputations and prolonged hospitalization yielded average mean costs of $31 716, or 80% of total expenditures. Thus, the severity of foot problems determines the costs of treatment. The overall costs of diabetic foot care were largely due to prolonged hospitalization and amputations. There appears to be a shift in major cost areas over time. For patients not requiring amputation, expenses were mainly related to outpatient care. When amputation was required, inpatient care became the major cost factor.

Databases (Health Insurance Companies)

In the US, Holzer et al. have found claims for foot ulcers in 5% of a working-age population (18–64 years) of

Table 6.1 Health care costs of diabetic foot ulcer and amputation: center-based studies

Study (country, year)	Study population and study aims	Outcomes	Costs
Apelquist et al. (Sweden, 1994) [13]	*n* = 314 diabetic patients with foot ulcers treated by a multidisciplinary foot care team Study aims: Short term costs and outcomes of diabetic foot ulcers	Primary healing: *n* = 197 (63%) Amputation: *n* = 77 (24%) Deceased: *n* = 40 (13%) Amputation: minor *n* = 27 (35%) major *n* = 50 (65%)	*Average costs (~ US$, range) in primarily healed patients:* Total costs per patient: $ 6 630 (390–105 040) In-patient care: $ 2 470 (0–10 700) Antibiotics: $ 130 (0–1 560) Outpatient care: Foot care team: $ 650 (260–2 860) Topical treatment: $ 2 990 (0–28 340) Orthop. appliances: $ 390 (0–2 470) *Average costs (~ US$, range) in amputated patients:* Total costs per patient: $ 44 720 (3 510–12 960) In-patient care: Hospital: $ 29 250 (780–66 820) Rehabilitation: $ 7 410 (0–55 380) Antibiotics: $ 390 (0–2 340) Outpatient care Foot care team: $910 (0–3 770) Topical treatment: $ 5 720 (0–2 570) Orthop. appliances: $ 1 170 (0–2 730)
Apelquist et al. (Sweden, 1995) [14]	*n* = 274 diabetic patients with healing from an initial foot ulcer (3 years follow-up) Study aims: Long-term costs and outcomes of diabetic foot ulcers stratified by critical ischemia (toe blood pressure < 45 mmHg, ankle: < 80 mmHg)	*n* = 197 patients with primary healing: Ulcer recurrences: *n* = 99 (50 %) New amputation: *n* = 21 (11 %) Died: *n* = 47 (24 %) *n* = 77 patients with primary amputation: New ulcers: *n* = 41 (53 %) New amputation: *n* = 21 (27 %) Died: *n* = 35 (45 %)	*Total average costs (US$) per patient for health care, home care, social services during three years (adjusted for survival rate, 5 % discount rate):* Primarily healed (without critical ischemia): $ 16 140 Primarily healed (with critical ischemia): $ 26 700 Minor amputation: $ 43 080 Major amputation: $ 63 080 *Total average costs per patient during follow-up:* Year 1: $ 12 470 Inpatient: 35 %, outpatient: 20 %; home care: 45 % Year 2: $ 9 760 Inpatient: 25 %, outpatient: 18%; home care: 57 % Year 3: $ 9 100 Inpatient: 29 %, outpatient: 17%; home care: 54 %

privately insured subjects with diabetes diagnoses (Table 6.**2**) [17]. The average costs per ulcer period of $4 600 were also mainly due to hospital treatment (80 %). Mean costs increased depending on the peripheral vascular status of the patients and the severity of the ulcers. Due to methodologic limitations, the actual magnitude of foot ulcer costs is most likely higher than estimated in this study.

In another study using data from a large health maintenance organization, Ramsey et al. observed an annual incidence of about 2 % of diabetic foot ulcers [18]. Excess care costs during the first year, estimated as the difference of total mean costs compared to subjects without foot ulcer, were substantial (e. g., in males aged 40–64 years: $21 400). The attributable costs for care of diabetic foot ulcers during the first two years after diagnosis were estimated to amount to $28 000 per average foot ulcer patient. Health care costs were already increased prior to the diagnosis, which may be related to comorbidities and diagnostic procedures.

Another economic study, using data from US private health insurance plans, estimated a duration of five weeks for an average episode of care for a diabetic foot

Table 6.**2** Health care costs of diabetic foot ulcer and amputation: results from studies using large administration databases

Study	Study population and study aims	Outcomes	Costs
Holzer et al. (US, 1998) [17]	Claims data for 59 000 diabetic enrollees in private health insurance plans (1991–1992)	n = 3013 diabetic patients with n = 3524 episodes of foot ulcers (episode duration > 7 days)	*Average annual expenditure per diabetic patient:* $ 2 687 Inpatient expenditures: 81% Outpatient expenditures: 18% Outpatient drug expenditures: 2%
	Study aims: Estimation of direct costs and duration of treatment of diabetic foot ulcers	Mean duration of episode: 58 ± 60 days Outcomes of episodes: Primary healing: 52% Osteomyelitis: 33% Gangrene/amputation: 14%	*Average total payments per episode:* $ 4 595 Primary healing: $ 1 929 Osteomyelitis: $ 3 980 Gangrene/amputation: $ 15 792
Ramsey SD et al. (US, 1999) [18]	Continuously enrolled patients of a health maintenance organization (1992–1995) Study aims: Incidence of foot ulcers, risk of serious complications and attributable costs	n = 8905 type 1 and type 2 diabetic patients n = 514 with new-onset foot ulcers Cumulative incidence of foot ulcers: 5.8 % over 3 years Lower extremity amputations: 11 % Amputation in osteomyelitis: 36 % 3-year-mortality (ulcer patients): 28 %	*Annual average direct expenditure (excess costs compared to controls) for representative foot ulcer patient (male, aged 40–64 years):* Before ulcer: $ 15 748 (excess costs: $ 10 821) First year: $ 26 490 (excess costs: $ 21 402) Second year: $ 17 245 (excess costs: $ 12 135) Total 2-year attributable costs of foot ulcers: $ 27 987
Mehta SS et al. (US, 1999) [19]	Claims data of > 200 fee-for-service private insurance plans (1993–1995) Study aims: Determining episodes of care for diabetic foot ulcers	n = 5149 diabetic patients with diagnoses of foot ulcer Average duration of episodes: 5 weeks	*Average incremental costs (compared to usual care)* for an episode of diabetic foot ulcers: Range: $ 900–2 600

ulcer, with an estimated range from 1 to 13 weeks [19]. The costs of care for one episode ranged from $900 to $2600.

Using Medicare claims data from 1995 to 1996, expenditures for diabetic lower extremity ulcer patients have been estimated to be on average three times higher than costs among Medicare patients in general ($15 309 vs $5226), accounting for $15 billion in 1995 for the whole US Medicare system [20]. In line with other studies, most of the costs accrued on the inpatient side (73.7 %).

Although these cost estimates were based on selected populations using less specific diagnostic data, they provide a useful impression of the enormous economic impact of diabetic foot ulcerations in the health care system.

Hospital-Based Studies

Because hospitalization is the major cost factor in diabetic foot care, a number of studies have investigated this sector in more detail. In the Netherlands, about 20 % of all hospitalizations in the diabetic population have been estimated to be related to diabetic foot complications, which was similar to the findings of a previous study from the US [21]. As expected, length of hospital stay (LOS) was the most important cost determinant. Average LOS for diabetic foot problems was 40 days in 1988 in Dutch hospitals, resulting in total costs of about 39 million ECU (US$53 million) (Table 6.**3**). Amputation was performed in one out of three of these elderly diabetic patients, mainly depending on the presence of osteomyelitis and on ulcer severity. LOS was significantly higher in patients who underwent an amputation (7.5 weeks), but was still five weeks on average even without amputation.

Another more recent study from the Netherlands found an average LOS of 42 days per hospitalization for diabetes-related lower extremity amputations in 1992, which was lower than in the previous study (50 days) [22]. Average hospital costs per amputation were estimated as US$15 330. Costs increased significantly with the age of the patients, a higher level of amputation, and the presence of multiple amputations.

In the US, about 60 000 diabetes-related amputations were performed per year [23]. The direct medical annual costs have been estimated at $300–$500 million. Direct mean hospital charges for primary amputations ranged from $20 000 to $28 000. The average LOS for diabetes-related amputations was shorter in the US (16–40 days) than in the Netherlands. It is note-

Table 6.**3** Health care costs for hospital treatment of diabetic foot ulcer and amputation

Study	Study population and study aims	Outcomes	Costs
Bouter et al. (Netherlands, 1993) [21]	National Dutch Information System on Hospital Care (1988–1989) Study aims: Number of hospitalizations due to diabetic foot, number of hospital days and amputations, discharge to rehabilitation center or nursing home	*n* = 3707 patients (1988) *n* = 3790 patients (1989) hospitalized for diabetic foot (20 % hospitalization in diabetic population; 32 % with amputations) Length of stay: 40 days With amputation: 53 days Without amputation: 34 days In-hospital mortality: 10 % Rehab. center, nursing home: 10%	*Total hospital costs in the Netherlands (1988, US$)* All patients: $ 46.3 million With amputation: $ 19.8 million Without amputation: $ 26.5 million
Van Houtum et al. (Netherlands, 1995) [22]	Nationwide data on diabetes-related lower extremity amputations (1992) Study aims: Duration of hospitalization and costs of diabetes-related lower extremity amputations	*n* = 1575 hospitalizations of diabetic subjects for *n* = 1810 diabetes-related amputations Total hospital days (diabetic population): 65 778 Average length of stay: 41.8 days	*Mean costs (US$) for a hospitalization for diabetes-related lower extremity amputation:* $ 17 674 *Total nationwide costs for amputations:* Diabetic population:$ 28 million Nondiabetic population: $ 24 million
Currie et al. (UK, 1998) [7]	Hospital admission among 408 000 people in Wales (1991–1995) Study aims: Relative risk of hospitalization for peripheral vascular disease, neuropathy, and amputations (diabetic vs nondiabetic) and related costs	*n* = 86 diabetic patients with hospital admission for chronic skin ulcer, average duration: 25.3 days *n* = 112 hospitalizations among diabetic patients with amputations of legs, feet, or toes	*Total hospital costs for chronic skin ulcer (4 years):* Diabetic population: $ 424 083 Percentage total costs: 22 % Mean costs per admission: $ 3301 Average costs per 1000 population: $ 1189

worthy that among African Americans the average LOS and costs of amputations were substantially higher, which can be explained by a higher prevalence of comorbidities (coronary heart disease, nephropathy) [23].

In the UK diabetic population, mean costs for hospital admission for chronic ulcer of the skin were estimated as US$3300, with an average LOS of 25 days [7]. In this population-based study, mean annual costs of $1190 were estimated per 1000 head of population for hospital care of chronic foot ulcer. Costs of hospital treatment for chronic skin ulcer in the US were higher than in the UK, e. g., average Medicare charges were $10 200 and private insurance charges amounted to $12 000, although LOS in the US was shorter (12vs18 days) [24].

Further Studies on Costs of Diabetic Foot Complications

The recently completed CODE-2 (Costs of Diabetes in Europe–Type 2) study, which aimed to assess direct and indirect costs of type 2 diabetic patients in eight European countries using comparable methodology, is expected to give further insights into the economic burden of diabetic neuropathy, foot ulcer, and amputation. The German part of CODE-2 indicated that amputation was the most costly complication in type 2 diabetes (mean annual costs per patient in 1998: US$11 640; range: $8760–14 830), followed by costs for patients with ulcer or gangrene ($8 130). Mean annual costs in type 2 diabetic patients with amputation were six times higher than costs in patients without complications (ulcer/gangrene carried four-fold higher costs) [25].

In New Zealand, nationwide hospital discharges for diabetic foot complications were estimated as 26 per 100 000 general population, accounting for about US$8 million per year [26].

In an attempt to provide cost estimates for various diabetic complications in the US, O'Brien et al. analyzed various data sources [27]. They estimated average acute hospital costs in 1996 of $9910 for foot ulcers, and about $18 600 for first and $19 000 for subsequent lower extremity amputations. The total event costs for an amputation including revisions, rehabilitation, and prosthesis were estimated as approximately $27 000.

There are a few studies from European countries; e. g., in France, nationwide annual costs of incident diabetic foot problems were estimated to amount to about $700 per year (4–6% of total diabetes-related costs) [28].

Economic Modeling: Benefits of Prevention

The costs of preventive strategies to avoid diabetic foot ulcerations and amputations in primary medical care are low compared to the enormous potential cost savings. Foot exams to detect high-risk patients can be easily performed with low technical costs, e. g., the costs of a monofilament are less than US$25 [29]. Debridement of nails and callus is also low-expenditure, and the costs for one pair of therapeutic shoes are up to US$500. The economic evaluation of a diabetic foot screening and protection program implemented at a local diabetes center in the UK showed that the program was cost-effective due to amputations averted [30].

The potential economic benefits of comprehensive lower extremity amputation prevention programs in diabetic patients have been assessed for the US health care system for a hypothetical cohort of 10 000 diabetic patients [31]. The model parameters were derived from a variety of studies, e. g., the annual cumulative incidence of first lower extremity amputation in patients with foot ulcer was assumed to be 4.8%. The potential economic benefits for prevention of lower extremity amputation were largest for educational interventions, followed by therapeutic shoe coverage and a multidisciplinary clinical approach (diabetologist, orthopedic and vascular surgeon, podiatrist, nurse). Economic benefits of various strategies ranged from $2.0 to $3.0 million, or $2 900 to $4 400 per person with history of foot ulcer over a study period of three years. Benefits were substantially higher in elderly diabetic patients above 70 years of age. Although the current evidence of effectiveness for some of these preventive efforts is relatively limited (e. g., education), this hypothetical model indicates an enormous cost-saving potential.

Cost-Effective Treatment of Diabetic Foot Ulcers

Economic analyses not only assess disease-related costs but also compare costs and outcomes of different treatment alternatives. Studies of cost-effectiveness or cost-utility (including quality of life) of the various treatment strategies for diabetic foot ulcers are rare, probably because they are subject to a number of methodologic problems. The prognosis of foot ulcers depends on a variety of factors, e. g., type of lesion, severity of infection, and extent of peripheral vascular disease, which makes valid comparisons of therapeutic strategies difficult. Randomized clinical trials are not ethical for solving some therapeutic controversies (e. g., amputation versus conservative treatment of deep infected foot ulcers).

One example of a comprehensive economic evaluation is a decision and cost-utility analysis of various diagnostic and therapeutic procedures in foot infections and suspected osteomyelitis in type 2 diabetes [32]. In patients with deep infected ulcers, a long course of antibiotic therapy following initial hospitalization for surgical debridement was predicted to be the preferred strategy. With respect to diagnostic tests, additional magnetic resonance imaging or scanning was not more cost-effective than roentgenography of the feet.

Another economic analysis of various topical treatments of diabetic foot ulcers indicated that the major factors were related to staff costs (nurses) and the travel expenses of the patients [33]. The costs of ulcer dressings mainly depended on the frequency of dressing changes per week (e. g., superficial ulcers: hydrocolloid dressing: two changes per week; dry saline gauze: nine changes per week).

There are few economic studies assessing the cost-effectiveness of growth factor treatment compared to conventional wound therapy in diabetic foot ulcers [34]. Recently, a cost-effectiveness analysis was performed comparing a recombinant growth factor preparation approved by the Food and Drug Administration and a platelet releasate with standard care [35]. Effectiveness was assessed as the percentage of ulcers healed at 20 weeks after the start of treatment. Under standard care ulcers healed in 31% of patients, compared to 43% with the growth factor and 37% with platelet releasate. The incremental costs of increasing the odds of healing by 1% over standard therapy were $37 for growth factor application and $414 for the releasate, which speaks in favor of growth factor therapy in diabetic foot ulcers.

The cost-effectiveness of living, metabolically active, tissue-engineered human dermis delivering growth factors for wound healing in diabetic foot ulcers was recently modeled for the French health care system [36]. Treatment costs were substantially higher compared to standard care; however, because of an increased healing rate, the average costs per healed ulcer were slightly lower when using graft treatment (FFr53 522 vs FFr 56687).

There are very few studies assessing the cost-benefit of preventive measures in diabetic foot care. With respect to therapeutic footwear, Medicare's evaluation of therapeutic shoes for diabetic patients found the provision to be cost-neutral [37]; studies in other health care settings have not been performed.

Conclusions

Although several studies have indicated that costs are high both for healed ulcers and amputations, comparisons are problematic because of differences in study designs and health care settings [38]. Because patients have often not been followed until the occurrence of complete healing in these investigations, the total cost related to diabetic foot ulcerations and amputations within the health care systems have even been underestimated. Future cost-effectiveness analyses of diabetic foot care also need to take into account long-term costs, e. g., those of rehabilitation, permanent disability, and recurrent ulcers or amputations. The most cost-effective management appears to be prevention of amputations [38]. Unfortunately, treatment of acute ulcers is reimbursed within the health care systems to a greater extent than preventive strategies such as foot care and protective shoes.

Indirect Consequences: Disability and Premature Death

From an economic perspective, the indirect costs of a disease are mostly estimated as loss of work time due to temporary or permanent disability or to premature death. There have been no efforts to estimate total indirect costs related to diabetic neuropathy or diabetic foot complications. It can be assumed that indirect costs (work absenteeism, loss of working years) comprise a smaller proportion than direct medical expenditures, because the majority of diabetic subjects with foot ulcerations, who are on average above 65 years of age, are already retired. Furthermore, intangible costs due to pain, suffering, and inconvenience are difficult to quantify, although they comprise the substantial part of the overall burden from the viewpoint of the affected individuals.

Diabetic neuropathy, especially cardiovascular autonomic neuropathy, is associated with increased mortality [39]. Diabetic foot ulcers were also associated with a poor prognosis, which could not be explained by factors directly related to the ulceration (e. g., infection), but was mainly due to cardiovascular events [40,41]. Mortality is even higher in subjects who have undergone an amputation. The standardized mortality rate compared to the general population was twice as high in foot ulcer patients with primary healing and four times as high among subjects who had undergone amputation. Mortality after lower extremity amputations is already high during the hospital stay, ranging from 5% to 23% of diabetic amputees [42]. This postoperative mortality is high compared to that associated with other major surgical procedures performed in elderly patients (e. g., 1.2% after total hip arthroplasty).

The five-year survival rate after lower extremity amputation in diabetic patients has been reported to be only 40–60% [43]. Coronary heart disease is the most frequent cause of death [44]. A significant number of diabetic patients die or require long-term care following amputation: in a study from the US, over 25% of diabetic amputees were discharged to an institutional care facility, including 19% to a nursing home [42]. Only 2% of these subjects were in a care facility before their amputation. Patients discharged to nursing homes were often elderly subjects living alone with high-level amputations and advanced cerebrovascular disease. In addition, many younger amputees are unable to return to full-time employment. The economic consequences of these conditions, both from the societal and the patient's perspective, have not been assessed.

Socioeconomic Status, Diabetic Neuropathy, and Foot Ulcer

There is growing evidence of a socioeconomic gradient in morbidity and mortality in the diabetic population. In general, persons with type 2 diabetes have less education and lower income levels than the nondiabetic population [45]. Low socioeconomic status (SES) as classified by job titles has been associated with a doubling of all-cause and cardiovascular mortality rates in diabetic patients [46]. This difference has been mainly explained by higher rates of smoking and higher blood pressure in the lowest socioeconomic groups; glycemic control had little impact. Furthermore, diabetic complications like proliferative retinopathy and macroalbuminuria are more prevalent in primary-educated than in college-educated male type 1 diabetic patients, even after glycemic control, diabetes duration, and blood pressure are taken into account [47].

The association of social factors and SES with diabetic neuropathy has not been intensively studied. SES has not been evaluated in prospective studies of risk factors for diabetic neuropathy. In a population-based cross-sectional study in adult type 1 diabetic patients, reduced vibration sensitivity (tuning fork) and foot complications were more prevalent in people with low SES, as assessed by an additive score of educational and employment level and household income [48]. Among known and potential risk factors for diabetic neuropathy, lower social class was associated with higher HbA_{1c} values, increased cigarette pack – years, and more uncontrolled blood pressure. Differential access to health care was not observed with respect to foot examinations in this study: there was no association between low SES and fewer foot examinations during the preceding year.

The results of this study in type 1 diabetic patients were not confirmed by a population-based survey in the Netherlands mainly including type 2 patients [49]. Diabetic subjects with a low level of education had a worse outcome of all complications combined. However, symptoms of sensitivity loss did not differ in the various educational categories. In line with this finding, no association of symptoms of sensory neuropathy among subjects with type 2 diabetes with low educational level was observed in a representative survey in the US [50]. However, diabetic subjects with neuropathy had a lower family income, another indicator of low SES. There are conflicting results about the association of SES with glycemic control, the major risk factor for diabetic neuropathy. Most studies, including data from the US National Health and Nutrition Examination Survey, found no relation between glycemic control and socioeconomic factors [51].

Social and racial factors have been found to be related to foot ulcer and amputation. Among minorities in the US (African Americans, Hispanic persons, Native Americans), the prevalence of type 2 diabetes and of diabetic patients with retinopathy and nephropathy was found to be two to six times higher than in the white American population [52]. African Americans with diabetes have higher amputation rates and a twofold increased mortality related to amputations than do whites. Pima Indians have about four times more amputations than the white population. Socioeconomic factors may be a strong underlying factor given that a large proportion of these minorities have low educational levels and are living in poverty.

There were few reports on the prevalence of diabetic neuropathy in minorities. In a national survey in the US, no association of prevalence of symptoms of sensory neuropathy with ethnicity was found [50]. This result was consistent with the San Luis Valley Study, in which, too, no effect of Hispanic heritage on prevalence of neuropathy was seen [53]. However, in these two studies the presence of neuropathy was not assessed using a detailed neurologic examination.

Among social factors, a lack of social connectedness was associated with an increased risk for amputation [29]. Diabetic patients with foot ulcer were more often living alone. It is conceivable that these mostly elderly subjects have impaired vision and limited mobility, increasing the likelihood of trauma by inappropriate self-performed foot care. In preventive care of foot ulcers and amputation, these social factors should be taken into account.

■ Health-Related Quality of Life and Diabetic Neuropathy

Quality of life increasingly influences every aspect of diabetes care. Basic elements of quality of life assessment include physical, psychologic, and social well-being, as well as the effects of disease on personal functioning. In persons with diabetes, daily treatment and acute and late complications have a major impact on quality of life [54].

Health-related quality of life can be evaluated using generic or disease-specific questionnaires. Global questionnaires like the Medical Outcomes Study SF-36 aim for comparisons across different diseases; however, to compare the impact of different therapeutic interventions within a particular disease, disease-specific measures are more appropriate. Diabetes-specific questionnaires and global tools may give complementary information [55].

The impact of diabetic neuropathy, diabetic foot ulcers, or amputation on quality of life has not been intensively investigated. Currently, no validated disease-specific questionnaire is available for these conditions; several attempts are currently under way to develop adequate instruments [56].

Quality of Life and Peripheral Neuropathy

The generic Medical Outcomes Study SF-36 questionnaire was used to assess self-rated health in the population-based longitudinal Wisconsin Epidemiologic Study of Diabetic Retinopathy [57]. In both younger-onset and older-onset diabetic patients, a higher sensory neuropathy score was strongly inversely related with the SF-36 scales for general health, physical functioning, and physical role. Other factors associated with diminished self-rated health included cardiovascular disease, proteinuria, end-stage renal disease, amputation, and retinopathy in young-onset diabetes, whereas in older-onset diabetes, in particular, cardiovascular disease and sensory neuropathy were important predictors of reduced self-perceived health. Elderly diabetic patients with symptomatic neuropathy in particular have a significant functional impairment in most areas of daily life [58].

Painful neuropathy has a considerable impact on quality of life. In a hospital-based study in the UK, type 1 and type 2 diabetic patients with symptomatic peripheral neuropathy were investigated using another generic tool, the Nottingham Health Profile [59]. Problems in patients with symptomatic nerve disorders were sleep disorders, loss of overall energy, and reduced physical mobility. This was not surprising, because pain is associated with anxiety, depression, and loss of mobility in general, all contributing to diminished perception of well-being. Painful diabetic neuropathy appears to have a substantial impact in particular on two quality of life items, sleep and enjoyment of life, whereas work, recreational, and social activities are less disrupted [60]. Substantial severity of pain interferes with all basic activities. Therefore, quality of life is an important outcome measure in clinical trials. Quality of life measures are increasingly used to assess the effects of pharmacologic treatment for painful diabetic neuropathy. Substances like gabapentin [61] or tramadol [62] have been shown to improve scores on SF-36 and other instruments to evaluate improved daily living.

Quality of Life, Foot Ulcer, and Amputation

The literature on diabetic foot complications often contain statements that the impact on the patient is devastating, a statement mostly based on clinical experience rather than quality of life research [63,64]. A high incidence of depressive symptoms has been observed in persons with lower limb amputations [65]. In particular, during the preoperative and immediate postoperative period, patients are at increased risk of depression [63]. After the return home, the physical and emotional impact of amputation on the primary caregivers, usually the patient's spouse, can be enormous. Subjects who are wearing a prosthesis often have a high level of social isolation and are at increased risk of psychiatric disorders [66].

The quality of life of diabetic patients with chronic foot ulcer may even be poorer than that of diabetic subjects who have undergone an amputation [65]. Patients with foot ulcers were more depressed and dissatisfied with their current situation. The emotional and functional adjustments of patients with active foot ulcers appear to be similar to those made by amputees. Using the generic SF-36, scores for subjects with foot ulcers were worse than for those with previous amputations [32].

In an attempt to develop a specific quality of life questionnaire for diabetic patients with lower extremity ulcers, the broad important domains were recently identified [67]. There was a major restriction on daily life due to the loss of mobility. Mobility limitations negatively influenced all domains of quality of life. The loss of mobility affected the ability to perform a number of daily activities such as shopping or bathing [64]. Foot ulcerations also made participation in leisure activities more difficult or even impossible. The major emotional reactions were anger and frustration, guilt about becoming a burden to others, and worry about the future compounded by the uncertainty surrounding the ulcer healing process. A completely different lifestyle affecting the whole social network of the patients was necessary. The requirement for the affected foot to be non-weight-bearing was the major burden. Other issues were tensions between the patient and their primary caregivers, e. g., the spouse, and the amount of planning involved in care because of the reduced mobility. Perceived dependence of patients on their family members was a constant source of tensions in family life [64]. It is noteworthy that there was a lack of platforms to express the emotional strains resulting from the foot ulcerations [67].

Finally, there are also adverse economic effects [64]. About half of the patients with foot ulcers who had not previously been retired were no longer in work, and the remaining subjects were aware of a loss of productivity limiting their career advancement, which resulted in diminished self-esteem. All patients had substantial additional expenses, e. g., travel costs due to frequent hospital appointments and contributory payments for medical devices (shoes, medications, wound care). This further contributed to the fact that diabetic patients with active foot ulcers expressed a negative attitude towards their feet [68].

Psychological Aspects of Preventive Care

A better understanding of the quality of life of patients with foot ulcers should result in improved support from physicians and other health care professionals. However, the effects of psychologic factors such as patients' attitudes and personality on their adherence to treatment recommendations and preventive measures against diabetic foot complications have not been intensively studied [69]. It appears that information alone is not sufficient to change patient behavior. Patients who have previously suffered foot ulceration follow foot care recommendations more closely, although they had the same level of information about preventive care as subjects without ulceration [69]. Patients' belief in their own vulnerability to this complication may deeply affect their adherence to medical treatment. Unfortunately, physicians, too, are more likely to provide preventive foot care in patients with a history of ulcerations; the presence of neuropathy alone was not sufficient to prompt intensive care [70].

Burden to the Patient

In considering the socioeconomics of diabetic neuropathy we must not overlook the significant unhappiness which occurs as a result of this disease. This unhappiness is best illustrated by statements from patients who have been involved in studies of lifestyle adjustments in diabetes (J. Ward; unpublished material):

"I am self-employed; my income has gone. There is no future."

"It worries me about what is going to happen in the future. By that I mean if they are going to chop off a few more parts" (neuropathic foot ulceration).

"You suffer in silence. You can't explain to some people how you are feeling some days."

"There is a big problem in that I sometimes worry about what is going to happen to me – I am my wife's full-time career."

"If I do go out, and they get a wheelchair for me this makes me feel terrible – I am reliant on somebody and feeling a burden."

"I can't examine my feet, for I am partially sighted due to the diabetes."

The expression of such emotions should spur diabetic professionals, not only to ensure adequate provisions of resources to help people with diabetic neuropathy, but also to stimulate deeper thought into the causation and prevention of nerve damage.

References

[1] American Diabetes Association. Economic consequences of diabetes mellitus in the U.S. in 1997. Diabetes Care 1998; 21:296–309.

[2] Jacobs J, Sena M, Fox N. The cost of hospitalization for the late complications of diabetes in the United States. Diabet Med 1991; 8: S23–S29.

[3] Huse DM, Oster G, Killen AR, Lacey MJ, Colditz GA. The economic costs of non-insulin-dependent diabetes mellitus. JAMA 1989; 262: 2708–13.

[4] Selby JV, Ray GT, Zhang D, Colby CJ. Excess costs of medical care for patients with diabetes in a managed care population. Diabetes Care 1997; 20: 1396–1402.

[5] Thomas PK. Diabetic peripheral neuropathies: their cost to patient and society and the value of knowledge of risk factors for development of interventions. Eur Neurol 1999; 41(suppl 1): 35–43.

[6] Gray A, Fenn P, McGuire A. The cost of insulin-dependent diabetes mellitus (IDDM) in England and Wales. Diabet Med 1995; 12: 1068–76.

[7] Currie CJ, Morgan CL, Peters JR. The epidemiology and cost of inpatient care for peripheral vascular disease, infection, neuropathy, and ulceration in diabetes. Diabetes Care 1998; 21: 42–8.

[8] Rathmann W, Haastert B, Roseman JM, Gries FA, Giani G. Prescription drug use and costs among diabetic patients in primary health care practices in Germany. Diabetes Care 1998; 21: 389–97.

[9] Rathmann W, Haastert B, Giani G. Drug prescriptions and costs in the treatment of diabetic polyneuropathy [in German]. Dtsch Med Wochenschr 1999; 124: 681–6.

[10] The Diabetes Control and Complications Trial Research Group. Lifetime benefits and costs of intensive therapy as practiced in the Diabetes Control and Complications Trial. JAMA 1996; 276: 1409–15.

[11] Eastman RC, Javitt JC, Herman WH, Dasbach EJ, Copley-Merriman C, Maier W, et al. Model of complications of NIDDM. II. Analysis of the health benefits and cost-effectiveness of treating NIDDM with the goal of normoglycemia. Diabetes Care 1997; 20: 735–44.

[12] Wake N, Hishige A, Katayama T, Kishikawa H, Ohkubo Y, Sakai M et al. Cost-effectiveness of intensive insulin therapy for type 2 diabetes: a 10-year follow-up of the Kumamoto study. Diabetes Res Clin Pract 2000; 48: 201–10.

[13] Apelqvist J, Ragnarson-Tennvall G, Persson U, Larsson J. Diabetic foot ulcers in a multidisciplinary setting. An economic analysis of primary healing and healing with amputation. J Intern Med 1994; 235: 463–71.

[14] Apelqvist J, Ragnarson-Tennvall G, Larsson J, Persson U. Long-term costs for foot ulcers in diabetic patients in a multidisciplinary setting. Foot Ankle Int 1995; 16: 388–95.

[15] Gibbons GW, Marcaccio EJ, Burgess AM, Pomposelli FB, Freeman DV, Campbell DR, et al. Improved quality of diabetic foot care, 1984 vs 1990. Reduced length of stay and costs, insufficient reimbursement. Arch Surg 1993; 128: 576–81.

[16] van Acker K, Oleen-Burkey M, de Decker L, Vanmaele R, van Schil P, Matricali G, Dys H, de Leeuw D. Cost and resource utilization for prevention and treatment of foot lesions in a diabetic foot clinic in Belgium. Diabetes Res Clin Pract 2000; 50: 87–95.

[17] Holzer SE, Camerota A, Martens L, Cuerdon T, Crystal-Peters J, Zagari M. Costs and duration of care for lower extremity ulcers in patients with diabetes. Clin Ther 1998; 20: 169–81.

[18] Ramsey SD, Newton K, Blough D, McCulloch DK, Sandhu N, Reiber GE, et al. Incidence, outcomes, and cost of foot ulcers in patients with diabetes. Diabetes Care 1999; 22: 382–7.

[19] Mehta SS, Suzuki S, Glick HA, Schulman KA. Determining an episode of care using claims data. Diabetic foot ulcer. Diabetes Care 1999; 22: 1110–15.

[20] Harrington C, Zagari MJ, Corea J, Klitenic J. A cost analysis of diabetic lower-extremity ulcers. Diabetes Care 2000; 23: 1333–8.

[21] Bouter KP, Storm AJ, de Groot RRM, Uitslager R, Erkelens DW, Diepersloot RJA. The diabetic foot in Dutch hospitals: epidemiological features and clinical outcome. Eur J Med 1993; 2: 215–18.

[22] Van Houtum WH, Lavery LA, Harkless LB. The costs of diabetes-related lower extremity amputations in the Netherlands. Diabet Med 1995; 12: 777–81.

[23] Ashry HR, Lavery LA, Armstrong DG, Lavery DC, van Houtum WH. Cost of diabetes-related amputations in minorities. J Foot Ankle Surg 1998; 37: 186–90.

[24] Reiber GE, Boyko EJ, Smith DG. Lower extremity foot ulcers and amputations in diabetes. In: National Diabetes Data Group. Diabetes in America. 2nd edition. NIH Publication No 95-1468, 1995: 409–28.

[25] Liebl A, Goertz A, Spannheimer A, Reitberger U, Renner R. Estimating costs of diabetes-related complications [abstract]. Exp Clin Endocrinol Diabetes 2000; 108(suppl 1): S163

[26] Payne CB, Scott RS. Hospital discharges for diabetic foot disease in New Zealand: 1980–1993. Diabetes Res Clin Pract 1998; 39: 69–74.

[27] O'Brien JA, Shomphe LA, Kavanagh PL, Raggio G, Caro JJ. Direct medical costs of complications resulting from type 2 diabetes in the U.S. Diabetes Care 1998; 21: 1122–8.

[28] Halimi S, Banhamou PY, Charras H. Incidence and cost of the diabetic foot in France: first data [in French]. Diabete Metab 1993; 19: 518–22.

[29] Mayfield JA, Reiber GE, Sanders LJ, Janisse D, Pogach LM. Preventive foot care in people with diabetes. Diabetes Care 1998; 21: 2161–77.

[30] McCabe CJ, Stevenson RC, Dolan AM. Evaluation of a diabetic foot screening and protection programme. Diabet Med 1998; 15: 80–4.

[31] Ollendorf DA, Kotsanos JG, Wishner WJ, Friedman M, Cooper T, Bittoni M, et al. Potential economic benefits of lower-extremity amputation prevention strategies in diabetes. Diabetes Care 1998; 21: 1240–5.

[32] Eckman MH, Greenfield S, Mackey WC, Wong JB, Kaplan S, Sullivan L, et al. Foot infections in diabetic patients. Decision and cost-effectiveness analyses. JAMA 1995; 273: 712–20.

[33] Apelqvist J, Ragnarson-Tennvall G, Larsson J. Topical treatment of diabetic foot ulcers: an economic analysis of treatment alternatives and strategies. Diabet Med 1995; 12: 123–8.

[34] Vogt PM, Peter FW, Topsakal E, Torres A, Steinau HU. Applications for polypeptide growth factors—experimental, clinical and financial aspects (in German). Chirurg 1998; 69: 1197–206.

[35] Kantor J, Margolis DJ. Treatment options for diabetic neuropathic foot ulcers: a cost-effectiveness analysis. Dermatol Surg 2001; 27: 347–51.
[36] Allenet B, Paree F, Lebrun T, Carr L, Posnett J, Martini J, Yvon C. Cost-effectiveness modeling of Dermagraft for the treatment of diabetic foot ulcers in the French context. Diabetes Metab 2000; 26: 125–32.
[37] Wooldridge J, Moreno L. Evaluation of the costs to Medicare of covering therapeutic shoes for diabetic patients. Diabetes Care 1994; 17: 541–7.
[38] Apelquist J, Larsson. What is the most effective way to reduce incidence of amputation in the diabetic foot? Diabetes Metab Res Rev 2000; 16(suppl 1): S75–S83.
[39] Ziegler D. Diabetic cardiovascular autonomic neuropathy: prognosis, diagnosis and treatment. Diabetes Metab Rev 1994; 10: 339–83.
[40] Apelqvist J, Larsson J, Agardh CD. Long-term prognosis for diabetic patients with foot ulcers. J Intern Med 1993; 233: 485–91.
[41] Boyko EJ, Ahroni JH, Smith DG, Davignon D. Increased mortality associated with diabetic foot ulcer. Diabet Med 1996; 13: 967–72.
[42] Lavery LA, van Houtum WH, Armstrong DG. Institutionalization following diabetes-related lower extremity amputation. Am J Med 1997; 103: 383–8.
[43] Frykberg RG, Arora S, Pomposelli FB, LoGerfo F. Functional outcome in the elderly following lower extremity amputation. J Foot Ankle Surg 1998; 37: 181–5.
[44] Faglia E, Favales F, Morabito A. New ulceration, new major amputation, and survival rates in diabetic subjects hospitalized for foot ulceration from 1990 to 1993. A 6.5 year follow-up. Diabetes Care 2001; 24: 78–83.
[45] Cowie CC, Eberhardt MS. Sociodemographic characteristics of persons with diabetes. In: National Diabetes Data Group. Diabetes in America. 2nd edition. National Institutes of Health Publication no. 95-1468; 1995: 85–101.
[46] Chaturvedi N, Jarret J, Shipley MJ, Fuller JH. Socioeconomic gradient in morbidity and mortality in people with diabetes: cohort study findings from the Whitehall study and the WHO multinational study of vascular disease in diabetes. BMJ 1998; 316: 100–5.
[47] Chaturvedi N, Stephenson JM, Fuller JH. The relationship between socioeconomic status and diabetes control and complications in the EURODIAB IDDM complications study. Diabetes Care 1996; 19: 423–30.
[48] Mühlhauser I, Overmann H, Bender R, Bott U, Jörgens V, Trautner C, et al. Social status and the quality of care for adult people with type I (insulin-dependent) diabetes mellitus – a population-based study. Diabetologia 1998; 41: 1139–50.
[49] van der Meer JBW, Mackenbach JP. The care and course of diabetes: differences according to level of education. Health Policy 1999; 46: 127–41.
[50] Harris M, Eastman R, Cowie C. Symptoms of sensory neuropathy in adults with NIDDM in the U.S. population. Diabetes Care 1993; 16: 1446–52.
[51] Harris MI, Eastman RC, Cowie CC, Flegal KM, Eberhardt MS. Racial and ethnic differences in glycemic control of adults with type 2 diabetes. Diabetes Care 1999; 22: 403–8.
[52] Carter JS, Pugh JA, Monterrosa A. Non-insulin-dependent diabetes mellitus in minorities in the United States. Ann Intern Med 1996; 125: 221–32.
[53] Franklin GM, Kahn LB, Baxter J, Marshall JA, Hamman RF. Sensory neuropathy in non-insulin-dependent diabetes mellitus. Am J Epidemiol 1990; 131: 633–43.
[54] Rubin RR, Peyrot M. Quality of life and diabetes. Diabetes Metab Res Rev 1999; 15: 205–18.
[55] Anderson RM, Fitzgerald JT, Wisdom K, Davis WK, Hiss RG. A comparison of global versus disease-specific quality-of-life measures in patients with NIDDM. Diabetes Care 1997; 20: 299–305.
[56] Vileikyte L, Bundy C, Tomenson B, Walsh T, Boulton AJM. Neuropathy-specific quality of life measure: construction of scales and preliminary tests of reliability and validity [abstract]. Diabetes 1998; 47(suppl 1): A44.
[57] Klein BEK, Klein R, Moss SE. Self-rated health and diabetes of long duration. The Wisconsin Epidemiologic Study of Diabetic Retinopathy. Diabetes Care 1998; 21: 236–40.
[58] Ahroni JH, Boyko EJ, Davignon DR, Pecoraro RE. The health and functional status of veterans with diabetes. Diabetes Care 1994; 17: 318–21.
[59] Benbow SJ, Wallymahmed ME, MacFarlane IA. Diabetic peripheral neuropathy and quality of life. Q J Med 1998; 91: 733–7.
[60] Galer BS, Gianas A, Jensen MP. Painful diabetic neuropathy: epidemiology, pain description, and quality of life. Diabetes Res Clin Pract 2000; 47: 123–8.
[61] Backonja M, Beydoum A, Edwards KR, Schwartz SL, Fonseca V, Hes M, et al. Gabapentin for the symptomatic treatment of painful neuropathy in patients with diabetes mellitus. JAMA 1998; 280: 1831–6.
[62] Harati Y, Gooch C, Swenson M, Edelman S, Greene D, Raskin P. Double-blind randomized trial of tramadol for the treatment of the pain of diabetic neuropathy. Neurology 1998; 50: 1842–6.
[63] Price P, Harding K. The impact of foot complications on health-related quality of life in patients with diabetes. J Cutan Med Surg 2000; 4: 45–50.
[64] Vileikyte L. Diabetic foot ulcers: a quality of life issue. Diabetes Metab Res Rev 2001; 17: 246–9.
[65] Carrington AL, Mawdsley SKV, Morley M, Kincey J, Boulton AJM. Psychological status of diabetic people with or without lower limb disability. Diabetes Res Clin Pract 1996; 32: 19–25.
[66] Thompson DM, Haran D. Living with an amputation: what it means for patients and their helpers. Int J Rehab Res 1984; 7: 283–92.
[67] Brod M. Quality of life issues in patients with diabetes and lower extremity ulcers: patients and care givers. Qual Life Res 1998; 7: 365–72.
[68] Tennvall GR, Apelquist J. Health-related quality of life in patients with diabetes mellitus and foot ulcers. J Diabetes Complications 2000; 14: 235–41.
[69] Vileikyte L. Psychological aspects of diabetic peripheral neuropathy. Diabetes Rev 1999; 7: 387–94.
[70] Del Aguila MA, Reiber GE, Koepsell TD. How does provider and patient awareness of high risk status for lower-extremity amputation influence foot-care practice? Diabetes Care 1994; 17: 1050–4.

7 Recommendations for Structured Care

F.A. Gries, P.A. Low, and D. Ziegler

Introduction

Diabetic neuropathy (DN) is as frequent as microvascular complications of diabetes mellitus. It includes manifestations in the somatic and autonomic parts of the peripheral nervous system [1,25]. Distal symmetric sensory or sensorimotor polyneuropathy (DSP) is the most important clinical manifestation, affecting approximately 30% of the hospital-based diabetic population and 20% of community-based samples of diabetic patients. DSP is related to both lower extremity impairments, such as diminished position sense, and functional limitations, such as walking ability [2]. Neuropathic symptoms are present in 15–20% of diabetic patients, 7.5% of whom experience chronic neuropathic pain [3]. Elevated vibration perception threshold predicts the development of neuropathic foot ulceration, one of the most common causes of hospital admission and lower limb amputation among diabetic patients [4] (Fig. 7.**1**). Autonomic neuropathy is similar in importance to DSP. There is accumulating evidence to suggest that markers of DN such as nerve conduction velocity, vibration perception threshold, and autonomic function tests predict mortality in diabetic patients [5,6].

Obviously the impact of DN on the quality of life and prognosis of the diabetic patient and its economic burden are important. However, while screening and monitoring of microangiopathies and macroangiopathy has become established as routine in diabetes care, DN is often neglected. Even the Saint Vincent Declaration of 1989 [7], which among other things has goals for prevention of amputations, myocardial infarction, and eye and kidney problems, and for improvement of fetal outcome in diabetic pregnancies, failed to consider DN. These deficiencies should urgently be corrected.

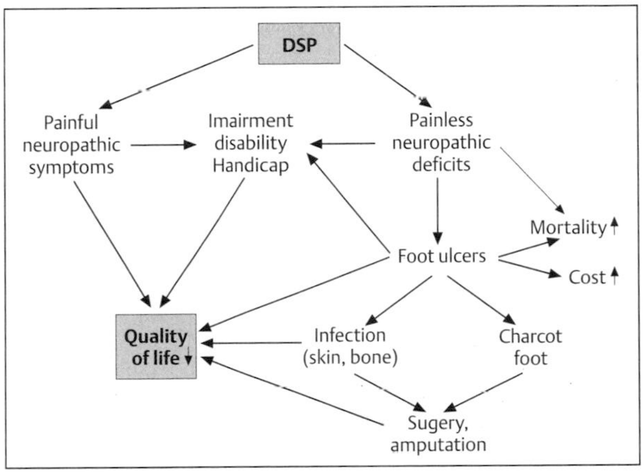

Fig. 7.**1** Clinical impact of diabetic distal symmetric polyneuropathy (DSP)

Outpatient Diabetes Care

Competent diabetes management includes correction of the metabolic disorder as well as prevention and treatment of the chronic complications of diabetes.

Well-educated and well-trained, self-motivated subjects with diabetes should take care of themselves on a day-to-day basis. Nevertheless, these persons should also regularly consult their doctor and their diabetes team for metabolism monitoring, physical health check-up, teaching, and, if necessary, psychologic support.

For the majority of diabetic people outpatient care is in the hands of general practitioners. The American Diabetes Association [8] recommends daily contact for the initiation of insulin treatment or a change in regimen, weekly contact for initiation of oral diabetic therapy or a change in regimen, three-monthly routine visits for patients who are not meeting the goals, and six-monthly visits for other patients. For the aims of treatment see pages 19–20. An annual physical examination is recommended, but previous abnormalities on physical examination should be checked up on at each regular diabetes-related visit. Patients with high risk foot conditions (see pages 295–300) should be seen more often.

The European type 2 diabetes policy group guide of 1993 [9] made precise proposals for what to do at the initial visits and at quarterly and annual follow-up (Table 7.**1**). Recent updates of the European guidelines on type 1 and type 2 diabetes mellitus [10,11] allow for more individual schedules for both types of diabetes. There seems to be a consensus on the recommendation of an annual physical examination and on frequent follow-ups of previous abnormalities. Proper diabetes care requires close cooperation between patients, the diabetes care team, diabetologists, and specialists in various fields [12].

Table 7.1 Clinical monitoring protocol[a] [9]

At initial visit[b]	*At second visit*
Complete history and examination: Weight, height (BMI; kg/m^2) Blood pressure Search for neuropathy Peripheral pulses Foot inspection Fundoscopy (dilated pupils) or fundus photography and visual acuity	Continue teaching program Weight Blood pressure Postprandial blood glucose
	Every 3 months[c]
Biochemical tests: Blood glucose HbA_1 or HbA_{1c} Serum triglycerides, cholesterol, HDL cholesterol (calculate LDL cholesterol if possible) Plasma creatinine Urine glucose, urine protein, microalbuminuria, urine ketones	Continue teaching program Weight Blood pressure Postprandial blood glucose HbA_1 or HbA_{1c} Lipids (if abnormal) Urine protein and microalbuminuria (if previously abnormal) Foot inspection in those at risk (peripheral pulses and/or peripheral neuropathy)
	Annually
Start teaching program Nutritional advice Start self-monitoring	Physical examination and biochemical tests as in initial visit Re-evaluate treatment and nutritional program Check self-monitoring technique Refer to specialist if progress is unsatisfactory Continue teaching

[a] Data can usefully be recorded on the St. Vincent International Care Card
[b] Can be spread over more than one visit
[c] More frequently for poorly controlled patients

Screening and Early Detection of Diabetic Neuropathy

Screening should detect DN at an asymptomatic stage. Therefore, the patient cannot contribute much more than asking for appointments at the appropriate time.

Screening requires practicable methods that can be applied to a large number of people. Physical examination is necessary but not sufficient. The rational selection of additional tests is difficult, because DN is a very complex disorder. Among the sensorimotor neuropathies, distal polyneuropathy (DSP) is the most frequent, and the most common form of autonomic DN is cardiovascular autonomic neuropathy (CAN), but other clinical manifestations of sensorimotor and autonomic neuropathy may develop first. Measurement of nerve conduction velocity, vibration perception threshold, and pressure perception by monofilament and other methods have been used to screen for asymptomatic DSP, and measurement of heart rate variability (HRV) has been recommended for detection of asymptomatic autonomic neuropathy, but there is still no generally accepted consensus on the battery of tests which takes into consideration the selection of nerves and functions and the conditions for HRV tests. This lack of standards is an impediment to regular screening.

Another reason why screening for DN has so far not been implemented in clinical routine is the lack of practicability. General practitioners will usually be unable to measure nerve conduction velocity. They could measure HRV, but determining HRV under different conditions "by hand" is time consuming and imperfect. With proper PC-based equipment it can easily be determined by technical assistants or even the doctors' receptionists. However, the equipment and software are expensive, and for these reasons patients usually have to be referred to a diabetologist or neurologist.

Thus, either general practitioners must be enabled to practice existing screening methods or more practicable tests must be developed (see below).

Outpatient Care of Diabetic Neuropathy

Early detection of symptomatic neuropathy is an urgent aim of quality assurance today. The interval between annual visits may be much too long for early detection. Therefore, the patients must be integrated

Table 7.**2** Symptoms of diabetic neuropathies

On extremities or trunk:
Deafness, numbness, tiredness
Tingling, clumsy fingers
Cold, numb, burning feet
Pain: shooting, radiating around the body
Abdominal pain, scrotal pain
Tenderness of nerves and muscles
Hyperalgesia, hyperesthesia
Itching, tingling of the feet/hands
Diminished pinprick, hot/cold sensation
Painless injury
Muscle cramps, especially at night,
Muscle weakness and atrophy
Foot ulceration, new nontraumatic foot deformities
Other:
Weight loss, early satiety, postprandial fullness, vomiting, constipation, paroxysmal or nocturnal diarrhea, incontinence, impotence, abnormal micturition
Tachycardia, postural hypotension
Delayed light–dark adaptation
Altered sweat distribution, anhidrosis, gustatory sweating

into early detection strategies. It is very important that they are aware of all the symptoms that may possibly indicate neuropathy (Table 7.**2**). Any such symptom should prompt a visit to the doctor's office or a diabetes center.

It is not expected that the general practitioner or diabetologist will always be able to make a final diagnosis, but they should be able to exclude or confirm a neuropathy and perform staging. The differential diagnosis may be difficult (Table 7.**3**) and will frequently require consultation with a neurologist or another specialist.

The Diabetes Neuropathy Study Group (Neurodiab) of the European Association for the Study of Diabetes (EASD) has developed international guidelines for the outpatient management of diabetic peripheral neuropathy [15] (see Appendix). The term "diabetic peripheral neuropathy" is used synonymously with "symmetric distal neuropathy," and "symmetric sensorimotor polyneuropathy." It should be mentioned that these guidelines are not evidence-based and need updating, especially with regard to therapy.

Evidence-based guidelines for diagnosis, treatment, and monitoring of DSP have recently been published by the German Diabetes Association [16]. These guidelines lay down the definition, stages, characteristics, and assessment as well as risk factors for the development and progression of DSP and foot ulceration, physical examination of the patient, and additional assessment. Diagnosis is based on the Young score [17], which uses generally available, simple, and standardized instruments such as the neuropathy symptom score (NSS) and the neuropathy disability score (NDS).

The guidelines for management are specified for each stage of peripheral neuropathy. Patient education is a key management tool. Referral of the patient to a diabetologist or neurologist should be considered in acute painful neuropathy. Painless injury or loss of sensation should prompt early referral to a neurologist and a member of the foot care team for prevention measures. All nondiabetic (or suspected nondiabetic)

Table 7.**3** Differential diagnosis of diabetic neuropathy

Inherited: Genelocus	
Hereditary motor and sensory neuropathies (HMSN):	
HMSN Ia	(17p11.2–12)
HMSN Ib	(q21.2,23)
HMSN X	(Xq13)
HMSN II	(1p 35) (autosomal dominant, heterogenous)
HMSN III	(PMP 22 locus)
Tomaculous neuropathy	(17p11.2,12)
Metabolic neuropathies:	
Familial amyloid polyneuropathy (heterogenous, associated with paraproteins (18q11.2,q12.1, 9q33, and 11q33–q24)	
Metachromatic leukodystrophy (22 q–13 q ter)	
Abetalipoproteinemia (Bassen-Kornzweig syndrome)	
Analphalipoproteinemia (Tangier disease)	
Fabry disease	
Refsum disease	
Acquired:	
Inflammatory:	
Guillain–Barré syndrome	
Associated with connective tissue disease:	
Sjögren syndrome	
Sicca syndrome	
Paraneoplastic:	
Paraproteinemias:	
Waldenström macroglobulinemia	
Cryoglobulinemia	
Primary amyloidosis	
Infectious:	
Tabes dorsalis	
Lyme disease	
Leprosy	
Human immunodeficiency virus (HIV)	
Metabolic:	
Uremia	
Hypothyroidism	
Nutritional:	
Vitamin B deficiency	
Alcohol	
Toxic:	
Drugs	
Heavy metals	
Industrial agents	

Modified after [13,14]

neuropathies and all types of neuropathy other than chronic symmetric sensorimotor neuropathy should be referred early to a specialist. The primary care doctor should provide all available information which may be useful for differential diagnosis.

The diabetic foot syndrome is a major problem. For this, as many as possible of the following specialists should be available for care: diabetologists, diabetes specialist nurses, chiropodists, podiatrists, and surgeons. Complications constituting the diabetic foot syndrome, such as ulcers, blisters, bleeding callus, cellulitis, and acute ischemia, may need referral the same day or the next available day.

Detailed proposals for the structure, equipment, staff, and organization of foot clinics have been published [18,19]. The guidelines of the German Diabetes Association [16] give detailed recommendations for the treatment of peripheral DN.

The American Diabetes Association [1,20], the American Academy of Neurology [21], and others have published consensus statements on diabetic neuropathy that are more directed at neurologists than at general practitioners and diabetologists. Various consensus statements and standards on diagnostic tests have also been published [20,22–25].

Guidelines for structured care of neuropathies other than DSP have been published by the German Diabetes Association [16]. With the exception of compression syndromes, these are rare conditions and in any case require a neurologist's care.

An evidence-based guideline on diagnosis and therapy of diabetic autonomic neuropathies has been brought up for discussion by the German Diabetes Association [26]. It distinguishes nine groups of organ manifestations (Table 7.**4**) and deals with the diagnosis and treatment of each group. A main emphasis is directed towards cardiovascular autonomic neuropathy (CAN). The structure of care is not addressed. Obviously, in many cases diagnosis, treatment, and monitoring all require cooperation with specialists (gastroenterologist, urologist, cardiologist, neurologist, and others).

In summary, an awareness of the broad spectrum of problems of DN is of the utmost importance. Patients and primary care physicians should take any symptoms or signs of DN seriously, because (1) DN is an indicator of poor prognosis, (2) early detection of DN offers the best chance for reversal of the disorder, and (3) spontaneous subjective improvement of symptoms must not lull anybody into a sense of security, since it may be a sign not of healing but of progression of DN. For these reasons, early objective quantification of the disorder is essential.

Frequently the management of DN and its sequelae requires teamwork between specialists. In these cases it is a sign of competence to arrange consultations as early as reasonable.

Table 7.**4** Organ manifestations of diabetic autonomic neuropathy [26]

Cardiovascular system	Reduced heart rate variability, tachycardia at rest, loss of diurnal variation of heart rate and blood pressure, orthostatic hypotension, perioperative instability, exercise intolerance, silent myocardial ischemia
Gastrointestinal tract	Gastroparesis, cholecystopathy, diarrhea, constipation, incontinence
Urogenital tract	Neurogenic bladder, erectile impotence, retrograde ejaculation, sexual dysfunction in women
Neuroendocrine system	Hypoglycemia unawareness, abnormal hypoglycemic counterregulation, reduced catecholamine reaction to standing and work load
Sudomotor	Dyshidrosis, anhidrosis, gustatory sweatening
Vasomotor	Warm skin, edema, rubeosis pedis, orthostatic hypotension
Trophic	Neuropathic ulcer, neuro-osteoarthropathy (Charcot foot)
Respiratory system	Sleep apnea
Pupillary reactions	Diminished dark adaptation

References

[1] American Diabetes Association. American Academy of Neurology: Consensus statement: report and recommendations of the San Antonio Conference on diabetic neuropathy. Diabetes Care 1988; 11: 592–7.

[2] Resnick HE, Vinik AJ, Schwartz AV, Leveille SG, Brancati FL, Balfour J, Guralnik JM. Independent effects of peripheral nerve dysfunction on lower-extremity physical function in in old age. The Women's Health and Aging Study. Diabetes Care 2000; 23: 1642–7.

[3] Chan AW, MacFarlane IA, Bowsher DR, et al. Chronic pain in patients with diabetes mellitus: comparison with non-diabetic population. Pain Clin 1990; 3: 147–59.

[4] Abbott CA, Vileikyte L, Williamson S, Carrington AL, Boulton AJM. Multicenter study of the incidence of and predictive risk factors for diabetic neuropathic foot ulceration. Diabetes Care 1998; 21: 1071–5.

[5] Forsblom CM, Sane T, Groop PH, Tötterman KJ, Kallio M, Saloranta C, Laasonen L, Summanen P, Lepäntalo M, Laatikainen L, Matikainen E, Teppo A-M, Koskomies S, Groop L. Risk factors for mortality in type II (non-insulin-dependent) diabetes: evidence of a role for neuropathy and a protective effect of HLA-DR4. Diabetologia 1998; 41: 1253–62.

[6] Coppini DV, Bowtell PA, Weng C, Young PJ, Sönksen PH. Showing neuropathy is related to increased mortality in

diabetic patients—a survival analysis using an accelerated failure time model. J Clin Epidemiol 2000; 53: 519–23.
[7] World Health Organization (Europe) and International Diabetes Federation (Europe). Diabetes Care and Research in Europe: the St. Vincent Declaration. Diabet Med 1990; 7: 360.
[8] American Diabetes Association. Clinical Practice Recommendations 2000. Diabetes Care 2000; 23(suppl): S32-S42.
[9] European NIDDM Policy Group. A desktop guide for the management of non-insulin-dependent diabetes mellitus (NIDDM): screening, diagnosis, monitoring, education, treatment, self-monitoring. Mainz: Kirchheim. 1993.
[10] European Diabetes Policy Group 1998. Guidelines for diabetes care: a desktop guide to type 1 (insulin-dependent) diabetes mellitus. Brussels: International Diabetes Federation, 1998.
[11] European Diabetes Policy Group 1998–1999. Guidelines for diabetes care: A desktop guide to type 2 diabetes mellitus. Brussels: International Diabetes Federation, 1999.
[12] Bending JJ, Keen H. Organisation of care: the diabetes care centre: a focus for more effective diabetes treatment and prevention. In: Alberti KGMM, DeFronzo RA, Keen H, Zimmet P, editors. International textbook of diabetes mellitus. Chichester, UK: John Wiley & Sons, 1992: 1593–600.
[13] Ziegler D, Claus D. Diagnostik und Therapie der peripheren Neuropathie bei inneren Erkrankungen. In: Peter H, Pfreundschuh M, Philipp T, Schölmerich J, Schuster H-P, Sybrecht GW, editors: Klinik der Gegenwart. München, Urban und Schwarzenberg 1998, Kapitel 25: 1–35.
[14] Grant JA, Dyck PJ. Differential diagnosis of diabetic neuropathies. In: Dyck PJ, Thomas PK, editors. Diabetes neuropathy, 2nd edition. Philadelphia: W.B. Saunders Co, 1999: 415–44.
[15] Boulton AJM, Gries FA, Jervell JA. Guidelines for the diagnosis and outpatient management of diabetic peripheral neuropathy. Diabet Med 1998; 15: 508–14.
[16] Haslbeck M, Redaelli M, Parandeh-Shab F, Luft D, Neundörfer B, Stracke H, Ziegler D. Diagnostik, Therapie und Verlaufskontrolle der sensomotorischen diabetischen Neuropathien. In: Scherbaum WA, Lauterbach KW, Renner R, editors. Evidenzbasierte Diabetes-Zeitlinien DDG. 1. Aufl. Bochum: Deutsche Diabetes Gesellschaft, 2000.
[17] Young M, Boulton A, McLeod A, Williams D, Sonksen P. A multicenter study of the prevalence of diabetic peripheral neuropathy in the United Kingdom hospital clinic population. Diabetologia 1993; 36: 150–3.
[18] Ward JD. Essential requirements for diabetic foot care. In: Connor H, Boulton AJM, Ward JD, editors. The foot in diabetes. Chichester, UK: John Wiley & Sons Ltd, 1987: 151–8.
[19] Edmonds M, Foster AVM. Diabetic foot clinic. In: Leonie ME, O'Neal LW, Bowker JH, editors. The diabetic foot. St. Louis, Mo.: Mosby Year Book, 1993.
[20] American Diabetes Association. Proceedings of a consensus development conference on standardized measures in diabetic neuropathy. Diabetes Care 1992; 15: 1080-1107.
[21] American Academy of Neurology. Assessment: clinical autonomic testing report of the Therapeutics and Technology Assessment Subcommittee of the American Academy of Neurology. Neurology 1996; 46: 873–80.
[22] Peripheral Neuropathy Association. Quantitative sensory testing. A consensus report from the Peripheral Neuropathy Association. Neurology, 1993; 43: 1050–2.
[23] Peripheral Nerve Society. Diabetic polyneuropathy in controlled clinical trials: consensus report of the Peripheral Nerve Society. Ann Neurol 1995; 38: 478–82.
[24] Task Force of the European Society of Cardiology and the North American Society of Pacing and Electrophysiology. Heart rate variability. Standards of measurement, physiological interpretation, and clinical use. Circulation 1996; 93: 1043–65.
[25] Consensus Statement C. Report and recommendations of the San Antonio Conference on diabetic neuropathy. Diabetes 1988; 37: 1000–4.
[26] Haslbeck M, Luft D, Neundörfer B, Stracke H. Ziegler D for Deutsche Diabetes Gesellschaft: Diagnose und Therapie der autonomen diabetischen Neuropathien – Diskussionsentwurf. Diabetes Stoffw 2001; 10: 113–32.

*Guidelines for the Diagnosis and Outpatient Management of Diabetic Peripheral Neuropathy**

AJM Boulton, FA Gries and JA Jervell

Guidelines on the out-patient management of diabetic peripheral neuropathy have been developed from an international consensus meeting attended by diabetologists, neurologists, primary care physicians, podiatrists and diabetes specialist nurses. A copy of the full document follows this summary (Appendix 1). The document arose out of suggestions from Neurodiab, a subgroup of the European Association for the Study of Diabetes, that there was a need for guidelines developed by consensus, for the outpatient management of patients with diabetic neuropathy. An international consensus group was created, chaired by two of the authors. A pilot working party met in 1995, followed by a full working party of 39 experts, neurologists and diabetes physicians (Appendix 2). This compiled a draft guideline document which was circulated to a number of international bodies. After consultation with its members, the final guidelines were approved by Neurodiab (chairman F.A. Gries) towards the end of 1997.

Definition

Diabetes peripheral neuropathy: the presence of symptoms and/or signs of peripheral nerve dysfunction in people with diabetes, after exclusion of other causes (Table 1).

■ Assessment as Part of the Annual Review of the Patient

Patient history: age, diabetes, physical factors, lifestyle, social circumstances, symptoms, other possible aetiological factors.

Examination should include:

- Inspection of both feet (Table 2): skin status, sweating, infection, ulceration, calluses/blistering, deformity, muscle wasting, arches; palpation for temperature, pulses, joint mobility; examine gait/shoes
- Vascular examination – foot pulses
- Other investigations, e. g. thyroid function, to exclude non-diabetic aetiologies
- Inspection for the presence or absence of characteristics of the "at risk" foot (Figure 1).

Table **1** Stages of diabetic peripheral neuropathy

Stage of neuropathy	Characteristics
No neuropathy	No symptoms or signs
Clinical neuropathy	
Chronic painful	Burning, shooting, stabbing pains ± pins and needles; increased at night; absent sensation to several modalities; reduced/absent reflexes
Acute painful	Severe symptoms as above (hyperaesthesia common); may follow initiation of insulin in poorly controlled diabetes; signs minor or absent
Painless with complete/ partial sensory loss	Numbness/deadness of feet or no symptoms; painless injury; reduced/absent sensation; reduced thermal sensitivity; absent reflexes
Late complications	Foot lesions; neuropathic deformity; non-traumatic amputation

1. Types of diabetic neuropathy: frequent, sensorimotor symmetrical neuropathy (mostly chronic, sensory loos or pain), autonomic neuropathy (history of impotence and possibly other autonomic abnormalities); rare, mononeuropathy (motor involvement, acute onset, may be painful), diabetic amyotrophy (weakness/wasting usually of proximal lower limb muscles).
2. Staging does not imply automatic progression to the next stage. The aim is to prevent, or at least delay, progression to the next stage.

* The above material has been reprinted from Boulton AJM, Gries FA, Jervell J: Guidelines for the Diagnosis and Outpatient Management of Diabetic Peripheral Neuropathy. Diabet Med 15:508–514, 1998. Reproduced with kind permission from John Wiley & Sons, Chichester, U.K.

Table **2** Foot tests

Pin prick test	• Use a disposable instrument, e.g. a disposable pin • Ask "Is it painful ?" not "Can you feel it ?"
Light touch	• Use a consistent method, ideally a cotton wisp
Vibration test	• Use a 128 Hz tuning fork, initially on the big toe
Pressure perception	• Absence of sensation in the foot to a 10 g monofilament
Ankle reflex	• Compare the ankle reflex with the knee reflex

Management

Education of people with clinical neuropathy and referral of people with late complications to a diabetologist or neurologist are the key factors in the prevention of amputation (Table 3). Prompt referral (same day/next available day) of the person with the following lesions will usually prevent amputation: ulcer, blister, bleeding callus, cellulitis, acute ischaemia.

Table **3** Management of the stages of neuropathy

Stage	Objectives	Key element	Referral
No clinical neuropathy	Education to reduce risk of progression; maintenance of near-normoglycaemia	Education; glycaemic control; annual assessment	As required
Clinical neuropathy	Management of symptoms; prevention of foot ulceration		
Acute/chronic painful		Stable glycaemic control; symptomatic treatment (simples analgesics or tricyclic drugs or carbamazepine). Consider referral of actute sensory neuropathy	Diabetologist/neurologist
Painless/loss of sensation		Education, especially footcare; glycaemic control according to needs	Appropriate member of foot care team
Other types of diabetic neuropathy		Early referral	Neurologist/diabetologist
Late complications	Prevention of new/recurrent lesions and amputation	Emergency referral if lesions present; otherwise referral within 4 weeks	Diabetologist/neurologist/chiropodist/podiatrist/diabetes specialist nurse/diabetic foot clinic if available

Appendix 1: International Guide on the Outpatient Management of Diabetic Peripheral Neuropathy

Developed form discussions at a meeting of a Pilot Working Party held in Brussels, Belgium, on 13 April 1995 and a meeting of a full Working Party held in London, UK, on 20-22 October 1995.

Introduction

Lack of awareness and inappropriate management of diabetic peripheral neuropathy leads to unnecessary morbidity and substantial healthcare costs. At least half of the foot ulcers, the end stage of such neuropathy, should be preventable, by appropriate management and patient education. However, lack of time and inadequate knowledge and information may lead, in many cases, to suboptimal management.

There is a clear need for a set of simple, practical, international guidelines to be used by primary care physicians (in many countries, 80-90% of people with diabetes receive care from general practitioners) and by hospital physicians for the clinical assessment and management of neuropathy. The guidelines should be applicable in day-to-day practice and should use readily available methods.

The neuropathy study group (Neurdiab) of the European Association for the Study of Diabetes (EASD) has identified the need for three sets of guidelines for diabetic peripheral neuropathy. These will cover the following areas:

- studies of the epidemiology of peripheral and autonomic diabetic neuropathy (DN)
- conduct of clinical trials in DN
- management of diabetic peripheral neuropathy by practising clinicians.

The International Guidelines on the Outpatient Management of Diabetic Peripheral Neuropathy have been developed to fulfil the third need.

The purpose of this document is to provide clear, internationally acceptable guidelines on the clinical diagnosis and management of diabetic peripheral neuropathy in primary or hospital care, the widespread adoption of which would bring about earlier diagnosis, better management, and a reduction in the late sequelae of this complication of diabetes.

The guidelines provide recommendations on methods of assesment and management of diabetic peripheral neuropathy and patient education, all of which should form part of the annual review of people with diabetes. A simple staging system has been developed for diabetic peripheral neuropathy to provide a framework for risk assessment and decisions on treatment and referral of those with diabetes. The emphasis is on simplicity and practicality to facilitate maximal adoption. It is intended that the guidelines should be used by physicians involved in the outpatient management of the person with diabetes. In addition, the guidelines emphasize the concept of a multidisciplinary diabetes footcare team and it is expected that the team members would use those sections that are applicable to their discipline. Clearly, there are variations in the epidemiology of diabetes, economic and cultural factors and healthcare personnel in different geographical regions; therefore, the guideline should be adapted to meet local needs and conditions.

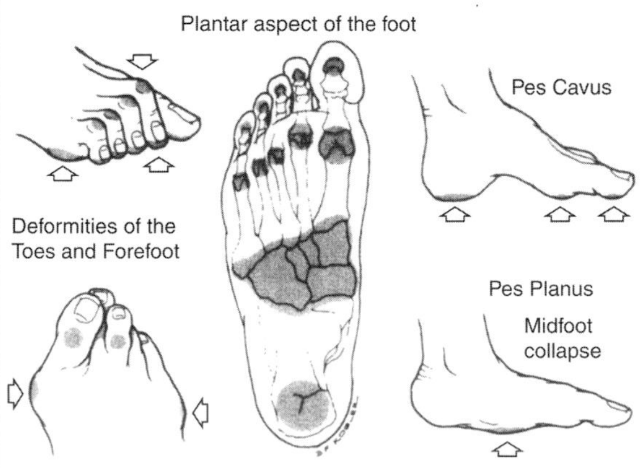

Shaded areas and arrows indicate primary regions 'at risk' for developing ulcers.

Fig. 1 The "at risk" diabetic foot (illustration by G. Kogler).

Peripheral Neuropathy in Diabetes

People with diabetes mellitus develop several types of peripheral neuropathy, including a distal sensory motor polyneuropathy, autonomic neuropathy, and mononeuropathy. The sensory motor polyneuropathy is the most common form of diabetic peripheral neuropathy and is the main focus of these guidelines. Estimates of its prevalence vary, although it is generally accepted that clinical diabetic peripheral neuropathy is found in approximately 30% of people with diabetes. In the USA, the risk of fool ulceration, a late complication of neuropathy, has been estimated to be 3% per patient per year. Neuropathy is also a major contributory factor in amputation. The incidence of amputation varies from country to country, owing to differences in the management of diabetes and diabetic foot disease. It is estimated, however, that 40% of non-traumatic foot and leg amputations in adults are due to diabetes.

There is an urgent need for improvement of the clinical management of neuropathy in primary care. At least half of the amputations in people with diabetes are believed to be preventable, yet there are still reports of people presenting with foot ulcera in whom diabetes, let alone neuropathy, has not been diagnosed. Neuropathy also has a major impact on healthcare costs. In the USA it is estimated that the cost of the sequelae of neuropathy, foot ulcers, and amputations is equal to the entire cost of the remainder of diabetes management.

Guidance for the primary care physician is lacking. In addition, the physician has limited time available for consultation with the patient with diabetes. It is the objective of this document, therefore, to provide clear and simple guidelines for the diagnosis and management of neuropathy on an outpatint basis, in particular during the annual review of the patient. The emphasis is on simple diagnostic testing, using equipment that is readily available. Although much can be done in primary care to manage and educate people with diabetes, guidance is also given on when it is appropriate to refer the patient to a member of the multidisciplinary diabetes footcare team. The availability of resources will vary in different locations and it is possible that some reorganization or modification of referral procedures may be required to achieve optimal management.

Adoption of the guidelines should lead to improvements in the management of neuropathy and this should be documented. Systems should, therefore, be established to monitor the implementation of the recommended practices and to assess their impact, in terms of reduction of the incidence of foot ulceration and amputation, in people with diabetes.

Definitions

Diabetic peripheral neuropathy is the presence of symptoms and/or signs of peripheral nerve dysfunction in people with diabetes, after exclusion of other causes.

Stages of Neuropathy

A staging system has been developed for neuropathy to provide a framework for diagnosis and management. Staging does not imply automatic progression ot the next stage and the aim is to prevent, or at least delay, progression (Table A1).

Table **A1** The stages of neuropathy

Stage	Characteristics
Stages 0/1: no clinical neuropathy	• No symptoms or signs
Stage 2: clinical neuropathy Chronic painful	• Positive symptomatology (increasing at night): burning, shooting, stabbing pains ± pins and needles • Absent sensation to several modalities and reduced or absent reflexes
Acute painful	• Less common • Diabetes poorly controlled, weight loss • Diffuse (trunk) • Hyperaesthesia may occur • May be associated with initiation of glycaemic therapy • Minor sensory signs or even normal peripheral neurological examination
Painless with complete/partial sensory loss	• No symptoms or numbness/deadness of feet; reduced thermal sensitivity; painless injury • Signs of reduced or absent sensation with absent reflexes
Stages 3: late complications of clinical neuropathy	• Foot lesions e. g. ulcers • Neuropathic deformity e. g. Charcot joint • Non-traumatic amputation

1. Subclinical neuropathy (Stage 1). This can only be diagnoses in special neurophysiological laboratories and such tests are not recommended for day-to-day clinical practice. Thus, Stage 1 cannot be differentiated clinically from Stage 0.
2. Diabetic amyotrophy. This is a predominantly motor disorder, usually encountered in elderly patients with undiagnosed or poorly controlled Type 2 diabetes. There is muscle weakness and wasting, mainly affecting the proximal lower limb muscles with a subacute onset. Sensory loss is slight, but pain, particularly at night, is common.

Assessment

Clinical assessment of neuropathy should form part of the annual review of the person with diabetes. The objective is to detect the presence of clinical neuropathy. Risk factors for the development and progression of neuropathy and the development of neuropathic foot ulceration are shown in Table A2.

Patient History

Questions should be adjusted according to the age of the patient, type of diabetes and symptomatology, although in general the following areas should be covered:

- Age
- Diabetes: type; duration; therapy; level of glycaemic control; knowledge of diabetes and its complications
- Physical factors: inability to see well or reach the feet.
- Lifestyle: smoking; alcohol intake; nutrition; employment; sport/leisure activities; footwear
- Social circumstances; social support; access to care
- Symptoms

Table **A2** Risk factors for development and progression of neuropathy and development of neuropathic foot ulceration

Risk factors for the development and progression of neuropathy	Risk factors for the development of neuropathic foot ulceration
• Poor glycaemic control	• Loss of pain sensation
• Undiscovered Type 2 diabetes	• Undiscovered Type 2 diabetes
• Smoking	• Smoking
• High alcohol intake	• High alcohol intake
• Low socio-economic status	• Low socio-economic status
• Renal failure	• Patient lives alone
	• Lack of flexibility/suppleness
	• Ill-fitting footwear
	• Poor foot hygiene/footcare
	• Denial of condition
	• Lack of diabetes education
	• History of previous ulceration or amputation
	• Poor glycaemic control
	• Peripheral vascular disease
	• Decreased vibration sensitivity

Symptomatology differs according to the stage and type of neuropathy (see above). Patients should be asked about the following:

- presence/absence of symptoms
- nature of symptoms, i. e. positive or negative symptomatology
- duration and progression of symptoms
- noctural exacerbation
- patients with chronic pain: ask if the pain is insidious, intermittent, bilateral, related/unrelated to treatment, does it occur on walking or at rest; presence of foot ulcers in the past; presence of autonomic symptoms
- patients with acute pain: presence of neuropathic pain or contact hyperaesthesia.

Other medical conditions/therapies which may be aetiological factors for neuropathy: vascular disease, HIV, vitamin B12 deficiency, hypothyroidism, weight loss, cancer, leprosy, syphilis, drug therapy, toxic exposure, paraproteinaemia.

Atypical features not usually related to diabetic neuropathy include rapid progression, foot drop, back or neck pain, weight loss (per se) and family history.

Examination of the Patient

Inspection of the Feet

The patient should be asked to remove shoes and socks on both feet. The feet should be inspected for the following:

- skin status: colour, thickness, dryness, cracking, trophic changes
- sweating
- infection (interdigital fungal infection)
- ulceration
- calluses/blistering
- deformity, e.g. Charcot joint or clawed toes
- muscle atrophy
- arches (standing/lying)

Table **A3** Neurological tests

Pin prick test	• Use a disposable instrument, e. g. a disposable dressmaker's pin • Do not use a hypodermic needle • Ask "Is it painful?" Not "Can you feel it?"
Light touch	• Use a consistent method, ideally a cotton wisp
Vibration test	• Use a 128 Hz tuning fork, initially on the big toe
Ankle reflex	• Compare the ankle reflex with the knee reflex
Pressure perception	• Absence of sensation in the foot to a 10 g monofilament may be used to assess the risk of foot ulceration

The feet should be palpated to assess temperature, foot pulses and joint mobility. The patient's gait and shoes should also be examined.

Neurological Examination

Four tests are recommended (see Table A3). All should be done bilaterally and the result should be a simple yes/no or normal/abnormal answer. For the first three, a proximal site should be compared with a distal site (vibration test – only if the result is abnormal). A simple temperature assessment may also be made by placing a cold tuning fork on the patient's legs.

To determine whether the patient has diabetic amyotrophy, look for proximal muscle wasting and weakness and loss of knee jerks, often with little sensory loss.

Vascular Examination

Systemic blood pressure and pulses (posterior tibial and dorsalis pedis) should be recorded.

Other Investigations

Appropriate investigations, e.g. thyroid function tests, serum B12, serum paraprotein, assessment of metabolic control should be considered for medical conditions, other than diabetes, which may be aetiological factors for the neuropathy. The need for such investigations will vary according to local circumstances. Possible aetiological factors as listed above. Other tests may be suggested as a result of the clinical examination.

The "At Risk" Foot

The characteristics of the „at risk" diabetic foot are shown in Figure 1. Attention should be paid to the absence/presence of these during examination of the patient.

Management

Education of people with Stage 2 neuropathy and referral of people with Stage 3 neuropathy are key factors in the prevention of amputation. For optimal care of people with neuropathy, a local multidiciplinary footcare team should be established. Although the structure of the team will vary according to local healthcare resourcing, as many as possible of the following should be included:

- diabetologist
- diabetes specialist nurse
- chiropodist
- surgeon

No Clinical Neuropathy (Stage 0/1)

Objective: education to reduce the risk of progression.

In Stage 0/1 the person does not have clinical neuropathy and, therefore, the emphasis is on education with respect to lifestyle, footcare, and metabolic control. At this stage there is no need for referral to a neurologist but referral to specialists in footcare, i.e. chiropodist, podiatrist or diabetes specialist nurse, may occasionally be indicated. A yearly foot examination has an important educational function. If, in future, specific therapies become available for the treatment of early neuropathy, the guidelines will require amendment to provide advice on the separate diagnosis and management of people with no neuropathy (Stage 0) and those with subclinical disease (Stage 1).

Clinical Neuropathy (Stage 2)

Objective: prevention of primary lesions and progression to late complications of clinical neuropathy (Stage 3)

Chronic Painful Neuropathy

For people whose daily lifestyle is not impaired by their neuropathy, there is no need to treat the symptoms. Attention should be given to maintenance of optimal glycaemic control, as assessed by glycated haemoglobin levels.

People who are disabled or whose quality of life is impaired should be referred to a diabetologist or neurologist with an interest in diabetes. In the interim, optimal glycaemic control should be maintained. Pain should be treated with tricyclic drugs (e.g. imipramine) as first-line therapy, starting with a low dose at night and increasing as necessary. If tricyclic drugs are contraindicated or ineffective, the person could be referred. New agents are available in some countries but these should be considered only if their efficacy has been demonstrated in more than one controlled clinical trial.

Acute Painful Neuropathy

These patients should be referred to a diabetologist or neurologist. In the interim, optimal glycaemic control should be maintained. The pain should be treated with simple analgesics, progressing to NSAIDs or tricyclic drugs. Other stronger agents may occasionally be necessary. The person should then be managed in accordance with the specialist's advice.

Diabetic Amyotrophy

People with suspected diabetic amyotrophy should be referred either to a neurologist or a diabetologist for a further evaluation.

Painless Neuropathy with Complete/Partial Loss of Pain Sensation

Patient education, particularly in relation to the risks of progression, is important for this group. Maintenance of optimal glycaemic control is recommended. Specific foot management may be required, including advice on footcare (see below) and treatment of fungal infections.

Referral will depend upon whether it is possible to manage the person adequately in the primary care setting and upon the need of the individual. It may be necessary to refer the person to a diabetologists or diabetes specialist nurse if there are problems with glycaemic control or other complications of diabetes. The patient may be referred to a neurologist if the picture is atypical or the neuropathy may have a cause other than diabetes. If the foot is at risk, e.g. because of deformity or the person's inability to reach his/her toes, the patient may be referred to a chiropodist or podiatrist for footcare, including the provision of special footwear.

Late Complications of Clinical Neuropathy (Stage 3)

Objective: prevention of new/recurrent lesions and amputation. At this stage, the key management issue is onward referral and its urgency. Advice and counselling, which involves the care giver or partner, is also important (see Patient Education).

Emergency Referral

The person should be referred to the specialist diabetes footcare team immediately (same day or next available day) if he/she has any of the following:

- ulcer
- blister
- bleeding callus
- cellulitis
- acute ischaemia

Prompt referral at this stage will usually prevent amputation. Vascular problems may have contributed to ulceration but, if peripheral pulses are present, the primary process is neuropathy with possible secondary infection.

The possibility of osteomyelitis should be considered; differentiation of this condition from a Charcot joint is difficult and requires referral for further investigation.

Ideally, the person should be referred with his/her care giver or partner. The specialist team should be provided with notes on the person's social circumstances, as a basis for risk assessment, and confirmation should be obtained that the patient has attended the consultation.

If the patient cannot be seen immediately, e.g., because of a national holiday, then treatment with a broad-spectrum oral antibiotic should be started.

Drugs such as clindamycin or Augmentin (amoxycillin and clavulanic acid in combination) are useful agents.

Subacute Referral

People with a Stage 3 diagnosis but no ulcera should be referred to the specialist diabetes footcare team but with less urgency. They should attend an appointment within 4 weeks.

Patient Education

Education of people with diabetes should be started before clinical neuropathy is present (Stage 0) and should be customized to the individual's circumstances and ability to understand. The content of the education will change according to the stage of neuropathy; for example, while glycaemic control should be stressed throughout, the emphasis on footcare and footwear will increase in clinical neuropathy (Stage 2) and late complications of clinical disease (Stage 3). It is recommended that there should be separate programmes for people with Type 1 and Type 2 diabetes, as more extensive advice is likely to be required for the elderly Type 2 than for the young person with Type 1 diabetes.

Initially, it is important to assess the patient's level of knowledge about his/her condition and then to implement a measure of whether the educational messages have been understood. Care givers/partners should be involved throughout.

Who Should Provide Patient Education ?

The providers of patient edcuation will vary according to local cirumstances and may include:

- primary care physician (primary health care team members in the UK)
- diabetes specialist nurse
- chiropodist/podiatrist
- patient support groups (e.g. through diabetes associations).

It is essential that these healthcare personnel have received adequate training on neuropathy and its management. Patient education may be provided at structured primary health care clinics, diabetes education centres or meetings of support groups. It is also possible to introduce elements of education during examination of the patient. For example, vibration sensation in a normal area of skin may be compared with impaired sensation in the neuropathic foot.

What methods should be used ?

The methods used will depend upon local circumstances, e.g. availability of equipment, such as video recorders, or patient literacy. Methods that involve personal interaction are preferred by patients. Four commonly used methods are:

- one-to-one personal training sessions
- video: ideally with opportunity for discussion
- literature/pamphlets; only validated material should be used, e. g. the EASD Survival Kit for older people with Type 2 diabetes
- group sessions: often very effective.

What elements should the education programme contain ?

Footcare and Footwear

Ongoing surveillance of the feet by the patient is important. The following points should be emphasized:

- change hosiery every day; check for thickened seams
- wear well-fitting comfortable shoes, with insoles as appropriate
- wear new shoes for brief periods (2–4 hours per day) until adaptation has occured
- examine feet each night for lesions, red spots, breaks in the skin
- cut and file nails carefully, with help from chiropodist/podiatrist/trained carer if unable to see or reach feet

Short written guidelines about footcare may be provided, containing information about whom to contact if a particular circumstance arises.

Metabolic Control

At all stages, the importance of optimal metabolic control (glycaemia and lipids) should be stressed.

Blood Pressure

Control of blood pressure should be discussed, if necessary.

Liftstyle Modification

The following lifestyle changes should be discussed, as appropriate:

- weight control/dietary modification
- reduction in alcohol intake
- cessation of smoking
- exercise: appropriate for the individual; should not impair foot hygiene or aggravate the neuropathic foot. In certain people, running or even excessive walking may be inadvisable.

General Information about diabetic neuropathy

Patients should be informed about the natural history of diabetic neuropathy and risk factors for progression. They should be told about likely interventions for pain,

Table **A4** Management of the stages of neuropathy

Stage	Key elements	Referral
No clinical neuropathy (Stage 0/1)	Education; glycaemic control[a] Annual assessment	Chiropodist/podiatrist/diabetes specialist nurse
Clinical neuropathy (Stage 2) Chronic painful	If disabled, treatment with tricyclic drugs; glycaemic control[b]	Diabetologist/neurologist
Acute painful	Simple analgesics/tricyclic drugs/NSAIDs/ opiates; glycaemic control[b]	Diabetologist/neurologist
Painless/loss of sensation	Education, especially footcare; glycaemic control	Appropriate member of footcare team according to needs
Diabetic amyotrophy	Early referral	Neurologist/diabetologist
Late complications	Emergency referral if lesions present; otherwise referral within 4 weeks	Diabetologist/neurologist/chriopodist/ podiatrist/diabetes specialist nurse

a If, in futrure, specific therapies become available for the treatment of early neuropathy, the guidelines will require amendment to provide advice on the separate diagnosis and management of people with no neuropathy (Stage 0) and those with subclinical disease (Stage 1)
b Editors comment: For detailed list of drugs used for treatment of painful neuropathy see pages 211–224

impotence, etc. For people with chronic painful neuropathy, it should be explained why the pain is occuring, i.e. nerve damage, and that if it disappears it does not necessarily mean that the neuropathy has improved. If tricyclic drugs are prescribed, the patient should be told that pain relief may not occur for up to 3 weeks and that they should continue to take the tablets. Patients with acute painful neuropathy should be told that the pain will improve with time.

Patients with sensory loss must be made aware of the lack of sensation and hence the risks of injury to the foot.

The advice of a psychologist may help to deal with problems of denial of the condition, particularly in the later stages of neuropathy.

Summary of the Management of Neuropathy

Key elements for the management of each stage of neuropathy are shown in Table A4.

Acknowledgement

The consensus meetings were supported by an educational grant from F. Hoffmann La Roche, Ltd.

Appendix 2 List of Participants

Pilot Working Party, Brussels, Belgium 13 April 1995

Professor A.J.M. Boulton Manchester, Uk[a], Dr. M. Pfeifer Illinois, USA, Dr. V. Bril Toronto, Canada, Prof. G. Said Paris, France, Professor F.A. Gries Düsseldorf, Germany, Dr. G. Sundkvist Malmö, Sweden, Professor J. Jervell Oslo, Norway Professor P.K. Thomas London, UK

Full Working Party, London, UK, 20–22 October 1995

Professor J.R.Attali Paris, France; Dr K. Bakker Heemstede, Netherlands; Professor A.J.M. Boulton Manchester, UK[b]; Dr. V. Bril Toronto, Canada; Dr. P.S. van Dam Utrecht, Netherlands; Dr. K. Dawson Vancouver, Canada; Dr. M. Falkenberg Kisa, Sweden; Dr. R. Forresst Luleå, Sweden; Dr. R. Gadsby Warwick, UK; Dr. D. Gelber Illinois, USA; Professor F.A. Gries Düsseldorf, Germany; Ms S. Hamilton London, UK; Dr. L. Harkless Texas, USA; Dr. K. Hosokawa Tokyo, Japan; Dr. I. Illa Barcelona, Spain; Professor J. Jervell Oslo, Norway[b]; Professor I. Kalo Copenhagen, Denmark; Dr. G. Kogler Illinois, USA; Dr. A. de Leiva Barcelona, Spain; Ms E. Liljeblad Kisa, Sweden; Dr L. Litwak Buenos Aires, Argentina; Professor G. Menzinger Rome, Italy; Professor B. Neundörfer Erlangen, Germany; Dr. K. Paterson Glasgow, UK; Dr. V. Petrenko Kaunas, Lithuania; Professor F. Santeusanio Perugia, Italy; Professor A. Serhiyenko Lviv, Ukraine; Dr. G. Sundkvist Malmö, Sweden; Professor P.K. Thomas London, UK; Dr. J.A. Touminen Helsinki, Finland; Dr. G. Valk Amsterdam, Netherlands; Dr. B. Vandeleene Brussels, Belgium; Dr. C. Vermigli Perugia, Italy; Dr. A. Veves Boston, USA; Dr. L. Vileikyte Manchester, UK; Professor J. Ward Sheffield, UK; Professor D. Ziegler Düsseldorf, Germany

[a] Chairman
[b] Co-chairman

Index

A

B

C

D

G

H

I

O

P

Q

R

U

V

W

Y

Z